THE NURSING EXPERIENCE

TRENDS, CHALLENGES, AND TRANSITIONS

THE NURSING EXPERIENCE

TRENDS, CHALLENGES, AND TRANSITIONS

FIFTH EDITION

Lucille A. Joel, RN, EdD, FAAN

Professor, College of Nursing
Rutgers–The State University of New Jersey
Newark, New Jersey

McGraw-Hill
Medical Publishing Division

New York   Chicago   San Francisco   Lisbon   London   Madrid   Mexico City
Milan   New Delhi   San Juan   Seoul   Singapore   Sydney   Toronto

The **McGraw·Hill** Companies

The Nursing Experience: Trends, Challenges, and Transitions, Fifth Edition

2 3 4 5 6 7 8 9 0   DOC/DOC   0 9 8 7

ISBN 0-07-145826-3

This book was set in Palatino by Keyword Group Ltd.
The editors were Michael J. Brown and Mary E. Bele.
The production supervisor was Sherri Souffrance.
Project management was provided by Keyword Group Ltd.
The cover designer was Aimee Nordin.
RR Donnelley was printer and binder.

This book is printed on acid-free paper.

Cataloging-in-Publication data for this title is on file at the Library of Congress.

Contents

PART 1: THE EVOLUTION OF NURSING

PART 2: NURSING IN THE HEALTH CARE SCENE

PART 3: NURSING PRACTICE

Preface

The fifth edition of the *The Nursing Experience* builds on the proud tradition of earlier versions. You will find the history, trends, and issues of contemporary nursing in one succinct and readable volume. A major objective of this text is to endow you with an intellectual curiosity that goes beyond this book and is, in fact, insatiable. The history of nursing is rich; the trends and issues are complex and open to endless interpretation. It is these characteristics that complicate what to keep and what to remove from an earlier edition; how much fact and how much opinion to include. I feel confident that my decisions have been sound and that you will be both well informed by this text and motivated to search for additional answers beyond these pages.

Each chapter and appendix has been updated, including information that readers might have difficulty accessing themselves. Each chapter includes study questions that will help you to synthesize the content. Helpful websites, which are invaluable given the computer sophistication of most students, have also been identified throughout the text.

Chapters 1 and 2 provide an orientation to the history of nursing, and include a chronological exhibit that traces the social context of nursing in the United States from 1865 to contemporary times. "Distinguished Nurses of the Past" (Appendix 7) adds to your historical perspective by familiarizing you with some of the giants in nursing's past. In developing this appendix, I aimed for a broad cross-section of significant personalities from the history of nursing, some well known and others of lesser notoriety. What could have been an endless list was purposefully limited, in the hope that you would be motivated to hunt for more personalities on your own.

The topics of Chapter 3 always prove to be a formidable challenge, a search for the best way to describe the evolving health care delivery system and the men and women who make it function due to their sheer effort. Nurses fill a unique role, standing at the center of this maelstrom. Each edition calls for reorganization of material for a better understanding of the infrastructure you will deal with on graduation. In some ways, the message is that there cannot be any assumption about form or function, only that there are societal needs for health, wellness, and peaceful death that must be met in some manner.

Chapter 4 presents the essence of nursing: who the nurses are, what they do, the theory that guides their work, the classification systems that describe the phenomena they deal with, and the results of their interventions. In a very few pages, you are given a comprehensive orientation to nursing at the beginning of the twenty-first century.

Nursing education is an intricate tapestry of several different routes to becoming a registered nurse. It is essential to know and respect these differences. These educational programs, described in Chapter 5, create flexibility and opportunity for nurses. The mission of research is also introduced here, showing the pragmatism of our scholarship and the vehemence with which nurses have fought to have nursing recognized as a scholarly discipline. Traditional, new, and emerging career opportunities are presented in Chapter 6, as well as an analysis of the periodic shortage and surplus cycles that nursing has found so painful and disruptive.

To control our work life and future more successfully, leadership skills are essential, and they are introduced in Chapter 7. Classic situations that have served to facilitate and deter our progress are discussed to a degree to motivate further reading. Among these are the women's movement, physician/nurse relationships, and the reality that most nurses are employees in bureaucracies. Such circumstances persist, but there is hope of progress through increased mentoring among nurses, a sense of professional pride and unity, and success in political action where our numbers and work ethic count for much.

Chapters 8 through 12 focus on "Nursing Ethics and Law." We are living in times when most of our actions as nurses have ethical or legal implications. There are issues of informed consent, the right to die, advance directives, the rights of the helpless and of patients in research, confidentiality, employee protections, and civil rights, to name a few. The use of principles for ethical decision making and knowledge of the law are basic protections in practice, but the content of this section is more than defensive. Nurses are formidable advocates for both themselves and their patients in the public policy arena. Chapter 10 offers serious advice on political action and information on legislation that has been significant to nursing.

Chapters 13, 14, and 15 facilitate the "Transition to Practice." These chapters define the role of professional organizations and point out both the hazards of practice and the continuing obligation to remain current and committed. Chapter 14 focuses on the work of finding a job and the mechanics of interviewing and résumé development that are part of the process. Chapter 15 highlights resocialization from the role of student to that of graduate nurse, which seems to be accomplished less stressfully when one anticipates the "reality shock." And there are rights and responsibilities of the workplace to understand and appreciate. You are not treading on unfurrowed ground, many have gone this route before you, and you will find many there to help in this exciting passage.

This book is unique, giving a great amount of important information in a compact edition. It is intended to have continuing use as you become a nurse and grow in sophistication and professional experience. It should stimulate thinking and discussion, pique curiosity, and make nursing your passion.

Lucille A. Joel

Author Profile

Lucille A. Joel is a Professor at Rutgers–The State University of New Jersey College of Nursing, and was Director of the Rutgers Teaching Nursing Home from 1982 to 1998. Dr. Joel is a past president of the American Nurses Association (ANA) and former First Vice-President of the International Council of Nurses (ICN), headquartered in Geneva. She holds official status as ICN's representative to UNICEF and the UN. Dr. Joel is author of Kelly's *Dimensions of Professional Nursing* and *The Nursing Experience*, both published by McGraw-Hill, and an international advisor to the *American Journal of Nursing*.

Dr. Joel has served as a professional-technical advisor to the Joint Commission on the Accreditation of Health Care Organizations (JCAHO), and chaired the FDA's steering committee on nursing and medical devices. She served as the ANA representative to the board of the Computer-Based Patient Record Institute, and as the association's liaison to HCFA (now CMS) in work on quality and case mix reimbursement for long-term care. She is currently Vice-President of the Commission on Graduates of Foreign Nursing Schools (CGFNS).

Lucille Joel is the recipient of many honors, including honorary doctorates from Villanova, Georgetown, Thomas Jefferson, and Medical College of Pennsylvania/Hahnemann Universities.

Acknowledgments

The Nursing Experience is critically dependent on those who are well positioned inside the profession for its "state of the art" information. Many gave generously of their time and knowledge for Kelly's *Dimensions of Professional Nursing* and again for *Experience*. Special thanks to Rita Munley-Gallagher of the American Nurses Association, and Diane Mancino of the National Student Nurses' Association. So many others would have been willing to give of themselves and their expertise, but the magic of the Internet has been able to fill in innumerable gaps in information. One who has been a constant source of consultation on the law is my husband, Dick Joel; thanks again.

Friends who deserve my appreciation have generously donated the incredible photographs that appear in this text. They are Nancy Valentine, formerly of the U.S. Department of Veterans Affairs, Toni Fiore of Hackensack University Medical Center, Linda Cuoco of the Valley Hospital, Nancy Holecek of the St. Barnabas Health Care System, Kathi Sengin of Robert Wood Johnson University Hospital, Barbara Davey of Christ Hospital, Jane Wandel of Beth Israel Deaconess Medical Center, Joyce Clifford of the Institute of Nursing Healthcare Leadership in Boston, Lyle Churchill of the Visiting Nurse Service of New York, Eurice Rojas and Lissette Andrews of Palisades Medical Center, Mary Ann Christopher and Susan Kline of the Visiting Nurse Association of Central Jersey, Ken McNulty and Casey Cuthbert-Allman of the Visiting Nurse Association of Boston, Judith Ryan and Patrice Meier of the Evangelical Lutheran Good Samaritan Society, Elaine Dolinsky of Rutgers College of Nursing, and Andrea Aughenbaugh of the New Jersey State Nurses Association.

PART 1

THE EVOLUTION OF NURSING

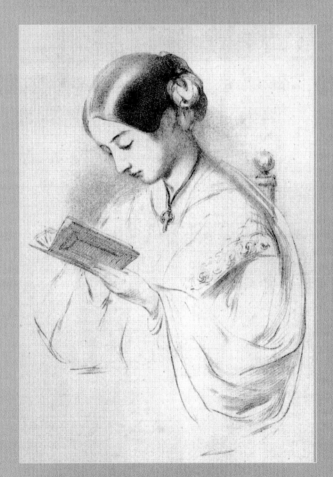

The young Florence Nightingale. (*Courtesy of Lucie Kelly, private collection*)

Chapter 1

Care of the Sick: How Nursing Began

OBJECTIVES

After studying this chapter, you will be able to:

1. Recognize the contributions of early civilizations to the care of the sick.
2. Discuss how various nursing religious orders influenced the evolution of nursing.
3. Describe at least three ways in which Florence Nightingale influenced the development of nursing.

What does it matter whether or not we know anything about nursing history? A lot of nursing today was formed by its history. Its development since ancient times, within the social contexts of those times, explains many things: its power or lack of power, its educational confusion, and the makeup of its practitioners. The changing relationships between nursing and other health care professions, nursing and other disciplines, and nursing and the public can be traced and better understood with the knowledge of past history. The impact of social and scientific changes on nursing and nursing's impact on society are ongoing processes that need to be studied; nursing does not exist in a vacuum.

Sometimes there is a repetition of history. For instance, 100 years ago, there were many arguments within and without the nursing profession about nursing education; this scenario is being repeated today. In that

3

same era, the question of nursing licensure was hotly debated; today, it is again a major concern. For over 75 years, studies have documented reasons for nurses' discontentment with their jobs; only recently were some changes made. These issues affect the practice of every nurse; in some cases, they are a factor in determining whether the nurse even chooses to stay in the profession. Understanding the past can be very useful in making decisions that shape the future.

CARE OF THE SICK IN EARLY CIVILIZATIONS

Undoubtedly, some form of nursing activity has existed since earliest civilization. Although for thousands of years concepts of health and illness were closely related to belief in the supernatural, there is evidence that plants were used as medicine, as well as heat, cold, and even some types of primitive surgery. In primitive times there were medicine men and women, but nursing care probably fell to the women of the family unit.

Records of the early known civilizations were sometimes written by the physicians of the time and provide interesting information on the care of the sick. There were also occasional references to nurses. In *Babylonia* for instance, one of the great civilizations that lay between the eastern Mediterranean and the Persian Gulf, a legalized medical system existed. There were even laws that punished physicians for malpractice. Some of the treatments included diet, rest, enemas, bandaging, and massaging (with or without incantations), and care was given by some type of lay nurse.

Although the ancient *Hebrews* attributed their illnesses to God's wrath, under the leadership of Moses they developed principles of hygiene and sanitation. The Mosaic Code contained a comprehensive set of public health practices, which were very advanced for the day: prohibitions on eating pork, the expectation that individuals having communicable diseases be isolated, and so on. They performed various kinds of surgery and dressed wounds, using sutures and bandages. Nurses are mentioned in the *Old Testament*, but other than visiting and possibly caring for the sick in the home, their role is not clear.

Ancient *Egypt*, located along the Nile, also was noted for its laws on health and sanitation, which included regulations about food use, preservation, personal hygiene, and a variety of aspects of primary health care. A pharmacopeia including over 700 drugs was authored.[1] There were medical schools and at least one school of midwifery for women, whose graduates taught physicians about "women's conditions." There is history of nurses being used by the aristocracy to care for

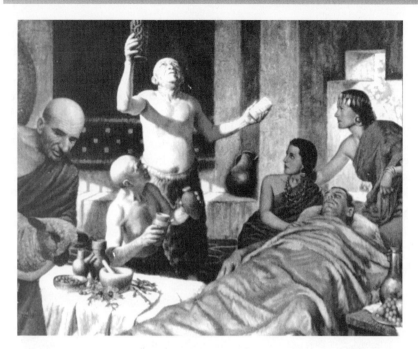

Physicians in ancient Babylon treated the sick with a mixture of medicine and charms; nurses were probably the women in the family. (*Courtesy of Parke, Davis and Company*)

children, the aged, and the sick. Excavated medical papyri have descriptions of nursing procedures, such as dressing wounds, but again, the nurses' duties are not clear.

The first hospitals were probably established in pre-Christian *India*. Records identify the first special nursing group: men who staffed the hospitals and performed some nursing functions. Actually, they may have been more like physicians' assistants. The Indian physicians were exceptionally skilled in surgery and used many drugs in their treatments, although, as in other civilizations, magic and evil spirits were part of medical belief.

In ancient *China*, both acupuncture and drug therapy were used. These were incorporated into the theory of Yang and Yin. Yang, the male principle, is light, positive, and full of life; Yin, the female principle, is dark, cold, and lifeless. When the two are in harmony, the patient is in good health. The Chinese also refined ancient measures of hydrotherapy, massage, and other physical techniques, and promoted systematic exercise to maintain physical and mental well-being. Many of these treatments are still used effectively today.

Greece, too, had its demons, spirits, and gods related to illness, with Asclepios (Roman version: Aesculapius), the classic god of medicine, honored by the founding of temples for the sick, which were actually more like health spas. The staff of Asclepios, intertwined with the snakes or serpents of wisdom and immortality, are thought to be the basis of today's medical caduceus. The greatest name in Greek medicine is *Hippocrates* (about 400 B.C.), who developed patient assessment and recording and rejected the supernatural origins of disease. His establishment of high ethical standards is reflected in the Hippocratic oath still taken in some medical schools. For centuries after his death, the medical books he had written were the basis of medical knowledge. There is no account of nurses here.

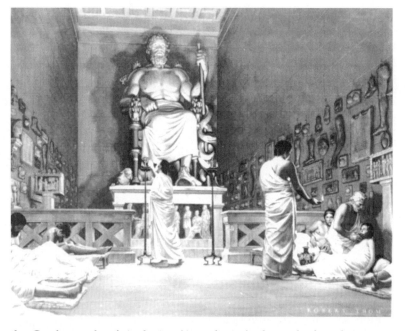

In the Greek temple of Asclepios (Aesculapius), the god of medicine, priests combined prayers and rituals with various treatments. (*Courtesy of Parke, Davis and Company*)

Rome's most lasting contribution to medicine may have been the founding of hospitals, at first primarily for the military as they conquered new territories. Both male and female attendants (nurses?) were used. Medical care was in the hands of the Greeks, like the great *Galen* (about 200 to 130 B.C.), who lived in Rome.

CHRISTIANITY'S IMPACT ON NURSING

In the early Christian era, bishops were given responsibility for the sick, the poor, widows, and children, but the deacons and deaconesses carried out the services. It appears that there was a group of specially designated women (deaconesses, widows, virgins, and matrons) who cared for the sick. *Phoebe*, mentioned in the Bible by Paul, was the first deaconess actually identified as giving nursing care. There were other noted women in the first centuries of Christianity, frequently designated as saints later. *Olympias*, a rich aristocratic widow of Constantinople, erected a convent and with 40 deaconesses cared for the sick. *Marcella*, a wealthy Roman, converted her palace into a monastery and, among other things, taught the care of the sick to her followers. *Fabiola* was one of Marcella's group and became a Christian convert. Also wealthy, she founded the first free hospital for the poor and personally nursed the sickest and filthiest people who came to her. St. Jerome wrote letters of praise about both women.

The Middle Ages (about A.D. 500 to 1500) has a mixed record in sick care. During the first half, called the *Dark Ages*, medical and nursing care, though needed, was barely available as wars, ignorance, famine, and disease flourished. The Christian church was obsessed with its belief that the main purpose of human beings on earth was to prepare for a future life and thus saw little need for science and philosophy. The teachings of hygiene and sanitation from earlier civilizations were discarded. Except for the eastern Roman and Moslem empires, medical knowledge stagnated.

During the Middle Ages, the deaconesses, suppressed by the Western churches in particular, gradually declined and became almost extinct. As the deaconesses declined, the *religious orders* grew stronger. Known as *monastic orders* and composed of monks and nuns (though not in the same orders), they controlled the hospitals, running them as institutions concerned more with the patients' religious problems than with their physical ailments. However, monks and some nuns were better educated than most people in those times, and their liberal education may well have included some of the medical writings of Galen.

Lay citizens banded together to form *secular orders*. Their work was similar to that of the monastic orders in that it was concerned with the sick and needy, but they lived in their own homes, were allowed to marry, and took no vows of the church. They usually adopted a uniform, or habit. Nursing was often their main work.

The *military nursing orders*, known as the *Knights Hospitallers*, were the outcome of the Crusades, the military expeditions undertaken by Christians in the eleventh, twelfth, and thirteenth centuries to recover the

Holy Land from the Moslems. The most prominent of these three types of orders—religious, military, and secular—were the Order of St. Benedict, Knights Hospitallers, Hospital Brothers of St. Anthony, Third Order of St. Francis, Beguines of Flanders, Order of the Holy Ghost (Santo Spirito), Grey Sisters, and Alexian Brotherhood.

NURSING CARE IN EARLY HOSPITALS

Gradually, more hospitals in which the sick received care were established as the need increased. At the close of the Middle Ages, there were hospitals all over Europe, particularly in larger cities such as Paris and Rome. In England, too, several hundred were established, some of which still remain. Hospitals in England during the Middle Ages differed from those on the Continent in that they were never completely church controlled, although they were founded on Christian principles and accepted responsibility for the sick and injured. The oldest and best-known English hospitals from a historical point of view are St. Bartholomew's, founded in 1123; St. Thomas's, founded in 1213; and Bethlehem Hospital, founded in 1247, originally as a general hospital, which later became famous as a mental institution, referred to frequently as *Bedlam*.

The Hotel Dieu of Paris, founded about 650, had an unfavorable record as far as nursing was concerned. Staffed by Augustinian nuns who did the cooking and laundry as well as the nursing, and who had neither intellectual nor professional stimulation, the hospital was not distinguished for its care of patients. The records of nursing kept by this hospital were well done, however, and have been a source of enlightenment for historians.

The nursing care in most early hospitals was essentially basic: bathing, feeding, giving medicines, making beds, and so on. It was rarely of high quality, however, largely because of the retarded progress of nearly all civilization and the shortsighted attitude toward women that was typical of the Dark Ages. Even after the Renaissance (1400 to 1550), during which Paracelsus, Vesalius, and Paré made major contributions in pharmaceutical chemistry, anatomy, and surgery, hospital nursing remained at the same basic level.

During the Reformation (beginning about 1500), which resulted in the formation of various Protestant churches, the Protestant leaders saw the vacuum in the care of the sick and urged the hiring of nurse deaconesses and elderly women to do nursing. By the end of the eighteenth century, nurses of some kind functioned in hospitals. Conditions were not attractive, and much has been written about the drunken, thieving women who tended patients. However, some hospitals made real efforts to set standards. Already a hierarchy of nursing personnel had begun, with aides and watchers assigned to help the *sisters*, as the early English nurses were called.

In other parts of Europe, nursing was becoming recognized as an important service. Diderot, whose *Encyclopedia* attempted to sum up all human knowledge, said that nursing "is as important for humanity as its functions are low and repugnant." Urging care in selection, since "all persons are not adapted to it," he described the nurse as "patient, mild, and compassionate. She should console the sick, foresee their needs, and relieve their tedium."[2]

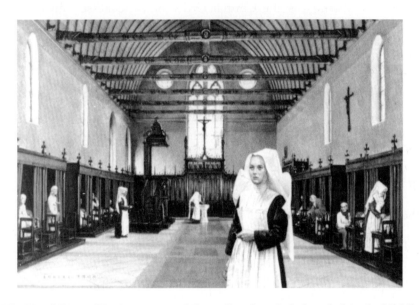

The Hotel Dieu of Paris was one of the earliest hospitals founded in the Middle Ages. (*Courtesy of Parke, Davis and Company*)

The dreary picture of secular nursing is not totally unexpected, given the times. Because proper young women did not work outside the home, nursing had no acceptance, much less prestige. Even those nurses not in Dickens's Sairy Gamp mold (Charles Dickens created Sairy Gamp as a fat, old, totally disreputable nurse with a hoarse voice and a red nose) or those desiring to nurse found themselves in competition with workhouse inmates, who were cheaper workers for hospital administrations. (Actually, most care was still given at home by wives and mothers.) It was acceptable to nurse as a member of a religious order, when the motivation was, of course, religious and the cost to the hospital was little or nothing.

A startling development during the Reformation was the disappearance of male nurses. The Protestant nursing orders were female, and except for a few male orders like the Brothers Hospitallers of St. John of God, the Catholic nursing orders after 1500 were primarily made up of women. Among the most noted were the Sisters of Charity (France), the Irish Sisters of Charity, and the Sisters of Mercy.

During the nineteenth century, several nursing orders were revived or originated that had substantial influence on modern nursing. In most instances, these orders cared for patients in hospitals that were already established, in contrast to the orders of earlier times, which had founded the hospitals in which they worked. Among the most influential orders was the Church Order of Deaconesses, an ancient order revived by Theodor Fliedner, pastor of a small parish in Kaiserswerth, Germany. (Florence Nightingale later obtained her only formal training there.) The Protestant Sisters of Charity, under Sister Elizabeth Fry, worked among prisoners and the physically and mentally ill.

Of the nursing orders established by the Church of England, the most noted were the Sisters of Mercy in the Church of England and St. Margaret's of East Grinstead, both of whom were involved with "district" or home nursing. The Anglican order that did the most for hospital nursing in this period was St. John's House, founded in 1848 in London, whose purpose was to train members of the church "to act as nurses and visitors to the sick and poor."[3] The original plan required the order to be associated with a hospital in which women under training or those already educated could gain experience and exercise their calling. The program was very successful.

Many of the Catholic and Protestant orders went to the New World, founding hospitals in Canada, the United States, and Mexico. Cortez is credited with founding the first hospital in the New World, located in Mexico City, and within 20 years, most major Spanish towns had one. Hospitals in the New World were no better than those in Europe, and given the hard living conditions, there were numerous health problems.

Progress in medicine and science during these centuries (Exhibit 1.1) was accompanied by accelerated interest in better service and nurses' training. Neither was achieved to a significant degree, however, despite the fine work of dedicated men and women who belonged to the nursing orders of the time. Limited in number and inadequately prepared for their nursing functions, the members of these orders could not begin to meet the need for their services. Such care as patients received in the majority of institutions was grossly inadequate.

In the mid-nineteenth century, therefore, the time was right—perhaps overdue—for the revolution in nursing education that originated under

Exhibit 1.1 Three Centuries of Scientific Landmarks

William Harvey (1578–1657), England	First to describe completely (except for the capillary system) and accurately the circulatory system.
Thomas Sydenham (1624–1689), England	Revived the Hippocratic methods of observation and reasoning and in other ways restored clinical medicine to a sound basis.
Anton van Leeuwenhoek (1632–1723), Holland	Improved on Galileo's microscope and produced one that permitted the examination of body cells and bacteria.
William Hunter (1718–1783) and his brother John (1728–1793), Scotland	Founded the science of pathology.
William Tuke (1732–1822), England	Reformed the care of the mentally ill.
Edward Jenner (1749–1823), England	Originated vaccination against smallpox.
René Laennec (1781–1826), France	Invented the stethoscope.
Oliver Wendell Holmes (1809–1894), United States	Furthered safe obstetric practice, pointing out the dangers of infection.
Crawford W. Long (1815–1878), United States	Excised a tumor of the neck under ether anesthesia in 1832 but did not make his discovery public until after Dr. William T. Morton announced his in 1846.
Ignaz P. Semmelweis (1818–1865), Austria-Hungary	Recognized that infection was carried from patient to patient by physicians and instituted preventive measures for puerperal fever in new mothers.
Louis Pasteur (1822–1895), France	Founder of microbiology and developer of pasteurization; developed preventive inoculations against anthrax, chicken cholera, and rabies.
Lord Joseph Lister (1827–1912), England	Developed and proved the theory of bacterial infection of wounds.
Robert Koch (1843–1910), Germany	Founded modern bacteriology; identified the tubercle bacillus.
Wilhelm Röntgen (1845–1923), Germany	Discovered x-rays in 1895 and laid the foundation for the science of roentgenology and radiology.
Pierre Curie (1859–1906), France, and his Polish wife, Marie (1867–1934)	Discovered radium in 1898.

the leadership of Florence Nightingale and that influenced so greatly and so quickly (from a historical point of view) the nursing care of patients and, indeed, the health of the world.

THE INFLUENCE OF FLORENCE NIGHTINGALE

It has been said that Florence Nightingale, an extraordinary woman in any century, is the most written-about woman in history. Through her own numerous publications, her letters, the writings of her contemporaries, including newspaper reports, and the numerous biographies and studies of her life, there emerges the picture of a sometimes contradictory, frequently controversial, but undeniably powerful woman who probably had a greater influence on the care of the sick than any other single individual.

Called the founder of modern nursing, Nightingale was a strong-willed, intelligent woman who used her considerable knowledge of statistics, sanitation, logistics, administration, nutrition, and public health not only to develop a new system of nursing education and health care but also to improve the social welfare systems of the time. The gentle, caring lady of the lamp, full of compassion for the soldiers of the Crimea, is an accurate image, but no more than that of the hard-headed administrator and planner who forced changes in the intolerable social conditions of the time, including the care of the sick poor. Nightingale knew that tender touch alone would not bring health to the sick or prevent illness, so she set her intelligence, her administrative skills, her political acumen, and her incredible drive to achieve her self-defined missions. In the Victorian age when women were almost totally dominated by men—fathers, husbands, brothers—and it was undesirable for them to show intelligence or profess interest in any-thing but household arts, this indomitable woman accomplished the following:

1. Improved and reformed laws affecting health, morals, and the poor.
2. Reformed hospitals and improved workhouses and infirmaries.
3. Improved medicine by instituting an army medical school and reorganizing the army medical department.
4. Improved the health of natives and British citizens in India and other colonies.
5. Established nursing as a profession with two missions: sick nursing and health nursing.[4]

The new nurse and the new image of the nurse that she created, in part through the nursing schools she founded, in part through her writings, and in part through her international influence, became the model that persisted for almost 100 years. Today, some of her tenets about the "good" nurse seem terribly restrictive, but it should be remembered that in those times not only the image but also the reality of much of secular nursing was based on the untutored, uncouth workhouse inmates for whom drunkenness and thievery were a way of life. It was small wonder that each Nightingale student had to exemplify a new image above reproach.

EARLY LIFE

Florence Nightingale was born on May 12, 1820, in Florence, Italy, during her English parents' travels there. The family was wealthy and well educated, with a high social standing and influential friends, all of which later would be useful to Nightingale. Primarily under her father's tutelage, she learned Greek, Latin, French, German, and Italian, and studied history, philosophy, science, music, art, and classical literature. She traveled widely with her family and friends. The breadth of her education, almost unheard of for women of the times, was also considerably more extensive than that of most men, including physicians. Her intelligence and education were recognized by scholars, as indicated in her correspondence with them.

Nightingale was not only bright but, according to early portraits and descriptions, slender, attractive, and fun-loving, enjoying the social life of her class. She differed from other young women in her determination to do something "toward lifting the load of suffering from the helpless and miserable."[5] Apparently, the encouragement of Dr. Samuel Gridley Howe and his wife, Julia Ward Howe (who wrote "The Battle Hymn of the Republic"), during a visit to the Nightingale family home in 1844 helped to crystallize Florence's interest in hospitals and nursing. Nevertheless, her intent to train in a hospital was strongly opposed by her family, and she limited herself to nursing family members.

Although remaining the obedient daughter, Nightingale found her own way to expand her knowledge of sick care. She studied hospital and sanitary reports and books on public health. Having received information on Kaiserswerth in Germany, she determined to receive training there—which was more acceptable because of its religious auspices. On one of her trips to the Continent, she made a brief visit and was impressed enough to spend three months in training and observation there in 1851. Her later efforts to study with various Catholic orders were frustrated. However, she got permission to inspect the hospitals in various cities during her tours. She examined the general layout of the hospital, as well as ward construction, sanitation, general administration, and the work of the surgeons and physicians.[6] Apparently, these observational techniques and her analytical abilities then and later were the basis of her unrivaled knowledge of hospitals in the next decades. Few of her contemporaries ever had such knowledge.

In 1853, Nightingale assumed the position of superintendent of a charity hospital (probably more of a nursing home) for ill governesses run by titled ladies. Although she had difficulties with her intolerant governing board, she did make changes considered revolutionary for the day and, even with the lack of trained nurses, improved the patients' care. And she continued to visit hospitals. Just as Nightingale was negotiating for a superintendency in the newly reorganized and rebuilt King's College Hospital in London, England and France, in support of Turkey, declared war on Russia in March 1854.

CRIMEA: THE TURNING POINT

The Crimean War was a low point for England. Ill-prepared and disorganized in general, the army and the bureaucracy were even less prepared to care for the thousands of soldiers both wounded in battle and prostrated by the cholera epidemics brought on by worse than primitive conditions. Not even the most basic equipment or drugs were available, and, as casualties mounted, Turkey turned over the enormous but bare and filthy barracks at Scutari, across from Constantinople, to be used as a hospital. The conditions remained abominable. The soldiers lay on the floor in filth, untended, frequently without food or water because there was no equipment to prepare or distribute either. Rats and other vermin came from the sewers underneath the building. There were no beds, furniture, basins, soap, towels, or eating utensils, and

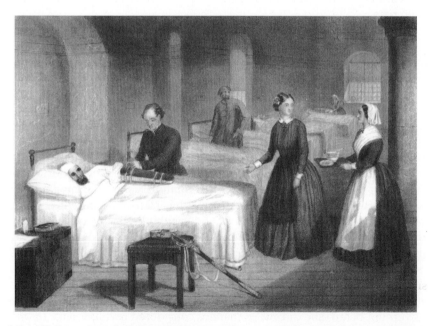

Miss Nightingale in the hospital at Scutari. (*Courtesy of Lucie Kelly, private collection*)

few provisions. There were only orderlies, and none of these at night. The death rate was said to be 60 percent.

In previous wars, the situation had not been much different, and there was little interest on the battle sites, for ordinary soldiers were accorded no decencies. However, now, for the first time, civilian war correspondents were present and sent back the news of these horrors to England with a newly aroused social conscience. The reformers were in an uproar; newspapers demanded to know why England did not have nurses like the French Sisters of Charity to care for its soldiers, and Parliament trembled. In October 1854, Sidney Herbert, Secretary of War and an old friend of Florence Nightingale, wrote, begging her to lead a group of nurses to the Crimea under government authority and at government expense. Nightingale had already decided to offer her services, and the two letters crossed. In less than a week, she had assembled 38 nurses, the most she could find who met her standards—Roman Catholic and Anglican sisters and lay nurses from various hospitals—and embarked for Scutari. One nurse who was not accepted was Mary Grant Seacole, who had nursed British soldiers in Jamaica. At her own expense she traveled to the Crimea, built and opened a lodging house for the comfort of the troops, and nursed sick officers with medicines, some of which were her own concoctions.[7]

Even under the miserable circumstances found there, Nightingale and her contingent were not welcomed by the army doctors and surgeons, who refused the nurses' services. Nightingale chose to wait to be asked to help. To the anger of her nurses, she allowed none of them to give care until one week later, when scurvy, starvation, dysentery, exposure, and more fighting almost brought about the collapse of the British army. Then the doctors, desperate for any kind of assistance, turned to the eager nurses.

Modern criticisms of Florence Nightingale frequently refer to her insistence on the physician's overall authority and her own authoritarian approach to nursing. The first criticism may have originated with her situation in the Crimean War. In mid-century England her appointment created a furor; she was the first woman ever to be given such authority. Yet, despite the high-sounding title that Herbert insisted she have—General Superintendent of the Female Nursing Establishment of the Military Hospitals of the Army—her orders required that she have the approval of the Principal Medical Officer "in her exercise of the responsibilities thus vested in her."[8] Although no "lady, sister, or nurse" could be transferred from one hospital to another without her approval, she had no authority over anyone else, even orderlies or cooks. What she accomplished had to be done through sheer force of will or persuasion. Her overt deference to physicians was probably the beginning of the doctor–nurse game.

Whatever the limitations of her power, Florence Nightingale accomplished miracles at Scutari. Even in the week of waiting, she moved into the kitchen area and began to cook extras from her own supplies to create a diet kitchen, which for five months was the only source of food for the sick.

Nightingale had powerful friends and control over a large amount of contributed funds—a situation that gained her some cooperation from most physicians after a while. Through persuasion and the use of good managerial techniques, she cleaned up the hospital: the orderlies scrubbed and emptied slops regularly; soldiers' wives and camp followers washed clothes; and the vermin were brought under some control. Before the end of the war, the mortality rate at Scutari declined to 1 percent.

When the hospital care improved, Nightingale began a program of social welfare among the soldiers—among other things, seeing to it that they got sick pay. The patients adored her. She cared about them, and the doctors and officers reproached her for "spoiling the brutes." News correspondents wrote reports about the "ministering angel" and "lady with the lamp" making late rounds after the medical officers had retired—which inspired Longfellow later to write his famous poem "Santa Filomena." England and America were enthralled, and she was awarded decorations by Queen Victoria and the Sultan of Turkey.

However, all did not go well. The military doctors continued in their resentment and tried to undermine her. There were problems in her own ranks, dissension among the religious and secular nurses, and problems of incompetence and immorality. No doubt Nightingale was high-handed at times. Despite praise of her leadership, she was also called "quick, violent-tempered, positive, obstinate, and stubborn."[9] Certainly she drove herself in all she did.

When the situation at Scutari was improved, she crossed the Black Sea to the battle sites and worked on the reorganization of the few hospitals there—with no better support from physicians and superior officers. There, she contracted Crimean fever (probably typhoid or typhus) and nearly died. However, she refused a leave of absence to recuperate and stayed in Scutari to work until the end of the war. She supervised 125 nurses and forced the military to recognize the place of nurses.

On her return from the Crimea, Nightingale took to her bed, or at least to her rooms, and emerged only on rare occasions. There is much speculation on this illness—whether it was a result of the Crimea fever, neurasthenia, a bit of both, or whether she simply found it useful to avoid wasting time with people she did not want to see.[10] For she was famous now and had been given discretion over the so-called Nightingale Fund, to which almost everyone in England had subscribed, including many of the troops.

From her experiences, and to support her recommendations for reform, Nightingale wrote a massive report entitled *Notes on Matters Affecting the Health, Efficiency, and Hospital Administration of the British Army,* crammed with facts, figures, and statistical comparisons. On the basis of this and her later well-researched and well-documented papers, she is often credited with being the first nurse researcher.[11] Reforms were slow in coming but extended even to the United States when the Union consulted her about organizing hospitals. In 1859 she wrote a small book, *Notes on Nursing: What It Is and What It Is Not,*[12] intended for the average housewife and printed cheaply so that it would be affordable. These and other Nightingale works are still amazingly readable today—brisk, down-to-earth, and laced with many a pithy comment. For instance, in *Notes on Hospitals,* written in the same year, she compared the administration of the various types of hospitals and characterized the management of secular hospitals under the sole command of the male hospital authorities as "all but crazy."[13]

Her knowledge was certainly respected, and she was consulted by many, including the Royal Sanitary Commission on the Health of the Army in India.

THE NIGHTINGALE NURSE

In 1860, Nightingale utilized some of the £45,000 of the Nightingale Fund to establish a training school for nurses. She selected St. Thomas's Hospital because of her respect for its matron, Mrs. S. E. Wardroper. The two converted the resident medical officers to their plan, although apparently most other physicians objected to the school. The students were chosen; the first class in the desired age range of 25–35 years and with impeccable character references numbered only 15. It was to be a one-year training program, and the students were presented with what could be called terminal behavioral objectives that they had to reach satisfactorily. Students could be dismissed by the matron for misconduct, inefficiency, or negligence. However, if they passed the courses of instruction and training satisfactorily, they were entered in the "Register" as certified nurses. The Committee of the Nightingale Fund then recommended them for employment; in the early years, they were obligated to work as hospital nurses for at least five years (for which they were paid).

The students' time was carefully structured, beginning at 6 A.M. and ending with a 9 P.M. bedtime, which included a semimandatory two-hour exercise period (walking abroad had to be done in twos and threes, not alone). Within that time there was actually about a nine-hour work and training day (a vast difference from future American schools).

This included bedside teaching by a teaching sister or the Resident Medical Officer and elementary instruction in "Chemistry, with reference to air, water, food, etc.; Physiology, with reference to a knowledge of the leading functions of the body, and general instruction on medical and surgical topics"[14] by professors of the medical school attached to St. Thomas's, given voluntarily and without payment.

The Nightingale school was not under the control of the hospital and had education as its purpose. The Nightingale Fund paid the medical officers, head nurses, and matron for teaching students, beyond whatever they earned from the hospital in carrying out their other duties. Both the head nurses and the matron kept records on each student, evaluating how she met the stated objectives of the program. The students were expected to keep notes from the lectures and records of patient observation and care, all of which were checked by the nurse-teachers. At King's College Hospital, run by the Society of St. John's House, an Anglican religious community, midwifery was taught in similar style and with similar regulations, again under the auspices of the Nightingale Fund Committee. Also, at the Royal Liverpool Infirmary, nurses were trained for home nursing of the sick poor under a Nightingale protocol but were personally funded by a Liverpool merchant–philanthropist. As Nightingale said in 1863, "We have had to introduce an entirely new system to which the older systems of nursing bear but slight resemblance. . . . It exists neither in Scotland nor in Ireland at the present time."[15]

The demand for the Nightingale nurses was overwhelming. In the next few years, requests also came for them to improve the workhouse (poorhouse) infirmaries and to reform both civilian and military nursing in India. In response to these demands, Nightingale wrote many reports, detailing to the last item the system for educating these nurses and for improving patient care, including such points as general hygiene and sanitation, nutrition, equipment, supplies, and the nurses' housing conditions, holidays, salaries, and retirement benefits. (For India, she suggested that they had better pay good salaries and provide satisfactory working and living conditions, or the nurses might opt for marriage, because the opportunities there were even greater than in England.) She constantly reiterated that she could not supply enough nurses but, when possible, she would send a matron and some other nurses, who would train new Nightingale nurses.[16]

Maintaining standards was a constant struggle. Even St. Thomas's Hospital slipped, and Nightingale, who had been immersed in the Indian reforms, had to take time to reorganize the program. What evolved over the years, from the first program, was one of preparation for two kinds of nursing practitioners: the educated middle- and upper-class ladies who paid their own tuition and the still carefully selected poor women who were subsidized by the Nightingale Fund. The former were given an extra year or two of education to prepare them to become teachers or superintendents; the latter were prepared to be hospital ward nurses. A third choice was district nursing. "This nurse must be of a yet higher class and of a yet fuller training than a hospital nurse, because she has not the doctor always at hand and because she has no hospital appliances at hand."[17] All of these special probationers were expected to enter the profession permanently.

In Nightingale's later years, she came into conflict with the very nurses who had been trained for leadership. In 1886, some of these nurses, now superintendents of other training schools, wanted to establish an organization that would provide a central examination and registration center, the forerunner of licensure. Nightingale opposed this movement for several reasons: nursing was still too young and disorganized; national criteria would not be as high as those of individual schools; and the all-important aspect of character could not be tested. She fought the concept with every weapon at her disposal, including her powerful contacts, and succeeded in limiting the fledgling Royal British Nurses' Association to maintaining a "list" instead of a "register."

Nightingale's prolific writings on nursing have survived, and some of them are still surprisingly apt. Often they reflected her concern about the character of nurses and her own determination that their main focus be on nursing. One principle from which Nightingale did not swerve was that nurses were to nurse, not to do heavy cleaning ("if you want a charwoman, hire one"); not to do laundry ("it makes their hands coarse and hard and less able to attend to the delicate manipulation which they may be called on to execute"); and not to fetch ("to save the time of nurses; all diets and ward requisites should be brought into the wards"). Then, as in many places now, status and promotion came through assumption of administrative roles, but Nightingale recognized that "many are valuable as nurses, who are yet unfit for promotion to head nurses." Her alternative, however, would not be greeted favorably today—a raise after 10 years of good service!

Nightingale also commented on other issues considered pertinent today. Continuing education was a must, for she saw nursing as a progressive art, in which to stand still was to go back. "A woman who thinks of herself, 'Now, I am a full nurse, a skilled nurse. I have learnt all there is to be learned,' take my word for it, she does not know what a nurse is, and she will never know: she has gone back already."[18] Although there is no evidence that she took any action to help end discrimination against women, Nightingale believed that women should be accepted into all professions, but she warned them, "qualify yourselves for it as a man does for his work."[19] She believed that women should be paid as highly as men, but that equal pay meant equal responsibility. In a profession with as much responsibility as nursing, she said, it was particularly important to have adequate compensation, or intelligent, independent women would not be attracted to it.

Until the end of her life, she was firm on the need for nurses to obey physicians in medical matters. However, she stressed the importance of nurse observation and reporting because the physician was not constantly at the patient's bedside, as the nurse was. She was adamant that a nurse (and woman) be in charge of nursing, with no other administrative figure having authority over nurses, including physicians. She knew the importance of a work setting that gave job satisfaction. In words that are a far-off echo of nurses' complaints today, she wrote:

> Besides, a thing very little understood, a good nurse has her professional pride in results of her nursing quite as much as a medical officer in the results of his treatment. There are defective buildings, defective administrations, defective appliances, which make all good nursing impossible. A good nurse does not like to waste herself, and the better the nurse, the stronger this feeling in her.[20]

Planner, administrator, educator, researcher, reformer, Florence Nightingale never lost her interest in nursing. At age 74, in her last major publication on nursing, she differentiated between sick nursing and health nursing, and emphasized the primary need for prevention of illness, for which a lay "Health Missioner" (today's health educator?) would be trained.

When Nightingale died on August 13, 1910, she was to be honored by burial in Westminster Abbey. However, she had chosen instead to be buried in the family plot in Hampshire, with a simple inscription: "F.N. Born 1820, Died 1910."

KEY POINTS

1. A certain amount of the ritual, mysticism, and belief in spirits or gods pervaded care of the sick in early civilizations.
2. Records of early civilizations emphasize treatment given by those designated as physicians or healers, and there also appear to have been men and women fulfilling nursing roles of some sort.
3. In early Egypt, India, China, Greece, and Rome, as well as in the lands of the Hebrews, setting rules of hygiene and sanitation, using herbs, and performing surgery were part of the care of the sick.
4. The Romans are generally credited with building the first hospitals, but in the Christian period, "houses for the sick" were available for the sick poor, often tended by men or women in religious and secular orders.

5. In 1860, Florence Nightingale founded modern nursing at St. Thomas's Hospital in London with organized training programs that included both theory and practice, careful selection of students, and freedom from hospital control.
6. In her careful observations and recording and her use of statistics in matters affecting health care and administration in the British army, in hospitals throughout Europe, and in the community, Nightingale is often credited with being the first nurse researcher.
7. Nightingale made many pertinent observations and recommendations on nurses and nursing practice, such as the need for nurses to be free from other duties so that they could concentrate on nursing, for holistic care, for home care, for continuing education, for adequate compensation, and for a satisfactory working environment.

STUDY QUESTIONS

1. What value does the study of nursing in early civilizations hold for us today?
2. In what ways did the evolution of modern nursing depart from the principles fostered by Florence Nightingale?
3. What circumstances during the Crimean War created a unique opportunity for the success of the Nightingale reforms?

REFERENCES

1. Ellis JR, Hartley CL. *Nursing in Today's World: Challenges, Issues and Trends*, 8th ed. Philadelphia: J.B. Lippincott, 2004.
2. Bullough B, Bullough V. *The Care of the Sick: The Emergence of Modern Nursing*. New York: Prodist, 1978, p 69.
3. Moore J. *A Zeal for Responsibility: The Struggle for Professional Nursing in Victorian England, 1869–1883*. Athens, GA: University of Georgia Press, 1983, p 3.
4. Barritt ER. Florence Nightingale's values and modern nursing education. *Nurs Forum* 12(4):7–47, 1973.
5. Bullough and Bullough, op cit, p 86.
6. Gillian G. *Nightingales: The Extraordinary Upbringing and Curious Life of Miss Florence Nightingale*. New York: Ballantine Books, 2004.
7. Griffon P. "A somewhat duskier skin": Mary Seacole in the Crimea. *Nurs Hist Rev* 6:115–127, 1998.
8. Seymer LR. *Selected Writings of Florence Nightingale*. New York: Macmillan Publishing, 1954, p 28.
9. Barritt, op cit, p 8.
10. Dossey B. Nightingale's Crimean fever. *J Holistic Nurs* 16:165–201, June 1998.

11. McDonald L. Florence Nightingale: Passionate statistician. *J Holistic Nurs* 16: 267–277, June 1998.
12. Nightingale F. *Notes on Nursing*. London: Harrison (Bookseller to the Queen), 1859.
13. Seymer, op cit, pp 222–223.
14. Ibid, p 244.
15. Ibid, p 234.
16. Ibid, p 316.
17. Pavey, AE. *The Story of the Growth of Nursing*. London: Faber and Faber, 1938, p 296.
18. Ibid.
19. Ibid.
20. Seymer, op cit, p 276.

Updates can be found at

 http://www.JoelTheNursingExperience.com

Chapter 2

Nursing in the United States: American Revolution to Nursing Revolution

OBJECTIVES

After studying this chapter, you will be able to:

1. *Explain how early nursing schools in the United States were established and functioned.*
2. *Name at least five early nursing leaders and their contributions to nursing.*
3. *Identify factors that influenced major changes in the education of nurses in the period between the Civil War and the current day.*
4. *Describe major changes in the practice of nursing in the period between the Civil War and the current day.*
5. *Identify the key findings of major studies and reports about nursing.*
6. *Determine the amount of change achieved by these studies.*
7. *Compare and contrast community and hospital practice over the years: its origins, nature of the work, and skills and demands of the practitioner.*

The first 100 years of American nursing show an interesting pattern. At the close of the nineteenth century and the dawn of the twentieth, there was rapid expansion of new training schools for nurses.

Many exciting developments unheard of for a largely woman's occupation occurred just as rapidly, thanks to the intelligence, initiative, and risk taking of an extraordinary group of women. Then for most of the next 50 years, progress seemed slow, with tedious chipping away at the many obstacles to quality education and practice. However, after World War II, another rapid series of events moved nursing into a new era. We continue to live through a revolution in process that creates both opportunities and risks, and the promise of rich gains and significant losses.

THE VOLUNTEERS

Just as the Crimean War spotlighted the activities of Florence Nightingale and the importance of nursing, the Civil War was an impetus for the development of training programs for nursing in the United States. There had never been an organized system for the care of the sick and wounded in wartime. During the American Revolution, some basic care was given by camp followers, wives, women in the neighborhood, and "surgeon's mates" who may have been employed by the army.[1]

When the Civil War began in 1861, untrained women quickly volunteered to become nurses. Dorothea Dix, well known by then, was appointed by the Secretary of War to supervise these new "nurses." Meanwhile, members of religious orders also volunteered, and nursing in some of the larger government hospitals was eventually assigned to them because of the inexperience of the lay volunteers.[2]

Except for that group, almost none of the thousands of Northern women who served as nurses during the war had any kind of training or hospital experience. They can be categorized as follows:

1. The nurses appointed by Miss Dix or other officials as legal employees of the army for 40 cents and one ration a day.
2. The sisters or nuns of the various orders.
3. Those employed for short periods of time for menial chores.
4. Black women employed under general orders of the War Department for $10 a month.
5. Uncompensated volunteers.
6. Women camp followers.
7. Women employed by the various relief organizations.[3]

Because of the prejudice against the idea of Southern women as nurses in the terrible conditions in Confederate hospitals, only about 1000 served, mostly as volunteers, and they performed valiantly. As in the North, many nuns gave nursing care.

Some of the information on what the Civil War nurses did comes from the diaries of Northern and Southern women and the writings of Louisa May Alcott and Walt Whitman, both Northern volunteers. In her journal, Alcott described her working day, which began at 6:00 A.M. After opening the windows, because of the bad air in the makeshift hospital, she spent her time "giving out rations, cutting up food for helpless boys, washing faces, teaching my attendants how beds are made or floors are swept, dressing wounds, dusting tables, sewing bandages, keeping my tray tidy, rushing up and down after pillows, bed linens, sponges, and directions . . . ."[4] Volunteers also read to the patients, wrote letters, and comforted them. Apparently, even the hired nurses did little more except, perhaps, give medicines. But so did the volunteers, sometimes giving the medicine and food of their choice to the patient, instead of what the doctor ordered. However, many of these women were very strong, and were outspoken about incompetence and corruption; sometimes one carried her complaints to the Secretary of War and got action.

By 1862, enormous military hospitals, some with as many as 3000 beds, were being built, although there were still some makeshift hospitals— former hotels, churches, factories, and almost anything else available. Floating hospitals were also inaugurated and served as transport units, with nurses attending the wounded. According to one army hospital edict, the nurses, under the supervision of the "Stewards and Chief Wardmaster," were responsible for the administration of the wards, but many of their duties appeared to be related more to keeping the non-medical records of patients and reporting their misbehavior than to nursing care. If the patient needed medical or surgical attendance, the doctor was to be called.

Georgeanna Woolsey wrote that the often incompetent contract surgeons treated the nurses without even common courtesy because they did not want them and tried to make their lives so unbearable that they would leave. The formidable nurse Mary Ann (Mother) Bickerdyke attacked the surgeons and officers who were drunk, refused to attend the wounded, or injured them further because of their incompetence. She managed to have a number of them dismissed (in part because of her friendship with General Grant and General Sherman).[5] Another fighter was Clara Barton. One story told about her is that while supervising the delivery of a wagonload of supplies for soldiers, she neatly removed an ox from a herd intended for the Union Army, so that some starving Confederate wounded would have food.[6]

Only in recent years has attention been given to the black nurses of the Civil War or before. Harriet Tubman, the "Moses of her people," not only led many black slaves to freedom in her underground railroad activities before the war but also nursed the wounded when she joined the Union army. Similarly, Sojourner Truth, abolitionist speaker and activist in the women's movement, also cared for the sick and wounded. Susie King Taylor, born to slavery and secretly taught to read and write, met and married a Union soldier and served as a battlefront nurse for more than four years, although she received no salary or pension from the Union Army.[7]

There were other heroines, untrained women from the North and South, caring for the sick and wounded with few skills but much kindness, and, as in the Crimea, the soldiers were sentimentally appreciative, if not discriminating. On the other hand, given the circumstances, what they accomplished was amazing. Altogether, some 10,000 women served.

Even when paid, Civil War nurses had little status and no rank. An investigative report by the United States Sanitary Commission noted that nurses had not been well treated or wisely used. Nevertheless, the Civil War opened hospitals to massive numbers of women, well-bred "ladies," who would otherwise probably not even have thought of nursing. Some of these, such as Abby, Jane, and Georgeanna Woolsey, later helped lead the movement to establish training schools for nurses.

NURSING EDUCATION: THE FIRST 60 YEARS

The nursing role of women in the Civil War, however unsophisticated, and the fame of Florence Nightingale brought to the attention of the American public the need for nurses and the desirability of some organized programs of training.

More physicians became interested in the training of nurses and, at a meeting of the American Medical Association (AMA) in 1869, a committee to study the matter stated that it was "just as necessary to have well-trained, well-instructed nurses as to have intelligent and skillful physicians." The committee recommended that nursing schools be placed under the guardianship of county medical societies, although under the immediate supervision of lady superintendents; that every lay hospital should have a school; and that nurses should be trained not only for the hospital but for private duty in the home.[8]

Although a number of training programs for nurses and midwives existed before the Civil War, what is considered the first American school to offer a graded course in scientific nursing, based on guidelines set by Florence Nightingale, began in 1872 at the New England Hospital for Women and Children. Women physicians gave the twelve lectures that comprised the formal education of the 12-month course. The students, who received a small allowance after three months, worked from 5:30 A.M. to 9:00 P.M. and slept in rooms near the ward so that they

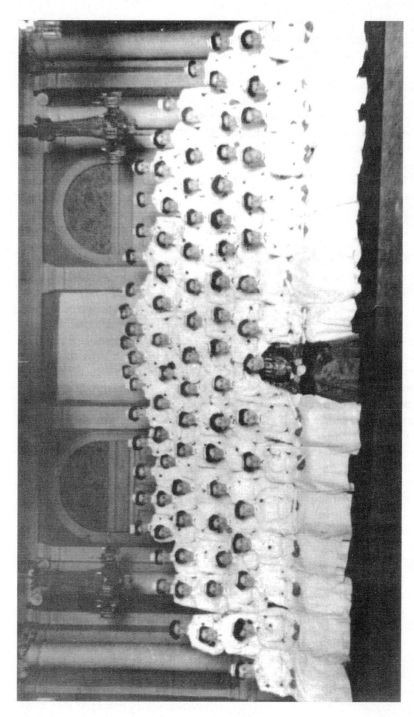

The Philadelphia Hospital (to change to Philadelphia General Hospital) Class of 1902 with Clara Barton as commencement speaker. (*Courtesy of the Museum of Nursing History, Inc., Philadelphia*)

were available when needed.[9] One of the first graduates was Melinda
Ann (Linda) Richards, thereafter called America's first trained nurse
(probably because, of all the nurses who graduated from this primitive
early program, she moved on to be a key figure in the development
of nursing education). Richards, like some of the other students in the
schools that evolved, had already been a nurse in a hospital. Some
schools would not accept these students because they wanted to set a
new image. Another outstanding graduate of the New England Hospital
for Women and Children (1879) was Mary Mahoney, the first trained
black nurse.

In 1873, three schools were established that were supposedly based
on the Nightingale model. The Bellevue Training School in New York
City was founded through the influence of several society ladies who
had been involved in Civil War nursing, including Abby Woolsey.
Although the school attempted to follow Nightingale principles and
reported that it was attracting educated women, its overall purpose
was to improve conditions in a great charity hospital, and much of the
learning occurred on a trial-and-error basis. Nevertheless, Bellevue had
a lot of interesting firsts: interdisciplinary rounds where nurses reported
on the nursing plan of care; patient record keeping and writing of
orders, initiated by Linda Richards, who became night superintendent;
and the first uniform, by stylish and aristocratic Euphemia Van
Rensselaer, which started a trend.

The Connecticut Training School was started through the influence of
another Woolsey, Georgeanna, and her husband, Dr. Francis Bacon.
Through negotiation with the hospital, the superintendent of nurses
was designated as separate from, and not responsible to, the steward
(administrator) of the hospital, and teaching outside the wards was
permitted. Good intentions notwithstanding, the students were soon
sent to give care in the homes of sick families, with the money going
to the School Fund—and the school could boast that for 33 years it
was not financed or directed by the hospital.

The Boston Training School was the last of that first famous trio. Again,
a group of women associated with other educational and philanthropic
endeavors spearheaded its organization, but this time their goal was to
offer a desirable occupation for self-supporting women and to provide
good private nurses for the community. After prolonged negotiations
that allowed the director of the school rather than the hospital to
maintain control, the Massachusetts General Hospital assigned "The
Brick" building to the school because it (The Brick) "stands by itself;
represents both medical and surgical departments; and offers the hard
labor desirable for the training of nurses."[10] Apparently, there was rather
poor leadership, and nurses continued to do menial tasks, with little
attention given to training. When Linda Richards became the third

director, she reorganized the work, started classes, and set out to prove that trained nurses were better than untrained ones.

Other major training schools that were to endure into the next century were founded in the next few years, somewhat patterned after Nightingale's precepts. Their success and the popularity of their graduates resulted in a massive proliferation of training schools. In 1880, there were 15; by 1900, 432; by 1909, 1105 hospital-based diploma schools. Hospitals with as few as 20 beds opened schools, and the students provided almost totally free labor. Usually, the only graduate nurses were the superintendent and perhaps the operating room supervisor and night supervisor. Students earned money for the hospital, for after a short period they were frequently sent to do private nursing in the home, with the money reverting to the hospital, not the school. Except for the few outstanding schools, all Nightingale principles were forgotten: the students were under the control of the hospital and worked from 12 to 15 hours a day—24 if they were on a private case in a home. Lessons, if any, were scheduled for an hour late in the evening when someone was available to teach. (It was not necessary for all students to be available.) Moreover, if the "pupils" lost time because of sickness, which was almost always contracted from patients or caused by sheer overwork, the time had to be totally made up before they could graduate.

Why then did training schools draw so many applicants? Because the occupational opportunities for untrained women were limited to domestic service, factory work, retail clerking, or prostitution. Higher education for women was limited to typewriting or teaching, but these were seldom taught in universities. Those colleges and universities that did admit women rarely prepared them for professions. Even with the strict discipline, hard work, long hours, and almost no time off, after a year or two of training (the second year consisting of unabashedly free labor to the hospitals), the trained nurse could do private duty at a salary ranging from $10 a week to the vague possibility of $20 (if she could collect it), a far cry from the $4 to $6 average of other women workers. Of course, on these cases, she was a 24-hour servant to the family and patient, lucky to have time off for a walk. Also, because there were necessarily months with no employment, even an excellent nurse was lucky to gross $600 a year.[11] The more famous hospital schools, in particular, had hundreds and even thousands of applicants a year. On the other hand, there was a multitude of hospitals and sanitoria of all kinds that were looking for students to meet their staffing needs, and for these, high-quality applicants were frequently lacking. Consequently, application standards were rapidly lowered. Apparently, most schools admitted a class of 30 to 35[12] (in some cases determined by their staffing and financial needs). Attrition, caused in part by the extremely high rate of student illness and the unpleasant working and living conditions, was often 75 percent.

Student admission requirements varied, but all nurse applicants were female. Some hospitals accepted men in programs but gave them only a short course and frequently called them *attendants*. In 1888, at Bellevue Hospital, the Mills School for men was established with a two-year course, but for a long time its graduates were also called *attendants*. Other schools admitting men followed. Blacks were also generally silently excluded. Over the years, formal programs for the education of black nurses were founded, the first, funded by the Rockefeller Foundation, in 1886 at Spelman Seminary (now Spelman College) in Atlanta. In 1891 the first hospital school exclusively for black women was established at the Provident Hospital in Chicago.[13] Progress was slow for both of these groups and the environment resistant.

The minimum age for all students was generally 21 years. Eight or fewer years of schooling were common, but usually good health and good character were absolute prerequisites. Obedience in training was essential, and a student could be dismissed as a troublemaker if the

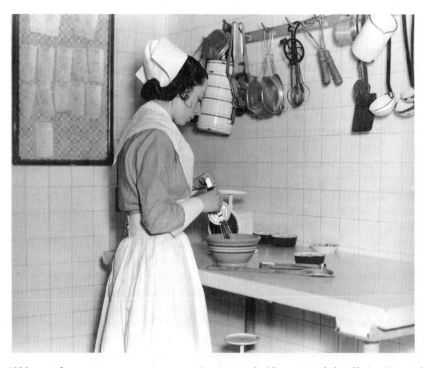

1930—student nurse preparing a patient's meal. (*Courtesy of the Christ Hospital School of Nursing, Jersey City, New Jersey*)

overworked girl grumbled, talked too much, was too familiar with men, criticized head nurses or doctors, or could not get along wherever placed. Married women and those over 30 were frequently excluded because they could not "fall in with the life successfully"; and, of course, if they were divorced, they were totally unacceptable.

In the 1890s, only 12 percent of nurse training was theory, consisting of some anatomy and physiology, materia medica, perhaps some chemistry, bacteriology, hygiene, and lectures on certain diseases. The leading schools developed their own institutional manuals, but a few pioneering texts were also written by nurses before 1900.[14]

Even into the twentieth century, students continued to live a slavelike existence, without outward complaint, and were poorly housed, over-worked, underfed ("rations of a kind and quality only a remove better than what we might place before a beggar," said a popular magazine), and unprotected from life-threatening illness (80 percent of the students in the average hospital graduated with positive tuberculin tests). If they survived all this, it was no wonder that they were expected to graduate as "respectful, obedient, cheerful, submissive, hard-working, loyal, pacific, and religious."[15] It was not professional education; it was not even a respectably run apprenticeship, because learning was not derived from skilled masters, but rather from their own peers, who were but a step ahead of them.

These principles of sacrifice, service, obedience to the physician, and ethical orientation are embodied in the Nightingale Pledge, written in 1893 by Lystra E. Gretter, superintendent of the school at Harper Hospital in Detroit, a pledge still sometimes recited by students today:

> I solemnly pledge myself before God and in the presence of this assembly;
> To pass my life in purity and to practice my profession faithfully; I will abstain from whatever is deleterious and mischievous and will not take or knowingly administer any harmful drug; I will do all in my power to maintain and elevate the standard of my profession, and will hold in confidence all personal matters committed to my keeping and all family affairs coming to my knowledge in the practice of my calling;
> With loyalty will I endeavor to aid the physician in his work, and devote myself to the welfare of those committed to my care.[16]

Although the passage of the first licensure laws in 1903 (discussed later) set standards for nursing education, there was little improvement. The laws were not mandatory. Most training schools remained under the control of hospitals, and the needs of the hospital took priority over those of the school. For instance, it was not until 1912 that an occasional nurse received time from hospital responsibilities in order to organize and teach basic nursing, and superintendents were warned not to "neglect" patient care in favor of the school or they would face punishment. The hours were still long, and the students continued to give free service, with "book learning" as an afterthought. Only in California, where an Eight-Hour Law for Women was passed in 1911, was there any movement to include student nurses (not even graduate nurses). Yet, when a bill was introduced in 1913, it was fought bitterly not only by hospitals, as might be expected, but also by physicians and nurses.[17]

While the Flexner Report of 1910 was bringing about reform in medical schools, eliminating the correspondence courses and the weaker and poorer schools, Adelaide Nutting and other leaders were agitating for reform in nursing education. In 1911, the American Society of Super-intendents of Training Schools for Nurses presented a proposal for a similar survey of nursing schools to the Carnegie Foundation. Ignoring nursing, the foundation directed a considerable amount of its funds to such studies in dental, legal, and teacher education.

Although women were having a little more success in being accepted in colleges and universities, there was only limited movement to make basic nursing programs an option in academic settings. The University of Minnesota program, founded in 1909 by Dr. Richard Olding Beard, a physician who was dedicated to the concept of higher education for nurses, became the first enduring baccalaureate program in nursing. Even this was more similar to good diploma programs than to other university programs. Although eventually the students had to meet university admission standards and took some specialized courses, they also worked a 56-hour week in the hospital and were awarded a diploma instead of a degree after three years. Similar programs were started by other universities that took over hospitals, in part to obtain student services for their hospitals. Just before World War I, several hospitals and universities, such as Presbyterian Hospital of New York and Teachers College, Columbia University, offered degree options. These developed into five-year programs with two years of college work and three years in a diploma school. This became a common pattern that lasted throughout the 1940s.

One of the more daring experiments of the time was the Vassar Training Camp for Nurses. In the summer of 1918 a preparatory course in nursing was offered at Vassar College in Poughkeepsie, New York, to 439 college graduates who would then complete their education for nursing in two additional years at a school of nursing of their choice. A large percentage of the women completed the program and entered the nursing schools they had selected. Students wore the uniform of the nursing school with which they would become affiliated following the "Vassar Camp" experience, and so became known as the "Vassar Rainbow Division."[18] Many of nursing's leaders arose from this group. Because this and similar programs were generally of considerably higher quality than the usual training schools, the movement of nursing education toward an academic setting received another nudge.

By the end of World War I, nursing had serious problems. There was a shortage of nurses, because many who had switched careers "for the duration" returned to their own field, and others appeared not to be attracted. In part, it was an image problem, one that was to continue to haunt nursing, but another important factor was that nursing education was in trouble. As Isabel Stewart said, "The plain facts are that nursing schools are being starved and always have been starved for lack of funds to build up any kind of substantial educational structure."[19] Later, this problem was clearly pinpointed by prestigious study committees (see Appendix 1).

In 1918, Adelaide Nutting had approached the Rockefeller Foundation to seek endowment for the Johns Hopkins School of Nursing, stressing the need for improvement in the education of public health nurses. The meeting resulted in a committee to investigate the "proper training" of public health nurses, an investigation that quickly concluded that the problem was nursing education in general. The finding of the 1923 Goldmark Report concluded that schools of nursing needed to be recognized and supported as separate educational components with not just training in nursing, but also a liberal education. Moreover, "Superintendents, supervisors, instructors, and public health nurses should in all cases receive special additional training beyond the basic nursing course."[20]

Although the report had little immediate impact, it did result in Rockefeller Foundation support for the founding of the Yale School of Nursing (1924), the first in the world to be established as a separate university department with its own dean, Annie Goodrich. Although a few other such programs followed, progress lagged, for many powerful physicians reached the public media with their notions that nurses needed only technical skills, manual dexterity, and quick obedience to the physician. Charles Mayo, for instance, deciding that city-trained nurses were too difficult to handle, too expensive, and spent too much time getting educated, wanted to recruit 100,000 country girls.[21]

This attitude was not new. Almost from the beginning, there were physicians who objected to so much education for nurses and devoted considerable medical journal space to raging about the "overtrained nurse." One physician even suggested a correspondence course for training nurses to care for the "poor folks," and a New York newspaper editorial proclaimed, "What we want in nurses is less theory and more practice."[22] But then, this was at a time when a leading Harvard physician insisted that serious mental exercise would damage a woman's brain or cause other severe trauma, such as the narrowing of the pelvic area, which would make her unable to deliver children.[23]

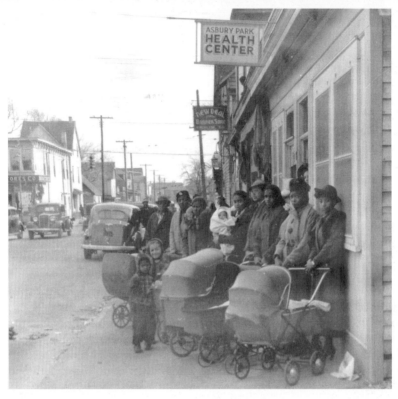

Health centers sponsored by community health nursing agencies were critical to public welfare during the depression. Asbury Park, New Jersey, 1933. (*Courtesy of the Visiting Nurse Association of Central Jersey, Red Bank, New Jersey*)

However, there were also farsighted physicians who supported not "teaching a trade, but preparing for a profession," as Dr. Richard Cabot noted in 1901. Even popular magazines recognized that student nurses were being exploited by hospitals and that the kind of student being encouraged into nursing by school principals was one seen as not too bright, not attractive enough to marry, and too poor to be supported at home.

A study following close on the heels of the Goldmark Report soon reaffirmed the inadequacy of nursing schools and practicing nurses. *Nurses, Patients, and Pocketbooks* pointed out that the hasty postwar nurse-recruiting efforts had not improved the lot of the patient or the nurse.[24] In 1928, problems included an oversupply of nurses, geographic maldistribution, low educational standards, poor working conditions, and some critically unsatisfactory levels of care.

NURSING'S EARLY LEADERS (see also Appendix 7)

In many ways, early nursing education and nursing leaders were intertwined. After graduating from one of the better training programs, these nurses often assumed dual positions as both superintendent of nursing in hospitals and superintendent of the training school. Since students provided almost all of the nursing service, with the exception of a few supervisors, the training school received much of the leaders' attention. They took the responsibility seriously. They were concerned with the quality of the students and the program, and much of what they did was directed at improving nursing education. In a male-dominated society, working in what was barely becoming an accepted, respectable occupation, these unusual women were not only talented but were also determined risk takers.

Before the new century was far along, they were responsible for setting nursing standards, improving curricula, writing textbooks, starting two enduring professional organizations and a nursing journal, inaugurating a teacher training program in a university, and initiating nursing licensure. They were a mixed group, but with certain commonalities: usually unmarried but, except for Lavinia Dock, not feminist. Almost all were involved in the early nursing organizations. Fortunately, most were also great letter writers and letter savers as well as authors, so that there are many fascinating insights into their lives. (See, in particular, the Christy series in *Nursing Outlook*, mentioned in the Bibliography.) Some highlights follow.

America's first trained nurse, Linda Richards, had a continuing impact on the training schools because she spent much of her career moving from hospital to hospital in what seems to have been an improvement campaign. In those earliest days, almost any graduate was considered a prime candidate for starting another program. Some undoubtedly lacked the intellectual and leadership qualities needed, so that the new schools, if not actual disasters, were frequently of poor quality. Linda Richards apparently had the skill and authority to upgrade both the school and the nursing service, which were, after all, almost inseparable. However, she seemed willing to accept school management that tied the economics of the hospital to student education, usually to the detriment of the latter.

One of the most noted nursing figures was Isabelle Hampton, who left teaching to enter Bellevue Training School in 1881. Not only was she attractive and charming, but she was "in every sense of the word a leader, by nature, by capacity, by personal attributes and qualities, by choice, and probably to some extent by inheritance and training; a follower she never was."[25] In her two major superintendencies, she made a number of then radical changes—cutting down the students' workday to 10 hours and eliminating their free private duty services. For the Johns Hopkins program, which she founded, she recruited feisty Lavinia Dock, who was still at Bellevue, to be her assistant. They must have made an interesting pair, for Lavinia, also a "lady," was outspoken and frequently tactless, particularly with physicians.

Adelaide Nutting graduated in that first Hopkins class, and the three became friends.[26] Nutting followed Hampton as principal of the school when in 1894 Isabel married one of her admirers, Dr. Hunter Robb, and, as was the custom, retired from active nursing. (Letters of the time reveal the anger, dismay, and even sadness of her colleagues at her marriage. They were sure Dr. Robb was not nearly good enough for her; besides, she was betraying nursing by robbing the profession of her talents.) Nevertheless, Isabel Hampton Robb maintained her interest in nursing and continued to be active in the development of the profession. In 1893, she had been appointed chairman of a committee to arrange a congress of nurses under the auspices of the International Congress of Charities, Correction, and Philanthropy at the World's Fair (Columbian Exposition) in Chicago. There, before an international audience of nurses, she voiced her concern about poor nursing education and stated that the term *trained nurse* meant "anything, everything, or next to nothing" in the absence of educational standards. At the same time, Lavinia Dock pointed out that the teaching, training, and discipline of nurses should not be provided at the discretion of doctors. Similar themes were repeated in other papers, as well as the notion that there ought to be an organization of nurses. Shortly after the Congress, 18 superintendents organized the American Society of Superintendents of Training Schools for Nursing, which was to become the National League of Nursing Education (NLNE) in 1912. Its purpose was to promote the fellowship of members, establish and maintain a universal standard of training, and further the best interests of the nursing profession. The first convention of the society elected Linda Richards president.[27]

Another attendee at those early meetings was Sophia Palmer, descendant of John and Priscilla Alden, and a graduate of the Boston Training School, who, after a variety of experiences, organized a training school in Washington, DC, over the concerted opposition of local physicians who wanted to control nursing education. She approved the actions that were taken by her colleagues but was impatient with what seemed to be the blind acceptance of hospital control of schools. "She had a very intense nature and, like all those who are born crusaders, had little patience with the slower methods of persuasion.... She was like a spirited racehorse held by the reins of tradition."[28]

Within a short time, Palmer and some of the others in the Society, including Dock and Isabel Hampton Robb, recognized the need for another organization for all nurses. Although some of the training schools had alumnae associations, they were restrictive; in some cases, their own graduates could not be members, and any "outsider" could not participate. Therefore, if a nurse left the immediate vicinity of her own school, there was no way in which she had any organized contact with other nurses. In a paper given in 1895, Palmer stressed that the power of the nursing profession depended on its ability to organize individuals who could influence public opinion. Dock also made recommendations for a national organization. In 1896, delegates representing the oldest training school alumnae associations and members of an organizing committee of the Society selected a name for the proposed organization: Nurses' Associated Alumnae of the United States and Canada (which became the American Nurses Association in 1911). They also set a time and place for the first meeting (February 1897 in Baltimore) and drafted a constitution. At the end of that February meeting, held in conjunction with the fourth annual Society convention, the constitution and by-laws were adopted, and Isabel Hampton Robb was elected president. Among the problems discussed at those early meetings were nursing licensure and the creation of an official nursing publication.[29]

There were a number of nursing journals: the *British Journal of Nursing*, established by one of England's nursing leaders, Ethel Gordon Fenwick; and, in the United States, the short-lived *The Nightingale*, started by a Bellevue graduate; *The Nursing Record* and *The Nursing World*, also short-lived; and *The Trained Nurse and Hospital Review*, which Palmer edited for a time and which continued for 70 years. However, the leaders of the new organizations wanted a magazine that would promote nursing, owned and controlled by nursing.

For several years there was discussion, but no action, until another committee on the ways and means of producing a magazine was formed. In January 1900, they organized a stock company and sold $100 shares only to nurses and nurses' alumnae associations. By May, they had a promise of $2400 in shares, and almost 500 nurses had promised to subscribe. Admittedly, they had overstepped their mandate. They reported to the third annual convention of the Nurses' Associated Alumnae, and were given approval to establish the magazine along the lines formulated. The J. B. Lippincott Company was selected as publisher, and Sophia Palmer became editor, which she did on an unpaid basis for the first nine months. (She had become director of the Rochester City Hospital in New York.) As the first issues went for mailing in October, it was discovered that the post office rules prevented its being mailed because the journal's stockholders were not incorporated. M. E. P. Davis (business manager) and Sophia Palmer assumed personal responsibility for all liabilities of the new *American Journal of Nursing*, and it went out. The *Journal* was considered the official organ of the nursing profession, but the stock was still held by alumnae associations and individual nurses. It was Lavinia Dock who donated the first share of stock to the association, and by 1912 the renamed American Nurses Association (ANA) had gained ownership of all the stock of the American Journal of Nursing Company.[30] The ANA retained ownership of the *Journal* until the mid-1990s, when it was sold to the Lippincott Company.

One other major organization, the American Red Cross, was established by a nurse, Clara Barton, the schoolteacher who had volunteered as a nurse and directed relief operations during the Civil War and served with the German Red Cross during the Franco-Prussian War in 1870. (The establishment of the International Red Cross as a permanent international relief agency that could take immediate action in time of war had occurred in Geneva in 1864 with the signing of the Geneva Convention guidelines.) After her return to the United States, Barton organized the American Red Cross and persuaded Congress in 1882 to ratify the Treaty of Geneva so that the Red Cross could carry on its humanitarian efforts in peacetime. Clara Barton, however, was not an active part of the nursing leadership that was molding the profession.[31]

The Society had another immediate aim. It recognized that the nurses were at a disadvantage because they had no postgraduate training in administration or teaching, so a committee consisting of Robb, Nutting, Richards, Mary Agnes Snively, and Lucy Drown was formed to investigate the possibilities. At the sixth Society convention, they reported their success. James Russell, the farsighted dean of Teachers College, Columbia University, in New York, had agreed to start a course for nurses if they could guarantee the enrollment of 12 nurses, or $1000 a year. The Society agreed. Members of the Society screened the candidates, contributed $1000 a year, and taught the course—hospital economics. Later, the students were also allowed to enroll in psychology, science, household economics, and biology. Anna Alline, one of the two graduates of the first class, then took over the total administration of the course of studies.

There was one more major goal to be reached: licensure of nurses. Not only did the hundreds of hospital-based schools vary greatly in quality, but the market was also flooded with "nurses" who had been dismissed from schools without graduating, "nurses" from six-week private and correspondence courses, and a vast number of those who simply called themselves nurses. It was inevitable that people became confused, for when they hired nurses for private duty in their homes, the "nurse" could present one of the elaborate diplomas from a $13 correspondence course which guaranteed that anyone could become a nurse, a real or forged reference, or a genuine diploma from a top-quality school. How could they judge? Therefore, because of the dreadful care given by individuals representing themselves as nurses, the public was once more disenchanted with nurses. Nursing's leaders were determined that there must be legal regulation, both to protect the public from unscrupulous and incompetent nurses and to protect the young profession by establishing a minimum level of competence, limiting all or some of the professional functions to those who qualified. Medicine already had licensing in some states, and many aspiring professions were also moving in that direction.

In September 1901, at the first general meeting of the newly formed International Council of Nurses, which was held in Buffalo, a resolution was passed, stating that "it is the duty of the nursing profession of every country to work for suitable legislative enactment regulating the education of nurses and protecting the interests of the public, by securing State examinations and public registration, with the proper penalties for enforcing the same."[32]

Despite considerable opposition to nurse licensure from untrained nurses, managers, and proprietors of poor training programs, and some physicians, licensure was achieved and basic educational standards were set. In 1903, North Carolina, New Jersey, Virginia, and New York passed laws. However, New York's law was the strongest. For instance, New Jersey's law omitted a board of any kind; North Carolina had a mixed board of nurses and doctors and allowed a nurse to be licensed without attending a training school if vouched for by a doctor. It should be remembered, though, that all nurse licensure laws in those times were permissive, not mandatory. That is, only the registered nurse (RN) title was protected. Untrained nurses could continue to work as nurses as long as they did not call themselves RNs.

One of the key figures in community health nursing was Lillian Wald. After graduating from the New York Hospital School of Nursing and working a short time, she decided to enter the Women's Medical College. When she and another nurse, Mary Brewster, were sent to the Lower East Side to lecture to immigrant mothers on the care of the sick, they were shocked at what they saw; neither had known that such abject poverty could exist. Wald left medical school, moved with Mary Brewster to a top-floor tenement on Jefferson Street, and began to offer nursing care to the poor. After a short while, the calls came by the hundreds from families, hospitals, and physicians. People were cared for, whether or not they could afford to pay. The concern of these nurses was not just giving nursing care but seeing what other services could be made available to meet the many social needs of the poor.

After two years of such success, larger facilities, more nurses, and social workers were needed. In 1895, Wald, Brewster, Lavinia Dock, and other nurses moved to what was eventually called the Henry Street

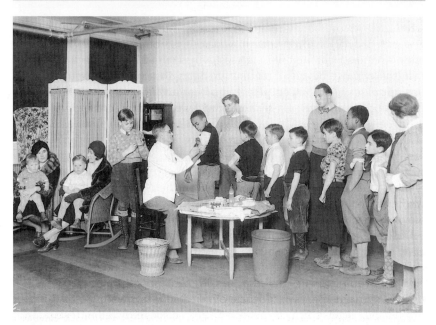

A child health center of the 1930s brought primary health care to the neighborhoods. (*Courtesy of the Visiting Nurse Association of Central Jersey, Red Bank,
New Jersey*)

Settlement, a house bought by philanthropist Jacob H. Schiff. By 1909, the
Henry Street staff had 37 nurses, all but five providing direct nursing
service. Each nurse was carefully oriented to the customs of the immigrants she served and was able to demonstrate the value of understanding
the family and the environment in giving good nursing care. Each nurse
kept two sets of records, one for the physician and another recording
the major points of the nurse's work. School nursing was also started
by Lillian Wald, who suggested that placing nurses in schools might
help solve the problem of the schools having to send home so many ill
children.[33]

Another outstanding public health nurse was Margaret Higgins
Sanger. She became interested in the plight of the poorly paid industrial
workers, particularly the women. She herself was married and had three
children when she decided to return to work in public health. She was
assigned to maternity cases on the Lower East Side of New York, where
she found that pregnancy, often unwanted, was a chronic condition.
In 1912, one of her patients died from a repeated self-abortion after
begging doctors and nurses for information on how to avoid pregnancy.
That was apparently a turning point for Sanger. After learning everything she could about contraception, she and her sister, also a nurse,

opened the first birth control clinic in America in Brooklyn. She was arrested and spent 30 days in the workhouse but continued her crusade. She fought the battle for free dissemination of birth control information for decades, against all types of opposition, until today, birth control education is generally accepted as the right of women and as one nursing role. Margaret Sanger went on to establish the Planned Parenthood Association of America, and promote family planning throughout the world.[34]

In the 23 years between World Wars I and II, nursing was affected by the Great Depression and by adoption of the Nineteenth Amendment to the Constitution in August 1920, granting women the right to vote. Of the two, the latter had less immediate impact. Nurses showed relatively little interest in fighting for women's rights, and only one, Lavinia Dock, can be called an active feminist. "Dockie" was a maverick of the times. A tiny woman who loved music and was an accomplished pianist and organist, she also seemed to take on the whole world in her battle for the underdog. Early on, she decided that nurses could have no power unless they had the vote. Her speeches and writings were brilliant, but she did not move her colleagues. Nevertheless, she devoted a good part of her life to working for women's rights. In England, she joined the Pankhursts and landed in jail. Back in the United States, she picketed the White House. Her colleague, Isabel Stewart, wrote, "They all went into the cooler for the night. I think it just pleased her no end."[35]

For all her devotion to women's rights, Dock remained committed to nursing. She was editor of the *Journal's* Foreign Department from 1900 to 1923, during which she quarreled regularly with editor Sophia Palmer and managed to ignore World War I because she was a pacifist. She was also involved with the International Council of Nurses and was the author of a number of books, including *Health and Morality*, published in 1910, in which she discussed venereal disease. She was equally outspoken on this forbidden subject in open meetings. A number of nurses had become infected because physicians frequently refused to tell nurses when patients had the disease. Dock also regularly criticized her profession for withholding its interest, sympathy, and moral support from "the great, urgent, throbbing, pressing social claims of our day and generation."[36]

There were other nurses who put their mark on nursing in its first 60 years. Anne Goodrich reported on the poor nursing conditions in military camps during World War I, which resulted in the establishment of the Army School of Nursing. She became its first dean, and the high quality of the educational program, with only six to eight duty hours (unlike civilian hospitals), made it an overwhelming success. Isabel Stewart, who succeeded Adelaide Nutting (the first nurse to receive a professorship at Columbia University), in her 39 years at Teachers College set up a respected graduate program. In 1922, six nursing students at Indiana University founded Sigma Theta Tau, nursing's honor society, now an international organization. Another pioneer, Mary Breckenridge, then founded the Frontier Nursing Service in 1925; its staff was a mixture of British and British-trained American midwives.[37]

Little is known about either black or male nurses. However, after the Civil War, recognized black nurse leaders included Mary Mahoney, the first black nurse to graduate from a training program; Jessie Scales, the first district nurse; and Martha Franklin, founder of the National Association of Colored Graduate Nurses (NACGN). Adah Thomas led the fight to gain acceptance of black nurses by the army. She had corresponded extensively with Jane Delano, chairman of the national committee of the American Red Cross through which army nurses were enrolled at the time, and urged black nurses to enroll in the American Red Cross. Finally, a month after the armistice was signed in 1918 and in the midst of the influenza epidemic, the first black nurses were assigned to army camps in Ohio and Illinois, with other assignments following. (However, it was not until World War II that black nurses were accepted into the military service.)[38]

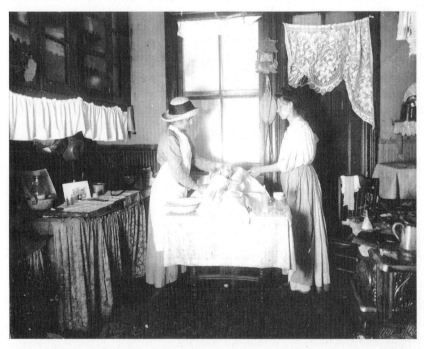

Turn of the century home care visits often included instructing parents in the care of their children. (*Courtesy of the Visiting Nurse Service of New York*)

THE NURSE IN PRACTICE

In the late nineteenth and early twentieth centuries, the graduate trained nurse had two major career options: she could do private duty in homes or, if she was exceptional (or particularly favored), gain one of the rare positions as head nurse, operating room supervisor, night supervisor, or even superintendent. In private duty, trained nurses often competed with untrained nurses who were not restrained from practicing in many states until the middle of the twentieth century. Also, given the long hours and taxing physical work in home nursing, most private nurses found themselves unwanted at 40, with younger, stronger nurses being hired instead. Some of the more ambitious and perhaps braver nurses chose to go west to pioneer in new and sometimes primitive hospitals. There were a few in industrial nursing, and a limited but gradually increasing number in public health nursing.

The practice of nursing was scarcely limited to clinical care of the patient. Job descriptions of the time appear to have given major priority to scrubbing floors, dusting, keeping the stove stoked and the kerosene lamps trimmed and filled, controlling insects, washing clothes, making and rolling bandages, and other unskilled housekeeping tasks, as well as edicts for personal behavior (see Exhibit 2.1). Nursing care responsibilities included, in addition to carrying out the orders of the physician,

> making beds, giving baths, preventing and dressing bedsores, applying friction to the body and extremities, giving enemas, inserting catheters, bandaging, dressing blisters, burns, sores, and wounds, and observing secretions, expectorations, pulse, skin, appetite, body temperature, consciousness, respiration, sleep, condition of wounds, skin eruptions, elimination, and the effect of diet, stimulants, and medications.[39]

At the end of the nineteenth century, there was a marked growth of large cities in the United States. Although the cities had their beautiful public buildings, parks, and mansions, they also had their seamy sides—the festering slums where the tremendous flow of immigrants huddled. Between 1820 and 1910, nearly 30 million immigrants entered the United States, with a shift in numbers from Northern European to Southern European by the early 1900s. Health and social problems multiplied in the slum areas. Somehow, Americans did not seem to feel a great need to serve the sick poor in their homes; after all, there were public dispensaries and charity hospitals. Some visiting nurse groups were formed, but by 1900 it was estimated that only 200 nurses were engaged in public health nursing.

In 1912, the Red Cross established the Rural Nursing Service. Lillian Wald, at a major meeting, on infant mortality, had cited the horrible

Exhibit 2.1 Wanted: A Very Special Nurse to Care for 50 Patients at a Local Hospital

Duties and requirements:

- Daily sweep and mop the floors of your ward. Dust the patients' furniture and windowsills.
- Maintain an even temperature in your ward by bringing in a scuttle of coal for the day's business.
- Light is important to observe the patient's condition. Therefore, each day fill kerosene lamps, clean chimneys, and trim wicks. Wash the windows once a week.
- The Nurses' notes are important in aiding the physician's work. Make your pens carefully. You may whittle nibs to your individual taste.
- Each nurse on duty will report every day at 7:00 A.M. and leave at 8:00 P.M. except on the Sabbath on which you will be off from 12:00 noon to 2:00 P.M.
- Graduates in good standing with the Superintendent of Nurses will be given an evening off each week for courting purposes, or two evenings a week if you go to church regularly.
- Each nurse should lay aside from each pay day a goodly sum of her earnings for her benefit in her declining years, so that she will not become a burden. For example, if you earn $30 a month, you should set aside $15.
- Any nurse who smokes, uses liquor in any form, gets her hair done at a beauty shop, or frequents dance halls will give the Superintendent of Nurses a good reason to suspect her worth, intention, and integrity.
- The nurse who performs her labors, serves her patients and doctors faithfully without fault for a period of five years will be given an increase by the Hospital Administration of five cents a day, provided there are no hospital debts that are outstanding.

Source: Reportedly an ad in a Western newspaper in 1887.

health conditions of rural America, the high infant and maternal mortality rates, the prevalence of tuberculosis, and other serious health problems and suggested that the Red Cross operate a national service, similar to that of Great Britain. (Red Cross involvement gradually decreased until, with increased government involvement in public health, it discontinued the program altogether in 1947.)

However, in 1915, it is estimated that no more than 10 percent of the sick received care in the hospitals, and the majority of people could not afford private duty nurses. From this need, a public health movement emerged that increased the demand for nurses. At first, most of these nurses concentrated on bedside care, but others, like those coming from the settlement houses, took broader responsibilities. Nevertheless, there were no recognized standards or requirements for visiting nurses. Therefore, in June 1912, a small group of visiting nurses, representing unofficially some 900 agencies and almost four times that many colleagues, founded the National Organization for Public Health Nursing (NOPHN), with Lillian Wald as the first president. It was an organization of nurses and lay people engaged in public health nursing and in the organization, management, and support of such work. The leaders of the group selected the term *public health nursing* as more inclusive than *visiting nursing*; it was also reminiscent of Nightingale's health nursing, which had focused on prevention. One of its first goals was to extend the services to working- and middle-class people, as well as to the poor.[40]

By 1916, public health nurses were being called on to be welfare workers, sanitarians, housing inspectors, and health teachers as well. A number of universities began offering courses to help prepare nurses to fulfill this multifaceted role, and Mary Gardner, one of the founders of NOPHN and an interim director of the Rural Nursing Service, authored the first book in the field, *Public Health Nursing*. One of the observations she made was that although broad-minded physicians recognized that public health nurses helped them produce results that would not have been possible alone, the more conservative feared interference by nurses and were resentful of them. She noted that a service had a better chance of success if it was started with the cooperation of the medical profession, and pointed out ways nurses could avoid friction with physicians and still be protected from the incompetents.

Gradually, various other nursing specialties developed, such as anesthesia, industrial nursing, and nurse midwifery. However, it was the Great Depression, which followed the stock market crash in 1929, that helped alter nursing practice drastically. This was a period of high unemployment for nurses. As financial crises hit their clientele, private duty nurses found that there was little demand for their services. The situation worsened as nurses who were laid off in offices and industry, as well as married nurses, also looked for private duty cases. Both the Goldmark Report and *Nurses, Patients, and Pocketbooks* (Appendix 1) had warned that the overproduction and maldistribution of nurses would soon cause a problem, but no action had been taken. Now a reevaluation of nursing and nursing education was imperative. The result was the closing of many small schools and an increased concern for high standards, the setting of an eight-hour day for private duty nurses, and the employment of graduate nurses in hospitals. Unfortunately, the last also had long-lasting bad effects. By 1933, some nurses worked in hospitals for little more than room and board. It took many years for nurses to earn reasonable wages and to gain some autonomy in their practice.

Some help finally came with the Roosevelt Administration, when relief funds were allocated for bedside care of the indigent, and nurses were employed as visiting nurses under the Federal Emergency Relief Administration (FERA). Ten thousand unemployed nurses were put to work in numerous settings under the Civil Works Administration (CWA) in public hospitals, clinics, public health agencies, and other health services. The follow-up Works Progress Administration (WPA) then continued to provide funds for nurses in community health activities.[41]

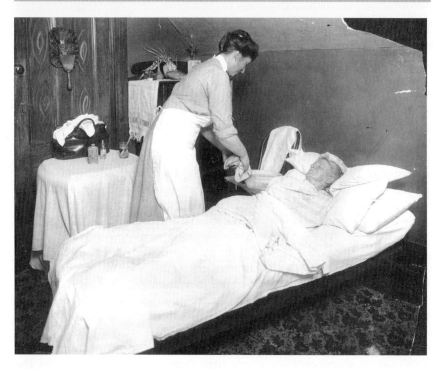

Home care has always included personal care of the sick as shown here in a picture dating back to the turn of the century. (*Courtesy of the Visiting Nurse Service of New York*)

Of all the entrants into nursing, two groups got particularly short shrift—men and blacks. As the distorted view of the female nurse evolved, men did not seem to fit the image held by powerful figures in and out of nursing. Therefore, although men graduated from acceptable, usually totally male nursing schools and attempted to become active members of the ANA, even forming a men's section, their numbers and influence remained small until the post-World War II era.

Black nurses were caught in the overall common prejudice against their race. Individual black nurses, as noted earlier, broke down barriers in various nursing fields. As early as 1908, they organized the National Association of Colored Graduate Nurses (NACGN), both to fight against discriminatory practices and to foster leadership among black nurses. Although the ANA had a nondiscriminatory policy, some state organizations did not, and a rule that the nurse must have graduated from a state-approved school to be an ANA member eliminated even more black nurses. Finally, in 1951, the NACGN was absorbed into the ANA, which required nondiscrimination policies and practices for all state associations as a prerequisite to ANA affiliation.[42]

In 1924, it was reported that only 58 state-accredited schools admitted blacks, and most of these were located in black hospitals or in departments caring for black patients in municipal hospitals. Of these schools, 77 percent were located in the South. Twenty-eight states offered no opportunities in nursing education for black women. Most of the southern "schools" that trained black nurses were totally unacceptable, and many of those approved barely met standards. Moreover, there were some 23,000 untrained black midwives in the South, but no one made the effort to combine training in nursing and midwifery, which would have been a distinct service. In 1930, there were fewer than 6000 graduate black nurses, most of whom worked in black hospitals or public health agencies that served black patients. Neither were opportunities in other fields often open to them because they did not have the educational prerequisites. Middle-class black women were usually not attracted to nursing, because teaching and other available fields offered more prestige and better opportunities.

It was not until a 1941 executive order and the corresponding follow-through that any part of the federal government made any effort to investigate the grievances and deal with the complaints of Blacks. Later, the Bolton Act opened the doors of participating nursing schools to Blacks. Yet, overt and covert methods were used in both the North and the South to prevent the more able black nurses from assuming leadership positions—some as simple as advancing the least aggressive, and for all the desperate need for nurses, the armed forces balked at accepting and integrating black nurses. Not until the end of World War II and after some aggressive action by the NACGN and the National Nursing Council for War Service did this situation change.

WARTIME NURSING

Another influence on nursing was nurses' participation in American wars. Ironically, although the military was not prepared to care for its sick and wounded in the short but deadly Spanish–American War, once more the military physicians objected to the presence of women nurses. Finally, when men lay dying of malaria, dysentery, and typhoid, women from the training schools took over. Their letters and journals relate the horrible conditions under which they worked. Some literally worked themselves to death in the army hospitals in the South. One of the most serious diseases that nurses contended with was yellow fever, about which little was known. In testing the theory that the disease was caused by a certain type of mosquito, nursing gained its first martyr. Twenty-five-year-old Clara Maas of East Orange, New Jersey, volunteered to be

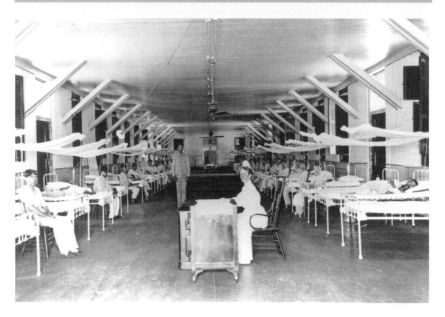

1898 (Spanish–American War)—Army contract nurse on a ward at the First Reserve Hospital, Manila, the Philippines. (*Courtesy of Center of Military History, Department of the Army*)

bitten by a carrier mosquito. After being bitten several times, she died of yellow fever and is still considered a heroine in helping to prove the source of the disease.

The value of nurses in wartime was clear after the Spanish–American War, and recommendations were made that a regular corps of nurses ready for wartime duty be formed. Yet some military authorities were still hostile. So, although the number of women army nurses had reached 1158 by September 1898, by the next July there were only 202. Despite this setback, a group of influential women, including some prominent nurses, eventually lobbied through a bill, and the Army Nurse Corps was established on February 2, 1901.[43] It took longer for the Congress to act on a Navy Nurse Corps, although it had the support of the Navy's Surgeon General, but finally it, too, became a reality in 1908.

World War I was different from other wars the United States had fought, both because of its international dimensions and the kinds of weapons that were used. The service of the nurse in the nightmarish battle conditions of World War I, coping with the mass casualties, dealing with injuries caused by the previously unknown shrapnel and gas, and then battling influenza at home and abroad, is a fascinating and proud piece of history.[44]

Both the Army and Navy Nurse Corps were expanded during this time, but not enough nurses were available and recruitment standards dropped. (Even though there were male nurses who volunteered, they, like black nurses, were not accepted in the nurse corps.) Nursing leaders then formed a committee to devise methods of dealing with the problems related to care of the sick in the military, in hospitals, and in homes. Later this committee was given governmental status, but very limited funding. The members found once more what had been true before and would be again: in wartime there are not enough nurses to meet the need. While efforts were made to recruit and produce nurses more rapidly, and they succeeded to some extent for the duration, there was inevitably a shortage afterward. When patriotic fervor faded away, the unpleasant conditions while "in training" and afterward, at a time when other working conditions were improving, made nursing a less desirable occupational choice. The high quality of students in the Rainbow Division of the Vassar Training Camp mentioned earlier was more the exception than the rule. The Army School of Nursing that emerged from World War I was also highly unusual.

In World War II, the role of nurses was even more extensive and perhaps even more dangerous. Once more nurses proved themselves able and brave in military situations.[45] Many were in battle zones, and some became Japanese prisoners of war.[46] Their stories have been told in films, books, plays, and historical nursing research and are well worth reading (see Bibliography). The war created opportunities, freedom, and also problems for nurses that proved to be long-lasting in both nursing education and practice. Some related to the nursing shortage that was again critical. There were not enough nurses for both the home front and the battlefield, even with stepped-up efforts to encourage women to enter nursing programs.

Finally, legislation was passed in 1943 establishing the Cadet Nurse Corps. The Bolton Act, the first federal program to subsidize nursing education for schools and students, was a forerunner of future federal aid to nursing. For payment of their tuition and a stipend, students committed themselves to engage in essential military or civilian nursing for the duration of the war. The students had to be between 17 and 35 years old, in good health, and with a good academic record from an accredited high school. This new law brought about several changes in nursing. For instance, it forbade discrimination on the basis of race and marital status and set minimum educational standards. The first standard, theoretically accepted, was not always implemented in good faith. The second, combined with the requirement that nursing programs be reduced from the traditional 36 months to 30, forced nursing schools to reassess and revise their curricula.[47]

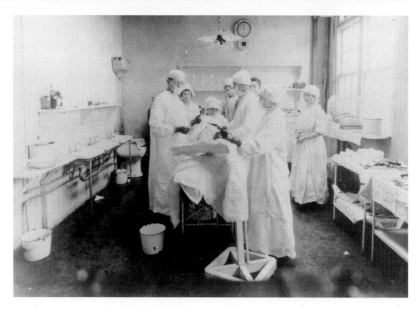

Army nurses are part of the operating room team at a base hospital in Savenay, France, 1919. (*Courtesy of The Center of Military History, Department of the Army*)

Two other major efforts to relieve the nursing shortage had long-range effects in the practice setting. One was the recruitment of inactive nurses back into the field. For the first time, married women and others who could work only on a part-time basis became acceptable to employers and later became part of the labor pool. The other change was the training of volunteer nurses' aides. Although such training was initiated by the Red Cross in 1919, it was discouraged later by nurses, particularly during the Depression. During World War II, both the Red Cross and the Office of Civilian Defense trained more than 20,000 aides. At first, they were used only for nonnursing tasks, but the increasing nurse shortage forced them to take on basic nursing functions. After the war, with a continued shortage, trained aides were hired as a necessary part of the nursing service department. Their perceived cost effectiveness stimulated the growth of both aide and practical nurse training programs and eventually increased federal funding for both.

Periodic shortages, some associated with the war efforts and others not as easily explained, have been common throughout nursing's history. No fewer than ten studies have been conducted in the last two decades dealing with this issue. The dynamics of these cyclical shortages and surpluses are discussed more fully in Chapter 6.

Finally, major changes occurred within the armed forces. Nurses had held only relative rank, meaning that they carried officers' titles but

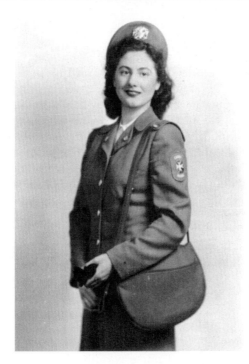

The Cadet Nurse program during World War II, which provided federal money to train nurses, was responsible for major changes in nursing education.

had less power and pay than their male counterparts. In 1947, full commissioned status was granted, giving them the right to manage nursing care. At the same time, as noted previously, discrimination against black nurses ended but, oddly enough, in the male-controlled armed services, it was not until 1954 that male nurses were admitted to full rank as officers.

When the Korean War broke out in 1950, the army again drew nurses from civilian hospitals, this time from their reserve corps. War nursing on the battlefront was centered to an extent on the Mobile Army Surgical Hospitals (MASH), located as close to the front lines as possible. Flight nurses, who helped to evacuate the wounded from the battlefront to military hospitals, also achieved recognition. When that war was over and nurse reservists returned to their civilian jobs, it is possible that their military experiences increased their discontent with working situations at home.

Each of this country's wars have had a profound effect on nursing. Constantly rising to the public need without prompting, a draft was never instituted for nurses, although it was a topic of public consideration on several occasions. The Vietnam War was a particularly important event in the relationship between nursing and war. There are estimates that anywhere from 4000 to 15,000 military nurses served; however, records are imprecise. In World War I we had "shell shock," in World War II "battle fatigue," Vietnam gave us posttraumatic stress disorder (PTSD). Our longest, most unpopular military action, and many say our first military defeat, Vietnam wreaked havoc with the altruism nurses bring to their work and their patients.[48] From a more positive perspective, the Cold War, the race for mastery of space, and Vietnam contributed significant scientific and technological advances which ultimately enriched nursing practice and promoted a sophistication in specialization.

TOWARD A NEW ERA: STUDIES AND ACTION

The usual postwar nurse shortage occurred after World War II, but this time for different reasons. Only one of six army nurses planned to return to her civilian job, finding more satisfaction in the service. Poor pay and unpleasant working conditions discouraged civilian nurses as well. In 1946, the salary for a staff nurse was about $36 for a 48-hour week (and much less for male nurses), less than that for typists or seamstresses. Salaries were supposed to be kept secret, and hospitals, in particular, held wages at a minimum, with such peculiarities as a staff nurse earning more than a head nurse. Split shifts were common, with nurses scheduled to work from 7:00 to 11:00 and from 3:00 to 7:00, with time off between the two shifts. The work was especially difficult, because staffing was short and nurses worked under rigid discipline. Small wonder then that in one survey only about 12 percent of the nurses queried planned to make nursing a career; more than 75 percent saw it as a pin-money job after marriage or planned to retire altogether as soon as possible. Unions were beginning to organize nurses, so in 1949 the ANA approved state associations as collective bargaining agents for nurses. However, because the Taft–Hartley Act excluded nonprofit institutions from collective bargaining, many hospitals and health care agencies did not need to deal with nurses. In addition, the ANA no-strike pledge took away another powerful weapon. As noted previously, one answer that administrators saw was the hiring of nurses' aides. The use of volunteers and auxiliary help—that is, anyone other than licensed nurses (practical nurses, aides, and orderlies)—increased tremendously.

One group of workers that proliferated in the postwar era was practical nurses, defined by ANA, NLNE, and NOPHN as those trained

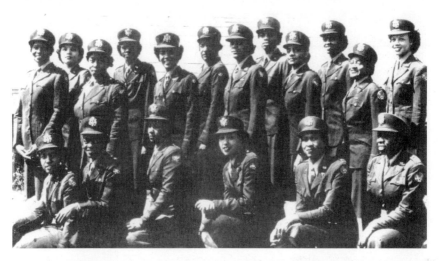

Black nurses' Army unit, World War II. (*Courtesy of the Museum of Nursing History, Inc., Philadelphia*)

to care for subacute, convalescent, and chronic patients under the direction of a physician or nurse. Thousands who designated themselves as practical nurses had no such skills, and their training was simply in caring for their own families or, at most, aide work. Although the first school for training practical nurses appeared in 1897, by 1930 there were only 11, and in 1947 there were still only 36. With the new demand for nurse substitutes, 260 more practical nurse schools opened by 1954, mostly in hospitals or long-term care institutions and a few in vocational schools. Aiding the movement was funding under federal vocational education acts. There were, unfortunately, also a number of correspondence courses and other commercial programs that did little more than expose the student to some books and manuals and then present a diploma. By 1950, there were 144,000 practical nurses, 95 percent of them women, and, although their educational programs varied, their on-the-job activities expanded greatly—to doing whatever nurses had no time to do. By 1952, some 56 percent of the nursing personnel were nonprofessionals, and some nurses began to fear that they were being replaced by less expensive, minimally trained workers.

Nevertheless, with working and financial conditions not improving, the nursing shortage persisted. Soon, a team plan was developed with a nurse as a team leader, primarily responsible for planning patient care, perhaps caring for patients with more complex problems, and less prepared workers carrying out the care plan for other patients. Although the team plan has persisted for years, it has done little to improve patient care, since generally it has not been carried out as originally conceived.

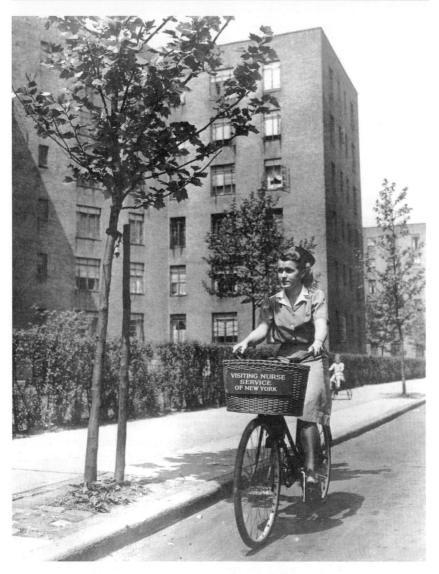

The postwar demand for health services saw nurses turning to nontraditional methods of transportation. (*Courtesy of the Visiting Nurse Service of New York*)

Rather, it has kept the nurse mired in paperwork, away from the patient or required to make constant medication rounds. Often practical nurses have carried the primary responsibilities for patient units on the evening and night shift, with the few nurses available stretched thin, "supervising" these workers.

There were more nurses than ever at mid-century, but there were also tremendously expanded health services, a greater population to be served, growth of various insurance plans that paid for hospital care, a postwar baby boom with in-hospital deliveries, new medical discoveries that kept patients alive longer, and a growing need for nurses to move into less traditional areas of practice. Although hospitals were not the most desirable places to work, and economic benefits were slow in coming, they continued to be the most common place for nurses to be employed. Moreover, there were now more married nurses who chose to stay home to raise families. Studies done in 1941, 1948, and 1958 (Appendix 1), all of which pointed out some of the economic and status problems of nurses, particularly in hospitals, went largely ignored by administrators.

Nursing for the Future was a study conducted by Esther Lucile Brown, a social anthropologist, and related to both nursing education and nursing service. The report received mixed reviews. Many nurses felt threatened, and some physicians and hospital administrators considered it a subversive document, fearing that it had economic security implications for nurses. (Nor did they appreciate the fact that the authoritarianism of hospitals was pinpointed, as was the dilemma of the nurse caught between the demands of physicians and administrators.)

In the 1950s, Frances Reiter began to write about the *nurse clinician*, a nurse who gave skilled nursing care on an advanced level. This concept developed into that of the clinical specialist, a nurse with a graduate degree and specialized knowledge of nursing care, who worked as a colleague of physicians. At the same time, the development of coronary and other intensive care units called for nurses with equally specialized technical knowledge, formerly the sole province of medical practice. In Colorado in 1965, a physician, in collaboration with a school of nursing, was pioneering another new role for nurses in ambulatory care. As the nurses easily assumed responsibility for well-child care and minor illnesses, they called upon their nursing knowledge and skills, as well as a medical component. What emerged was the *nurse practitioner.* (These roles are described in Chapter 6.)

Nursing education was also going through a transition period in those decades. In the years immediately after World War II, the quality of nursing education was under severe criticism. There was no question that in the diploma schools, where most nurses were educated, there was frequently poor teaching, inadequately prepared teachers, and major dependence on students for services; often two-thirds of the hours of care were given by students. These were also the findings of Esther Lucile Brown, who had gathered her data by visiting nursing schools and health care facilities and consulting with many key people in the health care field, including nurses. Her findings were not much different from those in earlier reports, and 22 years later, in another national study, *An Abstract for Action,* the author noted that many of the recommendations in *Nursing for the Future* were still valid but unfulfilled. Brown particularly cited the poor quality of many schools and the fact that many diploma schools were operated for the staffing benefit of the hospital. (Even in the years of the Great Depression, when hospital administrators complained bitterly about the cost of nursing programs, their economic benefit was clear and most were kept.) One strong recommendation of the Brown report was "that effort be directed to building basic schools of nursing in universities and colleges, comparable in number to existing medical schools, that are sound in organizational and financial structure, adequate in facilities and faculty, and well-distributed to serve the needs of the entire country."[49]

The slow rate of growth of collegiate programs, even into the next decade, resulted in part from the uncertainty of nurses about what these programs should be and how they should differ from diploma education. Another factor was the anticollegiate faction in nursing that saw no point in higher education—a faction that was cheered and nurtured by a large number of physicians and administrators. While the Brown report did result in a reexamination of beliefs and attitudes about educational practices, it was also viewed as a threat to the comfortable status quo by hospital administrators, some doctors, and diploma nurses. However, both this report and the 1950 report *Nursing Schools at the Mid-Century,* a follow-up report sponsored by six nursing organizations, are credited with being the impetus for an established process of accreditation in nursing. Those schools that chose to go through the voluntary process and that met the standards were placed on a published list, which for the first time gave the public, guidance counselors, and potential students some notion of the quality of one school compared with another (Appendix 1).

Eventually accreditation proved a significant force in improving good schools and closing poor ones (although it has also been accused of rigidity throughout the years). Actually the NLNE, which, as the National League for Nursing (NLN), later assumed responsibility for accreditation, had been involved in curriculum study and development since the publication of its 1917 *Standard Curriculum for Schools of Nursing* and its 1929 *A Curriculum for Schools of Nursing.* By 1937, these works were considered extremely helpful to those responsible for nursing programs, but their curricula were perhaps too inflexible. Out of this came *A Curriculum Guide for Schools of Nursing,* which was greatly influenced by a study directed by Isabel Stewart that had looked at "the most progressive ideas and practices" in basic nursing education. The new guide, intended, according to Stewart, for students of professional caliber preparing themselves for a profession, placed much greater emphasis on application of the sciences. The role of the clinical instructor was stressed, and all faculty members were encouraged to use newer and more creative methods of teaching. The guide was never revised again, but it was used in many schools for another quarter-century.

The study that probably changed nursing education more dramatically than any other was the doctoral research of Mildred Montag at Teachers College in New York. *Community College Education for Nursing*, published in 1959, was the report of a five-year project based on her dissertation. In this "action research" project, seven junior community colleges cooperated by establishing two-year associate degree (AD) programs for nursing. It was the right time for such programs with the rapid growth of community colleges and the availability of new types of students— mature men and women and the less affluent, who seized this opportunity for a college degree and a career. The project evaluation, including follow-up of the 811 graduates, presented persuasive arguments for the development of more such programs. Forty years later, AD programs prepare more nurses for RN licensure than any other educational program. AD education also had an effect on other nursing programs. It was probably partially the influence of the AD programs, which were nondiscriminatory and generally nonpaternalistic in their relations with students, that helped loosen the tight restrictions on nursing students' personal lives.

Federal funding of nursing education also had a major impact on nursing education. As noted earlier, nursing education was first subsidized during World War II with enactment of the Bolton Act in 1943. However, it was in effect only for the duration of the war, since its intent was to overcome the serious nursing shortage. There was no further funding of nursing education until the Health Amendments Act of 1956 provided traineeships, which did not have to be paid back, to prepare nurses for administration, teaching, supervision, and public health through both short-term and full-time study. However, useful as this was, even more far-reaching was the 1963 report *Toward Quality in Nursing, Needs and Goals*. It was prepared by a group of nurses, other health professionals, and members of the public appointed by the Surgeon General of the U.S. Public Health Service to advise him on nursing needs and the role the government should take in providing adequate nursing service for the public. The report, which cited major deficits in the number of nurses adequately prepared to meet the health needs for the future, had great influence. An obvious problem was the lack of qualified teachers; even in so-called university programs, nurses did not meet the usual requirements for teaching. Another was the almost total lack of educational background in management on the part of nurses who held administrative and managerial positions. The consequent enactment of the Nurse Training Act of 1964 not only provided funding for students and schools for the next five years, but in its later forms, continues to provide a varied amount of support to nursing education and research.

Such federal assistance was particularly important in the development of graduate programs in nursing education. Few such programs existed, and often nurses who sought graduate degrees turned to other disciplines such as education. However, even with the growth of graduate nursing programs, it was not until the 1960s that graduate education in clinical nursing was more readily available. This may have been due to the forms of federal funding. In fact, one outcome of such funding is the tendency for schools to develop educational programs according to the funding available—a great problem for the continuity of programs for minorities, continuing education, and clinical specialties when this "soft money" later diminishes or evaporates altogether.

Nursing research also tended to make slow progress. Although there were studies of nursing service, nursing education, and nursing personality, most were done with or by social scientists. When nurses assisted physicians and others in medical research, it was just that— assisting. Nursing leaders realized that nursing could not develop as a profession unless clinical research focusing on nursing evolved and was disseminated. One of the first major steps in that direction was the 1952 publication of *Nursing Research*, a scholarly journal that reported and encouraged nursing research. Another was the ANA's creation of the American Nurses Foundation in 1955 for charitable, educational, and scientific purposes. Of course, federal funding also had a considerable impact, and most especially the establishment of the National Institute of Nursing Research.

With all of these changes, the professional organizations of nursing took varied and sometimes uncoordinated action. A study to consider restructuring, reorganizing, and unifying the various organizations was initiated shortly after World War II. In 1952, the six major nursing organizations—ANA, NLNE, NOPHN, NACGN, the Association of Collegiate Schools of Nursing (ACSN), and the American Association of Industrial Nurses (AAIN)—finally came to a decision about organizational structure. Two major organizations emerged: the ANA, with only nurse members, and the renamed National League for Nursing (NLN), with nurse, nonnurse, and agency membership. The AAIN decided to continue, and the National Student Nurses' Association was formed. Practical nurses had their own organization. (See Chapter 13 for details of the organizations.) Although there was an apparent realignment of responsibilities, the relationships between the ANA and NLN ebbed and flowed: sometimes they were in agreement, and sometimes they were not; sometimes they worked together, and at other times each appeared to make isolated unilateral pronouncements. Some nurses wanted one organization, but there seemed to be mutual organizational reluctance to go in that direction. Yet, each had some remarkable achievements: NLN in educational accreditation, and ANA in its lobbying activities, its development of a model licensure law in the mid-1950s, and its increased action regarding nurses' economic security.

Licensing and the broader area of credentialing have been the focus of two significant studies since the late 1970s. The first, *The Study of Credentialing in Nursing*, defined the profession's responsibility to protect and advise the consumer on its practitioners. More lately, beginning in 1991, the Pew Charitable Trust funded a series of studies which focused on the competencies required for current-day practice and the role relationships between provider professionals, and which challenged existing licensing laws as being too inflexible for the public good (see Appendix 1).

In 1965, ANA precipitated (or inflamed) an ongoing controversy. After years of increasingly firm statements on the place of nursing education in the mainstream of American education, ANA issued its first *Position Paper on Education for Nursing*. It stated, basically, that education for those who work in nursing should be in institutions of higher learning; that minimum education for professional nursing should be at least at the baccalaureate level; for technical nursing, at the AD level; and for assistants, in vocational education settings.

Although there had been increasing complaints by third-party payers about the financial burden to hospitals created by diploma education, and diploma schools had declined as AD and baccalaureate degree programs increased, there was an outpouring of anger by diploma and practical nurses and those involved in their education. It was a battle that persisted and became another divisive force in nursing. The history of this controversy over education for "entry into practice" is presented in more detail in Chapter 5.

An additional volatile topic of the 1960s was the appearance of nurse practitioners. Many nursing leaders initially labeled this advanced practice role as pseudomedicine, and saw it as detracting from the professionalism of nursing. Quite the contrary, both the clinical nurse specialist and nurse practitioner were logical responses to the evolving times. The "Great Society" reforms created an increased demand for primary health care services. Nurses were the best choice to fill this need, even though the original plea was to respond to the shortage of physicians who overwhelmingly began to choose specialty practice. So too did nursing specialization become a necessity to complement the

(continued on page 72)

Exhibit 2.2 U.S. Nursing in the Context of the Times

1865 to 1885

Society at Large

- U.S. population (1870): 39.8 million; life expectancy 38–42
- 1865: End of Civil War: Union restored; President Lincoln assassinated
- Ku Klux Klan founded
- Westward expansion; railroads, land boom
- National trade union movement; labor unrest
- Wars against Indians in the West
- Purchase of Alaska
- Continuation of "old immigration" (Scandinavian, Irish, German)
- Chinese immigrant labor; other contract labor
- Beginning of petroleum industry
- Numerous political and financial scandals
- Panic of 1873 affects national income and leads to substantial unemployment
- Public schools free for all
- Booker T. Washington founds Tuskegee Institute for Blacks
- Spelman College opens to educate black women
- Illiteracy rate (1870) at 20 percent

Government, Legislation, Supreme Court Decisions

- 1863–65: Reconstruction Proclamation and Acts (ends 1877)
- 1865: 13th amendment abolishing slavery, ratified
- Freedman's Bureau established
- 1875: Civil Rights Act bestows citizenship upon the "Negro"
- 1875: Civil Rights Act guarantees equal rights in public places; declared invalid by Supreme Court in 1883
- Supreme Court upholds Congress's power to punish as crime, private interference with right of citizen to vote (against Ku Klux Klan)
- Chinese Exclusion Act, prohibiting immigration of Chinese laborers for 10 years
- Contract Labor Act forbids importation of all but skilled, professional, and domestic labor
- Garfield becomes 20th president (assassinated)

Medicine, Public Health, Science, Technology	Nursing
• First practical intercity telephone lines	• Volunteer nurses in Civil War include Dix (superintendent of nurses), Bickerdyke, Barton, Tubman, Truth, Taylor, and three Woolsey sisters (later influential in development of nurse training programs)
• Pioneer stages of motion pictures	
• Practical application of electric arc lamps and incandescent bulb (Edison)	
• Phonograph patented by Edison	• 1872: First training school—New England Hospital for Women and Children; first graduate, Linda Richards
• Advances in cameras and films	
• Development of automobiles	
• Various electrical home appliances and industrial equipment invented	• 1873: Three schools founded on Nightingale principles: Bellevue Training School (New York); Connecticut Training School for Nurses (New Haven, CT); Boston Training School for Nurses at Massachusetts General (Boston); Richards, first superintendent
• Advances in surgery, including methods for antiseptic surgery; advances in anesthesia	
• Specialized medical journals published	
• First state board of health established in Massachusetts	• First uniform designed
• Increased number of medical schools founded	• Sister Mary Bernard (nurse) gives anesthesia at St. Vincent's Hospital (Erie, PA)
• American Public Health Association founded (1872)	• First black trained nurse: Mary Mahoney
	• 1880: 15 nurse training programs
• Osteopathy established	• 1881: Robb heads training school at Johns Hopkins
• Index Medicus and Index-Catalogue founded	• 1881: American National Red Cross founded under leadership of Clara Barton
• Sanitarium for tubercular patients opened at Saranac Lake, NY	• 1885: First district nurse (Buffalo, NY)
	• Weeks writes textbook on nursing care for nurses and families.

(continued)

Exhibit 2.2 (Continued)

1886 to 1906

Society at Large

- U.S. population (1900): 76 million; life expectancy 48–51
- North Dakota, South Dakota, Montana, Washington, and Utah admitted to Union
- "Coxey's Army" of jobless men march on Washington for work; disbanded when leaders arrested
- Panic of 1893: lasts 4 years; stock market crash; decline of U.S. gold reserve
- Jane Addams founds Hull House in Chicago—settlement house for immigrants
- Klondike gold rush
- 1890: Women in the labor force, 3.7 million; 14 percent married
- 1900: Illiteracy rate at 10.7 percent
- 128 women's colleges founded by 1901
- Women make up about 25 percent of all undergraduate students
- 1898: Spanish–American War; won by U.S. Spain cedes Philippines to U.S. for $20 million; also Puerto Rico and Guam (become territories)
- "New immigration" from eastern and southern Europe develops. Over one million immigrants in 1905
- Bureau of Immigration established
- Scott discovers Antarctic Plateau
- Carrie Nation leads crusade against liquor and saloons
- 1906: San Francisco earthquake

Government, Legislation, Supreme Court Decisions

- Sherman Antitrust Act; declares restraint of trade illegal
- Various legislation creates early conservation measures
- Plessy v. Ferguson (1896) rules that separate but equal facilities do not deprive Negroes of equal protection under 14th Amendment; legalizes segregation
- Blacks deprived of vote in the South
- 1906: Pure Food and Drug Act enacted
- Meat Inspection Act enacted
- National Child Labor Council established
- 25th president: McKinley (assassinated)
- Vice-president Roosevelt becomes 26th president and is reelected; appoints Blacks and Jews to office, against Congressional pressure
- American Federation of Labor (AFL) established

Medicine, Public Health, Science, Technology	Nursing

Medicine, Public Health, Science, Technology

- Early stages of motion pictures
- Wright brothers make first "heavier-than-air" flight
- Rayon and Bakelite (plastic) patented
- Radio, flat-disk phonograph, vacuum tube, telegraphy, and battery invented
- Roentgen discovers x-rays
- Curies discover radium
- English physician Ross determines Anopheles mosquito transmits malaria; Dr. Reed determines Aedes mosquito transmits yellow fever
- Three biologists, working separately, rediscover Mendel's law of heredity
- X-rays used to treat breast cancer
- First Nobel prize awarded
- Introduction of rubber gloves in surgery
- Mayo Clinic founded
- Rockefeller Institute for Medical Research founded
- Chiropractic founded (1895)
- American Hospital Association founded
- 112 medical schools founded (1873–95)
- States tighten medical licensure exams
- "Typhoid Mary" seen as evidence that typhoid can be carried by healthy people

Nursing

- Nursing journal, *The Nightingale*, edited by Bellevue graduate (dies for lack of support 1891)
- *The Trained Nurse and Hospital Review* considered first real nursing journal; lasts 70 years
- Dock writes *Materia Medica* textbook for nurses; Kimber writes anatomy book; Robb writes first substantial clinical nursing book
- First nursing school for men established (Mills School of Nursing at Bellevue), followed by others
- First nursing program for Blacks founded (Spelman Seminary) in 1886, followed by others, including diploma program at Howard University (1893)
- Jessie Sleet (Scales) first Black public health nurse
- 1893: American Society of Superintendents of Training Schools of Nursing founded: Richards, first president
- 1897: Nurses' Associated Alumnae of the United States and Canada founded (later to become the American Nurses Association); Robb, first president
- Wald and Brewster establish Henry Street Visiting Nurse (NY) which eventually evolves into the Visiting Nurse Service of New York City.
- First industrial nurse, A. Stewart, employed by Vermont Marble Co.
- First school for training practical nurses
- Nurses, including Black nurses, serve in Spanish–American War
- Nurse Clara Maas dies: martyr to yellow fever research
- International Council of Nursing founded; Fenwick, first president (1899)
- Teachers College, Columbia University, first to offer college course to nurses (hospital economics)
- School nursing begins
- Permanent Army Nurse Corps established; headed by Kinney
- 1900: *American Journal of Nursing,* first nursing journal owned by nurses published; Palmer is editor
- 432 training schools in 1900; most graduates do private duty with few hired by hospitals
- 1903: First nurse licensure laws (NC, NJ, NY, VA)

(continued)

Exhibit 2.2 (Continued)

1907 to 1927

Society at Large

- U.S. population (1910): 92 million
- U.S. population (1920): 106 million
- Life expectancy 53–59
- Panic of 1907: stock market drop and business failures
- White House Conference on Conservation to educate public on importance of forest and water resources
- Arizona, Oklahoma, and New Mexico admitted to Union
- First woman elected to Congress (Montana, 1916)
- First woman elected governor (Wyoming, 1925)
- Du Bois founds NAACP
- 1909: Peary flies American flag over North Pole
- 1914: Panama Canal opens to traffic
- Outbreak of World War I
- 1917: U.S. declares war on Germany
- 1918: War ends; signing of armistice
- National League of Nations: no U.S. government representation
- Number of Ku Klux Klan exposés: membership down
- Women in labor force 1920: 8.4 million; 23 percent married
- International Ladies Garment Workers Union founded
- Beginning of labor setbacks with recession of 1920
- Exposure of dishonesty in banking, railroads, finance, environment
- First nonstop flight, New York to Paris
- First transcontinental flight
- 1916: Fundamentalist religions gain converts
- Beginning of decolonialization

Government, Legislation, Supreme Court Decisions

- Mann Act (White Slavery Traffic Act) prohibits interstate transportation of women for immoral purposes
- Social legislation in states re: wages and hours, employment of women and children. Public assistance for women with children (1911); first state workmen's compensation law (MD)
- 16th amendment establishes income tax (1913)
- 17th amendment ratified: direct election of senators
- Workmen's Compensation Act for federal employees
- Selective Service Act (1917)
- 1920: Prohibition Act (18th amendment) goes into effect, prohibits manufacture and sale of liquor
- 1920: 19th amendment ratified (women's suffrage)
- First seriously restrictive immigration law passed; set quotas
- Veterans Bureau established
- Soldiers Bonus Act passed
- Army Air Corps established
- Japanese Exclusion Acts limit immigration of Japanese laborers

Medicine, Public Health, Science, Technology	Nursing
• Flexner Report exposes abuses in medical education and proposes reforms	• 1105 diploma schools in 1909
• Number of medical schools and graduates decline	• 1908: National Association for Colored Graduate Nurses founded
• Mental health movement founded	• 1909: First collegiate nursing program established at University of Minnesota
• Schick skin test for diphtheria developed	• 1909: The nursing service of the American Red Cross is funded with Jane Delano as chief
• Basic research in preventive medicine expands	
• Vitamins discovered; increased research in deficiencies and related diseases	• Nutting becomes first nurse appointed to professorship in a university (Teachers College, Columbia)
• Studies on hereditary conditions and traits; term "genes" first used	• First public health nursing course given at Teachers College, Columbia
• Influenza epidemic (1918–19); 500,000 deaths in U.S.	• National Organization for Public Health Nursing founded; Wald, first president
• Iron lung invented (used for polio)	• Public health nursing journal published
• First commercial radio transmission (Pittsburgh)	• National League of Nursing Education publishes first *Standard Curriculum for Schools of Nursing*
• Einstein discloses theory of relativity	
• Color photography, sound films invented	• Nurses serve in World War I
• First telephoto pictures sent over telegraph wires	• Army School of Nursing established; Goodrich, superintendent
• First Model T auto introduced	• Vassar Training Camp (1918) provides preliminary course for college graduates for later shortened diploma programs
• First television images transmitted (London)	
• World's first helicopter flight (France)	• Breckinridge establishes Frontier Nursing Service in 1925, including midwifery school
• Scopes Trial: teacher convicted of teaching evolution	• Sanger arrested for distributing birth control information; founds predecessor of Planned Parenthood
	• Dock writes first nursing history book and book on venereal diseases; also active in women's suffrage movement
	• Red Cross establishes rural nursing service
	• Public health nursing section established in APHA
	• 1917: Forty-five states have enacted nursing practice acts and adopted the term "registered nurse"
	• Sigma Theta Tau, first national nursing honor society, founded (1922) (later international)
	• Yale School of Nursing, first autonomous collegiate school, opens; Goodrich, dean (1924)

(continued)

Exhibit 2.2 (Continued)

1928 to 1948

Society at Large

- U.S. population (1930): 122.7 million
- U.S. population (1940): 131.6 million
- Life expectancy 59–67
- "Bonus Army" of veterans march on Washington to demand bonuses promised after World War I
- 1929: Stock market crash; beginning of the Great Depression with serious unemployment
- Manufacturing declines during Depression
- President Roosevelt initiates "Good Neighbor" policy for improved relations with Latin America
- Jehovah's Witnesses founded
- Educational testing developed
- Junior Colleges beginning to spread
- Illiteracy rate (1930) at 4.2 percent
- Illiteracy rate (1947) at 2.7 percent of population; rural 5.3 percent
- Earhart is first woman to fly Atlantic
- First woman elected to U.S. Senate (Tennessee, 1932)
- Perkins becomes first woman Cabinet member (Labor, 1933)
- Hitler invades Poland: beginning of World War II (1939)
- Japanese bomb Pearl Harbor (1941); Germany declares war on U.S.
- U.S. declares war on Axis (Japan, Germany, Italy)
- Race riots erupt in Los Angeles and Detroit
- D-Day invasion of Normandy (1944); greatest amphibious assault ever
- U.S. drops atomic bombs; destroy two Japanese cities
- Concentration camps in Europe liberated
- World War II ends (1945)
- United Nations Charter adopted; First General Assembly (1946); WHO established
- Churchill's "Iron Curtain" speech marks the beginning of the "Cold War" (1946)

Government, Legislation, Supreme Court Decisions

- Prohibition (Volstead Act) repealed (1933)
- National Housing Act insures home mortgages
- Number of "New Deal" laws passed to provide jobs; e.g. Works Project Administration (WPA), Federal Employment Relations Agency (FERA); Federal Relief Administration (FRA); Civil Works Administration (CWA)
- National Labor Relations Act passed; recognizes workers' right to organize and bargain collectively (1935)
- Fair Labor Standards Act passed
- Social Security Act becomes law (1935)
- Food, Drug and Cosmetic Act passed
- Selective Service Act makes men 21–35 eligible for military service
- 1943: Bolton Act creates Cadet Nurse Corps
- Executive order to intern 120,000 Japanese on West Coast
- GI bill provides variety of benefits for veterans, including higher education subsidies and tuition
- Marshall Plan to rebuild postwar Europe
- Occupation of Japan
- First Clean Air Act passed
- Truman proclaims independence of Philippines
- 32d president: Roosevelt (4 terms, died in office)

Medicine, Public Health, Science, Technology	Nursing
• Effectiveness of sulfanilamide and related drugs for variety of infections	• 1929: 2200 diploma programs
• Use of insulin and electric shock for schizophrenia	• Nursing schools close; Depression affects nurse employment in private duty; hospitals begin to employ more nurses at a minimum wage
• Advances in psychotherapy	• New Deal agencies provide work for nurses in communities and governmental settings
• Fleming discovers penicillin; other antibiotics follow	
• Massive attacks on crippling and killing diseases through research	• American Association of Nurse-Midwives and American Association of Nurse Anesthetists founded
• Antihistamines discovered	• First Nurse-Midwifery school founded at Maternity Center in New York City
• Cortisone synthesized	
• Patent issued for Nylon and other synthetics	• Association of Collegiate Schools of Nursing founded
• First binary calculating machine and other precursors to computers	• USPHS employs first public health nurse
• Instant camera, long-playing records and microwave oven	• 1936: 1500 diploma schools; 70 "collegiate"
• Frozen food industry develops	• 1938: A nurses' monument (Spirit of Nursing) is dedicated in Arlington National Cemetery
• Polaroid glass invented	
• Transistor and solar battery invented	• Nurses serve in all fronts in World War II
• First jet engine produced	• Army and Navy nurse officers awarded permanent commission
	• Chi Eta Phi sorority, American Association of Industrial Nurses; Association of State and Territorial Directors of Nursing, and Nurses' Christian Fellowship founded
	• The U.S. Cadet Corps is formed
	• Major postwar nursing shortage

(continued)

Exhibit 2.2 (Continued)

1949 to 1969

Society at Large

- U.S. population (1950): 150.7 million
- U.S. population (1960): 179.3 million
- Life expectancy 66–75
- Baby boom peaks (1955)
- Suburbs expand
- Interstate highway system begins
- Korean conflict begins (1950); ends 1953
- Rosa Parks refuses to give up seat to white person in Montgomery, AL; bus boycott begins
- "Freedom Riders" test segregation laws in deep South
- Voter registration drive begins in South
- King leads civil rights march to DC, later to Selma, AL.
- Major racial unrest in American cities
- Truman orders development of hydrogen bomb
- Alaska and Hawaii join the Union (49th and 50th States)
- Early gay rights organization founded in California
- Carson's *Silent Spring* launches environmental movement
- National Organization for Women (NOW) founded
- Overcrowding in schools
- Expansion of higher education; major growth of community colleges
- President's Commission on the status of women recommends new educational opportunities for women
- Number of American troops in Vietnam escalated; opposition grows
- Postwar European refugees are the new immigrants
- Increase in Ku Klux Klan membership; about 40,000 in 1960s
- Gains in churches' rolls seen
- Authorine Lucy, first Black to be enrolled in University of Alabama

Government, Legislation, Supreme Court Decisions

- Immigration and Naturalization Act passed (1952), lifts last racial and ethnic barriers to naturalization
- Refugee Relief Act (1953) provides for entry into U.S. on emergency basis outside regular immigration quota
- Brown v. Bd. of Education (1955); outlaws "separate but equal" educational systems; and begins the unraveling of U.S. racial segregation
- 22d amendment ratified (presidential terms limited to two)
- Federal Nurse Traineeship Act; authorizes funds for baccalaureate and graduate education; also short-term continuing education
- Peace Corps established (1961)
- Johnson signs Civil Rights Act of 1964 and antipoverty bill prohibiting discrimination in voting, public housing, employment
- Beginning of "Great Society" and "War on Poverty"
- Medicare and Medicaid
- Clean Air Act
- Supreme Court holds that "right of privacy" covers use of contraceptives
- Supreme Court bans prayer in school
- 35th President: Kennedy (assassinated 1963)

Medicine, Public Health, Science, Technology	Nursing
• Advances in medical technology create changes in diagnosis and treatment of diseases	• Two practical nurse organizations founded
• Hill–Burton Act for support of hospital construction	• Air Force gives nurse officers permanent commissions
• Mechanical heart first used in human (1952)	• Male nurses granted full rank in armed services
• Reported increase in incidence of lung cancer due to cigarette smoking	• Code of ethics adopted by ANA
• New discoveries in genetics	• 1952: Associate degree programs in nursing begin
• Various hormones synthesized	• Nurses serve in Korean War, including MASH units
• Oral Orinase for diabetes developed	• Structure study of nursing organizations results in two large nursing organizations (ANA, NLN), founding of National Student Nurses' Association, and dissolving of NACGN after ANA forbids membership discrimination against Black nurses
• Tranquilizers synthesized; widespread use by 1955	
• Salk develops vaccine for polio	
• Sabin develops oral vaccine for polio	
• First birth control pills sold	
• Pandemic of Asian flu	• American Nurses Foundation created, devoted to research
• Dawn of space age: Russia launches Sputnik I, first artificial satellite (1957) and puts first man in space (1961)	• *Nursing Research* published
	• *Nursing Outlook* published
	• Reiter writes about clinical nurse specialist
• U.S. launches first satellite into orbit (1958)	• Some increase in nursing doctoral programs
• Shepard travels on first U.S. manned space flight (1961)	• Nurse practitioner role developed in Colorado
• Glen is first American to orbit earth (1962)	• 1965: ANA publishes *Educational Preparation for Nurse Practitioners and Assistants to Nurses: A Position Paper*, recommending baccalaureate education for professional nurses, AD education for technical nurses, and short preservice education for aides
• Armstrong is first man to walk on the moon	
• "Mariner" completes first successful interplanetary mission	
• Shortage of physicians	
• Albert Schweitzer wins Nobel Peace Prize	
• First human pregnancy induced with frozen sperm (1953)	• More than 5000 military nurses serve in Vietnam
• First color TV sold; videotapes and stereo recorders	
• Microprocessor and silicon chip	
• First commercial computers	
• First transatlantic television transmission by satellite	

(continued)

Exhibit 2.2 (Continued)

1970 and on

Society at Large

- U.S. population (1970) 203.3 million; (1980) 226.5 million; (1990) 248.7 million; (2000) 275 million
- 1970: 4 students protesting the U.S. invasion into Cambodia slain by guardsmen at Kent State
- Accelerating anti-war demonstrations
- 1973: U.S. withdraws from Vietnam
- Draft evaders pardoned by President Carter
- UN seats Communist China, expels Nationalist China
- Watergate scandal; Nixon eventually resigns from the presidency
- Americans held hostage in Teheran
- Increased international terrorism, Lockerbie
- Progress on nuclear disarmament and limitations on nuclear testing
- Challenger explodes after launch
- First woman appointed to the U.S. Supreme Court
- Tiananmen Square; the power of communication informed the world
- 1989: Berlin Wall falls; end of the Cold War
- Apartheid ends in South Africa
- Break-up of the Soviet Union
- "Desert Storm" as it happened brought to you by CNN
- The Panama Canal reverts to control of the Republic of Panama
- Expansion of the European Union
- Growing popularity of distance education
- 1 out of every 3 Americans does some work at home instead of commuting
- Inflation slows
- Job insecurity; growing episodic and part-time work patterns
- Transition to a service economy
- Increasing cultural diversification
- 9/11/2001: The U.S. attacked on its own soil, over 3000 dead
- U.S. emerges as the primary world power
- Emergence of China as a world power
- A smaller world due to communication, travel, education, and limited natural resources
- Decline of unionization
- Globalization of business and industry

Government, Legislation, Supreme Court Decisions

- Weakening of Roe v. Wade by federal and state legislation
- Supreme Court rules that bussing of students may be ordered to achieve desegregation
- 29th Amendment, voting age lowered to 18
- Supreme Court rules death penalty unconstitutional in 1972, and overturns that ruling in 1976
- Government deregulation of the cable communication industry
- "Open Skies" allowing any U.S. company to use communication satellites
- "Healthy People 2000, 2010": a renewed emphasis on healthy living and disease and accident prevention
- World Trade Agreements
- The House of Representatives votes to impeach President Clinton
- Legislative reforms to control the cost of health care to the federal government
- Prospective Payment System (PPS) instituted for almost every segment of publicly funded health care
- Increasing government control of the health care delivery system

Medicine, Public Health, Science, Technology	Nursing
• Voyager space craft lands on Mars	• 1971: The National Black Nurses Association established
• The videodisk, floppy disks, camcorder, computerized laser printing, hologram technology, laptop computers, and cellular car phones make an appearance	• The ANA moves its national headquarters from Kansas City to Washington, DC
• Videotype for the hearing impaired	• The *American Journal of Nursing* Company is sold to Lippincott Publishers
• 1983: *Time* names "The Computer" as Man of the Year	• RN licensing exam given by a system of Computer Adaptive Testing (CAT)
• Nationwide programming by satellite	• The American Nurses Credentialing Center (ANCC) establishes the baccalaureate degree as the requirement for certification in a specialty area by 1998, and reverses that position in 2000
• AT&T forced to break up and the Baby Bells are born	
• International fax service available	
• 1995: Sony demonstrates flat TV set	
• 1995: Denmark announces plan to put much of the nation on-line within 5 years	• Advanced practice nurses (APNs) reimbursable for services to Medicare recipients
• 1995: Major U.S. dailies create national on-line newspaper network	• Legislation creates the National Institute for Nursing Research
• Smallpox eradicated	• The American Nurses Credentialing Center (ANCC) establishes Magnet programs for excellence in nursing services in hospitals, long-term care, and home health
• Scientists identify AIDS; by 2000 it becomes a long-term disease	
• Dramatic advances in diagnostics and therapeutics which decrease the need for intrusive procedures	
• Managed care dominates as the model for allocating health care resources	• Consumers identify the quality of nursing as the most important factor in determining their satisfaction with a hospital experience
• Tailoring of managed health care insurance to meet consumer preference	• The primary focus for graduate study in nursing has become clinical practice, as opposed to teaching or management
• The vast majority of health care services are provided in the community setting	
• A new appreciation for healthy life styles, but obesity and teenage smoking increase	• The average age of the RN is about 45 years of age; revealing an "aging" workforce
• 45 million uninsured in 2003	• By 1992, the majority of RNs had received their basic education in an academic rather than a service setting
• Increased employment of older Americans	
	• Several cyclical shortages and surpluses of nurses
	• Severe shortage of nurse faculty
	• APNs grow in their practice rights

knowledge explosion in medical science. The first coronary care unit was opened in 1962–63,[50] and set the stage for more autonomy and greater specialization. The 1970 government-funded study, *Extending the Scope of Nursing Practice,* proposed greater responsibilities for the nurse as a member of the health care team, and was the impetus for federal funding and growth of nurse practitioner programs.

It is the "Great Society" that also gave us Medicare and Medicaid (1965). In short order, the government became aware that it had probably underestimated the dollar amount necessary to sustain these programs. In response, legislative reforms were to reduce the cost and monitor the quality of public entitlement programs in health care. Specifics are presented in *Dimensions of Professional Nursing,* eighth edition. These events opened the door for managed care as a way to curtail health care spending. Nursing is once again being shaped by the economics of the times. It becomes a choice whether to be held hostage, or respond strategically.[51]

The past is prologue. There are many benchmark events and intermediate gateways which have caused dramatic change in the education of nurses and the practice of nursing. Our history has been a continuous revolution, and we have won most of the battles.

KEY POINTS

1. The work and ongoing interest of the volunteers who acted as nurses in the Civil War were influential in the establishment of the first training schools for nurses modeled (to some extent) on Nightingale principles.
2. Students in the early training schools worked long hours, did many menial nonnursing tasks, and gave almost all the nursing care in hospitals.
3. Twenty-five years after trained nursing had begun, nursing leaders in the United States were responsible for setting nursing standards, improving curricula, writing textbooks, starting two enduring nursing organizations and a nursing journal, inaugurating a teacher training program in a university, and initiating nursing licensure.
4. Before the Great Depression, most graduate nurses worked at private duty, but public health nursing, school nursing, industrial nursing, midwifery, and other specialties gradually emerged under the leadership of nursing pioneers
5. Studies about nursing that pointed out deficiencies in nursing education and practice were often ignored because of the students'

economic benefit to the hospital, but they seem to have had a cumulative effect that eventually brought about change.

6. Because of the shortage of nurses that occurred during and after wars, reforms in both nursing education and practice were instituted.
7. AD nursing, initiated in 1952 as an action research project, produced a new kind of nurse and changed nursing education.
8. Black nurses and men were often discriminated against in nursing but slowly gained status in the last half of the twentieth century.
9. War and the economics of health care have always exerted a significant effect on nursing.
10. The absence of agreement among nurses on education and practice issues has limited our growth as a profession; the nurse practitioner movement and debate over education for "entry into practice" are good examples.
11. Much change in our education and practice has come about through external forces, rather than internal decisions.

STUDY QUESTIONS

1. What social and health care trends can you identify that will change nursing in the future? What will be the nature of that change?
2. What do you see as the relationship between the women's movement and the development of modern nursing?
3. The influence of communication in the major events of the last decades is obvious. What does this mean for nursing?
4. It is often observed that the U.S.'s major products in the world market are information and technology. What does this mean to nursing?

REFERENCES

1. Selavan IC. Nurses in American history: The revolution. *Am J Nurs* 75:592–594, April 1975.
2. Wall B. Called to a mission of charity: The Sisters of St. Joseph in the Civil War. *Nurs Hist Review* 6:85–113, 1998.
3. Kalisch P, Kalisch B. *The Advance of American Nursing*, 3d ed. Boston: Little, Brown, 1995, p 53.
4. Kalisch P, Kalisch B. Untrained but undaunted: The women nurses of the blue and gray. *Nurs Forum* 15(1):4–33, 1976; see p 17.
5. Kalisch and Kalisch (1995), op cit, p 47.

6. Dolan JA, et al. *Nursing in Society: A Historical Perspective*, 15th ed. Philadelphia: W. B. Saunders, 1983, pp 173–174.
7. Carnegie ME. Black nurses at the front. *Am J Nurs* 84:1250–1252, October 1984.
8. Bullough V, Bullough B. *The Care of the Sick: The Emergence of Modern Nursing.* New York: Prodist, 1978, p 114.
9. Dolan et al, op cit, pp 194–197.
10. Ibid, p 202.
11. Kalisch and Kalisch (1995), op cit, pp 144–148.
12. Ibid, pp 109–110.
13. Carnegie ME. *Black Nurses: A Historical Perspective*, http://www.aetna.com/diversity/aahcalendar/2003/perspective.html, accessed January 29, 2005.
14. Flaumenhaft E, Flaumenhaft C. American nursing's first text books. *Nurs Outlook* 37:185–188, July–August 1989.
15. Kalisch B, Kalisch P. Slaves, servants, or saints: An analysis of the system of nurse training in the United States, 1873–1948. *Nurse Forum* 14(3):230–231, 1975; see p 228.
16. Kalisch and Kalisch (1995), op cit, p 114.
17. Ibid, p 206.
18. Dolan et al, op cit, p 290.
19. Kalisch and Kalisch (1995), op cit, p 243.
20. Kelly L. *Dimensions of Professional Nursing*, 5th ed. New York: Macmillan Publishing, 1985, p 71.
21. Bullough and Bullough, op cit, p 156.
22. Ingles T. The physician's view of the evolving nursing profession—1873–1913. *Nurs Forum* 15(2): 123–164, 1976; see p 148.
23. Bullough B, Bullough V. Sex discrimination in health care. *Nurs Outlook* 23:40–45, January 1975; see p 43.
24. Kelly L, Joel L. *Dimensions of Professional Nursing*, 8th ed. New York: McGraw-Hill, 1999, p 68.
25. Nutting MA. Isabel Hampton Robb: Her work in organization and education. *Am J Nurs* 10:19, January 1910.
26. Poslusny S. Feminine friendship: Isabel Hampton Robb, Lavinia Lloyd Dock and Mary Adelaide Nutting. *Image* 21:64–67, Summer 1989.
27. Benson E. Nursing and the World's Columbian Exposition. *Nurs Outlook* 34:88–90, March–April 1986.
28. Christy TE. Portrait of a leader: Sophia F. Palmer. *Nurs Outlook* 23:746–751, December 1975; see pp 746–747.
29. Flanagan L. *One Strong Voice: The Story of the American Nurses Association.* Kansas City, MO: American Nurses Association, 1976, pp 35–38.
30. Ibid.
31. Pryor EB. *Clara Barton, Professional Angel.* Philadelphia: University of Pennsylvania Press, 1987.
32. Kalisch and Kalisch (1995), op cit, p 193.
33. Christy TE. Portrait of a leader: Lillian D. Wald. *Nurs Outlook* 18:50–54, March 1970.
34. Ruffing-Rahal MA. Margaret Sanger: Nurse and feminist. *Nurs Outlook* 34:246–249, September–October 1986.

35. Christy TE. Portrait of a leader. Lavinia Lloyd Dock. *Nurs Outlook* 17:72–75, June 1969; see p 74.
36. Ibid.
37. Pletsch PK. Mary Breckenridge: A pioneer who made her mark. *Am J Nurs* 81:188–190, February 1981.
38. Carnegie ME. *The Path We Tread: Blacks in Nursing 1854–1984.* Philadelphia: J.B. Lippincott, 1986.
39. Kalisch and Kalisch (1995), op cit, p 137.
40. Stanhope M, Lancaster J. *Community and Public Health Nursing.* St. Louis: Mosby, 2004.
41. Fitzpatrick ML. Nursing and the great depression. *Am J. Nurs* 75:2188–2190, December 1975.
42. Flanagan, op cit.
43. Gourney C. Military nursing: 211 years of commitment to the American soldier. *Imprint* 34:36–45, February–March 1987.
44. Kalisch and Kalisch (1995), op cit, pp 228–235.
45. Curtis D. Nurses and war: The way it was. *Am J Nurs* 84:1253–1254, October 1984.
46. Norman EM. *We Band of Angels.* New York: Random House, 1999, pp 159–168.
47. Kalisch B, Kalisch P. Nurses in American history: The Cadet Nurse Corps. *Am J Nurs* 76:240–242, February 1976.
48. Norman E. *Women at War.* Philadelphia: University of Pennsylvania Press, 1990, pp 27–43.
49. Brown EL. *Nursing for the Future.* New York: Russell Sage Foundation, 1948, p 178.
50. Chitty KK. *Professional Nursing: Concepts & Challenges,* 3d ed. Philadelphia: W.B. Saunders, 2001, p 25.
51. Grando VT. The influence of economic forces on American nursing. *Reflections* 23:24–25, Fourth Quarter 1997.

Updates can be found at

 http://www.JoelTheNursingExperience.com

HELPFUL WEBSITES FOR PART 1

University of Pennsylvania, School of Nursing, The Center for the Study of the History of Nursing: http://www.nursing.upenn.edu/history

Boston University, The History of Nursing Archives: http://www.bu.edu/speccol/nursing.htm

American Association for the History of Nursing, *Nursing History Review*: http://www.aahn.org/nhr.html

Florence Nightingale Museum, London: http://www.florence-nightingale.co.uk/

The Lycos Network: http://members.tripod.com/~DianneBrownson/
    history.html
Army Nurse Corps: http://www.army.mil/cmh-pg/anc/anchhome.html
University of Virginia, School of Nursing, Center for Nursing Historical Inquiry:
    http://www.nursing.virginia.edu/centers/history.html
American Association for the History of Medicine (AAHM): http://www.
    histmed.org
American Historical Association: http://www.theaha.org
American Nurses Association Hall of Fame: http://www.ana.org/hof/index.htm
American Nurses Association Centennial Exhibit: Voices from the Past, Visions
    of the Future: http://www.ana.org/centenn/index.htm
Archives of Nursing Leadership: http://www.nursing.uconn.edu/
    ARCHIVE.HTML
Black Nurses in History: http://www4.umdnj.edu/camlbweb/blacknurses.html
Clendening History of Medicine Library—Florence Nightingale Resources:
    http://clendening.kumc.edu/florence
Frontier Nursing Service: http://www.achiever.com/freehmpg/kynurses/
    fns.html
Images from the History of Medicine: http://wwwihm.nlm.nih.gov/
Medical History on the Internet: http://www.anes.uab.edu/medhist.htm
Men in American Nursing History: http://www.geocities.com/Athens/Forum/
    6011/
Nurses in the U.S. Navy—Historical bibliography: http://www.history.navy.mil/
    faqs/faq50-1.htm
Royal College of Nursing Archives: http://www.rcnscotland.org/Archivuk.htm

PART 2

NURSING IN THE HEALTH CARE SCENE

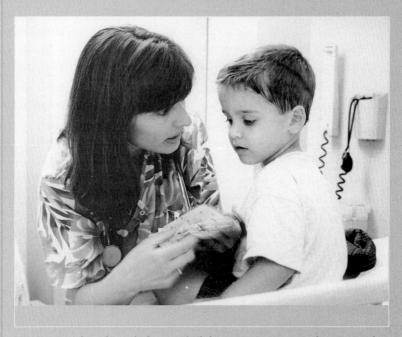

Nurses are often the only human link between patients and an intimidating experience in the health care delivery system. (*Courtesy of the Valley Hospital, Ridgewood, New Jersey*)

Chapter 3

The Health Care Delivery System

OBJECTIVES

After studying this chapter, you will be able to:

1. *Explain how social and economic factors have affected health care delivery.*
2. *Describe the impact of cost containment on health care.*
3. *Define self-care, primary care, secondary care, and tertiary care.*
4. *Identify the major settings in which health care is given.*
5. *Distinguish the roles of major personnel who are part of the health care team.*
6. *Recognize changes that are common to many health occupations.*
7. *Understand how predictions for future health care are related to current trends.*

Most people have no idea how complex health care is today, with its multiple settings and array of workers. Even those in the field often do not know much about what their colleagues do or how care is given in any place but their own. When a health "crisis" hits the headlines periodically, health workers are, naturally, more interested in how this affects them personally than in the larger picture. Yet, no part of health care is untouched when problems become big enough to be called a crisis. To remain ignorant or indifferent about what is going on is a luxury no one in health care can afford.

This chapter provides an overview of American health care, the settings, the people, the issues, and how outside factors influence the system.

WHAT INFLUENCES HEALTH CARE?

As a part of society and as one of the health professions, nursing is affected by the changes, problems, and issues of society in general, as well as those that specifically influence health care. Some changes, such as an emphasis on the civil rights of minority groups and women, have been with us for over 100 years. Others, such as changing social values and the growth of economic pressures, built up slowly and were largely ignored until the crisis was upon us. Still others, like new lifestyles and technological and scientific advances, emerged with a suddenness that caused the shattering stress and disorientation common in individuals when they are subjected to too much change in too short a time. Yet, even though it might be tempting simply to do your job and never mind the outside world, people (or professions) that do not pay attention to economic and social trends find themselves scrambling to catch up, rather than planning to move ahead—reacting, rather than acting. When the public accuses the professions of being unresponsive to their needs, it is, in part, because those professions have not been astute enough to observe patterns of change, or have been too self-centered to become part of them. Among the major factors to consider are changes in population, people's health, technology and scientific advances, education and employment, and social movements.

THE AMERICAN PEOPLE: A TIME OF CHANGE

A census has been conducted in the United States every ten years since 1790, as mandated by the Constitution. There are additional interim projections, the latest of which estimates the U.S. population at over 295 million in January of 2005. Although every attempt is made to be precise, there is undercounting which was verified by the Department of the Census, and at one point in time ranged from 4.5 percent for native Americans to 0.7 percent for Caucasians.[1] There are also socioeconomic lines which seem to be associated with undercounting, including people living in public housing projects and the homeless. The resident population grows even larger when we add undocumented aliens and migrant workers. The POPCLOCK maintained by the U.S. Census Bureau tells us that there is a net gain of one person every 12 seconds based on one birth every 8 seconds, one death every 12 seconds, and one international migrant (net) every 26 seconds. This represents a population increase of approximately 2.5 million people yearly since 1947.[2]

During the 1960s, population growth averaged 1.3 percent a year, but this reduced to 1.0 percent in the 1970s and 1980s. Even if growth continues at this modest level, by 2050 as predicted, a conservative population projection for that year is almost 420 million, an increase of 67 percent over 2000.[3] Other interesting comparisons are found in Exhibit 3.1. Numbers are an important ingredient in planning for health care needs, but only one aspect of the changing face of America.

The population will not be as white as before, and much less homogeneous. In the year 2000, almost one of every three Americans was a member of an ethnic minority, and by the middle of the twenty-first century, current minority peoples will become the numerical majority[4] (see Exhibit 3.1). The influx of immigrants has added to this diversity. Unlike the great European migration of earlier times, the new immigrants are primarily Hispanic, from the Americas, and Asian. This has affected the population mix in a number of states. The Asian population grew by 70 percent in the 1980s, and the Hispanic population is growing five times as fast as the rest of the population. Hispanic–Americans are

Exhibit 3.1 Projected Population of the United States, by Race and Hispanic Origin, 2000 to 2050 (In thousands except as indicated. As of July 1. Resident population.)

Population or % and race or Hispanic origin	2000	2010	2020	2030	2040	2050
Total Population	282,125	308,936	335,805	363,584	391,946	419,854
White alone	228,548	244,995	260,629	275,731	289,690	302,626
Black alone	35,818	40,454	45,365	50,442	55,876	61,361
Asian alone	10,684	14,241	17,988	22,580	27,992	33,430
All other races[a]	7,075	9,246	11,822	14,831	18,388	22,437
Hispanic (of any race)	35,622	47,756	59,756	73,055	87,585	102,560
White alone, not Hispanic	195,729	201,112	205,936	209,176	210,331	210,283
% of Total Population						
Total	100.0	100.0	100.0	100.0	100.0	100.0
White alone	81.0	79.3	77.6	75.8	73.9	72.1
Black alone	12.7	13.1	13.5	13.9	14.3	14.6
Asian alone	3.8	4.6	5.4	6.2	7.1	8.0
All other races[a]	2.5	3.0	3.5	4.1	4.7	5.3
Hispanic (of any race)	12.6	15.5	17.8	20.1	22.3	24.4
White alone, not Hispanic	69.4	65.1	61.3	57.5	53.7	50.1

[a] Includes American Indian and Alaska Native alone, Native Hawaiian and Other Pacific Islander alone, and two or more races.
Source: U.S. Census Bureau, 2004, U.S. Interim Projections by Age, Sex, Race, and Hispanic Origin: http://www.census.gov/ipc/www/usinterimproj/>. Internet release date: March 18, 2004.

the youngest population group. In March 2002, over 66 percent were under the age of 35, and over 34 percent under 18. Relatively few Hispanics (5.1 percent) were 65 years of age or over.[5]

Acceptance of the new immigrants has varied. One concern is their assimilation into the community. It has been noted that for the first time in our history, the majority of immigrants speak just one language— Spanish—and tend to live in ethnic enclaves served by media communicating in Spanish. Some Asians have also tended to cluster in ethnic neighborhoods and work in ethnic groups. The fact that foreign-born black and Hispanic people are more likely to have jobs than those native-born has caused resentment (although there is also resentment if the newcomers are receiving public assistance). The same is true of Asians, many of whom have the entire family working long hours to support a small shop or business and often pressure their children to perform well in school. There is no doubt that the diversity of our population enriches the nation. However, the American tradition of "one from many" is looking more like a mosaic than a melting pot (an analogy commonly made and not originating with the author). Each ethnic group is encouraged to retain its culture as a source of strength and identity. The implications for every aspect of life are staggering. Traditionalists who accept the reality of a multiracial society deplore a multicultural society, arguing that strong nations need a universally accepted set of values, and a common language. These patterns of cultural diversity give a mandate for nursing practice competencies. Health, illness, nutrition, caregiving, child rearing, and more all have differing cultural perspectives, and the nurse needs to be ready, willing, and able to deal with what the patient brings to their relationship.

The graying of America is considered the single most significant factor affecting the future of the United States, with special emphasis on health care. In the year 2003, there were almost 36 million Americans 65 years or older, and 4.7 million 85 and older.[6] Persons 85 or older are the fastest growing category of the U.S. population. More than 22 percent of Americans over 85 live in nursing and convalescent homes. On a given day such facilities are caring for one out of every 20 Americans over 65.[7] Those living in institutions are disproportionately women, generally unmarried or widowed. One major impact that the elderly, better educated than ever, have had is in influencing legislation. With organizations such as the American Association of Retired Persons (AARP) as their lobbyists, and with politicians' appreciation of their voting power, the elderly have clearly influenced legislation affecting them.

Each generation is a product of its times. The aged of 2005 faced the Great Depression as children, were the patriots of World War II, and knew economic deprivation in a period without social welfare programs. The major generations in the workplace are "baby-boomers" (1946–1961) and members of the "X" generation (1961–1980). Recent attention has been quick to focus on today's younger adults. They are alternately called the "X" generation because they originally defied classification, or the "13ers," being the thirteenth generation in American history. Their relationship with their parents, the baby-boomers, sets the stage for a generational crisis. They are a generation who inherited the repercussions of the excesses of their elders: a toxic environment, national debt, unemployment, economic recession, AIDS, recurrent tuberculosis (TB). The fact that the Cold War is over hardly seems an even exchange. Many were raised by grandparents of the silent generation of wartime America; while their parents, the boomers, were caught up in divorce or the "super-mom" phenomenon. Boomers have now turned their attention to public policy and the needs of the elderly. In contrast, the "X-ers" choose to strengthen the family, ask for very little governmental assistance throughout their lifetime, pursue conservative politics and investments, and favor the needs of the very young over the very old (mostly the boomers). Where the boomers were caught up in quick change and episodic relationships, the X generation looks to reestablish our traditional institutions and invest in our traditional social systems.[8] This portends a whole new brand of volunteerism, a movement from "adhocracy" to a more long-term commitment, but with a no-nonsense attitude about what should be accomplished. X-ers demand employment that is satisfying and complementary to their personal lives. The recent nursing workforce opposition to mandatory overtime in some way reflects this redefinition of priorities. X-ers are also more receptive to flexible work arrangements such as flex-time, home-based arrangements, and project and episodic assignments. They do not see "face time" as necessary to productivity, probably due to their comfort with electronic and computer systems. This is in contrast to the attitude of workers over 40, and has already revolutionized the American workplace.[9] The rising millennial generation, called generation Y, is the latest factor in the intergenerational equation, bringing with it attitudes and values more aligned with the baby-boomers than with generation X. Where the X-ers were disillusioned and pessimistic, generation Y seems to embody the optimism and idealism that baby-boomers themselves hold dear.[10] The reader should be alerted that these generational divisions are to some degree arbitrary, but the differences in communication styles, motivational needs, and career goals can be significant as we deal with people from different times.

A Department of Commerce report shows 500,000 fewer Americans living in urban areas at the end of 1997.[11] This also applies to northeasterners who tend to stay put more than most. Neither has migration been into rural America, where we still find significant poverty. Progress toward gentrifying inner cities, and a recent decline in urban crime, make future predictions worth watching.

American households have grown from an average of 2.62 family members in 1992, to 3.14 in 2000. Though there has been an increase, the frequency of one-parent families contributes to low family size. A single parent maintained over 27 percent of American households with children under 18, and this parent is usually a woman. Where children live with one parent, 38 percent of those parents are divorced, and 35 percent were never married.[12]

What had been a trend toward the declining size of households also slowed as younger members of the boomer generation began to start families, with women in their forties eager to take on parenthood. It is noteworthy that the National Center for Health Statistics has begun to collect information on births to mothers 50–54 years old. There has also been a dramatic increase in twin, triplet, and other higher order multiple births. Between 1980 and 2000, the number of twin births increased 74 percent, and the number of higher order multiples (triplets or more) has increased fivefold. Growth in these multiple births has been most marked in women over 30, with the twin rate increasing 63 percent for women aged 45–49. Low and very low birthweight and infant mortality are 4 to 33 times higher for twins and greater multiple births, respectively.[13] The health implications are obvious.

There has been an increase in the number of women working; 47 percent of households with children had two parents who were employed. Sixty-four percent of mothers with children under age six, and 78 percent of mothers with children ages six to 13, are in the labor force. Almost 60 percent of mothers with infants (under age one) are employed. In 1998, only 23 percent of families with children younger than six had one parent working and one parent who stayed at home. The majority (55 percent) of working women in the U.S. bring home half or more of the family income. Seventy-seven percent of women aged 30 to 44 returned to the workforce after the birth of their first child, sometimes because of necessity, sometimes because of career demands.[14] The disparity in pay between men and women working full time widened in 2003 for the first time in four years as women saw their incomes fall. For every dollar a man made in 2003, women made 75.5 cents. That was down from the record 76.6 cents that women earned vs. men's $1 in 2002.[15]

The national abortion rate was at its lowest in over two decades. The typical woman selecting abortion is likely to be young, low income, and unmarried with no previous live births, and having the procedure for the first time.[16] Additional children no longer guarantee more resources to families on public assistance given current welfare reforms. However, public dollars are not readily available for abortion services, making it more an option for women with money or insurance. Further, given the controversy around the procedure, fewer physicians are willing to risk the personal danger to those who continue to offer abortion services. In the midst of these circumstances, abortion continues to be a legal option, and is becoming de facto unavailable to many women. The reader is referred to the discussion of reproductive issues in Chapter 9.

The last 50 years have been an economic roller coaster in the United States, with more highs than lows. There have been several periods of unparalleled prosperity interspersed with periodic recession. Since 1995, there have been fewer poor people, and median family income has been higher. Still, in 2003, 12.9 million American children younger than 18 lived below the poverty line and more than one out of every six American children (17.6 percent) was poor. That is more children living in poverty today than 30 or 35 years ago. About one-half of the nation's poor are either under 18 or over 65. By race and ethnicity, 30.6 percent of poor children were Black, 28 percent were Hispanic, 14.4 percent were Asian and Pacific Islanders, and 12.9 percent were White. Poor children are twice as likely as nonpoor children to suffer stunted growth or lead poisoning, and to be kept back in school. They also score significantly lower on reading, math, and vocabulary tests when compared with other children. Two of five or 39.8 percent of children in families headed by a single woman were poor in 2000, whereas only 8.2 percent of children in married families were poor.[17] Further, the child poverty rate has been higher than the elderly poverty rate for the past three decades; but prior to 1973 the reverse was true. In 1959, the child poverty rate (27 percent) was well below the elderly poverty rate (35 percent). The improvement in the standard of living for older Americans is closely related to social policies such as Social Security and Medicare.[18]

About 3.4 million elderly persons (10.2 percent) were below the poverty level in 2000. Another 2.2 million or 6.7 percent of the elderly were classified as "near-poor" (income between the poverty level and 125 percent of this level). One of every twelve (8.9 percent) elderly Whites was poor in 2000, compared to 22.3 percent of elderly African-Americans and 18.8 percent of elderly Hispanics. Higher than average poverty rates for older persons were found among those who lived in central cities (12.4 percent), in rural areas (13.2 percent), and in the South (12.7 percent). Older women had a higher poverty rate (12.2 percent) than older men (7.5 percent) in 2000. Older persons living alone or with nonrelatives were much more likely to be poor (20.8 percent) than were older persons living with families (5.1 percent). The highest poverty rates (38.3 percent) were experienced by older Hispanic women who lived alone or with nonrelatives.[19]

There is a presumption that the poor have limited access to health care. Only 30.2 percent of the poor had no health insurance of any kind, but poor people or those with incomes below the poverty level comprise 27.1 percent of the uninsured. The group most likely to lack insurance coverage are 18 to 24 year olds. Additionally, the foreign-born population was without health insurance 32.5 percent of the time, as compared with the native-born population at 13.6 percent.[20] Further, there is a special population more correctly called the medically indigent. These folks are either uninsured or have inadequate insurance once confronted with medical necessity. The medically indigent are neither poor enough for Medicaid nor old enough for Medicare. They are middle-class people with little savings and commonly employed in part-time or episodic jobs that provide inadequate or no benefits.

Poverty is also associated with homelessness. Six hundred thousand people are homeless in this country at any one point in time, and 7 million people will be homeless at some point during their lifetime. Over two-thirds of the homeless are unattached men in their late thirties, and one-fifth are families with a woman in her early thirties as head of household.[21] Homelessness has become a way of life for some and is a transient incident for others. The circumstances that accompany homelessness are usually psychiatric disability, substance abuse, or just plain poverty. The homeless are at high risk for HIV/AIDS and tuberculosis. Thirty to forty percent of the male homeless are veterans. About 39 percent of the homeless have come from institutional living of some sort or were products of foster care as children.

The homeless have been caught in a vicious cycle—no home, no address, unsafe public shelters, no place to leave children while you look for a job, and much more. Recent public policy initiatives have begun to chip away at these problems. The homeless have been very successful in securing advocates who are vocal and influential. The homeless have gained a voice, and this is to our advantage. But they have also experienced significant backlash. They have lost the sympathy of middle America. Generational changes, problems with health care, and crime on the streets have all tested our patience and brought us back to basics. We seem to want more order in our lives, and we expect government to take charge. Citizens want their streets and public buildings back, and they want them clean and uncluttered. They want to move freely about their cities without fear of personal harm. The declining crime rates in many of our major cities are applauded. The homeless are a reminder of our shortcomings as a society, and we would prefer not to be reminded.

THE NATION'S HEALTH

Though Americans can boast about their scientific advancements in medicine and the specialists and subspecialists who constitute the workers in the delivery system, fewer positive things can be said about this nation's health. The major contributing factors to death in this

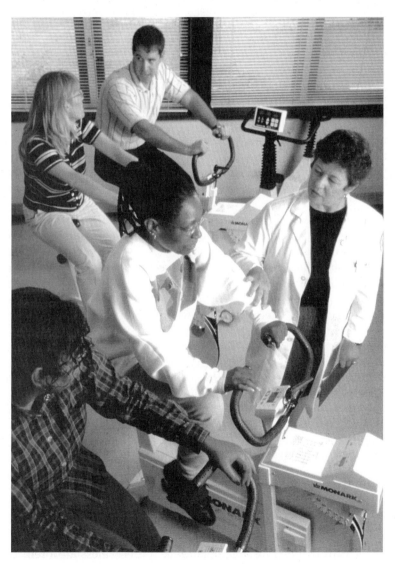

Nursing is more than illness. There is a large market for nurses in health promotion. *(Courtesy of the U.S. Department of Veterans Affairs)*

country are tobacco use, diet and activity patterns, substance abuse, firearms, risky sexual behavior, motor vehicles, and toxic agents. The status of the nation's health is the by-product of personal lifestyles, bad government, and a troubled social environment.

In 1979, the U.S. Department of Health and Human Services launched the first of three *Healthy People* initiatives in an effort to improve the health and well-being of the American people. Each of the *Healthy People* programs has included a set of objectives and measurable indicators to move the country toward very precise goals. The first program was *Healthy People: The Surgeon General's Report on Health Promotion and Disease Prevention*.[22] The goal was to decrease mortality for every age group in the population, and additionally to increase the independence of our oldest citizens. The 1990 targets for the first of the *Healthy People* programs were achieved with the exception of those for adolescents and seniors. It is disputable whether there was actually a lack of progress, or the monitoring and surveillance systems were faulty.

Healthy People 2000 benefited from this earlier experience and was built on an expanded science base allowing more sophisticated disease prevention and health promotion goals:[23]

- Increase the years of healthy life for all Americans.
- Reduce the disparities in health which exist among different populations in this country.
- Provide all Americans with access to disease prevention and health promotion services.

These broad goals were further developed into objectives and then organized into 22 priority areas as presented in Exhibit 3.2. After the mid-course review of 1995, objectives and some priority areas were revised. Progress was mixed and precise measurement hampered by the absence of baseline information in many areas and deficient surveillance systems. The process of *Healthy People 2000* has been as important as the content. This has been a true initiative of the American people. States and local communities have networked under this program, becoming aware of their deficiencies, and investing in programming for health and wellness. Government and private sector have partnered to make *Healthy People 2000* work, sharing the credit where there has been success and frustration where the absence of information or resistant patterns of living thwart progress. The latest phase of *Healthy People* began in January 2000. With *Healthy People 2010*, the emphasis is on health status and the nature of life—quality years, not just longevity. A broadened perspective has come from the development of the science of prevention, improved data systems and surveillance activities, consumer demand for promotion of health, and a renewed appreciation of the public health. *Healthy People*

Exhibit 3.2 Focus/Priority Areas—U.S. Department of Health and Human Services, Healthy People Programs

Healthy People 2000	Healthy People 2010
1. Physical activity and fitness	1. Access to quality health services
2. Nutrition	2. Arthritis, osteoporosis, and chronic
3. Tobacco	back conditions
4. Substance abuse: alcohol and other drugs	3. Cancer
5. Family planning	4. Chronic kidney disease
6. Mental health and mental disorders	5. Diabetes
7. Violent and abusive behavior	6. Disability and secondary conditions
8. Educational and community-based	7. Educational and community-based
programs	programs
9. Unintentional injuries	8. Environmental health
10. Occupational safety and health	9. Family planning and sexual health
11. Environmental health	10. Food safety
12. Food and drug safety	11. Health communication
13. Oral health	12. Heart disease and stroke
14. Maternal and infant health	13. HIV
15. Heart disease and stroke	14. Immunizations and infectious diseases
16. Cancer	15. Injury and violence prevention
17. Diabetes and chronic disabling conditions	16. Maternal, infant, and child health
18. HIV infection	17. Medical product safety
19. Sexually transmitted diseases	18. Mental health and mental disorders
20. Immunization and infectious diseases	19. Nutrition
21. Clinical preventive services	20. Occupational safety and health
22. Surveillance and data systems	21. Oral health
	22. Public health infrastructure
	23. Respiratory diseases
	24. Sexually transmitted diseases
	25. Substance abuse
	26. Tobacco use
	27. Vision and hearing

Source: U.S. Public Health Service: http://web.health.gov/healthypeople/

2000 put a participatory and decentralized process into operation; *Healthy People 2010* will capitalize on those dynamics. The agenda continues to be a variation on the theme: to increase quality and years of healthy life, and eliminate health disparities between America's people. *Healthy People 2010* consists of 27 focus areas (see Exhibit 3.2), each further defined by health indicators and targeted goals which were chosen because of their ability to motivate, their relevance as broad public health issues, and the availability of data to measure progress. All segments of American life have been personally involved in designing the goals, objectives and indicators, and in data collection and monitoring.[24] The information that comes from these programs is a rich source for understanding America's problems, strengths, and changing character. The student is encouraged to explore the websites associated with *Healthy People 2000* and *Healthy People 2010* for more detail. A good place to start

Exhibit 3.3 Interim Report on the Goals of *Healthy People 2010*

Priority area/focus	Baseline 1998–99	Target	Update (2002)
Access to health services			
Persons under 65 years old	83%	100%	83%
Regular exercise			
Persons over 18	32%	50%	33%
Young people grades 9 through12	65%	85%	63% (2003)
Overweight			
In adults 20 and over	23%	15%	31% (2000)
In children 6–19	11%	5%	15% (2000)
Fully immunized children and adolescents	73%	80%	75%
Cigarette smokers			
18 and over	24%	12%	22%
Grades 9–12	35%	22%	16% (2003)
Deaths from motor vehicle accidents	14.7	9.2	15.2
Alcohol-related auto vehicle accident injuries	113.0	65.0	
Alcohol use among youth 12–17	33%	12.6%	18%
Drug-induced deaths	6.8	1.0	9.0
Suicides	10.5	5.0	10.9
Homicides	6.0	3.0	6.1
Work-related injuries (per 100 full-time workers)	6.2	4.3	5.0
Low-birthweight babies	7.6%	5.0%	7.8%
Infant mortality (per 1000 live births)	7.2	4.5	7.0
Prenatal care (first trimester)	83%	90%	84%
Pregnant women abstaining from alcohol	86%	94%	
Pregnant women abstaining from cigarette smoking	87%	99%	89%
Breast-feeding (early post-partum)	64%	75%	70%
Deaths from:			
Coronary artery disease	203	166	180
Stroke	62	48	56
Cancer	200.8	159.9	193.5
Chronic obstructive pulmonary disease (over 45)	128.7	60.0	118.9

Statistics reported as a percentage or per 100,000 standard population unless noted otherwise.
Source: National Center for Health Statistics, Division of Health Promotion Statistics: http://wonder.cdc.gov/data2010/FOCUS.HTM. Retrieved February 14, 2005.

is http://www.healthypeople.gov. Select *Healthy People 2010* indicators, baseline data, targeted goals, and current progress are presented in Exhibit 3.3.

The list of the leading causes of death changed slightly over the years. The rank of leading causes of death showed heart disease being first, followed by cancer, stroke, chronic obstructive pulmonary disease, diabetes, pneumonia and influenza, and accidents in that order. Deaths from heart disease and cancer, except for smoking-related lung cancer, were slightly down. Death from heart disease, stroke, and diabetes were 20–60 percent more prevalent in minority populations. The life expectancy for Black males and females is 68.8 and 75.6 years, respectively, and for Whites 75.1 and 80.3 years—noticeable gains, but glaring inequities persist.[25] These distinctions should not be oversimplified nor can they be satisfactorily explained.

It is also apparent that compliance is better as government imposes controls. Some examples are the strictly imposed driving while intoxicated (DWI) penalties in many states; prohibitions against smoking in restaurants, public buildings, and public transportation; smoke and carbon dioxide detector requirements; lower speed limits on the nation's highways (which are now rising again); radon testing; safe water standards; mandatory seat belt and helmet use with cars, motorcycles, and bicycles; handgun laws, and so on. The cynic might say that we have to be protected from ourselves.

The shifting demographics in the U.S., the *Healthy People* agendas, and environmental concerns are all reflected in the data from the American Cancer Society:[26]

- Yearly, over 555,000 deaths are expected from cancer in the U.S., more than 1500 a day; cancer is the second leading cause of death.
- Approximately 9 million Americans alive today have a personal history of cancer.
- Seventy-seven percent of cancers are diagnosed in individuals 55 years of age or older.
- One of every two men and one of three women will develop cancer over the course of a lifetime.
- Over 1.2 million new cancer cases were diagnosed in 2002.
- Five to ten percent of cancers are attributable to heredity.
- In 2002, about 170,000 cancer deaths were caused by tobacco use.
- Cancer of the lung and bronchus is the leading cause of cancer deaths for both sexes, accounting for 31 percent of all deaths in men and 25 percent in women.
- The next most common cause of cancer death in men is the prostate (11 percent) and the breast in women (15 percent).
- Scientific evidence suggests that one-third of cancer deaths are related to nutrition, physical inactivity, obesity, and other lifestyle factors which could have been prevented.
- Certain cancers related to infectious exposures, such as hepatitis B virus (HBV), human immunodeficiency virus (HIV), heliobacter, and others, could have been prevented through behavioral change, vaccines, or antibiotics.
- Many of the more than one million skin cancers diagnosed in 2002 could have been prevented by protection from the sun's rays.
- The 5-year survival rate is 82 percent for those cancers detected by screening or self-examination, such as prostate, cervical, oral, breast, colon, rectal, testis, skin.

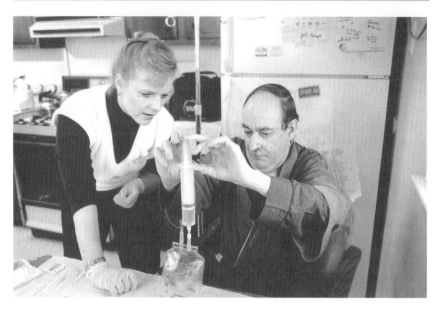

Teaching and self-care are necessary so that your patient with chronic disease can have as normal a life as possible. (*Courtesy of the Visiting Nurse Association of Central Jersey, Red Bank, New Jersey*)

○   Black Americans are more likely to develop and die from cancer than persons of any racial or ethnic group.

The major causes of death for Americans are for the most part incurable, but with lifestyle adjustments, a long and productive life is possible for most. For others, disability due to chronic disease is inevitable. By 2020, the number of Americans with chronic conditions is expected to increase to 157 million from 125 million in 2000. Further, the number of Americans with two or more chronic conditions is expected to grow from 57 to 81 million. People with chronic conditions accounted for 78 percent of health expenditure in 2000, and the amount is increasing geometrically.[27] Chronic disease and disability are not only the result of the way we live but also of the sophisticated medicine we practice.

Of all the diseases that affect Americans today, probably the most frightening is AIDS. Since AIDS was first identified in 1981, it has spread quickly and irrevocably. At the end of 2003, the Center for Disease Control (CDC) estimated 405,926 persons living with AIDS in the United States. Of these, 36 percent were white, 42 percent were black, 20 percent were Hispanic, and 77 percent were men. An estimated 1998 children were living with AIDS at this same time. Since the beginning of the

AIDS epidemic, an estimated 524,060 persons have died from AIDS in the United States.[28]

Many stereotypes about AIDS have been shattered in recent years. AIDS and HIV are no longer diseases restricted to the largest metropolitan areas. AIDS cases have increased dramatically for heterosexuals. The number of women and children infected is growing significantly. However, HIV infection as a cause of death has decreased substantially since 1996 and the widespread use of antiretroviral therapy. The age group 35–44 represents about 41 percent of all newly diagnosed AIDS cases in recent years. The number of females diagnosed with AIDS increased by 15 percent in 2003, while males only increased 1 percent. Those infected by both heterosexual and homosexual sex have increased in recent years, and infection in intravenous drug users has decreased, as has pediatric AIDS, reporting only 59 cases in 2003, less than one-third of those reported in 1999. This is attributed to new public health guidelines and treatment options.[29] Once the leading cause of death for 25 to 44 year olds, the rate of new infections has stabilized in the United States. This paints a picture of complacency. Those who are infected live longer, have a greater chance of infecting others, and eventually increase the chronic disease burden to the society. The rippling effect does not stop there. One-third of the increase in TB cases over the past five years has been as an opportunistic infection in HIV-infected people, most commonly multi-drug resistant TB which is a particular public health concern.

AIDS is not curable, but it is highly preventable. Because of the known relation between AIDS and substance abuse, as well as risky sexual practices, prevention programs have focused on the use of good-quality condoms as protection during sexual intercourse, discouraging needle-sharing among substance abusers, and establishing a rigorous standard in processing blood and blood products for transfusion. However, the human element remains. Many individuals are reluctant to demand the use of condoms in their sexual relationships, some religious groups object to publicizing safe sex, and drug users are often ignorant or indifferent. Teenagers continue to feel omnipotent and above harm and pursue risky behaviors. Given the length of time between infection and diagnosis, individuals with AIDS in their mid to late twenties were infected as teens.

Even in the midst of this tragedy there has been progress. Though there is no cure, great strides have been made in palliative drug therapy. Individuals with AIDS are living longer and experiencing better quality of life. Persons with AIDS are a protected class under the Americans with Disabilities Act, therefore allowing them to continue in the American mainstream. Compliance with CDC-approved universal precaution techniques is mandatory for every health care setting and provider.

The health care community has held the line to diffuse the public tendency to panic by opposing mandatory testing and disclosure for any group, including health care workers or patients.

A nation's health is often measured in terms of the health and wellness of its infants and children. In August of 2004, the Children's Defense Fund reminded us of the following key facts about America's children:[30]

- 3 in 5 preschoolers have their mothers in the labor force.
- 2 in 5 preschoolers eligible for Head Start do not participate.
- 1 in 2 never complete a single year of college.
- 1 in 2 will live in a single parent family at some point in childhood.
- 1 in 3 will be poor at some point in their childhood.
- 1 in 3 is behind a year or more in school.
- 1 in 5 is born to a mother who did not graduate from high school.
- 1 in 5 was born poor.
- 1 in 6 is born to a mother who did not receive prenatal care in the first three months of pregnancy.
- 1 in 7 never graduates from high school.
- 1 in 8 has no health insurance.
- 1 in 8 lives in a family receiving food stamps.
- 1 in 9 is born to a teenage mother.
- 1 in 12 has a disability.
- 1 in 13 was born with low birthweight.
- 1 in 13 will be arrested at least once before age 17.
- 1 in 14 lives at less than half the poverty level.
- 1 in 35 lives with grandparents (or other relative) but neither parent.
- 1 in 60 sees their parents divorce in any year.

The United States has the highest rates of teenage pregnancy and births in the western industrialized world. Thirty-four percent of young women become pregnant at least once before they reach the age of 20. Eight in ten of these pregnancies are unintended and 79 percent are to unmarried teens. The teen birth rate has declined slowly but steadily from 1991 to 2002, with an overall decrease of 30 percent for those between 15 and 19. This decline reverses the 23 percent rise in this birth rate from 1986 to 1991. The birth rates for black and Hispanic teens declined 42 and 20 percent respectively between 1986 and 1991. Most teenagers giving birth before 1980 were married, whereas most today are unmarried.[31] However, contrary to misconceptions, unwed motherhood is often a temporary status that leads to marriage. In contrast to other eras, fewer marriages take place because of pregnancy, abortions continue to decline, and fewer babies are given up for adoption.

Several government and private sector studies have attempted to understand the changing behaviors among America's teens. Results show that sexual activity among teens has sharply declined throughout the 1990s, and sexual activity is much more likely to include condom use.[32] Further, teens are more protected from a whole range of risky behaviors, including sexual activity resulting in pregnancy, where there are enhanced connections with the family and home, school, and community.[33] This has strong implications for health care.

Any chapter on today's health would be remiss by excluding a discussion of environmental factors. The issue of the effect of toxic agents on health has been very controversial in the last several decades. Much of this controversy probably derives from the fact that morbidity and mortality caused by such agents are often difficult to document. The effect on health may not be seen for decades, and there may not be a clear indication of which of the many interacting factors is clearly responsible for an illness or death. Some occupational illnesses have been identified, and to varying degrees, safety standards have been set and enforced by the Occupational Safety and Health Administration (OSHA) and the Environmental Protection Agency (EPA). Consumer groups and unions have claimed that such protection is generally insufficient, while industry complains that it is so over-regulated that expenses for compliance are unreasonable. Some conditions, such as byssinosis (brown lung disease), caused by cotton dust in the textile industries, and silicosis (black lung disease), caused by silica, particularly in mining, are clearly recognized as job-related diseases. It is generally accepted that other occupation-related disabilities are caused by benzine, formaldehyde, waste anesthesia gases, asbestos, ethylene oxide (a sterilizing agent in hospitals and medical products industries), diisocyanate (a chemical used to produce plastic products), vinyl chloride, lead, and radiation, to name a few. Clearly, some of these are particular hazards for nurses, along with the danger of AIDS, hepatitis B and C, and airborne pathogens, among others. The Nurses' Environmental Health Watch publishes information on hazards for nurses and how to avoid or minimize them.

Other environmental hazards are also cited by public health experts and environmentalists. The depletion of the stratospheric ozone layer caused by chlorofluorocarbons (CFCs) used in sprays, refrigeration, air-conditioning systems, industrial blowing agents, insulating foams, metal cleaning and drying, garment cleaning, sterilization of medical supplies, and liquid fast freezing causes skin cancer, cataracts, and potential changes in the world's climate. Limitations have been set by the Clean Air Act of 1990 and its Amendments of 1997, but there is a constant battle to determine what the limit should be.

Acid rain, resulting from emissions from coal-burning plants and factories—chiefly sulfur dioxide and nitrogen oxides that are chemically changed in the atmosphere—is suspected of destroying freshwater life, damaging forests and crops, and possibly threatening human health. Cited by the EPA as probably the most serious environmental problem in the United States is that of hazardous wastes. These are by-products of the manufacturing process of many products, but the large-scale generators are chemical manufacturers, petroleum refiners, and metal-production companies. Careless dumping of these wastes, for instance, in areas where they leak into a water supply or cause an explosion, has resulted in serious danger to whole communities. Scientists contend that it is possible to contain wastes safely if certain caveats are observed, and some manufacturers are making an effort to clean up sites. Meanwhile, dangerous old waste dumps are continually being discovered.

The deadly chemical dioxin, an unwanted by-product of herbicides, pesticides, and other industrial products, has been given considerable attention, beginning with its effect on soldiers and civilians in Vietnam, where it was a chemical contaminant of the defoliant Agent Orange. There is some belief that others, such as inhabitants of the Love Canal area and those exposed to dioxin in train wrecks or factory explosions, have suffered from a variety of conditions, including kidney and liver ailments, birth defects, and cancer.

Almost daily, there is some report in the media about product or environmental dangers, whether noise, food additives, safety failure of equipment, toys, autos, clothing, hazardous wastes, acid rain, radioactive leaks, unsafe drinking water, or even human destruction from nuclear weapons or plants. Some feel that this is a hysterical reaction to unproven claims. Others ignore the entire issue. Still others feel that with or without more definitive data, a stronger effort must be made to improve the environment. The EPA's website provides an excellent resource for state-of-the-art information on these issues: http://www.epa.gov/epahome.

TECHNOLOGICAL, SCIENTIFIC, AND MEDICAL ADVANCES

There is little question that the technological advances of the last century have been amazing and, combined with scientific advances in medicine, the health care delivery system in the United States has sustained a dramatic transformation. Some of the most significant technological and scientific changes affecting patient care can be categorized as follows:

1. *Developments in diagnosis and treatment* such as automated clinical laboratory equipment, artificial human organs, improved surgical techniques and equipment such as microsurgery, lasers, bloodless

surgery, an endless variety of nonintrusive techniques which reduce the need for surgery, and the use of computers to both diagnose and provide treatment options.

2. *Hospital information management*—the use of the computer and electronic systems for rate calculation, billing, accounting, transfer of information and funds, maintenance of databases, and record keeping and transmission of clinical documentation. The criteria for systems development have been speed, accuracy, and equity— ensuring that providers make their decisions based on information that is dependable and reflects the state-of-the-art of the science, that the least amount of effort possible is needed for coordination, and that all parties are paid promptly for what they do.

3. Developments affecting *health care supplies and services*, such as widespread adoption of plastic, other inexpensive and improved materials, and such equipment as specialized carts, conveyers, and pneumatic tubes.

4. Improvement in *the management processes and structural design* of health facilities all aimed at more efficient utilization of personnel, equipment, and space, and consumer satisfaction. This involves sensitivity to the needs and preferences of both the internal (employee) and external consumer (recipient of service).

5. *Mass communication*, which not only increases the opportunity to educate the consumer, but can be a powerful influence in molding public opinion. Consumers can be empowered on their own behalf and make more knowledgeable decisions about their choice of providers and treatment.

Clearly, technology plays an important role in health care. Scientific and medical advances have gone beyond the imagination of science fiction. Almost all progress raises ethical issues, and sometimes legal complications in relation to access, quality of life, and right to life. (Some of these issues are discussed in Chapters 8 and 9.) Even though life expectancy has increased, medical science has done little to increase the length of a healthy life. The rapidity of technological development has caught almost everyone unprepared. For instance, the progress of genomic medicine and the process of cloning are no longer a hypothetical and distant frontier, but today's reality.

In 1978, the birth of the first test-tube babies with the ovum fertilized outside the mother's body created worldwide controversy. The replacement of nonfunctioning human parts with artificial substitutes or human transplants has the potential of bringing a bionic era to reality. Implanted or attached titanium and polyethylene thigh bones; cords of woven Dacron for tendons; plastic, steel, and metal-alloy joints; Orlon and Dacron blood vessels; plastic and titanium heart valves; and artificial voice devices are commonplace. Moreover, progress has been made in electronic stimulation of the brain for hearing and seeing, and in developing miniaturized versions of the artificial kidney. Versatile lasers can remove the cloudiness from the eyes of the visually impaired, open clogged blood vessels, and break up kidney stones.

New diagnostic techniques are hailed because of both their effectiveness and the fact that they are noninvasive, sometimes eliminating the need for exploratory surgery. Among the newest techniques are monoclonal antibody imaging agents which increase the ability of doctors to detect and diagnose cancer, heart disease, and other conditions. These antibodies are linked to a radioactive isotope and injected into the patient; they flow through the blood and latch on to their targets, e.g., tumors. They show up as hot spots of activity when photographed by the usual means used in nuclear medicine. There is also hope that these might eventually be used as a "magic bullet" to treat disease.

The expense of developing and maintaining technology is frequently criticized as adding to the cost of health care. This cannot be denied, but as new diagnostics and therapeutics become accepted as common practice, the cost to the consumer or the insurer becomes less.

Computer applications to medicine and health care are particularly significant. Not only are computers used in almost every phase of business, the professions, and education but they have also become commonplace in the home. Children are taught to work with computers in elementary school; computer literacy is expected for high school graduation; and it is impossible to survive in college without basic computer skills—word processing, searching/using the Internet and library systems, communication by e-mail, etc.

Several immediate problems of current computer usage have alarmed the public. First is the question of security of information. In the last decade computer experts have made headlines with their ability to invade the computers of banks, hospitals, industry, and even the government, in some cases changing or erasing data. While others had already used the computer to commit crimes (and were not always caught and punished), this new danger reinforced earlier concerns about the confidentiality of computer-stored information. Would an employer, or simply a curious individual, be able to review another individual's credit record or health information? For that matter, would the record be accurate? Anyone who has had to deal with the unresponsive computers of businesses and the government knows the difficulty of catching and correcting errors; computer input still has a human component. Confidentiality is precisely the issue that is slowing progress on the electronic transfer of information in health care. For many years, there have been predictions that eventually each person would carry one "smart" card containing their personal demographics and a comprehensive health history. The technology exists, but fears about violations of privacy have slowed progress.

Most of the settings where nurses practice make extensive use of computer technology. Though the initial use was often for operations' purposes, clinical information was quickly integrated into these systems as the level of reimbursement became driven by observations about the patient's condition and the services provided. Nurses have always been positioned in the midst of clinical information, given their continual presence and comprehensive role.

Nursing Information Systems (NIS) are an integral part of the information system existing in every health care organization. There are Hospital Information Systems (HIS), as well as systems for long-term care facilities, home care agencies, and so on. These systems are designed to be easily adapted to computerization, but can also operate with paper and pencil. Information systems exist to promote efficiency, effectiveness, and accountability, and those qualities can be enhanced through the proper use of computers. Though quite to the contrary, often information requirements and their entry into computer systems may prove to be very disruptive and painful to employees. If the information is not relevant and both computer software and hardware are not friendly and useful, communication can be less effective than before.

Over the last several years, there has been a great deal in the nursing literature about the use of computers in education and practice. The variety of uses continually increases, and more nurses are becoming experts. Nurses, like others, must find fast, effective ways to turn raw data into useful organized information. Information systems can assist in patient assessment, designing care, monitoring progress, documentation and charting, discharge coordination, staffing and scheduling, and tracking acuity, cost, and quality. Computers can also enrich clinical decisions and offer alternative solutions for relatively common problems. Computer terminals at the patient's bedside, in the examining room, or even the patient's home can ease the burden of record keeping, improve accuracy, and eliminate duplication of information. If used properly, computers can also improve exchange of information between nurses and other health care professionals and staff. Critical paths are one example of a clinical information system that is exceptionally suited to computerization, although they may operate with paper alone. Ideally, critical paths (also known as caremaps) are the product of interdisciplinary consensus on the preferred course of treatment for a specific condition, the anticipated response of the patient, and the manner in which organizational systems should respond in support of the patient and provider. The path serves as a prompter to clinical decision making

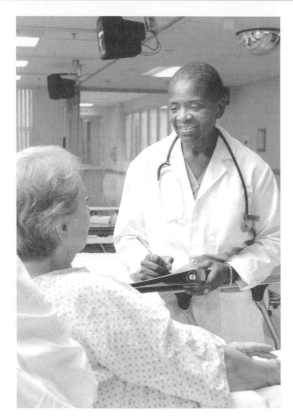

Today's technology threatens to depersonalize health care, creating the need to listen more and be more humane. (*Courtesy of Palisades Medical Center, New York Presbyterian Healthcare System*)

and alerts the provider to situations in which the patient is not responding as anticipated. The existence of the path documents the plan of care and allows the nurse to limit charting to exceptions to the path, thus reducing paperwork.

Computer technology is used widely in nursing education and research. Computer-assisted instruction (CAI) is used in such areas as drill and practice, simulations, and tutorials. Internet courses allow independent learning and self-pacing. Interactive television (ITV) broadcasting brings educational programming to many who would otherwise be absent opportunities. Nursing informatics is a component in every basic curriculum, and there is the expectation that students bring some computer skills. Nursing research is dependent on computer technology for data collection and analysis, retrieval of information, and communication between researchers with similar scientific interests.

This increased use of electronic media is demonstrated in the new Sigma Theta Tau Center for Nursing Scholarship International Library in Indianapolis, where just about all its holdings are in electronic format; it is a library without paper.

The ideal electronic system would be fully interactive and link the point at which care is given with every department and service from accounting to materials management, computer-assisted clinical prescribing, and monitoring drug interactions, ancillary services, clinical decision-making support, and computerized patient records, including bedside information systems. Such a system would provide multiple record correction from a single point of entry of data. More descriptively, the nurse enters an order for a diagnostic procedure which requires a preparatory regimen including medication and special diet. As the order is placed, the procedure is scheduled for the time of day that is most comfortable for the patient as identified in the nursing history, the pharmacy receives the order for medication, transport is notified when to pick up the patient, diet is changed, inventories are updated where supplies were used, the episode enters the quality assurance loop, and the nurse is alerted to any possible adverse reactions. Given the amount of nursing effort that is invested in coordination of services, the value of information technology is limitless. For nurses, this means learning to use the new technology for the benefit of the patient but continually maintaining the emphasis on individuality and human contact, which no machine can provide, as well as protecting the patient's privacy.

EDUCATION

Trends in education affect nursing in a number of ways: (1) the kind, number, and quality of students entering the nursing programs and the background they bring with them; (2) the introduction of new technology to respond better to the needs of the learner; and (3) the impact of social demands on education, which are eventually extended to education in the professions, including nursing. Usually it is not just one social or economic condition that brings about change in education, nor is there only one kind of change. For instance, over-expansion by most institutions of higher education when baby-boomer admissions were at their height created a large pool of unemployed college graduates in the early 1970s. Some of these, as well as college students with a worried eye to the future, looked for educational programs that seemed to promise jobs immediately on graduation, among them nursing. Thus, what had once been a trickle of mature, second-degree students into nursing became a steady stream. As the baby-boom group diminished, over-extended institutions of higher education and their nursing programs found it necessary to use marketing strategies of all kinds to attract enough students. They discovered the working adults in the community, who were a relatively untapped pool.

To attract and retain these nontraditional students, higher education had to make the college experience more flexible and individualized. Successful schools became innovative without sacrificing their integrity. This standard was applied to every aspect of the academic experience: fulfilling requirements for graduation, course scheduling, and more.

The more mature student brought a lot of life experience to college with them, and it became necessary to find approaches to award academic credit for what a person knows regardless of when, where, or how that knowledge was acquired. The concepts of independent study and credit by examination were explored by an increasing number of colleges, and a variety of mechanisms which have wide acceptance are being used to grant credit for life experience and self-study in all areas of scholarship, including nursing. These chiefly include teacher-made tests, standardized tests, and portfolio development. One example of standardized testing is the College Level Examination Program (CLEP), which was developed some time ago by the Educational Testing Service through funding by the Carnegie Corporation. It provides testing in a variety of general and specialized courses for which most colleges and universities award credit.

Over time, the higher education community has responded to public pressure for nontraditional routes to educational credentials. One model has been the "external degree" as an option to traditional college attendance. Some "external degree programs" are marginally legitimate operations that have given the whole concept a bad name with meaningless mail-order degrees. However, more and more respected, accredited educational institutions have established creative but rigorous processes to assure the quality of their graduates. The true "external degree" university does not give any courses itself, but functions as a clearing house to verify the competence of the degree recipient through testing and/or studies completed in a variety of acceptable settings. A particularly successful example of the "external degree" exists at Excelsior College, originally the New York Regents External Degree Program, which includes both associate, baccalaureate, and master's degree programs in nursing.

Other flexible educational options are programs which concentrate course work in weekends, evenings, summers, or a combination of these. We see more outreach programs for isolated geographic areas or even workplaces which have enough employees interested in course work. These satellite or outreach programs have thrived on the technology associated with distance education. Distance education is discussed at greater length in Chapter 5.

Equally significant are other happenings in higher education. Cost, to student and institution, is an ongoing controversy. As government aid declines, the cost to the student for higher education increases. Because there are not as many tax benefits to encourage charitable giving, colleges and universities have a major problem in balancing costs, quality, and service to students. Two-year colleges are under particular pressure because of their very low tuition fees. On the other hand, despite the cry for higher quality, there is less state interest. This translates to a lack of funding to improve public community colleges or public higher education in general. The public only seem ready to put their dollars where quality already exists and has become critical of providing remedial instruction in basic skills to students who come ill-prepared for college, but somehow were admitted. Though what may be needed is a reassessment of the mission of publicly funded colleges and universities, the response has been to raise tuition fees and vigorous marketing to attract new and different students. Nursing continues to be a very popular program for community colleges, offering occupational preparation in two years. Financial problems of private colleges are just as serious; many smaller colleges have been forced to close their doors, as have some nursing programs. College tuition cost is closely followed by student attitude, drug problems, and poor quality of academic programs, including lack of demonstrated faculty interest in teaching, as major concerns of the public. The cost of a college education is outpacing inflation.

Nontraditional students have found the cost of college particularly serious since they are often not eligible for financial aid, historically reserved for full-time students. Organized nursing's influence in Washington made government traineeship dollars available to nurses for part-time study as early as 1989. However, all students who rely on government funding may have problems in the next few years, since the standard has moved away from grants to loans that have to be repaid. Experts say that this may have a negative effect on students from low-income backgrounds, who are often reluctant to go into debt for education. Also, colleges and universities whose students have a poor record of repayment will be penalized.

Completing a bachelor's degree in 4 years is no longer guaranteed. Graduate study is also more drawn out and frequently part-time. Retention rates in higher education are also of concern, but the information is guarded. Many people believe that an institutional emphasis on research as opposed to teaching is part of the problem, since faculty, especially in universities, tend to be rewarded and promoted largely on the basis of their research productivity. Loudly voiced public discontent has forced such institutions to work on ways to reestablish teaching as a priority.

Today's undergraduate students consist of an almost equal number of men and women; Asians make up the vast majority of foreign students. Almost 83 percent of freshmen in the fall of 2001 were white, 12.7 percent black, 3.7 percent Asian–American, and 11 percent Hispanic. Where these students were not emancipated and parental income was an issue, families earned less than $50,000 a year. Lack of financial aid keeps 170,000 from college. Half of full-time students work 25 hours a week, which affects their academic performance. Almost 14 percent of students speak a language other than English at home. Almost 40 percent expected to eventually complete a graduate degree, and described themselves most often as politically "middle of the road." The motivation for higher education was closely associated with a future work life, and the financial security that represents, but there was also the inquisitiveness to learn more about things "that interest me." The college was selected because of its academic reputation and the observation that their graduates get good jobs. Freshmen believed that the government should do more to preserve the environment, that we should be less concerned about protecting the rights of criminals, employers should be allowed to require drug testing, handguns should be controlled, a national health care plan is necessary, wealthy people should pay more taxes, and racist/sexist speech should be prohibited on campus. Only slightly more than half thought that abortion should be legal (56 percent), and that undocumented immigrants should be denied access to public education (55 percent). For over 70 percent, a major objective in their life was to raise a family and be well-off financially.[34] Whether or not students' attitudes change during their college years has never been measured accurately, but it can be assumed that at least some changes will occur. Meanwhile, the data are, at the least, interesting to consider, and very much representative of the Y generation. One basic difference between nursing and non-nursing students is often their age. Many individuals select nursing for a midlife or later-life career change.

THE WOMEN'S MOVEMENT

Nursing, from its beginnings in America, has been primarily made up of women, and some nurses have always been involved in the women's movement. For example, Lavinia Dock was active and prominent in the early struggles for suffrage, and Margaret Sanger fought courageously to bring birth control to the poor. However, feminist women and nurses have historically had an "uneasy alliance." A group of nurse activists describe this relationship as follows:

> Much of the energy in the women's movement has been directed toward opening up nontraditional fields of study and work for women. Nursing has been seen as one of the ultimate female ghettos from which women should be encouraged to escape.... Feminists have sometimes failed to look beyond the inaccurate sexist stereotypes of nurses and to acknowledge the multiple dimensions of professional nursing.[35]

Being a suffragette was not easy in the late nineteenth and early twentieth centuries, and often women did not support the movement. That reaction may have been caused, in part, by the negative, even vindictive, portrait newspapers painted of those in the movement, as illustrated by a few typical quotes: "organized by divorced wives, childless women, and sour old maids," "unsexed women," "entirely devoid of personal attractions," "laboring on the heels of strong hatred towards men." Whether the opposition resulted from the fear of overthrowing "the most sacred of our institutions (marriage)"[36] or any other threat to the status quo is a moot point. For despite the success of the women's movement, most notably the passage of women's suffrage in 1921, discrimination against women has not ended. Women still face many formidable economic, social, and political barriers.

Women in all occupations, professions, and walks of life have encountered these barriers, and the success of the women's movement attests to the fervor and commitment with which they have fought to improve women's status. It is no surprise that the women's movement has been considered one of the major phenomena of the mid-twentieth century.

Over the years, there has been a proliferation of women's organizations concerned with women's rights. Among the most active groups is the National Organization for Women (NOW), founded in 1966 and made up of women and men who support full equality for women in truly equal partnership with men and ask for an end to discrimination and prejudice against women in every field of importance in American society.

The founding of NOW offered one of the most politically radical agendas of the twentieth century: men and women would share equally in public and private responsibilities—in paid work and in the rearing of children. NOW activities are directed toward legislative action to end discrimination, and it attempts to promote its views through demonstrations, research, litigation, and political pressure. It is interesting that the first president of NOW, Wilma Scott Heide, was a nurse and feminist, demonstrating that nursing and feminism can find common ground.

Another prominent women's organization is the National Women's Political Caucus (NWPC). It was founded in 1971 as the first national political organization to promote women's entry into politics at leadership levels. The main thrust of the NWPC is to ensure that women's issues are given more attention by facilitating the election of women to political office. EMILY's List (Early Money is Like Yeast) has a similar mission, and contributes dollars to women candidates during the early days of their political campaign.

Although many of the issues that women have confronted over the past 25 years are slow to be resolved, the women's movement has been the major catalyst in raising awareness and instigating action on sex discrimination and women's rights. The impact of the movement can be observed in both legal and social changes occurring, slowly but surely, in women's roles. However, children are still being socialized into stereotyped male and female roles by books, use of toys, and influence of parents, teachers, and others—a problem that feminists and others continue to address. According to NOW, "A feminist is a person who believes women (even as men) are primarily people; that human rights are indivisible by any category of sex, race, class or other designation irrelevant to our common humanity; a feminist is committed to creating the equality (not sameness) of the sexes legally, socially, educationally, psychologically, politically, religiously, economically in all the rights and responsibilities of life."[37]

Certainly these attitudes are not merely American. A 1974 UN report indicated that sexist attitudes were found around the world (and frequently held by UN delegates). In 1975, the International Women's Year culminated in a UN-sponsored conference in Mexico City, intended to develop a 10-year plan to improve the status of women, particularly stressing education and health care. More than 1000 UN delegates and 5000 other feminists and interested spectators attended, but despite a document of official recommendations, the highly politicized meeting was not as successful as had been hoped. Women were polarized by their special interests. The caucus of Third World women, for instance, showed little interest in the concerns of Western women. Equal pay and day-care centers were not issues in countries where most women have no voting or property rights. The recommendations that emerged were a mixture and focused on encouraging governments to ensure equality in terms of educational opportunities, training, and employment, to ameliorate the "hard work loads" falling on women in certain economic groups and in certain countries, and to ensure that women have equal rights with men in voting and participating in political life.

In 1979, the United Nations General Assembly adopted "... what is essentially an international bill of rights for women." However, the treaty, known as the United Nations Convention on Elimination of All Forms of Discrimination Against Women, has yet to gain worldwide recognition or acceptance. In 1994, 128 countries had ratified the treaty, and few had made any significant efforts to eliminate discrimination against women. Notably, although the United States was part of the General Assembly consensus in adopting the convention, the U.S. has yet to ratify it.

In 1985, a UN Third World Conference on Women was held in Nairobi, Kenya. It pulled together the disparate views that had kept women apart in Mexico a decade earlier and focused them into a document called "Nairobi Forward-Looking Strategies for Advancement of Women to the Year 2000." The strategies evolved from three basic objectives: equality, economic and social development, and peace.[38]

The Kenya focus on development was unable to ignite the spark to unify women and drive them on to some very challenging positions, which were certain to create personal jeopardy. Also, however eloquent the rhetoric in 1985, the resources to fund the platform were nonexistent at the international or national level. The 10 years between Kenya and Beijing, the site for the United Nations Fourth World Conference on Women, were unique and changed the dynamics of the international women's movement. Telecommunications came into its own, and though not penetrating every corner of the world, networks began to build and women began to realize that there was a common agenda. The barriers that had existed between women of the developing and industrialized worlds were realized for what they were, self-imposed limitations on our ability to join together and become a unified force. Digging beneath the surface, there was a common cause. The other variable which happened on the scene at the same time as telecommunications, and maybe was strengthened because of it, was the growing presence and power of nongovernmental organizations (NGOs). It is the NGO that can speak out boldly, rise above government in many instances, and often find the dollars to do what has to be done. It is the NGO that penetrates down to the grass-roots, cements the marriage of public/private sector resources, and knows the capacity for success in most ventures. The magic of women's networks fashioned and strengthened by NGOs, and the ability to sustain communications, brought 50,000 participants to Beijing. The agenda was also "right" for the times. The legal and legislative focus of 1985 gave way to discussions of personal security. The Platform for Action included issues on empowerment of women, reproductive health, valuing women's unpaid work, the equal right of women to inherit, women's rights as human rights, and violence against women. Particular attention was given to the "girl-child" and their right to nurturing and protection.[39] Though not surprisingly, the UN has lagged in follow-through. However, pieces of the platform are already being mobilized through the growing global web which has begun to connect women's groups.

In the United States, resistance to the women's movement was epitomized by the death of the proposed Equal Rights Amendment (ERA) to the Constitution, three states short of the 38 needed for ratification. Ten years after it was passed by Congress, and despite an extension of the deadline for ratification from 1979 to 1982, Indiana in 1977 was the last state to ratify. More than 450 national organizations endorsed the amendment, and polls showed that more than two-thirds of U.S. citizens supported it, but to no avail. The conservative opposition, including fundamentalist Christian churches, the so-called Moral Majority, the John Birch Society, the Mormon Church, and the American Farm Bureau, led a well-financed, smoothly organized, and politically astute campaign. Anti-amendment forces assured state legislators that the Fourteenth Amendment offered sufficient protection to women, and claimed that the ERA would cause the death of the family by removing a man's obligation to support his wife and children, would legalize homosexual marriages, lead to unisex toilets, and most damaging, result in the drafting of women for combat duty. Advocates of the ERA were later criticized as lacking political finesse and alienating women who were potential supporters—Blacks, pink-collar (office) workers, and housewives.

In the 1980s and early 1990s, feminists determined to concentrate women's new consciousness and resources in building legislative strength eventually to pass the ERA and to mount a campaign for reproductive freedom, including abortion and recognition of all human rights, including gay and lesbian rights, democratization of families, more respect for work done in the home, and comparable pay for the work done outside it. Since 1973, when *Roe v. Wade* was decided by the U.S. Supreme Court, women have had the right to seek an abortion, at least in the first trimester. The basis for this decision was a woman's right to privacy. Efforts to overturn *Roe* have not been successful, but anti-abortion forces have succeeded in eliminating Medicaid funding of abortion for poor women (Hyde amendment), and in some states, requiring a waiting period prior to abortion, and parental consent for minors who seek an abortion.

Three decades after Betty Friedan published *The Feminine Mystique* (called by the futurist Alvin Toffler "the book that pulled the trigger of history") changes can be clearly identified, even though some of the results have varied.

In terms of the ERA, Congress voted down another ERA bill in 1983. The bill was defeated by six votes. Yet, both friends and foes of equal rights note that the campaign for the amendment, along with other social forces, made a definite impact on American life.

The labor force participation of women can be viewed as a further disadvantage when one considers the many single mothers who have no choice but to work outside of the home because they are facing such difficult financial hardships. These problems seem to be intensifying as the proportion of families maintained by women alone has increased (see The Nation's Health earlier in this chapter).

Finally, despite the narrowing of the wage gap between women and men, 59 percent of women work in low-paying "pink-collar" jobs because they are trained for nothing else, some because such jobs tend to be more compatible with child rearing. It is harder to explain why the higher women advance, the larger the wage gap between men and women. Corporate women at the vice-presidential level and above earn 42 percent less than their male peers.

A growing number of lawsuits and union negotiations have challenged the male–female pay ratio based on the "comparable worth" theory. This theory, going beyond equal pay for equal work, calls for equal pay for different jobs of comparable worth. The intent is to revalue *all* jobs on the basis of the skills and responsibility they require. A landmark case resulted in the state of Washington being ordered in 1984 to pay female workers up to $1 billion in back wages and increases because of comparable worth inequities. However, shortly thereafter, the decision was reversed on appeal.

Generally, federal and state governments, as well as the courts, have not been supportive of comparable worth. For example, in 1985, the U.S. Civil Rights Commission rejected the comparable worth concept. That same year, a Court of Appeals ruling written by Judge Anthony M. Kennedy, who was later appointed to the Supreme Court, approved a state's relying on market rates in setting salaries even if it knowingly paid less to women as a result.

More recently, a federal judge in California ruled that California had not deliberately underpaid thousands of women in state jobs held predominantly by women, a serious blow to the country's largest lawsuit on this issue. Nonetheless, industry and business are becoming more interested in job evaluation studies, with presumably issues of comparable work and equal pay following.

The need to give equal attention to home and family and career along with a variety of other personal interests, once attributed to women, is becoming increasingly important to both sexes. Modern times call for the emergence of a new leadership style, which focuses on quick responses to change and the ability to bring out the best in people. This is not only a response to the values that women have brought to the workplace, but also totally consistent with what today's employees want for themselves.

The issue of women's rights is closely related to the problems, activities, and goals of women working in the health service industry. From 75 to 85 percent of all health service workers are women, and the largest health occupation, nursing, is almost totally female.

These female-dominated occupations are also expanding most rapidly, but men continue to dominate the positions of authority within the health care system.

The reasons for so many women in health care are that, first, they are an inexpensive source of labor; second, they are available; and third, they have been safe, no threat to physicians. The rise of nurses as autonomous practitioners certainly is a threat to that traditional power base.

More than any other factor, the absence of professional autonomy for nurses is considered a direct result of sex discrimination in nursing, with the end result that the patient and client ultimately suffer. The movement of nurses toward autonomy is seen partially as the result of the women's movement, and the struggles in achieving autonomy have certainly enhanced interest in the movement. The fight against sexual discrimination has gained new impetus in nursing, as well as in other segments of society, and has spilled over to include the consumer movement of women's health.

LABOR AND INDUSTRY

As nursing is part of the health care industry and as unions are making new efforts to organize nurses and others in health care, the status of labor unions is an important socioeconomic factor. Unions represented 13.5 percent of the workforce in 2001, significantly reduced from its high of 20.1 percent in 1983, the first year for which comparable data are available.[40]

Beginning with President Reagan's breaking of the air controllers' illegal strike in August 1981, by firing and subsequently replacing the air controllers, the unions have had special difficulties. Some employers simply threaten to file for bankruptcy, and the courts have supported their right to abrogate any existing union contract under those circumstances. Others find that they can withstand long strikes because they are legally permitted to make permanent job replacements, and the unemployed and workers in lesser paid fields are willing to take the strikers' jobs. (Note that President Clinton signed an executive order making it illegal for employers who participate in federal government contracts to permanently replace strikers.) Given the compromised position of most employees, employers are demanding (and getting) paybacks of benefits and pay in new contracts, citing competition as the reason. Union leadership has been blamed by many for not seeing the economic problems and being greedy in earlier years. What has also made it easier for management is the growing tendency of people to prefer to work part time, or in several part-time jobs. Although this is particularly true of women, including nurses, who have family care-giving responsibilities, there are also a surprising number of men who make this choice. Both women and men may be attending school, beginning their own business, testing out a different field, working at a second job, or simply looking for more flexibility and independence. Some like the variety and the fact that they need not get involved in the politics and problems of the workplace. On the other hand, wages may be lower (not necessarily true for nurses), there is little opportunity for career advancement, and some temporary workers complain of being "dumped on by regular employees." Industry has found these "contingency workers" economically advantageous. Employers do not usually pay for any benefits, which can be a considerable saving, and they can bring in these workers at busy times, while maintaining a minimum workforce. It provides a way around union work rules and, at times, a way to confront striking unions. The negative side is that part-time or short-term workers may not have the same commitment to the system that employs them, and unless they return to the same place frequently, need orientation and perhaps even training before they can be useful; and realistically, the existence of this temporary workforce and full-time replacements has made strikes a less powerful union tool.

Despite these problems, by the early 1990s, there was some optimism in the ranks of labor. For the first time in over a decade, younger, more sophisticated labor leaders had replaced nearly all the old guard. Also, both labor and industry were stressing the need for harmony. Union membership had grown, although with a greater overall growth in the workforce, the percentage continued to diminish. There was considerable growth in governmental unions, but the service industries, accounting for most of the growth in the labor force, had only 6 percent union participation. All seemed to be good candidates for organization. Because women are a large part of the latter group (they are also considered easier to organize), the unions are beginning to tackle "women's issues" such as abortion, and the safety of women on the job. However, their interest has not extended to placing women in the top echelon of the labor federation's hierarchy.

Management, criticized for its authoritarian approach, is trying new techniques to increase worker satisfaction. While far from widespread, there does seem to be growing interest in involving workers in decision making. Most American companies have reform programs in which workers and supervisors discuss operations. In industry these may be called quality circles; in health care they may be shared governance. Some labor experts say that these "reforms" (also known by such names as *job redesign, work humanization, employee participation, workplace democracy,* and *quality of work life*) are more cosmetic than real, since few workers participate in the companies' most important decisions, and that in a difficult situation most managers revert to an authoritarian stance.

In summary, American unions have been in decline since 1980, with the presence of a federal administration from 1980 to 1992 that favored big business and created incentives for the country's financial recovery to occur through the development of small business and industry. This anti-labor sentiment was acted out through management-friendly appointments to the Supreme Court and the National Labor Relations Board, the governmental unit critical to facilitating efforts at organizing and unionization. At the same time, more basic employee guarantees were being provided through legislation and regulations, decreasing the need for union protection. A more recent (1992–2000) pro-labor administration has done little to reverse this trend. A final observation is that the American union tradition has been built on an adversarial relationship between labor and management. This has proved to be inconsistent with the employee–employer relationships that have saved some of our largest and most productive industries.

THE CONSUMER REVOLUTION

The consumer revolution, said to have begun when Theodore Roosevelt signed the first Pure Food and Drug Act in 1906, has been an accelerating phenomenon since the 1950s. Although various interpretations are put on the term, it might be broadly defined as the concerted action of the public in response to a lack of satisfaction with the products and/or services they receive. The publics are, of course, different, but often overlapping. A man unhappy about the cost and quality of auto repairs might be just as displeased by the services of his dentist, the cost of hospital care, or the use of dangerous food additives.

There have probably always been dissatisfied consumers, but the major difference now is that many are organized in ad hoc or permanent organizations and have the power, through money, numbers, and influence, to force providers to be responsive to at least some of their demands. The methods vary but include lobbying for legislation, legal suits, boycotts, and media campaigns. One of the most noted, albeit highly criticized, consumer activists is Ralph Nader, whose Center for Study of Responsive Law produced a blitz of study group reports in the early 1970s that exposed abuses in a wide range of fields. Currently, his Health Research Group is one of the most influential in health consumerism. There is an increasingly strong force moving in that direction especially with the better educated and more aggressive baby-boomers. Consumers, who first concentrated their efforts against the shoddy quality of work and indifferent services offered on material goods, have now turned to the quality, quantity, and cost of other services, particularly in health care. Fewer patients and clients are accepting without protest the "I know best" attitudes of health care providers, whether physician, nurse, or any of the many others involved in health care. The self-help phenomenon, in which people learn about health care and help each other ("stroke clubs" and Alcoholics Anonymous, for instance), has extended to self-examination—sometimes through classes sponsored by doctors, nurses, and health agencies. Interest in health promotion and illness prevention has also been manifested by the involvement of consumers in environmental concerns.

The dehumanization of patient care, which is contrary to all the stated beliefs of the professions involved, is repeatedly castigated in studies of health care. Although complaints often are directed at the care of the poor, too often it is a universal health care deficiency. The concerted action of organized minority groups led to the development of the American Hospital Association's Patient Bill of Rights, which was followed by a rash of similar rights statements specifically directed to children, the mentally ill, the elderly, pregnant women, the dying, the handicapped, patients of various religions, and others. In some cases, presidential conferences and legislation have followed. The whole area of the rights of people in health care, which focuses to a great extent on patients' rights to full and accurate information so that they can make decisions about their care, has major implications for nurses.

An excellent example of the rise of a health consumer group is the Women's Health Movement, which emerged from women's disenchantment with their personal and institutional health relationships. Their complaints centered on physicians' attitudes toward women, which seem to be the result of both medical education and professional socialization. The fact that women's complaints of the health care system are neither isolated nor trivial is attested to by the attention given by lay and professional media to such problems as unnecessary hysterectomies and cesarean sections. However, the impetus toward organization is credited to the women's consciousness-raising groups of the 1960s, in which women shared their medical experiences and found support for taking action. Their activities are centered on changing consciousness, providing health-related services, and working to change established health institutions. Specific and well-known (as well as controversial) entities are the various feminist health centers and their know-your-body and self-help courses and books. The organization's scope of functions is increasing to include not only primary care, but nutritional, psychological, gerontologic, and pediatric services. Without doubt, those involved see the need for women to control their own essential femaleness as related to the wider issues of female equality and liberation.

The creation of the Agency for Healthcare Research and Quality (originally the Agency for Healthcare Policy and Research) is another example of the growth of consumerism in the health care industry. The Agency was charged by the Congress to work with the medical community to reach consensus on the preferred treatment of a select group of common conditions identified by the Institute of Medicine. This was a direct response to the frustration experienced by government and the public over inconsistencies in the medical management of these conditions, and that the absence of adequate explanations usually resulted in the patient deferring to the provider. These consensus statements were translated into consumer-friendly language and provided as public information.

The growth of managed care has created a consumer revolution of another type. With the current competition between hospitals and even nursing homes to fill their beds, consumer satisfaction has emerged as a significant outcome indicator. Institutions are placing a priority on the courtesy that employees show to consumers and conduct frequent surveys to identify where indignities and impatience may continue to exist. It is right and proper that the "customer" be treated with courtesy and respect, but the consumer cannot always be "right" where decisions often require knowledge and skill accrued over a lifetime of professional service. The goal is commendable, but caution must be exercised before we lose sight of the ultimate end of improving the human condition.

It has been hard for many Americans to adjust to the limited options provided by some managed care plans. Responding to the allegation that quality, and even safety, are often compromised, President Clinton established an Advisory Commission on Consumer Protection and Quality in the Health Care Industry which authored a "Patient's Bill of Rights." The following consumer protections continue to be major concerns, and they are repeatedly played out on both the federal and state scenes:[41]

- Holding managed care plans liable for decisions on withholding care that cause harm to patients.
- Ensuring that treatment decisions are made by the patient and their chosen health care provider.
- Ensuring that physicians and nurses can report quality problems with health plans or settings for care without retaliation.
- Preventing health care professionals from being rewarded for limiting a patient's care.
- Requiring hospitals to disclose publicly information on nurse staffing and adverse clinical outcomes in patients.
- Protecting nurses who voice concern about poor staffing from retribution.

○ Requiring health care institutions considering a merger or acquisition to report on the anticipated effect this would have on the community.

○ Ensuring patient access to clinical trials.

This list is not all inclusive, but provides an indication of the range of public concern over health care.

Other consumers are concerned with the power issue and are insisting, with some success, on increased representation on governing boards of hospitals and other health care institutions, accrediting boards, health planning groups, and licensing boards. What lies ahead in terms of more regulation, such as an overall federal consumer protection law and state laws that are really enforced, is not yet known. However, the consumer movement continues to gain strength, and some further action is inevitable. The nursing community has a history of supporting public policy that builds the strength of consumerism.

COST, QUALITY, ACCESS

The issues in U.S. health care have historically been access, cost, and quality. The "Great Society" of the mid-1960s wanted to guarantee health care as a right to every American. This was accomplished for a large segment of the population in 1965 through the creation of Medicare and Medicaid. Medicare is a federal program which funds health care for the elderly, and Medicaid pays for health services on behalf of the poor. The Medicaid program is administered at the state level with the contribution of federal dollars. These programs are discussed in more detail in Chapter 10.

National health care spending increased dramatically after establishment of the Medicare and Medicaid programs, as did the government's share in the total cost of health care. National spending has been 15.3 percent of the gross domestic product (GDP) in 2003; this is in stark contrast to 5.7 percent in 1965. In 2003, national spending, including both public and private sources, was 1.7 trillion dollars or $5805 per person. Over the years, government dollars as a percentage of total dollars spent on health care have also increased. In 1960, private funds, including private insurance and out-of-pocket dollars, paid for over three-quarters of health care in this country. By 1998, the government's share was almost half.[42] The GDP is the total value of goods and services produced in the United States and is an indicator of total economic production (or total economic output).

The magnitude of dollars spent forced government to search for some way to cut costs. In the beginning, both Medicare and Medicaid and most private health insurance plans paid for the "full and reasonable" cost of care retrospectively, that is, whatever the provider said it had cost, within certain limits, after the service was delivered. With the high cost of new technology used for both diagnosis and treatment, consumer demand for the biggest and the best, and the tendency of providers to over-order to protect themselves from being sued, costs soared. In 1983, because of fear that Medicare funds would run out, a new form of payment for hospital service was devised. Under this system, each Medicare recipient admitted is classified according to their medical diagnosis, the presence or absence of complications/comorbidity and surgery to one of hundreds of diagnosis related groups (DRGs). The hospital will receive a predetermined dollar amount for bundled services. The bundle of services consists of the usual length of stay for a patient with these clinical characteristics and the diagnostic and therapeutic services which would usually be ordered. Some hospitals are exempt from the system, and special provisions are made for patients who have needs that are extraordinary. This model is philosophically built on the principle of shared risk. Given enough patients in any DRG, there will be those who consume more resources and those who consume less, consequently adjusting the risk. In summary, the payment to health care providers for services to Medicare recipients will eventually all be based on patient assessment information which is then linked to a prospective payment system (PPS) model, setting the amount of dollars available before service is rendered. The model is consistent across settings, but the patient information needed and classification systems will differ. Hospitals were the first to be moved on to this system, because they are the more costly sector of the health care delivery system. It is also important to note that once methodologies prove useful at the federal level, they are considered for state adoption.

The more inclusive the PPS payment, the better for cost control. Hospital payment is based on the episode of hospitalization, but nursing home rates are still calculated on the day of service; the ideal would be an inclusive rate for the episode of illness. On the positive side, PPS is driven by the needs of the recipient of care, allows better budget control by anticipating revenue, and encourages more prudence in the use of resources. One negative is that payment can be denied retroactively, after the service has been given, if the service is not justified. Proper justification requires careful documentation. Another concern has been whether the severity of the patient's illness is considered, especially in regard to the nursing care needed. Many feel that the risk adjustment quality described earlier is not equitable, especially since patients differ so in their need for professional nursing.

If discharge occurs in a period shorter than anticipated or if fewer ancillary services are used, the facility may keep all or a portion of the unexpended dollars. This has resulted in accusations that hospital patients are being discharged "sicker and quicker," with more complex and highly technological care required in the home or nursing home. Hospital utilization has been greatly reduced, and patients are considerably sicker since there are no grace periods of early admission for tests, now to be done on an outpatient basis, and no leisurely postacuity or postsurgical recovery before discharge.

The creativity in cutting cost has been amazing. Although it is sometimes denied, administrators may encourage physicians to admit patients who are likely to be discharged early. Some hospitals have closed units that were costly and unlikely to be fully reimbursed, such as burn units and trauma units. "Patient dumping," transferring certain patients to public hospitals, was another cost-saving technique, although in 1989 a law was enacted penalizing hospitals that dump. Hospitals looked for other ways to fill beds with paying patients, such as those requiring long-term care. They developed subacute and skilled nursing units, satellite clinics, emergicenters, and surgicenters. These services were not subject to the DRG model, but have since been disallowed if they are in close proximity to the sponsoring hospital. They used helicopters to bring in emergency patients from distant areas and advertised their premier services in media campaigns. Some created profit-making components that included equipment rental, health promotion and teaching classes, and even hotels and contracts with noted fast-food companies. They merged or partnered with other hospitals or agencies to share services, or take advantage of the savings in group purchasing. Some even created health-care malls, which included doctors' offices, a hospital, ambulatory care, laboratory, pharmacy, optometry, physical therapy and physical fitness services, as well as home care services, restaurants, gift shops, banking, and parking. Despite their best effort, many small hospitals, especially in rural areas, have gone out of business. Those that have survived have undergone dramatic transformation, focusing on primary care, emergency services, and ambulatory and home care, with linkages to more distant hospitals for critical, acutely ill, and trauma patients. However, closures and downsizing continue, as the U.S. still remains overbedded with the average length of stay at 5.57 days in 2002,[43] and the average occupancy for all hospitals in 2000 at 65 percent.[44]

Another major problem for private hospitals is the number of people who cannot pay for their care. They are labeled medically indigent and create bad debt or uncompensated care. They consist of the uninsured, underinsured, illegal aliens, and the poor who have never been processed for Medicaid. Most of these people are not unemployed but are the working poor, neither old enough for Medicare nor poor enough for Medicaid, and unable to afford adequate private health insurance.

Hospitals have always given free care, and usually the cost was absorbed by increasing the bills of paying patients. Now this practice, called "cost shifting," is backfiring. In many states, the courts have made this cross-subsidization illegal. Health insurers have put a variety of strategies into place to control cost escalation which eventually means higher premiums. Preapproval of payment for an elective procedure is common. Many employers have become self-insured to control better the health care spending of their employees. Self-insured programs are not as tightly regulated by state laws. Smaller companies may simply drop this employee benefit, or increase the copayment and deductibles to keep premiums affordable.

By far the most common approach to the rising cost in health care has been managed care. Managed care plans are an option for employees who receive insurance through the workplace, and they are the mandated choice for the poor in many states. Managed care options are also available through Medicare. There are a number of versions, but the principle is for the insurer to enter into an agreement with a limited number of providers, hospitals, home care agencies, and so on, who will offer service to plan members at a discounted price. In some plans there is an all-inclusive periodic fee no matter how much service is used. This is called a capitation fee. Managed care is discussed in more detail later.

Managed care has reduced our freedom of choice, but forced us into more healthy living and personal responsibility. Many Americans have reevaluated their lifestyle, and become more self-sufficient in their decisions about their health, and economically prudent in their choices. Some companies reward healthy lifestyles by allowing the buyback of unused portions of health benefits. The Medical Savings Account (MSA) is a program which is enabled through federal or state legislation, and which also supports the philosophy of personal responsibility. Consumers are allowed to set aside pretax dollars to be used for medical expenses. This money can be used for copayments, deductibles, uncovered health expenses, and in some cases dependent care. Success is contingent on your ability to predict your expenses accurately, since unused dollars are usually forfeit.

A combination of these circumstances has rekindled the movement to guarantee basic health care services for everyone, but it seems this will happen incrementally, and not through any national health plan.

Massachusetts and Hawaii were the first states to provide near-universal access for their citizens, requiring employers to provide insurance while providing some state support. The federal government has allocated more dollars to provide health care to uninsured children under the age of 21. Other state initiatives have given hospitals the opportunity to develop managed care plans for the uninsured, and the 106th Congress (1999–2000) seriously considered extending Medicare coverage to young retirees from age 55. This proposal was defeated.

There are predictions that quality of care will be the issue of this new millennium. Beyond state licensing of hospitals and other health care facilities and agencies, which includes screening for adequacy, the Joint Commission on Accreditation of Healthcare Organizations (JCAHO), described later, puts its stamp of approval on institutions and agencies that meet specific criteria of quality. There are additionally "Magnet" awards for nursing services in hospitals and home care agencies which attain a standard of excellence; but all of these credentials are voluntary. The public also expect that health practitioners, be they provider professionals or administrators, will take responsibility for ensuring high-quality care. Although physicians, nurses, and administrators have peer review systems in place, to one extent or another, the warning is that unless improvements are made, government oversight will intensify. One existing example is the mandated peer review or peer review-like organizations (PROs) that monitor medical necessity, appropriateness, and quality of the hospital care provided to Medicare and Medicaid patients to determine if payment is justified.[45] Though on a voluntary basis, managed care plans seek accreditation by the National Committee for Quality Assurance (NCQA).

Meanwhile, the U.S. health care system continues to evolve, being shaped by its environment. It is a unique blend of public and private sector resources which is not to be belittled despite its flaws. There has been movement although it is incremental. Americans are making conscious decisions about the degree of personal health care risk they are willing to assume, and about the degrees of freedom they are willing to sacrifice for cost saving. More than ever before, their voices are heard and they are in control of decisions about their health. The growing prominence of managed care supports the use of nontraditional therapeutics, providers, and settings for care. Coordination and continuity of services has been proven to be a necessity and not a luxury. Women, children, and primary care have become our priorities, and we continue to fix the parts of the system that do not work as we had anticipated they would, never seeing the need to undo as failure. Our health care system is, as ever, as diverse and pluralistic as our population.

MANAGED CARE

It is impossible to speak of health care without giving significant attention to managed care. What it is. What it is not. What it hopes to accomplish.

Managed care is not a place, but an organizational structure. Neither is it one type of organization, such as a health management organization (HMO). It is based on specific principles that govern the relationship between insurers and providers, such as the observation *that cost and utilization are linked*. One nonnegotiable rule is to remove the temptation of using volume to increase profit. The technique of prepayment *shifts the risk* to the provider, although it is not used in every plan. Capitation means that the insured (or someone on their behalf, perhaps an employer) agrees to prepay periodically a fixed amount which is established independent of the actual service utilization practices of the enrollees. With capitation, *prudent utilization* can create profit for the provider, while overutilization can create a financial liability. In some models risk is even shifted to the insured, for example, in the choice to go to a provider outside of the network available to enrollees. The goal of managed care is to require the decision makers, who are the consumers, payers, and providers, to consider carefully the merit of services, procedures, and treatments in view of the resources available to them. In many instances, a *primary care provider* (PCP) is expected to assume the *responsibility for oversight* and become the "gatekeeper," ensuring that care is timely and necessary. Particular vigilance is directed toward the major drivers of cost: hospitalization, specialists, high technology.

Physicians and advanced practice nurses are definitely seen as the dominant influence since they generate cost through their clinical management. To offset this fact, the insurer moves to establish a level of control over them. This is done clinically by the existence of preferred approaches for the therapeutic management of a situation. The ultimate goal is standardization. Control is achieved financially by seeking a more or less exclusive relationship between the provider and the insurer, thereby creating a financial dependency. The most controlled model is the staff HMO where physicians and nurses are salaried and must usually agree to work exclusively for that HMO. Except for the staff HMO, most providers continue to see patients from a variety of plans. The need to assure coordination and avoid duplication is truly respected and has created a very prominent role for nurses in case management.

Many of the decisions internal to the managed care organization are based on observations of populations as opposed to individuals.

What works best for most of the people most of the time. Though contrary to our usual mind set, this could reap much benefit as we struggle to reverse our eroding public health.

Managed care includes the HMO, and an endless number of hybrids. The HMO is both an insurer and a provider. Two models are common: the staff model and the individual practice association (IPA). In the former the HMO operates its own facilities and provider professionals are employees. In the latter, service is delivered through a network of community-based physicians or APN offices, and the providers are independent contractors. The HMO is a prepaid health plan, and the consumer pays a single monthly or annual fee. In addition, small co-payments are usual for each visit or service. In HMOs primary care providers (doctors of medicine, doctors of osteopathy, APNs) act as "gatekeepers," managing common medical conditions and authorizing access to services and specialty care. It has been verified through extensive data collection that APNs are especially suitable for this role.

There are a variety of managed care models. With the exception of the HMO, there is little clarity on these other models, except that they differ in regard to:

- The ability to secure services from providers who are outside the plan's panel (point of service option).
- Direct access to specialists without going through a "gatekeeper."
- Payment on a fee-for-service or capitated basis.
- The amount of co-payment or deductible (if relevant).

Today, three-quarters of Americans with private health insurance, about 150 million people, are enrolled in an HMO or some other managed care plan. Numbers for Medicare and Medicaid beneficiaries are less current, but patterns are emerging. In 2001, 5.5 million Medicare recipients were enrolled in managed care entities, 20.8 million Medicaid eligibles, and 150.1 million covered by private plans, representing 61.3 percent of the U.S. insured population.[46]

Managed care organizations will have hit their stride when they compete on the basis of quality as opposed to cost. Many now seek accreditation by the National Committee for Quality Assurance (NCQA). The NCQA was established in 1979 by the trade associations for HMOs and managed care. It has become independent and conducts a very rigorous, voluntary accreditation of these plans. Many employers and state agencies require NCQA accreditation as a condition of doing business. Others look to the health-plan "report card" which provides data from the NCQA's HEDIS (Health Plan Employer Data and Information Set), showing measures of plan performance. The quality assurance infrastructure for managed care is taking shape.

HEALTH CARE DELIVERY: AN EXPANDING MAZE

Health care is big business, sometimes said to be the second or third largest industry in the United States with over $1.7 trillion spent each day. The industry employs one out of every 10 American workers, and is growing at a rapid pace. The settings for services are varied with hospitals, nursing homes, and home care agencies but a fraction of the places where service is delivered. Uncounted but growing are a wide variety of ambulatory care services, besides the physician's single and group practice. Among these are surgicenters and other "centers" for urgent care, mental health, alcohol/drug addiction, renal dialysis, women's health, childbearing, adult/geriatric day care, and holistic health, to name a few. Health maintenance organizations and hospices, more concepts than places, are also on the rise, while free clinics and community health centers may come and go, depending on the economy and support. The workers in the system represent as much variety. Given that a career in the health care industry of today requires an interdisciplinary perspective and team functioning, it is important to know who will be your colleagues and understand their work. The following sections will orient the student to where care is given and who gives it. Specific details on how the nurse may function in various settings are presented in Chapter 6.

SELF-CARE

Obviously, most people spend the greater portion of their lives in relative health. The constitution of the World Health Organization (WHO) defines health as a "state of complete physical, mental, and social well-being, and not merely the absence of disease or infirmity," which, although it serves as a broad philosophical declaration, is more an optimum goal than a reality.

On a practical level, the Public Health Service's National Center for Health Statistics defines health implicitly in its use of "disability days," when usual activities cannot be performed.

Self-care can be defined as "a process whereby a lay person can function effectively on his own behalf in health promotion, [and disease] prevention, detection and treatment at the level of the primary health resource in the health care system."[47] It is not new and ranges from a simple matter of resting when tired to a more careful judgment of selecting or omitting certain foods or activities, or the care activity of taking one or more medications self-prescribed or prescribed by a physician. Health care advice comes gratuitously from family, friends, neighbors, and the media (often with a product to sell). People also actively seek, although informally, information or advice from groups, a health professional acquaintance, or the Internet, but their self-care often becomes a matter of trial and error. Increasingly, a new consumer mentality has included the help of others with similar conditions or concerns, so that the individual has support and reinforcement as needed but can also detect at what point he or she needs professional help.

In some cases, a person may have had some level of professional care previously and may again, but a certain amount of informed self-diagnosis is not only less expensive for the public but may also serve a useful purpose for the individual. For instance, a mother who has been taught to take her child's temperature can give much more accurate information to a doctor or nurse practitioner, or avoid a call altogether if she also knows how temperature relates to a child's well-being. A blood pressure reading taken properly at home is more likely to identify a hypertension problem quickly than is a yearly physical examination. The sale of do-it-yourself medical tests, stethoscopes, blood pressure devices, and other medical devices for home use has become a rapidly expanding market. The Internet will allow us to interpret our data and weigh our options, or chat with others who have had the same problem.[48] Given adequate support systems, it has been said that 85 percent of health care could be self-provided. The knowledgeable consumer is the secret weapon of the new millennium, and a natural threat to provider professionals who are not comfortable in their role.

Besides consumerism, another factor that encourages self-care is cost and convenience. For instance, emergency rooms are frequently filled with patients who have minor conditions that could have been prevented or self-treated at home at an earlier stage.

Nursing incorporates a philosophy of holism and empowerment. It is empowering for individuals to be capable in taking charge of their own health and the health of those for who they are responsible, children, the elderly, the disabled. To be encouraged to be dependent is to be crippled. Approaching self-care with the best attitude and hoping for maximum benefits, the focus should be wellness and prevention of illness, and the nurses' greatest contribution should be educating and reeducating to healthful lifestyles. Many of the major causes of illness are learned behaviors, but these can be unlearned. The strongest support for this approach appears to come from business, the insurance industry, and union leaders (perhaps because of the increasing cost and overuse of health insurance that is often a workplace benefit). Education for self-care is well placed in schools, the workplace, and community programs of all types, and has historically been the forte of HMOs, where the relationship between cost and self-care has long been recognized and respected.

ALTERNATIVE/COMPLEMENTARY MEDICINE

Although alternative or complementary medicine may not fit correctly in this chapter, it does fit with self-care, and which term is used to describe this movement can also evoke emotional responses. Are we speaking of a rejection of traditional Western medicine or new strategies to augment that tradition? In 1997, 42 percent of respondents to a national survey said that they would look to an alternative if traditional medical treatment was not working.

Americans make more visits to alternative care providers than to primary care physicians, and most of the cost of this treatment is out of pocket. In response to public pressure, many health plans are beginning to recognize some of these options and even mainstream health facilities are establishing departments or clinics which specialize in complementary therapies.[49]

Whether disenchanted with the medical model, or searching for some way to regain control of their lives, in 2004 the Institute of Medicine

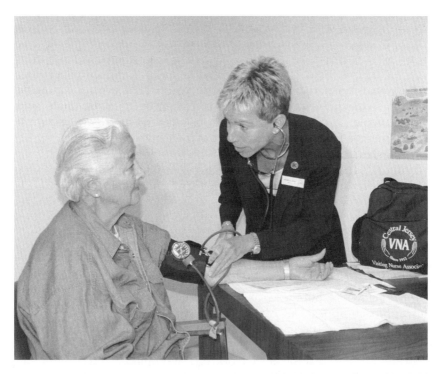

Community-based health promotion programs for the elderly are part of the role of the visiting nurse. (*Courtesy of the Visiting Nurse Association of Central Jersey, Red Bank, New Jersey*)

(IOM) reported annual sales of $16 billion for dietary supplements among the American public.[50] The frequency of use of alternative/complementary care services and products in rank order were herbal therapy, chiropractic, massage, vitamin therapy, homeopathy, yoga, acupressure, acupuncture, biofeedback, hypnotherapy, and naturopathy. A common observation was that alternative care practitioners spend more time with their patients, about four times more than a physician, and are more holistic. The most common reasons for seeking alternative therapy are chronic pain (specifically back pain), arthritis, anxiety, depression, allergies, insomnia, and menopause. Evidence is mounting that complementary therapy has made a difference in these conditions.[51] How much can be attributed to the mind/body connection is yet to be determined.

AMBULATORY CARE

It is not practical to discuss the institutions involved in the various types of health care delivery under the headings of primary care and so on (but these labels are still important and are presented in Exhibit 3.4), because there is considerable overlap of functions. For instance, hospitals and HMOs may deliver all levels and types of care, even encouraging or sponsoring self-care activities on the part of individuals and community groups. Therefore, institutions and agencies are presented as more traditional units of service, such as ambulatory care, hospitals, emergency services, and home care. Additionally, there are some venues for care which are better described as programs. They integrate and coordinate a wide variety of services on behalf of the patient. Such programs are considered separately and include, among others, long-term care, hospice, and managed care entities. Managed care is an insurer, but can also be a provider, and was included earlier in this chapter.

Ambulatory care consists of those health care services that do not require an overnight stay in any health care facility, and consequently are community based. The patient/client comes to the provider as compared with home care where the provider goes to the recipient of care. The shared characteristic between ambulatory services and home care is that they are both community based, but respecting their differences, home care is treated separately.

Ambulatory care is rapidly becoming the dominant mode of service delivery in this country. Once ambulatory care was almost exclusively provided in physicians' offices, hospital emergency rooms, and out-patient clinics. Today, ambulatory care is much more diverse, and

Exhibit 3.4 Definitions

Primary care: "(a) a person's first contact in any given episode of illness with the health care system that leads to a decision of what must be done to help resolve his problems; and (b) the responsibility for the continuum of care, i.e., maintenance of health, evaluation and management of symptoms, and appropriate referrals."[a]

Secondary care: the point at which consulting speciality and subspeciality services are provided in either an ambulatory, residential, or community hospital inpatient setting.

Tertiary care: the point at which highly sophisticated diagnostic, treatment, or rehabilitation services are provided, frequently in university medical centers or equivalent settings.

Acute care: those services used in the treatment of illness or disability that have as their purpose the restoration of normal life processes and function.

Long-term care: "those services designed to provide symptomatic treatment (palliative), maintenance, and rehabilitative services for patients of all age groups ..."[a]

Levels of prevention:
Primary: healthy actions taken to avoid illness or disease;
Secondary: screening or early detection and treatment of health problems;
Tertiary: occurs during rehabilitative phase of an illness to prevent complications and further disability; establishing a new self-concept and a new trajectory of wellness in chronic disease.

Vertical integration of services: arrangement between organizations that provide different services with the goal of creating a continuum of care.[b]

Horizontal integration: arrangement between organizations that provide similar services, such as a chain or network of hospitals.[b]

[a] U.S. Department of Health, Education, and Welfare: *Extending the Scope of Nursing Practice.* Washington, DC: The Department, 1971, pp 3–11.
[b] Sullivan EJ, Decker PJ. *Effective Leadership and Management in Nursing*, 4th ed. Menlo Park, CA: Addison Wesley Longman, 1997, p 21.

anything that can be conveniently and safely accomplished outside of a hospital has been moved to an ambulatory care setting.

PHYSICIAN OFFICE PRACTICE

Except for home care and nurse-managed centers (NMCs), most ambulatory services currently involve physician–patient contact. Various sources indicate that the vast majority of care given by physicians is on an ambulatory basis; only about 10 percent of the people seen are ever admitted to a hospital. Most patient visits for health (or sick) care have been made to health care practitioners in solo, partnership, or private group practice. This is the major mode of organization for physicians and other health care providers who are acknowledged to be licensed to practice independently, such as dentists, chiropractors, podiatrists, and optometrists. There is also a growing acceptance of advanced practice nurses practicing independently or in partnership with a physician.

NURSE PRIVATE PRACTICE

Nurses have been in private practice since formal nursing programs were started (see Chapter 2). In a manner of speaking, private-duty nursing was and is a private practice for which the individual nurse has professional and financial responsibility.

In a contemporary model of private practice, the nurse has an office where patients are seen, although he or she may also make house calls. In this form of independent practice, nurses have the same economic and managerial requirements as physicians, with the added concern that reimbursement by third-party payers may be limited and, even if legal, nurses often have to fight with intermediaries to start to establish their "track record." Also, in many states, advanced practice nurses (APNs), who are the most common candidates for independent practice, are required to establish a collaborative relationship with a physician to facilitate their prescriptive authority. Despite all this, there are many nurses in successful independent or group practices. Some may simultaneously hold other positions, such as teaching posts. There are also those in a nursing faculty who carry a private practice to enhance their faculty role and are not solely dependent on that income.

COMMUNITY HEALTH CENTERS

Out of the social unrest of the 1960s and early 1970s emerged the *neighborhood health center* (NHC), an ambulatory practice with mandated community involvement in both policy making and facility operations. The NHC movement was stimulated by funding from the Office of Economic Opportunity (OEO) during the Johnson administration. In many ways, NHCs were similar to early charitable dispensaries, which were established because of hospitals' lack of interest in ambulatory care and disappeared in the 1920s because of poor financing, poor staffing, and physician disapproval.

Now more commonly called *community health centers* (CHCs), and including migrant health centers, they serve some 6 million Americans, usually poor, in about 2000 locations nationwide. They may be free-standing, with a backup hospital for special services and in-patient care, or legally part of a hospital or health department, functioning under that institution's governing board and license, but with a community advisory board.

CHCs are primarily found in medically underserved urban areas, where the minority poor, the homeless, and various ethnic groups rely on hospital ambulatory services for primary care. In many cases, the hospital clinic service and the emergency service, often expensive, overcrowded, fragmented, and disease-oriented, are inappropriately used. Their ineffectiveness is a major reason for the rise of the CHCs, called by some "one-stop health shopping" at acceptable, affordable prices, with interest in providing holistic health care. Often, they are at least partially staffed by the ethnic group served, so that communication is improved, and a real effort is made to provide services when and where patients and clients need them in an atmosphere of care and understanding. Use of nontraditional workers such as family health workers and an emphasis on using a health care team have been characteristic.

Although much of the health care given by CHCs is excellent, their problems have caused a drop in number from the peak development of the 1970s. Problems include tensions between community advisory boards and administrators of the center and/or the backup hospitals, and funding. Maintaining CHCs is extremely expensive, and most patients can pay only through Medicare or Medicaid, if at all. Few centers are self-supporting. When external funds are not available, severe program and personnel cuts are often necessary. The future of CHCs remains uncertain, in part because of a sociological question: are they perpetuating a separate kind of care for the poor?

NURSE-MANAGED CENTERS

Nurse-managed centers (NMCs) are a variation on the theme of the CHC. They are introduced separately because of some details which set them apart. The NMC offers the ultimate in autonomous practice opportunities to nurses as managers and primary caregivers. NMCs may also be called nurse-run clinics, or designated as community nursing organizations (CNOs). They guarantee direct client access to nursing services, offer services that are reimbursable, place the accountability for both the services and the management of the center with nurses, and allow nurses to practice to the fullest extent of their legal scope of practice. They recognize that patient care must be interdisciplinary and refer to collaborating physicians when a presenting case exceeds that scope of practice.

NMCs are not new creations, but can trace their roots to the turn of the century and the tradition of the visiting nurse and public health nursing.

Neither must all NMCs be community based. A modern-day example of an NMC can be observed in the Loeb Center established at Montefiore Hospital in New York by Lydia Hall in the early 1960s. Hall characterized Loeb as a nursing center with the qualities of public health being offered in an institutional setting.

NMCs may be freestanding and entrepreneurial, or affiliated with a college of nursing or a health care institution. In any of these relationships, they may become part of a network as we move toward managed care. The services offered by an NMC may be narrow in scope or diverse. They can offer all of the traditional primary care services, and consequently serve as an excellent point of entry for managed care plans.

It should be noted that some of our most successful NMCs have been birthing centers established by certified nurse midwives (CNMs). Models for NMCs have also been developed by clinical nurse specialists (CNSs) within such areas as cardiovascular, oncology, low-birthweight babies, patients with chronic obstructive pulmonary disease, diabetics, and so on. The chronically ill need primary care too.

The future of NMCs will depend on their success as participants in managed care, and in making strategic decisions to diversify or focus their services. Further, our commitment to the underserved is consistent with our history, but to grow and flourish the vast middle class must become our consumers.

OTHER HEALTH CENTERS AND CLINICS

There are endless variations on CHCs, and nurses are responsible for knowing that they exist. *Rural health centers*, developed under federal financing such as regional health and the Appalachian projects or funded by communities or foundations, are the rural corollary to CHCs—existing to serve people, usually poor, in medically underserved areas (MUAs). Since few physicians are available, care is often given by nurse practitioners (NPs) and physician assistants (PAs) linked to physicians at other sites.

Mental health centers or *community mental health centers* are intended to provide a wide range of mental health services to a particular geographic "catchment area." They may be sponsored by state mental health departments, psychiatric hospitals or departments of hospitals, or the federal government. Staffed by teams of mental health personnel, they may consist of single physical entities or networks, but tend to focus on short-term care, including "crisis intervention."

A large portion of the mentally ill qualify for government entitlements. Seen as a group with special needs, their health care is frequently "carved out" or treated separately and differently from programs for the general population of the poor and disabled. In many instances psychiatric NPs have been designated as the primary care providers or case managers for these patients. These are nurses with a graduate degree and dual preparation as a psychiatric–mental health nursing clinical specialist and a nurse practitioner.

Women's clinics are usually owned and operated by women concerned about women's health problems and dissatisfied with the quality of care for women and the attitudes of many male health care providers. Most emerged out of the women's movement, along with the consumer and self-care movements. Services may include routine gynecological and maternity care and family planning, as well as some general health care. Emphasis is on self-help, mutual support, and noninstitutional personal care. Both nurse–midwives and lay midwives are used, as are NPs and supportive physicians, although many staff are lay people. In a number of cities and towns, the clinics have been harassed by conservative groups and medical societies, and some have had to become involved in lengthy and expensive legal suits. These should not be confused with women's health care centers developed and operated by hospitals to target this specific clientele.

Family-planning clinics, of which the clinics of Planned Parenthood are most notable, provide a spectrum of birth control and women's health services and information.

Abortion clinics are sponsored by community and other groups, as well as proprietary organizations, or may be located in a physician's private practice. There may also be abortion services offered in conjunction with a women's health or family-planning clinic. However, harassment by anti-abortion activists, including picketing and sometimes violent action, as well as some cutbacks in funding by the government and other external funding sources, have resulted in limitation of services and even closings in the last few years. A recent U.S. Supreme Court decision considered the harassment of patients and professionals and came down in favor of the public's right to access these facilities.

Renal dialysis centers were spurred into massive growth by their inclusion in the 1972 Medicare amendment. Once, the treatment of those with chronic kidney disease by using expensive artificial kidneys was a sensitive matter of "who shall live." When Congress decided that all should have that opportunity and funded it, the cost rose to unexpected millions of dollars. Many centers are freestanding, mostly physician owned or developed by proprietary organizations, but they also exist in hospitals. The desired emphasis now is on the less expensive home dialysis.

Another group of burgeoning facilities are those for rehabilitation of drug abusers. Most common are the *methadone maintenance programs* (substituting methadone for heroin, along with certain rehabilitative measures), which have had varying success. *Drug-free* programs include self-help and therapeutic residential programs, halfway houses, counseling centers, and "hot lines."

Adult day-care centers are agencies that provide health, social, psychiatric, and nutritional services to infirm individuals who are sufficiently ambulatory to be transported between home and center. Psychogeriatric day-care centers were first opened in 1947 under the direction of the Menninger Clinic. Studies ordered by Congress in 1976 showed day-care centers to be cost-effective, but no national policy on reimbursement followed. Funding now comes from uncoordinated disparate sources, and therefore some communities have set priorities as to who can use the services. Yet, day care has been shown to be superior to nursing homes to eligible individuals because of lesser cost, improved health and functional outcomes, and an increased quality of life. Unresolved issues are related to their use for young adults with debilitating diseases, the feasibility of rural centers, and the need for regulation and licensing. Currently, governmental distinctions exist between medical and social day care. The former requires some presence of health care personnel or some available health care services.

AMBULATORY CARE ALTERNATIVES TO INSTITUTIONS

The 1980s brought increased complaints about the expense of health care, particularly in hospitals, and ushered in the "competitive model." The core of the model is that consumer choice and market forces rather than regulation should be used to control health care costs.

As a result, alternative health care delivery modes, particularly in ambulatory care, developed and expanded. Among these are the *surgicenters*, independent proprietary facilities for surgery that do not require overnight hospitalization. The first was established in 1970 in Phoenix, Arizona, and their popularity has escalated. Some are specialized, such as the plastic surgery centers, but in general the centers can perform any surgery that does not require prolonged anesthesia. Surgicenters are said to be able to perform up to 40 percent of all surgical procedures, including face lifts, cataract surgery, vasectomy, breast biopsy, dilatation and curettage, knee arthroscopy, and tonsillectomy, among other procedures. Because of low overhead, surgicenters can charge as little as one-third of hospital costs for the same procedure, and patients like being able to return to home, or even work, the same day.

When it was evident that this new delivery mode was not only well accepted (some do as many as 6000 procedures a year) but reimbursable by insurance plans, many hospitals joined the movement and set up "day surgery" centers. Although greeted enthusiastically by payers at first because of the cost savings, in a few years the unregulated fees soared.

Emergicenters or *Urgicenters* may be for-profit or nonprofit, public or private, freestanding or owned by another entity. The term *freestanding* refers to the fact that this facility may be sponsored or affiliated with a hospital, but is not owned by it. They are designed to treat episodic, nonurgent health problems.

Closely related are *wound care centers* treating chronic nonhealing wounds, *pain clinics, incontinence clinics*, and so on. Staff may also coordinate access to other needed services. All these centers have the potential to be a lucrative business, and are natural markets for advanced practice nursing. Government regulation is still largely nonexistent.

Although some women are again turning to home births attended by midwives, a more popular and growing alternative to hospital births is the *childbearing center*, also called *birth center* or *childbirthing center*. These centers made their appearance in 1973, when the alienated and questioning middle class became disenchanted with hospital maternity care. The original nurse–midwifery model was the Maternity Center of New York. Now an increasing number of out-of-hospital centers are operating. Some are operated by or utilize nurse–midwives; others are sponsored by physicians and/or lay midwives.

There are both freestanding (autonomous) childbirthing centers and a variation of the concept in hospitals. Both allow for more humane care in a high-quality, homelike setting with the father and other children present—all costing considerably less than traditional hospital care. If only one in four pregnant women had access to and used birthing centers, millions and perhaps billions of health care dollars would be saved.

Another humanistically oriented as well as cost-saving mode of care is the *hospice*. The hospice movement was pioneered in Great Britain by Dr. Cicely Saunders at St. Christopher's Hospice in London. The first widely recognized hospice in the United States was established in 1971 in New Haven, Connecticut. Modeled after St. Christopher's, its concentration was on improving the quality of patients' last days or months of life so that they could "live until they die."

The Hospice Association of America estimates that there are between 1700 and 1900 hospice programs in the United States; about 1158 hospitals have certified hospice services. Medicare classifies hospices into four types: hospital-based; home health agency-based; skilled nursing facility-based; and independent. The first three are part of a larger institution; the independent, of which there are very few, are corporate entities. Hospices may offer inpatient care, home care, or a mix of the two, but whatever the setting, in reality it is a concept, an attitude, a belief that involves support of the family as well as the dying patient. It can be carried out in an ordinary hospital setting, with extraordinary perception. The hospice functions on a 24-hour, 7-days-a-week basis; backup medical, nursing, and counseling services are always available. The typical hospice team consists of a physician and some combination of nurses; medical social workers; psychiatrists; nutritionists; pharmacists; speech, physical, and occupational therapists; and clergy or pastoral counselors. The staff meets regularly both to discuss treatment plans and to provide support for one another. Because they are close to both patient and family, team members may suffer from burnout and stress, so counseling is available for them as well. Hospices frequently rely on well-trained volunteers, who provide respite care, companionship, transportation, patient teaching, and bereavement support. The family is also considered part of the team.

Most hospices serve cancer patients primarily, but many also care for patients with progressive neurological or chronic diseases and now AIDS. Except for the latter two groups, the majority of hospice patients are elderly. Any patient whose physician certifies that he or she has a life expectancy of less than six months is eligible for hospice care. Patients must be aware of their diagnosis and prognosis. Most patients die at home, surrounded by their families, and free of technological, life-prolonging devices. Symptom control is a vital step, and pain-relieving medications are dispensed at a level which will ensure that the patient is virtually pain-free at all times. Psychological comfort is considered as important as physical comfort, and the counseling, support, and companionship of hospice staff help relieve fear, depression, and anxiety.

A number of studies have shown that hospice care is less expensive than traditional care, and slowly reimbursement is being offered. Most major private insurance companies and some HMOs reimburse at least partially; however, since this can be an "add-on" benefit, very few patients receive full reimbursement. In 1986, hospices became a permanent Medicare benefit and an optional Medicaid benefit, but at least 80 percent of the care is supposed to be provided in the home and patients relinquish the right to curative therapy. Difficulties are surfacing as modern drug therapy extends life beyond that six months, and it additionally becomes difficult to determine whether a procedure or course of treatment is curative or palliative in its intent.

HOSPITALS

In 1946, at the close of World War II, there were 6000 American hospitals. With the passage of the Hill–Burton Act to fund hospital expansion and the burgeoning of hi-tech, the system grew to a high of 7200 acute care hospitals. In the current climate which discourages hospital use for anything but major illness, the number of community-based hospitals has been reduced to approximately 5000.[52]

Hospitals are generally classified according to size (number of beds, exclusive of bassinets for newborns); type (general, mental, tuberculosis, or other specialty, such as maternity, orthopedic, eye and ear, rehabilitation, chronic disease, alcoholism, or narcotic addiction); ownership (public or private, including the for-profit, investor-owned proprietary hospital or not-for-profit voluntary hospital, which may be owned by religious, fraternity, or community groups); and length of stay (short-term or long-term). Hospitals vary from fewer than 25 to more than 2000 beds. The most common type of hospital in this country is the nonprofit voluntary, general, short-term, community-based hospital. Many hospitals have been forced to close. Causes cited by the American Hospital Association (AHA) included financial cutbacks in federal funding, pressure by insurance companies and business to reduce health expenditures, and changing health care practices (such as those described earlier). If not closed, the small hospitals are likely to become part of a multi-institutional system, a major trend in health care delivery. These may comprise two or more hospitals owned, leased, sponsored, or contract-managed by a central organization. They can be for profit or nonprofit. Advantages can include improved access to capital markets, group purchasing, technology, economies of scale, shared use of technical and management staff, richer referral networks, and the opportunity to specialize among the facilities.

The terms teaching and nonteaching are also used to describe hospitals. Teaching hospitals are associated with medical schools and maintain accredited educational programs in which medical students, residents, and specialty fellows are taught. Teaching hospitals receive special government funding for educational purposes. The teaching designation does not derive from programs or experiences which the hospital may provide for other health professionals or allied health workers. These hospitals (about 9 percent) usually have more than 400 beds and are in medical centers proximate to the medical school (in which case they are often tertiary care centers). The extra funding that derived from the teaching hospital status is drying up quickly, and one of the most confounding questions in health care is where the money for medical education will come from.

Because of all these variations, it is difficult to draw one picture of the hospital as an entity. Exhibit 3.5 shows a common organizational pattern of a general hospital, which illustrates both the lines of authority and the kinds of services available. Larger and more diverse systems will have more complex organizational structures. A hospital that has

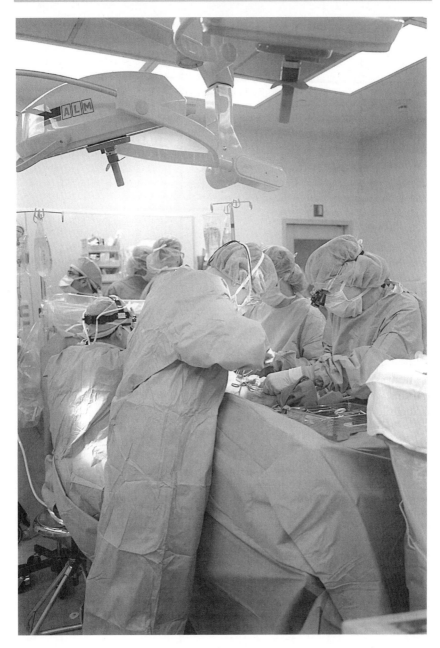

Today's operating rooms are centers of advanced technology. (*Courtesy of Beth Israel Deaconess Medical Center, Boston, Massachusetts*)

Exhibit 3.5 One Pattern of Hospital Organization

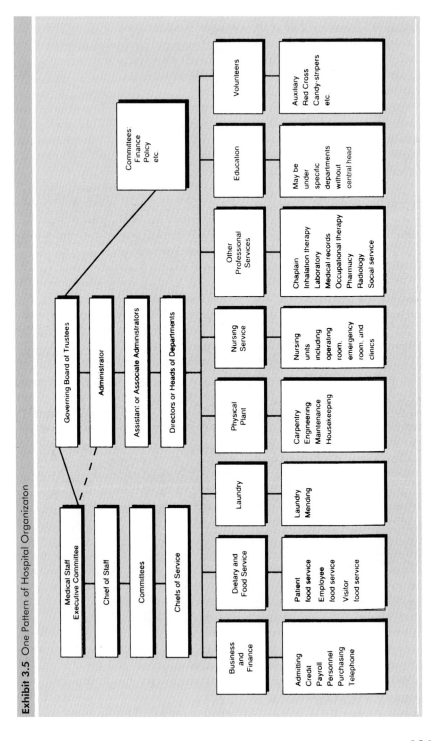

outreach programs, home health services, or a long-term care facility differs greatly from a 50-bed community hospital. Smaller hospitals may have fewer diverse clinical services and few, if any, education programs, but almost always there are business and finance departments, physical plant (maintenance of all kinds), laundry, supplies and storeroom, dietary and food services, clinical nursing units (inpatient and outpatient), and the other professional service units, such as laboratories, radiology, other diagnostic and treatment units, pharmacy, and perhaps social service. Some hospitals are now out-sourcing laundry and food services in the belief that this is less expensive than maintaining your own equipment and dealing with all of the human resource problems that inevitably come with the job.

The physical layout of a hospital varies from one-story to high-rise, and may include large or small general or specialized patient units, special intensive-care units, operating rooms, recovery rooms, offices (sometimes including providers' private offices), space for diagnostic and treatment facilities, storage rooms, kitchens and dining rooms, maintenance equipment, work rooms, meeting rooms, classrooms, chapel, waiting rooms, and gift and snack shops. Most hospitals have some form of emergency service, such as an emergency room, but many no longer maintain their own ambulance services. A great many have outpatient or ambulatory services, and perhaps an extended-care, subacute-care, or cooperative-care unit for patients who do not need major nursing service; some provide home care.

The nursing service department has the largest number of personnel in the hospital, in part because of round-the-clock, 7-days-a-week staffing. Other departments, such as radiology and clinic laboratories, may maintain some services on evenings and weekends, and may be on call at nights. There is a trend to have other clinical services available at least on weekends. For instance, a patient who needs rehabilitation exercises or other treatments in the physical therapy department lacks this necessary care in the evenings and weekends when that department follows the usual nine-to-five, Monday-through-Friday staffing pattern.

Hospitals are licensed by the state and presumably are not permitted to function unless they maintain the minimum standards prescribed by the licensing authority. ("Presumably" because the process of closing a hospital due to inadequate facilities and/or staff is long, difficult, and not always successful.) However, to be eligible for many federal grants and to be affiliated with educational programs, accreditation is necessary. Accreditation by the Joint Commission on the Accreditation of Health Care Organizations (JCAHO) is voluntary and is a stamp of quality. JCAHO accreditation is particularly necessary, because it holds "deemed" status with the Health Care Financing Administration

(HCFA); that is, if a hospital is accredited by JCAHO, HCFA accepts this credential as verification of quality and allows reimbursement for service to Medicare beneficiaries.

Voluntary hospitals are usually organized under a constitution and by-laws that invest the board of trustees with fiduciary responsibility. This governing board is generally made up of individuals representing various professional and business groups interested in the community. Although unsalaried and volunteer (except for proprietary hospitals, in which members are often stockholders), board members are usually extremely influential citizens and are often self-perpetuating on the board. This type of membership originated because at one time administrators of hospitals did not have a business background, and because of the need to raise money to support hospitals. (Most trustees still see recovery of operating costs as their most crucial hospital problem.) Some consumer groups have complained that most members are businessmen, bankers, brokers, lawyers, and accountants, with almost nonexistent representation of women, minorities, consumers in general, and labor. Physicians also complain of lack of medical representation, although they work closely with the board and are subordinate to it only in certain matters. Because of these pressures, boards are gradually acquiring broader representation.

Public hospitals usually do not have boards of trustees. Hospital administrators are directly responsible to their administrative super-visors in the governmental hierarchy, which may be a state board of health, a commissioner, a department such as the Veterans Administra-tion (VA), or a public corporation with appointed officials. Presumably, all are ultimately responsible to the public.

Although *administrator* is still the generic term for the managerial head of a hospital, in recent years this title has included a variety of designations such as *president* and *chief executive officer* (CEO). The hospital administrator, the direct agent of a governing board, implements its policies, advises on new policies, and is responsible for the day-to-day operations of the hospital. Some years ago, physicians and nurses frequently became hospital administrators, but increasingly this position is filled by a lay person with a management background and possibly a master's degree in hospital administration or business administration. Hospital or health administration, like any other, encompasses planning, organizing, directing, controlling, and evaluating the resources of an organization. In large institutions, the administrator (the vast majority of whom are men) has a staff of assistants or associates, each responsible for a division or group of departments. Forward-looking hospitals have recognized that the nurse executive should hold one of these positions in order to participate in the policy-making decisions that inevitably affect the largest hospital department. Department heads or supervisors are next in the line of authority; these individuals are also gradually becoming specialists by education and experience in their area of responsibility.

The *medical or professional staff* is an organized entity made up of provider professionals who are admitted to membership by the incumbents. Subsequently their appointment is approved by the Board of Trustees who are ultimately responsible for the welfare of the patients. Members of the staff are granted the privilege of using the hospital's facilities for their patients. A typical classification of medical staff includes honorary (not active), consulting (specialist), active (attending provider), courtesy (those not wishing full status but occasionally wanting to attend private patients), and resident (house staff of residents and fellows). Through their committees, including the Credentials Committee, the medical staff is an impressive power in the hospital, for it is often in a position to control not only medical practice, but also all patient care in the hospital. Professional staff privileges may be awarded to any licensed provider professional, including nurses. Many advanced practice nurses (APNs) hold staff appointments, although the nature of their privileges may be limited.

GOVERNMENT FACILITIES

In the federal government, at least 25 agencies have some involvement in delivering health services. Those with the largest expenditures in direct federal hospital and medical services are the Veterans' Administration, which operates the largest centrally directed hospital and clinic system in the United States, the Department of Defense (members of the military and dependants), and the Health Resources and Services Administration (HRSA) of the Department of Health and Human Services (DHHS). The HRSA operates one Public Health Service (PHS) hospital devoted to Hansen's disease, and provides care for federal prisoners and Coast Guard personnel. The Indian Health Service (IHS) operates hospitals, health centers, and satellite health clinics for Native Americans and Alaskan natives. A variety of DHHS agencies provide indirect funding or contracts for clinics, drug and alcohol rehabilitation centers, maternal-child and family planning, neighborhood health centers, and the National Health Service Corps.

State and local governments also have multiple functions and multiple services in health care delivery, directly through grants and funding to finance their own programs, and indirectly as third-party payers. Although most states have some version of a state health agency or department of public health, health services are often provided through other state agencies, a situation that creates territorial battles, duplication, and gaps. In most states, operation of psychiatric hospitals and the Medicaid program, two of the most important state health functions, is by departments other than an official state agency for health. In direct services, some states operate psychiatric, TB, or other hospitals, and alcohol and drug rehabilitation programs; provide noninstitutional mental health services; fund public health nursing programs and laboratories; and provide services for maternal and child health, family planning, crippled children, immunization, TB, chronic respiratory disease control, and venereal disease control. All are considered traditional public health services, in addition to environmental health activities.

On a local level, services offered by a health department depend a great deal on the size, needs, and demands of the constituency. There appears to be little information about local health departments or health officers. Those with considerable visibility are in large urban centers, where health problems are complex and generally unresolved.

Some large municipalities operate hospitals that provide for the indigent or working poor who are not covered by Medicaid or private insurance. Health departments may run school health services and screening programs. Some duplicate services are offered by the state. There are few data on how much state and local agencies coordinate their services to avoid duplication or omission, but lack of coordination or cooperation is not uncommon. Although there is a great deal of criticism of most local health services in relation to high cost, waste, corruption, and poor quality, attempts to terminate any of them, particularly hospitals in medically underserved areas, become political conflicts, with representatives of the poor complaining that no other services are available and that the loss of local jobs will create other hardships.

One emergent trend that may somewhat dilute these politics is the tendency to privatize governmental programs and facilities. In the U.S., the expectation has always been that the private sector can do it better and cheaper. Many states have given their Medicaid recipients a "voucher" to buy into the managed health care plan of their choice. Others are requiring that Medicaid recipients enroll in managed care plans offered for their use. Some public facilities have executed contracts for management services with private sector companies. All of this forces many public health care facilities, which have primarily served the poor, to rise to the cost-efficiency and attractiveness standard of the private sector, and substantially reduces the infrastructure that is directly under governmental control. In the same spirit of seeking simplification, talk on Capitol Hill questions whether the existing federal systems (VA, state-side military health care facilities) should continue to exist as separate entities or should continue to exist at all, the option being to award vouchers for use in the private sector to all individuals having a right to government entitlement programs.

EMERGENCY MEDICAL SERVICES

Ambulance services, originally a profit venture of funeral directors, are a vital link in transporting accident victims or those suffering acute overwhelming illnesses (such as myocardial infarctions) to a medical facility. In most cases, providing for such services, either directly or through contracts, has now become the responsibility of a community, a responsibility that is not consistently assumed.

With continued federal and state funding and regulation, the previous diverse ambulance and rescue services of volunteers, firefighters, police, and commercial companies are being coordinated and standardized within regional systems. Criteria include training of appropriate personnel, education of the public; appropriate communication systems, transportation vehicles, and facilities; adequate record keeping; and some participation by the public in policymaking.

Under these laws, a variety of emergency medical technicians (EMTs) have been trained and staff many ambulance services, including mobile intensive-care units, which have very sophisticated equipment.

HOME HEALTH CARE

Home health care is probably more of a nurse-oriented health service than any other, originating with Florence Nightingale's "health nurses" and the pioneer efforts of such American nurses as Lillian Wald. (Today the terms used also include public health nurse or community health nurse.) Nevertheless, what Wald worked for in the late nineteenth century—comprehensive services for the patient and family that extend beyond simple care of the sick—is even more pertinent today.

Home care includes a broad spectrum of services from home birthings to hospice care. Medical services are primarily provided by the individual's private or clinic physician or APN, although in some instances agencies will employ or contract for these services. In addition, home-maker–home health aide services may be required in conjunction with nursing and therapies. These consist of bathing, personal grooming, assistance with self-help skills, meal planning and preparation,

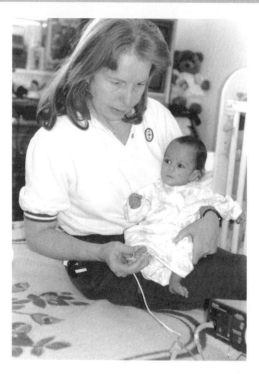

Home care is much more complex today as patients are sent home earlier, even the smallest ones. (*Courtesy of the Visiting Nurse Association of Boston*)

and general housekeeping services. Among the other home health services that may be available are medical supplies and equipment (expendable and durable), nutrition, occupational therapy, physical therapy, speech pathology services, and social work. Additional services may also be provided through coordinated efforts of the agency and the community.

Certified home health operates under various auspices. The major types are visiting nurse associations (VNAs), public agencies, hospital-based agencies, and proprietary agencies. In 2000, VNAs numbered 436 and represented less than 3 percent of all agencies, whereas there were 909 public home health agencies for about 9 percent of the national total. VNAs and public agencies have experienced significant decline in recent years. In 1975, they were 23 and 55 percent of the home care market, respectively. Freestanding proprietary (40 percent) and hospital-based agencies (30 percent) have grown the most in recent years since then.[53]

VNAs are freestanding, voluntary, nonprofit organizations governed by a board of directors (volunteers) and supported by contributions as well as by revenues received for care and services delivered. VNAs are the oldest and have been the classic providers of home care service. Depending on the location and resources, the spectrum of services may vary greatly but generally includes at least skilled nursing and other professional services. Many VNAs also operate adult day-care centers, wellness clinics, hospices, and Meals on Wheels programs. The mission of VNAs has always been to provide quality care to all people, regardless of their ability to pay. Volunteers have played a large role in assisting VNAs to accomplish their mission through fundraising, friendly visiting, telephone reassurance, and assistance with clinic and office work.

Public agencies are government entities operated by a state, county, city, or other unit of local government. In addition to providing home health care services, these agencies have a major responsibility for preventing disease and for community health education

Hospital-based agencies are operating units or departments of a hospital. The hospital-based agencies have grown substantially since the initiation of prospective payment for inpatient hospital services in 1983. The attraction of a hospital-based agency is particularly strong where consumers have had a positive inpatient experience. Although hospitals are required to give discharged patients several options to choose from, the myth or reality of continuity is a strong incentive.

Proprietary agencies are freestanding for-profit home health agencies. They have been characterized by aggressive development of new services, especially in the area of high-tech home care, and by brisk and sophisticated marketing activities. They have often provided the competitive impetus and organizational models for other home health agencies to rethink their service delivery patterns and structures.

Home care in the United States is in a state of crisis. The financial support of Medicare and Medicaid has been a major factor fueling the growth of the home care industry. Medicare is the largest single payer for services. In 2000, Medicare spending accounted for 26 percent of total home care revenue and Medicaid for 9.3 percent.[54] Although home care represents a relatively small percentage of total Medicare expenditures, it has been the fastest-growing category of expenses for this program. Government's need to keep a tight rein on health care costs and the anticipated growth of home care created an uncomfortable situation. The response was the Balanced Budget Act of 1997, designed to demand efficiencies by reducing the number of federal dollars to the program, and moving home care on to PPS by October 2000.

Growth in managed care plans and their desire to bundle payment for acute and post-acute services has influenced a number of freestanding agencies, especially VNAs, to affiliate with or become part of larger integrated health systems. Within these relationships the home health agency often relinquishes at least some autonomy in return for a secure and often expanded referral base.

LONG-TERM CARE

Long-term care (LTC) services for chronic conditions and functional dependency comprise one of the fastest-growing components of the industry. In part this is due to the success of medical science in saving those who might have died at any earlier stage of life, and in part to the fact that often the nuclear family has no place for the incapacitated who, years ago, were simply cared for at home with no public help. LTC signifies much more than the chronic disease hospital and the nursing home. A whole range of options have evolved with the intent of

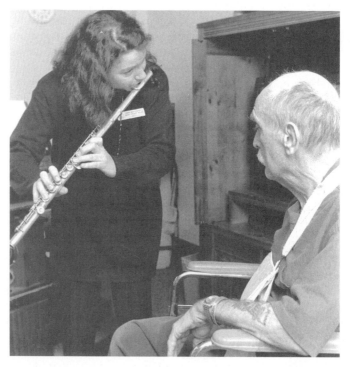

Music therapy can be a meaningful experience for the elderly. Sara Macdonald, a music therapy intern, plays the flute for John Geyer. (*Courtesy of the Evangelical Lutheran Good Samaritan Society, Sioux Falls, South Dakota. John Danicic Jr., Photographer*)

supporting consumer choice, maintaining self-care and independence, and avoiding institutionalization.

The concept of the hospice as originally conceived, a cluster of seamless services which support the patient's movement back and forth depending on comfort and ability, has found renewal in many life-care communities for older Americans.

Assisted living offers the frail elderly and disabled a comprehensive package of nontraditional services, such as personal care, chore services, or companionship. Assisted living is a social, not a medical, program. It rejects the concept of dependency and requires that the beneficiaries retain control of their lives. Independence, individuality, choice, privacy and dignity are its mantra. Assisted living assumes that care that requires a nursing home can be offered in the home and at lower cost. Given acceptance of that requirement, there is the opportunity to "age in place." There are also those who are able to do fine with long-term home care, medical or social day care, and a variety of other "stand alone" programs.

Even as we support a return to community and home care services, we know that for many it just is not enough. The multiple backup services, social and health related, that are needed are not easy to organize or to coordinate and even less likely to be reimbursed. Therefore, despite much rhetoric, institutional care, while considerably more expensive and often lessening the individual's quality of life, still appears to be necessary for part of the population.

There are two major categories of long-term care institutions: long-stay or chronic disease hospitals (e.g., psychiatric, rehabilitation, chronic disease, and TB) and nursing homes. There are only a few long-stay hospitals left in the United States. They are declining given the trend toward deinstitutionalization, and the development of subacute and special care units in hospitals and nursing homes.

In 2000, 15,371 licensed nursing facilities were reported with over 1.7 million beds. Special care units have become common for Alzheimers, AIDS, ventilators, special rehabilitation, and sometimes hospice. Most nursing homes have an average bed size of 107, and 33 percent are owned or operated by a chain. Forty-seven percent are independently operated and 65.5 percent are run for profit. The overwhelmingly greatest number of residents are Medicaid recipients. The reader is reminded that Medicare is an episodic program assuming some return to health and improvement in functional ability, while Medicaid is designed for continuing care.

Although about 12 percent of nursing home residents are under 65, the rapid growth of the over-85 population has made the care of the frail elderly and chronically ill a public concern. It has been noted that those over age 85, who are most apt to need LTC and financial assistance for such services, are increasing seven times as fast as the population as a whole, and elderly Americans who will need some sort of help, now over 6.5 million, will climb to 19 million by 2040. One expert said that actuarially, the odds are nearly one in two that an individual would need LTC between the age of 65 and death, largely because of chronic disabilities.

THE CAREGIVERS: A GROWING NUMBER

U.S. health care employs over 11.5 million people, and includes more than 200 acknowledged occupations and professions. These are positions in direct care, those involved in healthcare as a business, and others indirectly supporting the work of direct caregivers.

The overwhelming growth of personnel is in direct health services. Many of the health occupations and suboccupations have emerged because of increased specialization in health care, others on the peculiar assumption that several less-prepared workers can substitute for one scarcer professional. Some of these workers can be employed in almost any health setting—hospitals, nursing homes, clinics, doctors' offices, occupational health, and school health. Some work primarily in one setting. Most of these workers are not licensed; many are trained in on-the-job programs, and even more are trained in a variety of programs with no consistent standards. Others have standardized programs approved by the state or some private sector authority. A total of 1700 allied health educational programs are accredited by the Commission on Accreditation of Allied Health Educational Programs (CAAHEP), an independent entity originally developed under the auspices of the American Medical Association (AMA). *Allied health personnel* (AHP) as defined by the federal government includes almost any health worker engaged in activities that support, complement, or supplement the functions of the professional provider (nurse, doctor, and so on). Services rendered by AHP range across the entire spectrum of service delivery and include every aspect of patient care, as well as services provided as part of community health promotion and protection. AHP range from personnel with complex functions and the highest educational degrees, who have always had a great deal of autonomy, to those who function in relatively simple assisting roles and must be supervised, sometimes by others categorized as AHP.

The largest categories of health workers, in order, are nursing (all types, including aides), physicians, dentists and their allied services, clinical laboratory workers, pharmacists, and radiological technicians. As feminists are the first to point out, from 75 to 85 percent are

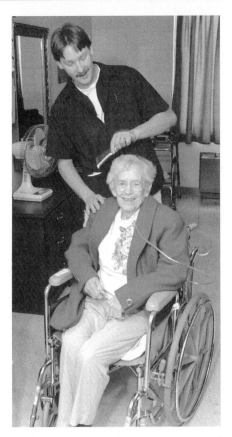

Nurses' aides and volunteers add a great deal to the well-being of patients in nursing homes. Elizabeth "Betsy" Wood gets her hair brushed by aide Britt Batterten. (*Courtesy of the Evangelical Lutheran Good Samaritan Society, Sioux Falls, South Dakota. John Danicic Jr., Photographer*)

women, and they are, or have been, in the lower-paid and less powerful positions.

It would be unrealistic to attempt to describe all the professional and technical workers with whom nurses work or interact. However, an introduction to the most prevalent health occupations should provide a better understanding of the complex relationships in health care. Details on education, salaries, and a broader range of occupational roles in health care are included in Appendix 2.

The organization of this section is primarily alphabetical, although two closely related groups may be placed in logical succession. The education of RNs, practical nurses, and nursing assistants is described in Chapter 5 and the practice of nursing in Chapter 6.

CHIROPRACTIC

Chiropractic is described by the American Chiropractic Association (ACA) as "a branch of the healing arts which is concerned with human health and disease processes. Doctors of chiropractic are physicians who consider man as an integrated being, but give special attention to spinal mechanics and neurological, muscular, and vascular relationships." Chiropractors use standard diagnostic measures, but treatment methods, determined by law, do not include prescription of drugs and surgery. Essentially, treatment includes "the chiropractic adjustment, necessary dietary advice and nutritional supplementation, necessary physiotherapeutic measures, and necessary professional counsel." Most chiropractors are in private practice. All 50 states, the District of Columbia, and Puerto Rico recognize chiropractic as a health profession and authorize these services for workmen's compensation. They are also reimbursable by Medicare and Medicaid. Practitioners in this area may be designated as Doctors of Chiropractic, Chiropractic Physician, or Chiropractor. They treat problems of the body's structural and neurological systems.

CLINICAL LABORATORY SCIENCES

There are a number of technicians or technologists working in the clinical laboratories in such specialties as immunohematology, hematology, clinical chemistry, serology, microbiology, and histology. The person in charge is usually a physician who is a pathologist, although technologists may have specific responsibilities for technicians. *Medical technologists* are prepared for all phases of clinical laboratory work. *Certified laboratory assistants* perform routine laboratory tests, and *histological technicians* prepare body tissues for microscopic examination by pathologists.

DENTISTRY

Dentists treat oral diseases and disorders. They may fill cavities, extract teeth, and provide dentures for patients. About 15 percent of dentists specialize, selecting orthodontics (straightening teeth), oral and maxillofacial surgery (operate on mouth and jaw), pediatric dentistry, periodontics (treating gums), endodontics (root canal therapy), oral pathology, public health dentistry, or prosthodontics (making artificial teeth). These specialties usually require two or more additional years of training and a specialty board examination. Nine out of ten dentists are in private practice; the others practice in institutions, the armed forces, and health agencies, teach, or do research. An increasing number of minorities and women are entering the field.

Dental hygienists, almost all women, provide dental services under a dentist's supervision. Many are self-employed and subcontract with dentists to provide their services. They examine and clean teeth, give fluoride treatments, take x-rays, and educate patients about proper care of teeth and gums. In many states, hygienists' responsibilities have been expanded to include duties traditionally performed by dentists, such as giving local anesthetics.

Dental assistants maintain supplies, keep dental records, schedule appointments, prepare patients for examinations, process x-rays, and assist the dentist at chairside, but their functions are also expanding.

Dental technicians or *denturists* make and repair dentures, crowns, bridges, and other appliances, usually according to dentists' prescriptions. They are lobbying to work directly with patients and have become licensed in some states.

DIETETICS AND NUTRITION

Nutritionist is a general occupational title for health professionals concerned with food science and human nutrition. They include dietitians, home economists, and food technologists.

Dietitians may have a *general dietary* background or preparation in *medical dietetics.* Medical or therapeutic dietitians are responsible for selection of appropriate foods for special diets, patient counseling, and sometimes management of the dietary service. More and more are becoming licensed and are seeking third-party reimbursement. *Therapeutic dietitians* work with patients not only in the hospital, but in clinics, neighborhood health centers, or in the patient's own home.

Dietetic technicians graduate from one of two kinds of American Dietetic Association (ADA)-approved technical programs with an associate degree. A program with food service management emphasis allows the individual to serve as a technical assistant to a food service director and, with experience, to become a director. The program with nutritional care emphasis enables the individual to become a technical assistant to the clinical dietitian.

Most *dietetic assistants* serve as *food service supervisors* in hospitals, schools, and nursing homes. However, a number of food service supervisors currently functioning in that position lack such preparation.

HEALTH EDUCATORS

Community health educators help identify the health learning needs of the community, particularly in terms of prevention of disease and injury.

They may then plan, organize, and implement appropriate programs, for example, screening, health fairs, classes, and self-help groups. Some health educators are employed by the state as consultants, others by insurance companies, voluntary health organizations such as the American Heart Association, the school system (school health educators), and, occasionally, industry.

A number of hospitals are employing *patient educators* or health educators to develop and direct programs of both patient education and community health education. Frequently, these people are nurses with or without training in health education and administration. In a few states, health educators are registered and/or certified.

MEDICAL RECORDS

Medical record administrators are responsible for preparation, collation, and organization of patient records, maintaining an efficient filing system, and making records available to those concerned with the patient's subsequent care. They may also classify and compile data for review committees and researchers.

Medical record technicians assist the provider professional and the administrator in preparing reports and transcribing histories and physicals. They also work closely with others using patient records.

Medical record transcriptionists have specialized courses in terminology, in addition to typing and filing.

MEDICINE

Doctors of medicine and osteopathy practice prevention, diagnosis, and treatment of disease and injury. Medicine is a licensed profession in every state, and some states require continuing education for relicensure. The licensure exam consists of three parts, two taken in medical school, and the third within the first year of an approved residency. The *Doctor of Medicine* (MD), awarded in 125 accredited allopathic medical schools, and the *Doctor of Osteopathy* (DO), awarded in 22 accredited osteopathic medical schools, are considered the first professional degree. Some physicians may later decide to acquire advanced degrees (master's or doctorates) in an advanced science or public health.

The formalized program of education after the MD degree is titled *graduate medical education* and consists primarily of the residency, which involves preparation for specialties, a period of generally two to seven years. On completion of the specified years of residency, the physician may take certification exams in the specialty and is board-certified. If exams are not taken (or failed), the physician is board-eligible. In some cases, continuing medical education is required for recertification. Ninety percent of American allopathic physicians choose specialties as their field of practice; however, this is changing slowly, since there is an oversupply of specialists and many are not being accepted into managed care plans because the need is for primary care physicians. In medical centers, a *fellow* is a postresidency physician who enters even more advanced, highly specialized, or research-oriented programs, although presumably still involved in patient care.

Physicians practice in every setting where medical care is provided, as well as in medical or public health education, public health practice, and research. About 65 percent are now employees (not in private practice), with the number increasing as HMOs enroll the physicians' patients, cutting down on their practice. Some positions, such as that of medical director, are primarily administrative and are beginning to be recognized as such.

The number of women in medical schools has increased and there has been a slight increase in under-represented minorities.

Doctors of osteopathy (DOs) are qualified to be licensed as physicians and to practice all branches of medicine and surgery. DOs graduate from colleges of osteopathic medicine, accredited by the Bureau of Professional Education of the American Osteopathic Association (AOA). After graduation, almost all DOs serve a 12-month rotating internship, with primary emphasis on medicine, obstetrics/gynecology, and surgery, conducted in an approved osteopathic hospital. Those wishing to specialize must serve an additional three to five years of residency. Continuing education is required by the AOA for all DOs in practice.

Osteopathic physicians are considered separate but equal to allopathic physicians in American medicine; they are licensed in all states and have the same rights and obligations. The "something extra" they claim is emphasis on biological mechanisms by which the musculoskeletal system interacts with all body organs and systems in both health and disease. They prescribe drugs, use routine diagnostic measures, perform surgery, and selectively utilize accepted scientific modalities of care. DOs comprise about 5 percent of all physicians; most are general practitioners who provide primary care, usually in small cities and towns and rural areas. Osteopathic physicians are chiefly located in states with osteopathic hospitals. In 1994, four out of five DOs were practicing in 16 states; most were in Michigan followed by Pennsylvania, Ohio, Florida, Texas, and New Jersey.

Medical assistants (MAs) are usually employed in physicians' offices, where they perform a variety of administrative and clinical tasks to help the doctor; however, some work in hospitals and clinics. They perform tasks required by the doctor and are supervised by the doctor. The MA, among other things, answers the telephone; greets patients and other callers; makes appointments; handles correspondence and filing; arranges for diagnostic tests, hospital admissions, and surgery; handles patients' accounts and other billings; processes insurance claims, including Medicare claims; maintains patient records; prepares patients for examinations or treatment; takes patients' temperature, height, and weight; sterilizes instruments; assists the physician in examining or treating patients; and, if trained, performs laboratory procedures.

PHYSICIAN ASSISTANTS (PAs)

In 1965 Dr. Eugene A. Stead, Jr., of Duke University inaugurated a program for *physician's assistants* (PAs), designed to assist physicians in their practice either to enable them to expand that practice or to give them time to pursue continuing education, or to have more time for themselves.

As defined in HRSA reports, PAs are skilled members of the health care team who, working dependently with physicians and under their supervision, provide diagnostic and therapeutic patient care. They take patient histories, perform physical examinations, and order laboratory tests. When medical problems are diagnosed, PAs develop treatment plans and explain them to patients. They are also permitted to diagnose illnesses. PAs are recognized in all states, the District of Columbia, and Guam. The requirement for physician supervision to practice varies greatly in interpretation. In 42 states, including the District of Columbia, physicians may supervise PAs without being on the premises. If PAs are necessary in underserved areas, this latitude is essential, and now "supervision from a distance" using electronic technology is also considered satisfactory. In 47 states, the District of Columbia, and Guam, PAs are authorized to prescribe.[55] In addition to specific technical procedures that PAs perform, which vary with the practice setting, they carry out a variety of minor surgical procedures. They also may provide pre- and postoperative care. PAs with surgical training often act as first or second assistants in major surgery.

As of 2002, 132 programs were accredited by the Accreditation Review Commission on Education for the Physician Assistant (ARC-PA). The typical PA program is 24–25 months long and requires at least two years of college and some health care experience prior to admission. The majority of students have a BA/BS degree and 45 months of health care experience before admission to a PA program. Of the 132 accredited PA programs, 76 award master's degrees, 57 award bachelor's degrees, 7 award associate degrees, and 56 award certificates.

(Some programs offer more than one option.)[56] The trend is toward graduate education.

PAs receive their national certification from the National Commission on Certification of Physician Assistants (NCCPA). Only graduates of an accredited PA program are eligible to take the Physician Assistant National Certifying Examination (PANCE). Every two years, a PA must complete 100 continuing education hours and reregister her/his certificate with the NCCPA (second and fourth years), and by the end of the sixth year, recertify by examination or documented experience. All states require passage of the PANCE for state licensure. Forty-seven states make provisions to license new physician assistant program graduates prior to availability of PANCE results.[57]

Concern about the relative status of advanced practice nurses (APNs) and PAs was, and is, an issue in certain situations. Although APNs can offer services to the public beyond any that the PA can offer, frequently nurse and PA may be competing for the same job. For a number of reasons, the PA not only may be the one employed but will also receive a higher salary than that offered to the APN. Despite the fact that most physicians tend to say that they prefer nurses to PAs, the truth is that too often doctors have inadequate or no knowledge about the APN's capabilities. What doctors are saying is that they want the nurse as a PA. A number of nurses have sought additional credentials to qualify for status as a PA. This has caused some negative reaction from other nurses and nursing associations.

There are still many unresolved issues related to PA practice, particularly in relation to role and functions. The American Hospital Association has published a statement on PAs in hospitals, which recommended that the medical staff and administration should formulate guidelines under which the PA can operate, and that any request for PA practice in hospitals should be handled by the medical staff credentials committee. Emphasis is on medical supervision; however, current reality has shown that PAs go unsupervised in busy urban hospitals where they handle many emergency and other ambulatory patients.

The following comments from the Ninth Report to the Congress on Health Personnel in the United States puts the often testy relationship between physicians, PAs, and APNs into perspective:

> Physicians conceived and fostered the idea of PA practice in the mid-1960s. It is not surprising, then, that physicians generally accept PAs. For their part, PAs are committed to the team approach to patient care in which each profession is recognized for its unique skills and contributions. Unlike nurse practitioners, who seek greater autonomy, PAs believe the most appropriate and logical individual to supervise the health care team is the physician.[58]

EMERGENCY MEDICAL TECHNICIANS

Emergency medical technicians (EMTs) recognize, assess, and manage medical emergencies involving acutely ill or injured persons in prehospital settings. They may administer cardiac resuscitation, treat shock, provide initial care to poison or burn victims, and transport patients to a health facility.

In addition to the EMT-Ambulance (EMT-A), the entry level worker, there are two other levels of EMTs, known in most places as EMT-Intermediates (EMT-Int) and EMT-Paramedics. The former may assess trauma patients, administer intravenous therapy, and use antishock garments and esophageal airways. They are widely used in rural areas. EMT-Paramedics are trained in advanced life support. Working in radio communication with a provider professional, they may, in most states, administer drugs, interpret EKGs, perform endotracheal intubation, and defibrillate.

EMTs are employed by community fire and police departments, by private ambulance services, and in hospital emergency departments.

PHARMACY

Pharmacists are specialists in the science of drugs and require a thorough knowledge of chemistry and physiology. They may dispense prescription and nonprescription drugs, compound special preparations or dosage forms, serve as consultants, and advise physicians on the selection and effects of drugs.

With the increase of prepackaged drugs and the use of pharmacy assistants, pharmacists in hospitals and clinics are becoming interested in a more patient-oriented approach to their practice. They may be involved in patient rounds, patient teaching, and consultation with nurses and physicians. Pharmacists working in (or owning) drugstores have also been encouraged to increase their client education efforts in terms of explaining medications.

In 2000, 82 colleges of pharmacy were accredited to confer degrees by the American Council on Pharmaceutical Education. Pharmacy programs grant the degree of Doctor of Pharmacy (Pharm.D.), which requires at least 6 years of postsecondary study and the passing of the licensure examination of a state board of pharmacy. This degree has replaced the Bachelor of Science (BS) degree, which will cease to be awarded after 2005. Pharmacists are licensed in all states and have reciprocity (simultaneous recognition) among all states with the exception of California and Florida.

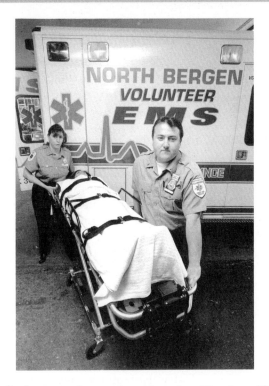

Emergency medical personnel are partners in caring. (*Courtesy of Palisades Medical Center, New York Presbyterian Healthcare System*)

Besides the traditional responsibilities of pharmacists, the doctor of pharmacy (Pharm.D.) or clinical pharmacist provides consultation with the physician, maintains patient drug histories and reviews the total drug regimen of patients, monitors patient charts in extended care facilities and recommends drug therapy, makes patient rounds, and provides individualized dosage regimens. In some states, such as California, clinical pharmacists may also prescribe, with certain limitations.

PODIATRY

Podiatrists, doctors of podiatric medicine (DPM) (once called *chiropodists*), are professionally trained foot-care specialists who diagnose, treat, and try to prevent diseases, injuries, and deformities of the feet. Treatment may include surgery, medication, physical therapy, setting fractures, and preparing orthodics (supporting devices that mechanically rearrange the weightbearing structures of the foot). Podiatrists may note symptoms of diseases manifested in the feet and legs and refer the patient to a physician. Most podiatrists are in private practice; others practice in institutions, agencies, the military, education, and research.

Podiatric assistants aid podiatrists in office management and patient care.

MENTAL HEALTH PRACTITIONERS

Besides the physician (the psychiatrist), clinical psychologists, psychotherapists, nurses, and social workers, a variety of semiprofessionals trained in mental health participate in individual and group therapy. Psychologists may also give and interpret various personality and behavioral tests, as might a *psychometrician*, who is skilled in the testing and measuring of mental and psychological ability, efficiency, potentials, and functions.

PUBLIC HEALTH: THE ENVIRONMENT

Industrial hygienists deal with the effects of noise, dust, vapor, radiation, and other hazards common to industry on workers' health. They are usually employed by industry, laboratories, insurance companies, or government to detect and correct these hazards.

Sanitarians, sometimes called *environmentalists*, apply technical knowledge to solve problems of sanitation in a community. They develop and implement methods to control those factors in the environment that affect health and safety, such as rodent control, sanitary conditions in schools, hotels, restaurants, and areas of food production and sales. Most work in government under the direction of a health officer or administrator.

Biostatisticians apply mathematics and statistics to research problems related to health. *Epidemiologists* study the factors that influence the occurrence and course of human health problems, including not only acute and chronic diseases but also accidents, addictions, and suicides.

RADIOLOGY

Radiologists are physicians who deal with all forms of radiant energy, from x-rays to radioactive isotopes; they interpret radiographic studies and prescribe therapy for diseases, particularly malignancies. A number of technicians work under the direction of a radiologist in radiology departments. They operate equipment, prepare patients, and keep records. These include the *radiologic technologist,* sometimes called *x-ray technician* or *radiology technician; radiation therapy technician* or *technologist;* and *nuclear medicine technologist.*

REHABILITATION SERVICES

Occupational therapy is concerned with the use of purposeful activity in the promotion and maintenance of health, prevention of disability, and evaluation of behavior. Persons with physical or psychosocial dysfunction are treated using procedures based on social, self-care, educational, and

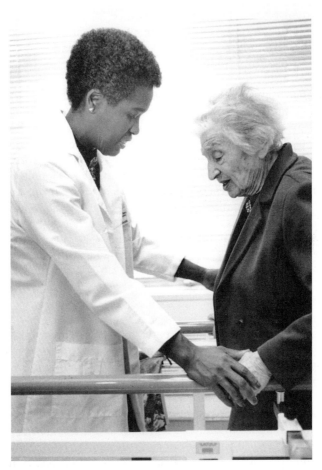

Rehabilitation services aim to restore independence. (*Courtesy of the American Nurses Association*)

vocational principles. One important responsibility is helping patients with activities of daily living. Adaptive tools such as aids for eating or dressing may also be provided.

Occupational therapists (OTs), the professional workers, and *occupational therapy assistants and aides* are usually employed in rehabilitation settings. However, OTs may also work in private practice or for nursing homes, community agencies, or hospitals.

Physical therapy is concerned with the restoration of function and the prevention of disability following disease, injury, or loss of a body part. The goal is to improve circulation, strengthen muscles, encourage return of motion, and train or retrain the patient with the use of prosthetics, crutches, walkers, exercise, heat, cold, electricity, ultrasound, and massage. Most *physical therapists* (PTs) and *PT aides* work in hospitals, but PTs may also work in private practice or for other agencies. The PT designs the patient's program of treatment. He or she may participate in giving the therapy and/or evaluate the patient's needs and capacities and provide psychological support. The aides work directly under the PT's supervision.

Rehabilitation counselors help people with physical, mental, or social disabilities begin or return to a satisfying life, including an appropriate job. They may counsel about job opportunities and training, assist in job placement, and help the person adjust to a new work situation. Others assisting in patient rehabilitation include *art therapists, dance therapists,* and *music therapists* who work primarily with the emotionally disturbed, mentally retarded, or physically handicapped. *Recreational therapists* or *therapeutic recreationists* may plan and supervise recreation programs that include athletics, arts and crafts, parties, gardening, and whatever else helps fulfill recreational needs.

RESPIRATORY THERAPY

Respiratory therapy personnel perform procedures essential in maintaining life in seriously ill patients with respiratory problems and assist in the treatment of heart and lung ailments. Under the supervision of a doctor or respiratory therapist, the *respiratory therapy technician* administers various types of gas, aerosol, and breathing treatments; assists with long-term continuous artificial ventilation; cleans, sterilizes, and maintains equipment; and keeps patients' records. The *respiratory therapist* may be engaged in similar tasks, but exercises more judgment and accepts greater responsibility in performing therapeutic procedures.

SOCIAL WORK

The *social worker* attempts to help individuals and their families resolve their social problems, using community and governmental resources as necessary. Social workers are employed by community and governmental agencies as well as hospitals, clinics, and nursing homes. If the social worker's focus is on patients and families, he or she may be called a *medical* or *psychiatric social worker*. When patients are being discharged to go home or transfer to another health care facility, these social workers assist the patient and family in making suitable arrangements.

Social workers also have assistants and aides, who sometimes carry a client load in certain agencies. There may be only on-the-job training available for these workers, but in order to move up, they must acquire additional education.

SPEECH PATHOLOGY AND AUDIOLOGY

Speech therapists and *audiologists* are specialists in communication disorders. Speech pathologists or therapists diagnose and treat speech and language disorders that may stem from a variety of causes. Speech therapists are particularly valuable in assisting patients whose speech has been affected by a cerebrovascular accident or patients with laryngectomies. Audiologists often work with children, and may detect and assist with the hearing disorder of a child who has been mistakenly labeled as retarded.

VISION CARE

Ophthalmologists are physicians who treat diseases of the eye and perform surgery, but they may also examine eyes and prescribe corrective glasses and exercises. *Opticians* grind lenses, make eyeglasses, and fit and adjust them. *Optometrists,* doctors of optometry (OD), are educated and clinically trained to examine, diagnose, and treat conditions of the vision system, but they refer clients with eye diseases and other health problems to physicians. They describe their focus as maximizing visual ability, and therefore often use therapeutic programs such as eye training. They may also prescribe corrective lenses and contact lenses. The majority of optometrists are in private office practice, but they are increasingly found in institutional settings. All of these professionals are aided by technicians and assistants.

OTHER HEALTH WORKERS

There are a number of other health workers not described in this chapter, such as those in science and engineering: anatomists, biologists, biomedical engineers (who design patient care equipment such as dialysis machines, pacemakers, and heart–lung machines), biomedical technicians (who maintain and repair the equipment), and technicians dealing with instrumentation. There are also diagnostic medical sonographers; electrocardiograph (EKG/ECG) technicians; electroencephalographic (EEG) technologists and technicians; clinical perfusionists, who operate equipment to support or replace temporarily a patient's circulatory or respiratory functions; specialists in dealing with the visually handicapped; biological photographers; medical illustrators; patient advocates; acupuncturists; health science librarians; and computer specialists, to name just a few. In addition, volunteers provide many useful services.

The fact that this list of services and providers is not complete and is expanding may help to explain why the public often becomes angered and confused. It is clear that, if the public is to receive the services it requires, expects, and deserves, direction must be given for negotiating the health care delivery maze. And optimistically, it is possible to make predictions for the new century given some careful observations of evolving patterns (see Exhibit 3.6).

KEY POINTS

1. The complexity of our human problems demands a social model for the delivery of health services, accepting the fact that health care, housing, education, workplace safety, and a host of other concerns interrelate in the search for quality of life and vie for the same resources.

2. Health care and its support systems exist within a cultural context and it becomes dangerous to impose an alien value system.

3. We are entering a period of social stabilization; social structures may not look the same, but there is a recommitment to traditional values.

4. In the U.S., demographics are our destiny; we are faced with an aging and chronically ill population.

5. Our most prominent health problems could be significantly reduced through more healthy living—diet, weight, exercise, stress reduction, rest.

6. No cure has been found for HIV/AIDS, but massive strides in managing the disease make a long and productive life possible.

Exhibit 3.6 Predictions for Health Care in a New Century

- Hospitals will continue to shrink, essentially becoming giant intensive care units
- Technology will have a dramatic impact:
  More accurate diagnoses
  Treatment based on history of effectiveness
  Less invasive procedures
  Genetic screening and engineering
- Ethical dilemmas associated with cost, quality, access, and use of certain technology will escalate
- There will be universal access to a minimum standard of health care through increased governmental programs for the poor, near poor, unemployed, and underserved
- There will be decreased federal control over health care with increased state involvement
- A two-tiered health care system will be even more apparent
- The medical domination of the delivery system will wane
- Personal responsibility for health care will grow and include over-the-counter diagnostics and therapeutics, Internet information sources, and self-help groups
- There will be industry emphasis on primary care, health promotion, and a basic standard of quality
- Consumers, even the poor, will have control over their health care choices; marketing will become critical and consumer satisfaction will become a major ingredient for success

- There will be increased concern over the effects of environment on health
- The decisive movement toward community-based integrated services will continue
- Alternative treatment for illness will challenge traditional medicine: behavioral and holistic medicine, biofeedback, meditation, acupuncture, homeopathy, therapeutic touch, herbal remedies, and more
- Disputes among health care providers about overlapping roles will create public intolerance of turf battles
- There will be better understanding of the relationship between cost and quality or value
- The age for Medicare eligibility will be raised, and a means test will be instituted for benefits (the well-to-do will get less)
- The public will demand guarantees of continued competency from provider professionals
- Dominance of the health care industry by managed care will escalate, but consumers will find it possible to work within that system and government will increase consumer protection
- There will be more private/public sector partnerships in delivering services, administering plans, and every other conceivable dimension of health care

7. A nation's health is often judged in terms of its infants and children. Despite recent efforts, America's children are still significantly needy.

8. The declining presence of the traditional family in this culture demands the creation of new services, programs, and public policy.

9. A fragile environment requires we take every precaution to prevent its further deterioration.

10. "High tech" advances will not stop, but must be counterbalanced by a conscious and generous dose of caring and humanism.

11. Nurses stand at the center of an information-rich environment, a most strategic position for the twenty-first century.

12. Americans are demanding personal expression in their work, hours that complement a private life, and participation in decisions that impact the quality of their workplace.

13. Suspicion of our most basic institutions has moved us to demand more accountability from professionals.
14. Americans are returning to self-reliance after a crippling period of dependence on institutions and government to make our decisions and do our bidding.
15. We are in a period of active consumerism, that will only intensify as Internet information increases in quality.
16. Health care is big business and the PPS system allows disbursement according to the needs of the recipient of care.
17. Health care services have moved into the community, and consumers are looking to complementary medicine and alternate providers as good options.
18. Integrated systems of health care delivery and continuity are not options, but necessary to maximize resources and decrease consumer frustration.
19. Health manpower needs are seldom predicted accurately, with a resulting cycle of shortage and oversupply.
20. Many of the common issues that concern health care providers are related to competition—the desire of some to expand their scope of practice and others to hold on to their territory
21. The public is demanding proof of competency from provider professionals, so credentials are taking on new importance and meaning.
22. Even if Americans have to live with less, they will never give up their right to choose.

STUDY QUESTIONS

1. The U.S. is no longer a cultural melting pot. Interpret that statement, and identify the implications for health care and nursing.
2. What are the implications for health care in the changing characteristics of the American family?
3. What changes would you make in the workplace to increase the job satisfaction and organizational commitment of generation-X employees?
4. Explain changes in the prognosis for people with HIV/AIDS, and the implications this holds for society.
5. What would you do to enhance the health and welfare of America's children?
6. What are the issues out of the women's movement that have particular significance to nursing, and why?
7. Identify the ways in which you practice self-care.
8. Describe the changes which you can predict for the U.S. delivery system in the next decade.

9. Discuss opportunities for upward mobility within health care occupations.

REFERENCES

1. Kovner A. *Health Care Delivery in the United States*, 5th ed. New York: Springer, 1995, p 39.
2. U.S. Census Bureau: http://www.census.gov/population/www/popclockus.html. Accessed February 1, 2005.
3. U.S. Census Bureau: http://www.census.gov/population/www/projections/popproj.html. Accessed January 20, 2005.
4. Ibid.
5. The Hispanic Population in the United States: http://www.census.gov/prod/2003pubs/p20-545/pdf. Retrieved January 20, 2005.
6. U.S. Census Bureau: http://www.census.gov/popest/national/asrh. Retrieved February 13, 2004.
7. Marshall RT. Nursing Home Issues: http://www.elderweb.com. Retrieved August 15, 2000.
8. Howe N, Strauss B. *13th Generation: Abort, Retry, Ignore, Fail?* New York: Vintage Books, 1993.
9. Cordeniz J. Recruitment, retention and management of generation X: a focus on nursing professionals, *J Healthcare Mgmt* 47(4), 237–245, 2002.
10. Northwestern University. Faces of the New Millenium: http://pubweb.acns.nwu.edu. Retrieved May 28, 2002.
11. U.S. Department of Commerce. *Department of Commerce News*. July 12, 2000.
12. Casper L, Bryson K. *Household and Family Characteristics*. Washington, DC: U.S. Department of Commerce, March 1998.
13. The March of Dimes. Multiples: Twins, Triplets and Beyond: http://www.marchofdimes.com/professionals/681_4545.asp. Retrieved February 7, 2005.
14. Children's Defense Fund: http://www.childrensdefense.org/familyincome/childsupport/default.asp. Retrieved February 4, 2005.
15. Women's pay suffers a setback. *USA Today*: http://www.usatoday.com/money/workplace/2004-08-26-women_x.htm. Retrieved August 26, 2004.
16. The Alan Guttmacher Institute: http://www.guttmacher.org/media, October 8, 2002. Retrieved February 15, 2005.
17. O'Hare WP. Trends in the Well-Being of America's Children. Population Reference Bureau: http://www.prb.org/Template.cfm?Section=PRB&template=/ContentManagement/ContentDisplay.cfm&ContentID=12039. Retrieved February 10, 2005.
18. Engelhardt G, Gruber J. *Social Security and the Evolution of Elderly Poverty*. Working Paper w10466. Washington, DC: National Bureau of Economic Research, issued May 2004.
19. Administration on Aging: http://www.aoa.gov/press/did_you_know/2003/april.asp. Retrieved January 25, 2005.

20. U.S. Census Bureau. Income and Poverty Status of Americans Improve, Health Insurance Coverage Stable, Census Bureau Reports: http://www.census.gov. Retrieved April 10, 2002.
21. Homelessness: Programs and the People They Serve: http://www.huduser.org/publications/homeless/homelessness/content.html. Retrieved June 17, 2002.
22. U.S. Public Health Service. *Promoting Health/Preventing Disease: Objectives for the Nation*. Washington, DC: U.S. Department of Health and Human Services, 1980.
23. U.S. Public Health Service. *Healthy People 2000*. Washington, DC: U.S. Department of Health and Human Services, 1990.
24. U.S. Public Health Service. *Laying the Foundation for Healthy People 2010—The First Year of Consultation*. Washington, DC: U.S. Department of Health and Human Services, 1999.
25. National Center for Health Statistics: http://www.cdc.gov/nchs/data/dvs. Retrieved February 14, 2005.
26. American Cancer Society. Cancer Facts and Figures 2002: http://www.cancer.org/statistics/cff2002/. Retrieved February 14, 2005.
27. Anderson GF. Physician, public, and policymaker perspectives on chronic conditions. *Arch Intern Med.* 163:437–442, 2003.
28. United States AIDS and HIV Statistical Summary: http:www.avert.org//statsum.htm. Retrieved February 15, 2005.
29. Ibid.
30. Children's Defense Fund: http://www.childrensdefense.org/data. Retrieved February 15, 2005.
31. The National Campaign to Prevent Teen Pregnancy: http://www.teenpregnancy.org/resources/data/genlfact.asp. Retrieved February 16, 2005.
32. Centers for Disease Control and Prevention. Trends in sexual risk behaviors among high school students—United States, 1991–1997. *MMRW* 47(36): 749–752, 1998.
33. Resnick NM, et al. Protecting adolescents from harm: Findings from the National Longitudinal Study on Adolescent Health. *JAMA* 278(10):823–832, 1997.
34. The Chronicle of Higher Education. The Nation: http://chronicle.com/free/almanac/2001. Retrieved June 20, 2002.
35. Vance C, et al. An uneasy alliance: Nursing and the woman's movement. *Nurs Outlook* 33:281–285, November–December 1985.
36. Christy T. Liberation movement: Impact on nursing. *AORN* 15:67–68, April 1972.
37. National Organization for Women. Resolved: The Pursuit of Feminist Ideals is Detrimental to the Achievement of Gender Equality, November 11, 1995: http://www.now.org/history/debate.html. Retrieved November 1, 2002.
38. United Nations: The Nairobi forward looking strategies for the advancement of women (as adopted by the World Conference to Review and Appraise the Achievement of the United Nations Decade for Women and Equality). *Development and Peace*, Nairobi, Kenya, July 1985, 15:26.

39. NGO Working Group on Girls. *Clearing a Path for Girls*. New York/Geneva: UNICEF, 1998.

40. U.S. Department of Labor, Bureau of Labor Statistics: http://www.bls.gov/news.release/union2.nr0.htm. Retrieved July 1, 2002.

41. The Patient's Bill of Rights, July 25, 2001: http://thomas.loc.gov/cgi-bin/query. Retrieved June 20, 2002.

42. *USA Today*, February 12, 2004.

43. DRGs as a Framework for Structural Reform in the Hospital: http://healthcare.siemens.com. Retrieved February 10, 2005.

44. Hospitals Facing Financial Headaches: http://www.lao.cagov/analysis_2002/health_ss. Retrieved February 10, 2005.

45. Quality Improvement Organizations: http://www.cms.hhs.gov/qio/4.asp. December 8, 2004. Retrieved February 15, 2005.

46. Joel LA. *Kelly's Dimensions of Professional Nursing*. New York: McGraw-Hill, 2003, p 140.

47. Lewin L. Self care: Towards fundamental changes in national strategies. *Int J Health Ed* 24:219–228, 1991.

48. Hafner K. Can the internet cure the common cold? *New York Times*, July 9, 1998, G1, G11.

49. Brody J. Alternate medicine makes inroads, but watch out for the curves. *New York Times*, April 28, 1998, p A3.

50. Institute of Medicine. *Dietary Supplements: A Framework for Evaluating Safety*. Washington, DC: The Institute, 2004.

51. Brody J. Americans gamble on herbs as medicine. *New York Times*, February 9, 1999, pp F1, F7.

52. Sultz H, Young K. *Health Care USA*, 3d ed. Gaithersburg, MD: Aspen, 2001.

53. Basic Statistics about Home Care: http://nahc.hcstats.html. Retrieved February 15, 2005.

54. Ibid.

55. American Academy of Physician Assistants. Facts at a Glance: http://www.aapa.org/glance.html. Retrieved June 20, 2002.

56. Ibid.

57. Ibid.

58. U.S. Department of Health and Human Services. *Health Personnel in the United States: Report to the Congress*. Washington, DC: The Department, 1993, p 27.

Updates can be found at

 http://www.JoelTheNursingExperience.com

Chapter 4

The Discipline of Nursing

OBJECTIVES

After studying this chapter, you will be able to:

1. Give a definition of nursing that is based on your beliefs.
2. Identify the essential qualities for a field of work to be considered a profession.
3. List nursing functions common to all nurses.
4. Describe the nursing process, nursing diagnosis, and classifications for interventions and outcomes.
5. Name five major nursing theorists.
6. Describe how today's image of nursing differs from the reality and how it might be accurate.

THE NEW–OLD QUESTION: WHAT IS NURSING?

If asked what a nurse does, probably most people entering nursing would, like the general public, say "Take care of the sick." That is a common dictionary definition, a common media image, and a large part of reality. That nurses do health teaching and want to keep people well is also part of the reality. So is the fact that they hold nursing positions in education, administration, research, and publication in many settings that are not too different in basic responsibilities from similar jobs in other fields. Also, more are becoming entrepreneurs. Yet the historical orientation of nursing has been one of mother surrogate, of tending and watching over a dependent ward, of a helping person. Perhaps because the caring, helping part of the role is basic to nursing, it is confusing to some that nurses can also be powerful, assertive professionals cutting out a piece of the health care pie for *nursing*, controlled by *nurses*.

Some nurses cherish a traditional image and are uncomfortable as they move into new roles. Others, as they enter this changing field, have more contemporary ideas about what nursing is, without discarding the caring concept, which is seen as the heart of nursing. Thus, there are many interpretations of nursing. Why not? There are many facets to nursing, and perhaps it is not logical or accurate to settle on one point of view. All nurses must eventually determine their own philosophies of nursing, whether or not these are formalized. The public and others outside nursing will probably continue to adopt an image that is nurtured by contact, hearsay, or media representations of the profession. The first may be the most powerful influence. This chapter presents an overview of the components of nursing, the theory, the image, and the reality.

PROFESSIONS AND PROFESSIONALISM

An ongoing debate centers on whether or not nursing as a whole is an occupation, rather than a profession, in the same sense that medicine, theology, and law have been called professions since the Middle Ages. The classic work on the topic was done in a 1915 study of medicine by Flexner.[1] Flexner proposed six criteria, characterizing professions as: intellectual, possessing an expanding body of knowledge, unique and socially necessary, taught through a system of professional education as opposed to an apprenticeship, internally organized in a manner which allows peer accountability and independence, and motivated through altruism. These statements ring just as true today as they did some 85 years ago, but they must be reinterpreted for contemporary use. Later scholars have added their own perspectives and enriched our understanding.[2–5] In total, there is little disagreement. Neither is there any profession, even the most historically recognized, that can claim to be untouched by our changing times. Synthesizing the best of thinking on the topic, professions are distinguished by the following qualities:

1. A profession utilizes in its practice a well-defined and well-organized body of knowledge that is intellectual in nature and describes its phenomena of concern.

2. A profession constantly enlarges the body of knowledge it uses and subsequently imposes on its members the life-long obligation to remain current in order to "do no harm."

3. A profession entrusts the education of its practitioners to institutions of higher education.

4. A profession applies its body of knowledge in practical services that are vital to human welfare, and especially suited to the tradition of seasoned practitioners shaping the skills of newcomers to the role.

5. A profession functions autonomously (with authority) in the formulation of professional policy and in the monitoring of its practice and practitioners.

6. A profession is guided by a code of ethics which regulates the relationship between professional and client.

7. A profession is distinguished by the presence of a specific culture, norms, and values that are common among its members.

8. A profession has a clear standard of educational preparation for entry into practice.

9. A profession attracts individuals of intellectual and personal qualities who exalt service above personal gain and who recognize their chosen occupation as a life's work.

10. A profession strives to compensate its practitioners by providing freedom of action, opportunity for continuous professional growth, and economic security

It has also been popular to use the term *semiprofession*, with the implication that there are steps that a group must go through to become professional. Caplow[6] describes a first step as the formation of a membership organization with explicit criteria for belonging. The name of the area of work is changed to create a new identity and begin to stake-off both the title and the area of service. A code of ethics comes next and the lobbying to secure legal recognition which eventually makes licensure mandatory. During this same period, education for the profession is being either directly or indirectly upgraded by the professional society. This scenario is highly descriptive of nursing. Each of the state nurses associations (the state affiliate of the ANA) was established for the express purpose of seeking regulation of nursing practice through licensure and title protection. The battle to increase nursing's presence in health care (for the public good) is the continuing governmental agenda: more nurses in nursing homes, direct access to nurses by the public without the physician's approval, the right to have nurses do school physicals. These are but a few examples. The *Code of Ethics* was completed in 1950. The ANA has been vigorously lobbying the profession since 1965 to standardize our system of education. All of these things will be discussed in more detail in subsequent chapters.

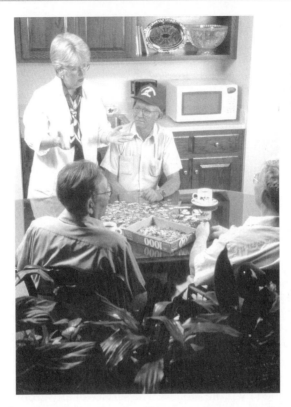

Professions change with the times, and nursing is no exception. The nurse's presence in a domiciliary or boarding home is not unusual. (*Courtesy of the U.S. Department of Veterans Affairs*)

Looking objectively at the criteria associated with the professions, nursing does not fulfill all of them. It has been pointed out that nursing's theory base is still developing, the public does not always see the nurse as a professional, not all nurses are educated in institutions of higher learning, not all nurses consider nursing a lifetime career, and in many practice settings, nursing does not control its own policies and activities. This lack of autonomy is considered the most serious weakness. Sociologists have long contended that an occupation has not become a profession unless the members of that occupation are the ones who make the final decisions about the services they provide.

The public expects that the professions will establish standards and monitor the practice of their own members. This is a courtesy given to experts in a complex area of work who exercise unquestioned integrity and respect the client–provider relationship above all others. This tradition has seriously eroded in recent years. Surveys tell us that Americans have developed a significant suspicion about professionals.

Given this discomfort with individuals who provide very essential services, the public has looked to government for more oversight. Some examples are: consumer presence on professional boards, setting of fee schedules for payment, the development of guidelines for the management of certain disease conditions, the governmental requirement to advise patients of their right to execute a living will.

Autonomy and immunity from governmental intrusion has always been the strongest in areas of specialty practice, where consumers feel least qualified to challenge the judgment of professionals. The credentialing of nurses in advanced or specialty practice, which is now in existence in all states and territories, is both an example of eroding autonomy and a cue that we are arriving too late to apply traditional models.[7]

Declining autonomy may well be associated with the changing client–provider relationship. For nurses that relationship is further challenged by a U.S. Supreme Court decision of May 1994.[8] In that opinion, the court creates the potential for any nurse who supervises assistive personnel to be considered management. This could rob nurses of their employee protections and of the autonomy that has enabled them to be patient advocates first and employees second. These critical incidents provide beginning evidence to cause us to rethink or at least reinterpret our criteria for professionalism.

A second point of debate is associated with the uniqueness of the services provided by professionals. The service of any group of providers must be timely, relevant, and offered with an appreciation of what each discipline can contribute. Resistance to change and refusal to move with the times is not only counterproductive but a violation of the public trust. The very public and negative response of physicians to the role of nurses as primary care providers is one example.

In recent years, there has been progress in both achieving autonomy and, perhaps more important, nurses' recognition that this is important to both the profession and to themselves in terms of how they practice. This mental turnaround has something to do with the fact that more nurses are seeking higher education and that more are planning nursing careers as opposed to taking nursing jobs. Nurses are also becoming more aggressive about getting recognition for what they *have* accomplished. Both nurses and others are convinced that the fact that nursing is predominantly female is also a factor in why nurses have had difficulty achieving high professional status. If nursing is not considered a profession in the strictest sense of the word, it is well on the way to becoming so.

Never forget that the term *profession* is essentially a social concept and has no meaning apart from the society it serves. That society observes a need, and awards individuals who will meet that need special privileges.

The expectation is that these individuals will honor that obligation, constantly reexamining and scrutinizing their functions for the best practice, and always maintaining competence. When they fail to honor these obligations and/or assume an overbearing and demanding attitude in areas that have no connection with their work, society may reconsider whether its trust was well placed.

Violation of this agreement eventually brings retribution from society, as seen today in the tightening of laws regulating professional practice and payment for services. Certain behaviors, such as unprofessional conduct, may be specifically punished by removal of the practitioner's legal right to practice—licensure (see Chapter 11).

The stereotype of idealized professionals who are guaranteed economic security by the public in exchange for a lifetime of dedicated service to their work is a rarity. This does not make these individuals any less, but only a product of their times. First, economic security is a relative term and open to a range of definitions. No group will be guaranteed income, most especially those in the health care field, as we move into models of managed care with providers as employees more commonly than as entrepreneurs. Perhaps even more telling is the trend for members of the American workforce to demand more personal and private time. More Americans are also enjoying the opportunity to change careers or at least enjoy some variety in their work life. Mid-life and later-life career changes are not rare, and the professions are not immune to these trends. Further collective bargaining, unionism, and strikes, once seen as unprofessional, have been gradually accepted as legitimate activities by professionals who are employed. One of today's challenges is for the professional employee to distinguish obligations as an employee from those as a professional.

So the debate continues, and we are lost in a sea of confusion over whether we have achieved some degree of professionalism. The danger lies in taking too much time to decide who we are, while much work remains to be done. In these changing times, the qualities of professionalism are being redefined. Rather than taking our cues from tradition, we may be better served by looking internally. Establish our own standard, herald our uniqueness, look to the public need and our own sense of purpose. There was a time when nurses never doubted their professionalism. Do we have more time to flail at windmills today?

WHAT DO NURSES DO???

Causing almost as much disagreement as the question of whether nursing is a profession is "How do you define nursing?" Definitions of

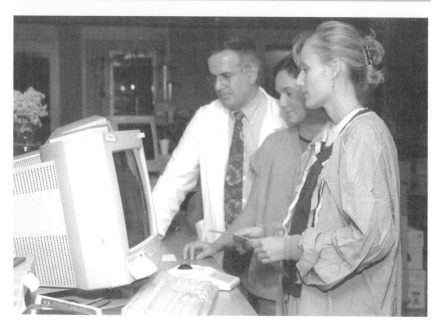

Multidisciplinary collaboration is an expected part of nursing practice. (*Courtesy of Beth Israel Deaconess Medical Center, Boston, Massachusetts*)

nursing vary according to the philosophy of an individual or group. And how people see the roles and functions of nursing is based on what they think nursing is. Exhibit 4.1 gives an overview of some of the best-known definitions. Most nurses would probably accept any of these in principle, although they might argue that some are more ideal than real. In the ANA position paper of 1965, the concepts *care, cure*, and *coordination* were part of a definition of *professional practice*, and have since become commonly associated with nursing.

As nurses expanded their functions into the nurse practitioner (NP) role, *cure* acquired a new meaning. Advanced practice nurses, including NPs, assumed responsibility for the diagnosis and treatment of medical conditions. Some nurses were adamant that medical (not nursing) diagnosis and treatment diminished the role of the nurse as nurse. In reality, the social contract described in the previous section requires role readjustment as the times change. Many of these same individuals opposed the title of nurse practitioner. Ford, a pioneer of the NP movement, immediately responded, calling this "semantic roulette" and added, "I'm not so concerned about the words. I'm convinced that nursing can take on that level of accountability of professional practice that involves the consumer in decision making in his care and also

Exhibit 4.1 Definitions of Nursing by Nurses

- "(to have) charge of the personal health of somebody...and what nursing has to do...is to put the patient in the best condition for nature to act upon him." (Florence Nightingale, 1859)

- Nursing in its broadest sense may be defined as an art and science which involves the whole patient—body, mind, and spirit; promotes his spiritual, mental, and physical health by teaching and by example; stresses health education and health preservation as well as ministration to the sick; involves the care of the patient's environment—social and spiritual as well as physical; and gives health services to the family and the community as well as to the individual. (Sister M. Olivia Gowan, 1944)

- The unique function of the nurse is to assist the individual, sick or well, in the performance of those activities contributing to health or its recovery (or to peaceful death) that he would perform unaided if he had the necessary strength, will, or knowledge; and to do this in such a way as to help him gain independence as rapidly as possible. This aspect of her work, this part of her function, she initiates and controls; of this she is master. In addition she helps the patient to carry out the therapeutic plan as initiated by the physician. She also, as a member of a medical team, helps other members, as they in turn help her, to plan and carry out the total program whether it be for the improvement of health or the recovery from illness or support in death. (Virginia Henderson, 1961)

- ...to facilitate the efforts of the individual to overcome the obstacles which currently interfere with his ability to respond capably to demands made of him by his condition, environment, situation and time. (Ernestine Wiedenbach, 1964)

- The essential components of professional nursing are care, cure, and coordination. (ANA Position Paper, 1965)

- Nursing's first line of defense is promotion of health and prevention of illness. Care of the sick is resorted to when our first line of defense fails. (Martha Rogers, 1966)

- Nursing is the diagnosis and treatment of human responses to actual or potential health problems. (New York State Nurse Practice Act, 1972)

- The first level nurse is responsible for planning, providing, and evaluating nursing care in all settings for the promotion of health, prevention of illness, care of the sick, and rehabilitation; and functions as a member of the health team. (International Council of Nursing, 1973)

- Nursing is an essential service to all of mankind. That service can be succinctly described in terms of its focus, goal, jurisdiction, and outcomes as that of assessing and enhancing the general health status, health assets, and health potentials of all human beings. (Rozella Schlotfeldt, 1978)

- A service of deliberately selected and performed actions to assist individuals to maintain self-care, including structural integrity, functioning and development. (Dorothea Orem, 1980)

- The "Practice of Nursing" means assisting individuals or groups to maintain or attain optimal health, implementing a strategy of care to accomplish defined goals, and evaluating responses to care and treatment. (Model Practice Act, National Council of State Boards of Nursing, 1994)

demands sophisticated clinical judgment to determine levels of illness and wellness and design a plan of management."[9]

Coordination and integration of the therapeutic regimen have historically been the province of nursing. We did it in the home and in the community within our early models of practice, and took these traditions into hospitals. Our 24-hour presence and holistic philosophy suited us well to this responsibility. Active coordination on behalf of our patients has always been a nursing hallmark and is more critical today as nurses are often the only human link between patients and an intimidating experience in the health care delivery system.

The day-to-day practice of nursing is shaped by legal, professional, and institutional definitions. Each may be different. Consistency one to the other is a goal. The institutional definition will most likely be incorporated in the introductory paragraph of your job description. The professional and legal definitions are promulgated by the ANA and the National Council of State Boards of Nursing (NCSBN), respectively. However, the ultimate decision on the legal definition and interpretations of that definition is the work of each State Board of Nursing. For the purpose of this section it is interesting to note the evolution of our professional definitions over the years, especially if we expect the profession's definition, in the true spirit of autonomy, directly or indirectly to drive practice. The 1965 definition was bold in its incorporation of the concepts "cure, care and coordination," but risked the ire of those opposed to any repositioning of the boundaries between professions. In the early 1970s, nursing was defined as "...the diagnosis and treatment of human responses to actual or potential health problems." The somewhat obscure definition made what we do less than totally clear to some nurses, and totally confusing to nonnurses.

The intervening years have rewarded us with more internal solidarity and the consequent ability to be flexible and live with uncertainty. The boundaries between professions will shift, with those things that were the exclusive domain of one group becoming the day-to-day work of another. To accommodate a rapidly changing world of practice, the 2003 revision of *Nursing's Social Policy Statement* avoids a precise definition of nursing, but cautions that "...nursing [has] been influenced by a greater elaboration of the science of caring and its integration with the traditional knowledge base for diagnosis and treatment of human responses to health and illness."[10] Given this environment, ANA does not offer any specific definition, but observes that definitions of nursing increasingly acknowledge four essential features of current practice:

1. Attention to the full range of human experiences and responses to health and illness without restriction to a problem-focused orientation.
2. Integration of objective data with knowledge gained from an understanding of the patient or group's subjective experience.
3. Application of scientific knowledge to the processes of diagnosis and treatment.
4. Provision of a caring relationship that facilitates health and healing.[11]

These statements allow flexibility and confer many liberties. They:

- Remove any restriction to a problem-focused relationship (nursing may be intervening in a good situation to make it better).
- Recognize subjective experience as a valid source of information on which to design care (a critical admission as we enter a multi-cultural era, and additionally open the door to give credibility to intuition as a quality in nursing practice).
- Use language which returns the profession to a recognition of our caring relationship, and link that caring to outcomes, building a case for a science of caring.
- Talk of diagnosis and treatment without the modifier "nursing," thereby recognizing that as we bridge the boundaries of other professions, new role functions are not only valid, but also required.

As a class, all of these definitions (personal, professional, legal) portray nursing as a comprehensive, holistic health service working to empower patients on their own behalf through teaching, counseling, surveillance of physical and mental status, intimate personal care, coordination of their health care experience, and participation in interdisciplinary practice. The most recent renditions infer diagnosis and treatment of illness, and remind us that we are also responsible for the environment in which we practice, including the performance of personnel who assist with nursing activities.

The degree of expertise with which a nurse carries out these functions depends on his or her level of knowledge and skills, but the profession has the responsibility of setting standards for its practitioners. In its 2004 revision of *Nursing: Scope and Standards of Practice*, the ANA continues to distinguish between Standards of Care (patient/client centered), a competent level of care as demonstrated by the nursing process, and Standards of Professional Performance (provider centered), a competent level of behavior in the professional role.[12] These standards serve as the basis for specialty standards as they are developed or updated and are recognized by 33 specialty associations.

THE NURSING PROCESS AND CLASSIFICATION SYSTEMS

The term *nursing process* was not prevalent in the nursing literature until the mid-1960s, with limited mention in the 1950s. Orlando was one of the earliest authors to use the term,[13] but it was slow to be adopted.

In the next few years, models of the activities in which nurses engaged were developed, and in 1967, a faculty group at the Catholic University of America specifically identified the phases of the nursing process as assessing, planning, implementing, and evaluating. In fact, the nursing process adheres to the steps in logical thinking or problem solving. The fact that it is used in nursing has gained it the label of the nursing process.

At this point, there is considerable information in the nursing literature about the use of the nursing process, and many schools of nursing use it as a framework for teaching. However, there are those who feel that other approaches are more suitable to today's complex care. More specifically, we are not proposing the abandonment of logical thought, but to incorporate in our educational systems and practice the most cutting edge of cognitive techniques. It would benefit nursing to look at recent work in critical thinking, diagnostic reasoning, and skill acquisition.

After 30 years of pioneering efforts, NANDA International (the North Atlantic Nursing Diagnosis Association) has succeeded in generating a scientifically based and tested classification system. This classification system or taxonomy is a collection of labels that represent conditions which nurses are licensed to treat. The NANDA system has gained broad acceptance in the profession.[14] Additionally, NANDA has entered into a formal arrangement with the International Council of Nurses (ICN) which solidly moves them into the work of the international classification of nursing practice. A *nursing diagnosis* is:

> a clinical judgment about individual, family or community responses to actual and potential health problems/life processes. Nursing diagnoses provide the basis for selection of nursing interventions to achieve outcomes for which the nurse is accountable.[15]

This definition establishes diagnosis as the linchpin in the diagnosis, intervention, outcome triad. There are currently 172 diagnoses, organized under nine broad categories; each diagnosis includes the label itself, a definition, defining characteristics, and related factors. Because the process of developing, validating, and reaching consensus on a diagnosis has evolved over time, not all the diagnoses are developed to the same extent. Some diagnoses have major and minor defining characteristics, major being the indicators that are present in 80–100 percent of clients with the diagnosis, and minor appearing in 50–79 percent of situations. Exhibit 4.2 presents one diagnosis.

The *Nursing Intervention Classification* (NIC) and the *Nursing Outcome Classification* (NOC) are of more recent origin and the products of the Center for Nursing Classification at the University of Iowa College of Nursing which has excelled in this work under the leadership of Joanne McCloskey Dochterman and Gloria Bulechek. Both NIC and NOC are organized at the broadest level of abstraction into six domains. These

Exhibit 4.2 Example of a Nursing Diagnosis

Coping, ineffective individual

Definition: A state in which the individual experiences, or is at risk of experiencing, an inability to manage internal or environmental stressors adequately due to inadequate physical, psychological, behavioral, and/or cognitive resources.

Defining Characteristics: **Major (one must be present)**: Verbalization of inability to cope or ask for help, inappropriate use of defense mechanisms, inability to meet role expectations. **Minor (may be present)**: Chronic worry, anxiety, alteration in social participation, high incidence of accidents, frequent illness, destructive behavior toward self or others, verbal manipulation; inability to meet basic needs, nonassertive response patterns, change in usual communication patterns, substance abuse. **Related factors**: May be pathophysiological, treatment-related, situational, maturational. **Diagnostic errors**: More appropriate as a diagnosis with prolonged or chronic coping problems. Overwhelming acute stress may be a *grieving response* or *impaired adjustment*. Cultural variations are particularly important to consider here. **Differential Diagnosis**: *Defensive coping, ineffective denial.*

Adapted from Vincent KG. The validation of a nursing diagnosis. *Nursing Clinics of North America*, 20:631–639, 1985.
Carpenito LJ. *Nursing Diagnosis: Application to Clinical Practice*, 9th ed. Philadelphia: Lippincott, 2003.

domains are subdivided into 24–27 classes or categories, under which 330 outcomes or 514 interventions cluster.[16,17] Though the domains are slightly different one classification to the other, each gives credibility to the holistic orientation of nursing. Each NOC outcome is accompanied by a 5-point scale to measure patient status for each of the indicators and subsequently for the outcome as a whole.

None of these systems will ever be complete. They will continue to evolve with the growing sophistication of nursing science. Examples from NIC and NOC are presented in Exhibits 4.3 and 4.4. NANDA diagnoses and NIC are labels, while NOC incorporates the capacity to indicate the direction and extent of change in the patient's condition. Students are referred to the primary works on diagnosis, intervention, and outcomes, and to the websites included at the end of this chapter, both to understand their own practice better and to appreciate the precision with which nursing treats its stewardship to the public.

Such a monumental work is not without its critics. It will remain to be seen whether these classification systems are a strategy to bring us to maturity as a profession, or a sign of our maturity. The trends in health care restructuring move us toward interdisciplinary practice. Should our language also reflect a unity of practice? There are others who believe that our own classifications are requisite for autonomy, and must be well developed before any move to a consolidated language.

In the late 1980s, the ANA initiated an era dedicated to recognition of the work nurses do as reflected in their classification systems. The

Exhibit 4.3 Nursing Interventions Classification (NIC)—Example of a Nursing Intervention

Coping enhancement
Definition: Assisting a patient to adapt to perceived stressors, changes, or threats which interfere with meeting life demands and roles.
Activities: (abridged, 51 activities proposed in primary source)
Appraise impact of patient's life situation on roles and relationships
Appraise patient's adjustment to body image, as indicated
Encourage patient to identify a realistic description of change in role
Appraise and discuss alternative responses to situation
Encourage verbalization of feelings, perceptions, and fears
Assist the patient to break down goals into small manageable steps
Encourage patient to identify own strengths and abilities
Evaluate patient's decision-making ability
Encourage relationships with persons who have common interests and goals
Arrange situations that encourage autonomy
Explore patient's previous achievements of success
Explore with the patient previous methods of dealing with life problems
Explore patient's reasons for self-criticism
Foster constructive outlets for anger and hostility
Encourage the identification of specific life values
Support the use of appropriate defense mechanisms
Appraise patient's need/desire for social support

Adapted from Dochterman J, Bulechek G (eds.). *Nursing Interventions Classification (NIC)*, 4th ed. Mosby, 2004, with permission from Elsevier.

diagnostic labels of NANDA, NIC, and NOC were accepted by the National Library of Medicine. A formal appeal to the World Health Organization asked for the NANDA classification to be included in the next revision of the International Classification of Diseases (ICD). This request was denied, based on the opinion that this language was not internationally useful, understandable, or relevant. Rejection provided the challenge to claim our practice internationally. The need to move nursing out of the shadows and formalize our presence proved to be a common cause which transcended national borders. Though Americans contributed the most advanced work in this area, they were not alone. There had been significant progress in other countries. Profiting from the mistakes of others and generous funding from the Kellogg Foundation, this international project was able to proceed more logically and strategically.

An international constituency presented new problems. There was a need to search for the most agreeable language if these labels were to be useful, and to avoid any negative cultural connotations. There was common agreement that the language must originate at the bedside. Local area work in Europe, South America, Asia, and Africa has allowed

Exhibit 4.4 Nursing Outcomes Classification (NOC)—Example of a Nursing Outcome

COPING

Definition: Actions to manage stressors that tax an individual's resources

Indicators of coping (abridged, 18 indicators in full scale)	Never demonstrated	Rarely demonstrated	Sometimes demonstrated	Often demonstrated	Consistently demonstrated
Reports decrease in stress	1	2	3	4	5
Verbalizes acceptance of situation	1	3	3	4	5
Uses available social support	1	2	3	4	5
Avoids unduly stressful situations	1	2	3	4	5
Employs behaviors to reduce stress	1	2	3	4	5
Identifies multiple coping strategies	1	2	3	4	5
Reports decrease in physical symptoms of stress	1	2	3	4	5
Reports increase in psychological comfort	1	2	3	4	5

Adapted from Moorhead S, Johnson M, Maas M. (eds.). *Nursing Outcomes Classification (NOC)*, 3d ed. Mosby, 2004, with permission from Elsevier.

the International Classification of Nursing Practice (ICNP) under the auspices of the International Council of Nurses (ICN) to forge ahead.

In 2005, NANDA and the ICN entered into an agreement that will allow them to join efforts, and proceed with this work in a harmonious rather than competitive fashion.[18]

MAJOR NURSING THEORIES

As nursing has developed in professionalism, nursing scholars have developed theories of nursing based on research, and the science of nursing is coming of age. A scientific body of nursing knowledge is important to provide a basis for clear differentiation between medicine and nursing, on the one hand, and nursing and nurturing on the other.

Research and theory building unique to a discipline are elements required for that discipline to be recognized as a profession.

Although Florence Nightingale identified a body of knowledge specific to the nursing of her time and used this as the basis for instruction in the Nightingale schools, it was not until the 1950s and 1960s that there was a proliferation of nursing concepts and theories. Nursing scholars argued that without research and theory building, nursing would be unable to carve out a role for itself in the future health care system, and would thus allow itself to be defined, instructed, and controlled by other disciplines.

A theory is a system of concepts and relationships that allows nurses to describe, understand, predict, and prescribe in their practice. Theory (for nursing or anything else) can take one of three forms, each with its distinct purpose. There are nursing philosophies or *philosophical theories* that give meaning to situations requiring nursing. This is accomplished through the cognitive skills of analysis, reasoning and often divergent thinking. *Grand theories* are the most comprehensive, able to be applied to the entire domain of nursing, and more properly called models because they are so all-encompassing. *Mid-range theories* are built on the work of supportive sciences (natural, behavioral), earlier nursing theories, or grand theories. Mid-range theories have a narrower focus, are more concrete, and target specific practice questions or patient populations. They are essential to the conduct of research and subsequent development of specialty knowledge. This knowledge will in turn filter down, allowing cutting-edge practice in general nursing and in education for entry into practice.

Each theory for nursing has its own concepts, definitions, and assumptions, and derives from different more basic scientific models or theories. Exhibit 4.5 provides an overview of selected nursing theories which have significantly influenced practice. The common theme of holism and patient/client empowerment through the nurse–patient relationship is noteworthy. Further, each theory is organized around its view of man (human beings), health, society (environment), and nursing. These four concepts are known as the metaparadigm elements, and when defined and viewed as a whole, create an individualized view of nursing.

Exhibit 4.5 is but a limited glimpse of a representative sample of grand, mid-range, and philosophical theories. A concept, definition, or assumption has been chosen for presentation because it shows the distinctiveness of each theorist's work. In some instances, a statement is a very subtle variation on a theme. There are other observations that are even more telling. Chronologically the early theorists were more philosophical, searching to give form and meaning to nursing, and they were successful. In many contemporary situations, we go back to their work for a clarity that has been lost over the years. Later theorists became highly abstract, taking behavioral, systems, and developmental approaches to nursing. For all the difficulty in sometimes translating their work to practice, they have given us credibility as scholars. Swept away as we have been in the allure of high technology and the search for precise scientific explanations for our practice, the humanness of nursing often became lost. Our most recent theorists bring us full circle to our roots, reminding us that health and illness are personal experiences and that nurses serve the public best by their commitment to caring.

ATTITUDES OF NURSES AND ABOUT NURSES

The variety of work in nursing guarantees that all nurses can find an area of practice that complements their personality and style. Those that like fast-paced action and the unpredictable may gravitate toward emergency or trauma. Others who prefer healing the mind and can use their own interpersonal and personal skills to advantage may find most satisfaction in psychiatric nursing. Order and precision are constants in operating room or special care units. Work with substance abusers or AIDS patients requires the ability to be nonjudgmental while refusing to accept antisocial behavior. In fact, every personality and style can find satisfaction within the discipline. The danger is to prejudge a person's suitability for an area of practice.

The last nursing shortage, which came to an abrupt halt in the early 1990s, prompted a series of studies about nurses and their job satisfaction. It became obvious that those factors that were dissatisfying to nurses in their work were not the same as those that created job satisfaction. Nurses were dissatisfied because of low pay and poor working conditions. Job satisfaction hinged on things like status, respect, pride in their work, and career mobility. Whether the technique was a summit meeting of nursing organizations, focus groups, or direct mail survey, nurses have consistently expressed the same priorities. The reason for choosing nursing as a career has not changed over the years. It continues to be a desire to help people and an interest in health care.

These same sentiments have been reiterated by nurses over the decades as they have suffered through surpluses, shortages, restructuring, job redesign, and downsizing. The largest survey of nurses, almost 7500, was conducted by the *American Journal of Nursing* partnering with Boston College in 1996. Job satisfaction was much more closely associated with pride in their work than salary and benefits. Pride in work

(*continued on page 190*)

Exhibit 4.5 Some Nursing Theorists and their Work

Theorist, theory, and date of early work[a]	Concepts/definitions assumptions	Influential models or sciences
Florence Nightingale: Patient/Environment, 1859	• Disease is a reparative process • Rejected germ theory • Imbalance between patient and their physical environment frustrates energy conservation and decreases the capacity for health	Environment/sanitation
Dorothy Johnson: Behavioral Systems Model, 1959	• Seven behavioral subsystems that can be analyzed in terms of structure and function • Structure includes the elements of drive (motivation), set (predisposition to act), choice (behavioral repertoire), and action (behavior) • Functional requirements are protection, nurturance, and stimulation • Attachment, or the affiliation subsystem, is the cornerstone of social organization	Ethological systems
Dorothea Orem: Self-Care Model, 1959	• Constituted from three related theories: self-care, self-care deficit, and nursing systems • People have a need for the provision and management of self-care actions on a continuing basis to sustain life and health and to recover from disease • When an individual's self-care agency is not adequate to their requirement or that of their dependants, deficit is created	Henderson

Nursing role	Theory type	Major contribution
• Manipulation of the external environment, such as ventilation, warmth, light, diet cleanliness, and noise, would contribute to well-being and the reparative process • Patient is relatively passive • Nursing places patients in the best condition for nature to act upon them • Saw nursing role in health as well as illness • Stressed nurses' use of observation	Philosophical	• Pioneered nursing's domain as the patient/environment relationship • Statistical analysis for health and nursing
• Maintain or restore balance and equilibrium, or • Help person achieve a more optimum level of function if possible or desirable	Grand	• Strong philosophical statements related to model • Strong influence on Roy, Neuman, and others
• Self-care deficit is the target of nursing • The nursing system is designed as wholly or partially compensatory or supportive–educative as dictated by the agency of the patient	Grand	• Pragmatic and comfortable concepts

(continued)

Exhibit 4.5 (continued)

Theorist, theory, and date of early work[a]	Concepts/definitions assumptions	Influential models or sciences
Virginia Henderson: Developmental Model, 1961	• The patient is a person who requires help toward independence	Thorndike Rehabilitation principles Orlando Maslow
Ida Jean Orlando: Theory of Deliberative Nursing Process, 1961	• Distinguishes automatic from deliberate action • Perception, thoughts, and feelings are not explored in automatic actions • Deliberate actions yield solutions and prevention of problems	Eclectic
Imogene King: Open Systems Model, 1964	• The dynamic nature of life assumes continuous adjustment of life's stressors • The self is a person's total subjective environment, and is a distinctive center of experience and significance for each • Adjustment entails the three open systems interacting with the environment: personal, individual, and social	Highly eclectic Piaget Erikson Etzioni Bennis (among others)

Nursing role	Theory type	Major contribution
• Acts in the patient's behalf to do those things that they would do for themselves had they the strength, knowledge, or willingness to do so	Philosophical	• Delineates autonomous functions
• Identifies 14 components of basic nursing care corresponding to Maslow's hierarchy of needs		• Stresses goals of interdependence with the patient
• Three levels of nurse–patient relationship: substituting, helping, partnering		• Self-care concepts that influenced later theorists
• Use of empathic understanding		
• Interdependence with other providers		
• A nursing situation consists of patient behavior, nurse reaction, and nursing actions	Mid-range (psychiatric nursing)	• Advanced nursing to a disciplined practice
• Nurse provides assistance to patients to deal with helplessness		
• Physician's orders directed to patient, and nurse helps patient comply or decide not to comply		
• Nursing's goal is to help individuals maintain their health so that they can function in their roles	Grand	• The Theory of Goal Attainment is a product of this model, and describes the nature of the nurse–client encounter
• The nurse enters the situation when the client can no longer perform their usual daily activities, yet . . .		• Emphasis on the derivation of nursing knowledge from other disciplines
• The domain of nursing includes health promotion and maintenance		
• Nursing is a process of human interaction with a patient, based on communication to set goals, and a means for achievement		

(continued)

Exhibit 4.5 (continued)

Theorist, theory, and date of early work[a]	Concepts/definitions assumptions	Influential models or sciences
Myra Levine: Conservation Model, 1966	• Focuses on holism, integrity, and conservation • The life process is characterized by unceasing change that has direction, purpose, and meaning • The organism retains integrity through adaptive capability • Loss of balance causes fear, inflammation, stress, or sensory response	Borrowed from a range of natural and behavioral sciences
Joyce Travelbee: Human-to-Human Relationship, 1966	• The self-actualization aspect of illness is a natural and commonplace life experience • Healing is based on empathy, sympathy, and emotional bonding	Peplau Orlando
Lydia Hall: Core, Care, and Cure Model, 1969 (clinical work dates to 1950s)	• Illness and rehabilitation are learning experiences	Carl Rogers
Martha Rogers: Science of Unitary Man, 1970	• The person is a unified energy field continually interacting and exchanging matter and energy with the environment • This exchange results in increased complexity and innovativeness of the person • Well-being is reflected in pattern and organization	• Systems • Electromagentic theory

Nursing role	Theory type	Major contribution
• The goal of nursing is promotion of wholeness • Nursing intervention provides help in adaptation based on the principles of conservation of energy, and structural, personal, and social integrity	Grand	• Distinctive and extensive vocabulary that makes it complex • Logically consistent and holistic • Great influence on later theorists
• A major goal of nursing is helping the patient find meaning in illness through building a therapeutic mutual relationship	Mid-range (psychiatric nursing)	• Early emphasis on caring
• Stressed the autonomous function of nurses • The nurse guides and teaches in the process of personal care-giving • The nursing role consists of therapeutic use of self (core), the treatment regimen within the health care team (cure), nurturing, and intimate bodily care (care)	Philosophical	• The eventual base for primary nursing • Applied to practice in a large metropolitan setting
• Acts to promote symphonic interaction between man and environment • Achieve maximum health potential by repatterning the human and environmental field	Grand	• Strong voice for the development of nursing as a basic science

(continued)

Exhibit 4.5 (continued)

Theorist, theory, and date of early work[a]	Concepts/definitions assumptions	Influential models or sciences
Sister Callister Roy: Adaptation Model, 1970	• Individual adapts behavior to cope with stimuli from environment that are stressors • Stressors disrupt dynamic state of equilibrium and illness results • Adaptive modes focus on physiological needs, self concept, role function, and interdependent relations • A positive response to stress is determined by whether the stimulation exceeds the level that can be accommodated by the individual	• Systems • Stress • Henson's Adaptation Theory
Betty Neuman: Systems Model, 1972	• Stressors as well as reaction and reconstitution can be viewed as intra-, inter-, and extrapersonal • Each individual has a usual range of responses to stress that maintains equilibrium and is called the normal line of defense • A flexible line of defense also exists to protect against unusual stress • Should stress break through the normal line of defense, lines of resistance attempt to stabilize the situation	• Gestalt theory • Levels of prevention • Systems theory • Stress theory
Jean Watson: Theory of Human Caring, 1979	• Caring is a universal social behavior • Care for the self is necessary before care for others • Care and love are the cornerstones of humanness	Leninger Existential phenomenology
Patricia Benner: Caring, 1984	• Describes caring as a common human bond	Dreyfus Model of Skill Acquisition

[a] As determined by published work.

Nursing role	Theory type	Major contribution
• Nurse assesses the adequacy of the patient's coping, and if needed changes the patient's response potential by holding the stimuli to the point where positive response is possible	Grand	• Excellent example of how knowledge can become unique in nursing; an eclectic view including stress, systems, and adaptation
• Nursing aims at the reduction of stress factors and adverse conditions which threaten optimal functioning in a given situation • This is accomplished by identifying stress factors and assisting individuals to respond by strengthening their normal and flexible lines of defense • Purposeful intervention with a total person approach	Grand	• Potentially useful in a variety of health care disciplines • Produced two separate theories: Optimal Patient Stability and Prevention as Intervention
• Emphasizes the humanistic dimension of nursing which can only be practiced interpersonally	Philosophical	• Makes the humanism in nursing scientific and credible
• Primary focus of the model is nursing • Through a qualitative process describes five stages of competency development: novice, advanced beginner, competent, proficient, and expert • A phenomenological theory describing caring	• Philosophical	• Recognizes the value of experience in a practice discipline • Gives credibility to the role played by intuition in practice

also means pride in patient care: feelings of personal competency, the ability to control the environment on behalf of your patients, and the absence of any "moral compromise."[19] The ethic of nursing has remained constant.

Nurses see their work as stressful, but anticipate the stress and are willing to live with it given a certain modicum of respect and support. The workplace stresses most mentioned by nurses are inadequate staffing, interruptions which keep them from their patients, paperwork, lack of support from peers, unattractive and disorganized work areas, high noise level, lack of supplies, absence of information or directions, no voice in decisions that affect them, lack of respect, conflict between the business orientation of the industry and the service orientation of the profession, and the death of "my" patient. Put eloquently by someone whom I cannot remember: "Nurses love their work, but hate their job."

The changing health care system, the proposal that nurses take on increased responsibility within any restructured system, and most lately the emphasis on consumer satisfaction have prompted a series of consumer surveys that provide some interesting public opinion about nurses.

In 1985, public opinion supported an expanded role for nurses, and identified them as an untapped resource for decreasing the cost of health care. A 1990 survey conducted by Peter Hart Associates funded by the Pew Charitable Trusts found similar public sentiment. The public saw nurses as respected, trustworthy, and underutilized. A poll conducted by the Gallup Organization in 1993 found the public supporting the use of nurses as primary care providers; 86 percent of the respondents would personally use a nurse for these purposes, and over half of the respondents were very willing. A Kellogg Foundation poll in 1994 found that half of their sample had been treated by a nurse practitioner in the last year; and in a Gallup poll of the same year respondents identified reductions in RN staffing as the most dangerous strategy for cutting costs in hospitals.[20] In 1996, motivated by the continued displacement of RNs from hospitals in favor of assistive personnel, the ANA began the public information campaign, "Every Patient Needs a Nurse." That campaign included a survey conducted by the Princeton Survey Research Associates to gage the true opinion of the American public. The public saw nurses as a vital ingredient in hospital care, and were apprehensive about their decreased presence at the bedside. They supported the right of nurses to take action if they observed unsafe conditions, and most were interested in knowing how hospital units were staffed and details about patient satisfaction surveys, morbidity, and infection rates.[21] A 1999 Harris poll commissioned by Sigma Theta Tau showed that an overwhelming majority of the public (92 percent) trusts information about health care coming from nurses as much as that coming from physicians, but most consumers were unaware that nurses prescribe medications and actually make decisions on treatment.[22] In 2004, Gallup's annual survey on the honesty and ethical standards of various professions found nurses again at the top of the list, as they have been in all but one year since they were first added to the poll in 1999.[23] To summarize the public attitude, consumers see nurses as advocates for their health and safety and an untapped resource for the nation's health.

THE MEDIA IMAGE OF NURSING

Set apart from public opinion on nurses as provider professionals is the media image, which often remains as a deadly undercurrent, being laden with all the stereotypes of generations. The thoughtfulness consumers have demonstrated in giving opinion on the value of expanded services delivered by nurses and of the RN as their advocate should eventually filter down and reshape the media image. In order to effect that change, a healthy dose of intolerance is necessary from the profession, and vigilance on our own behalf, to discourage destructive portrayals of the nurse. Though completed in 1987, a multicultural comparison of images of nurses and physicians in 30 geopolitical areas of the world found that "cross-culturally, nurses were viewed as positive, active, and kind, but not associated with power, independence and knowledge." This was in contrast to physicians who were viewed as powerful and strong. Clearly, the image problem is not confined to this country.

Presently, nurses are at a critical stage in changing this image. Periodic shortages have forced organized nursing to admit that nursing's public image can be an obstacle to recruitment. A mindless, subservient image of nurses will hold little attraction for the best and the brightest who are making career choices, and nurses contribute to the perpetuation of dysfunctional stereotypes by our silence.

In response, many organizations and health care professionals have been motivated to take a new look at the image issue. Nursing's mandate with regard to image is to educate the public that nurses make serious decisions about their health, and that a career in nursing requires intellectual talent, stamina, and dedication, but provides rewards commensurate with that investment.

An individual's image of the nurse is highly variable, depending on personal experiences, and when there is no personal experience, the media exerts a powerful influence. Interviews and research articles or news programs generally portray the nurse in a reasonably accurate way, when nursing is singled out to be in the limelight. As a rule, however, in fiction, the media have not, and still do not, correct a distorted image.

Comic strips, novels, and television tend to portray the nurse (almost always female) either as a very sweet and/or sexy young girl who plays obedient handmaiden to the doctor, or as a tough, starched older woman, efficient and brusque. The popularity of medically oriented television series is supposedly a reflection of the public's intense interest in the field, but the images of the nurses portrayed have been notoriously inaccurate, and even nursing advisers to the shows seldom get the script changed. On the screen, Nurse Ratched in the award-winning movie *One Flew Over the Cuckoo's Nest*, which was also a book and a play, was probably thoroughly hated by millions of people.

In the early 1990s, nurses did take a proactive stand against the NBC-TV show, *Nightingales*, which portrayed nurses as well-meaning, if promiscuous, and having no real stake in the care of patients. Nursing organizations and individuals offered to provide script consultation and were turned down. Eventually, the surge of protest against the show from nurses across the country led many of its commercial sponsors to back out, and eventually the show was canceled. Yet not all TV programs portray nurses in a negative manner. *China Beach* managed to depict realistically and sensitively the challenges of nursing during the Vietnam War. Several documentaries on nursing and health care have also been favorable to nurses.

The power of the media and the numerous shows that continue to portray nurses in a negative and unrealistic manner prompted the establishment of a group called Nurses of America (NOA) and their publication, *Media Watch*. NOA was funded by a grant from the Pew Charitable Trusts and administered by the National League for Nursing (NLN). NOA worked with a variety of media, ranging from newspapers and magazines to TV and community forums. A large component of their activities included monitoring the media for health-related issues and the portrayal of nurses and nursing practice, and developing a speaker's bureau of nurses who were media-prepared and had news-worthy stories to tell about their work. Suzanne Gordon provided important leadership for the NOA. She is not a nurse, but a journalist who was astounded at the invisibility of nursing given their powerful impact on the human condition. She has used the power of the pen to bring vivid descriptions of our work to gain public attention. Gordon has continued to be an eloquent spokesperson for nursing. She is our advocate in her most recent book, *Nursing Against the Odds*, describing how health care cost cutting, media stereotypes, and medical hubris undermine nurses and patient care.[24] In an earlier volume, *Life Support*, she shared her observations on the practice of three nurses that she followed for a three-year period. She describes their "tapestry of care" that is woven with such intimacy "... that many would choose to forget the weaver."[25]

This same phenomenon of invisibility is described in the final report of the Woodhull Study on Nursing and the Media, in 1998 completed under the sponsorship of Sigma Theta Tau. Though nurses are a critical mass in health care, the front-line care givers, and trends verify that their roles are critical and expanding, they are relatively invisible to the media.[26]

The best strategy to counter invisibility is visibility, visibility through involvement in community services and organizations, visibility through workplace committee participation, and making every nurse's practice visible to every other nurse. It would benefit the image of the profession if more nurses could converse easily on a wide range of issues, including those of colleagues in areas such as nurse anesthesia, nurse midwifery, occupational health, critical care, and so on.

One of the most widely applauded strategies to improve nursing's image was the advertising campaign launched between 1989 and 1992 by the National Commission on Nursing Implementation Project (NCNIP) and the Advertising Council of New York. The Ad Council guaranteed a minimum of $20 million in creative development and media exposure over a three-year period. The idea was to portray nursing as a "discipline that offers excitement, clinical substance, and authority and responsibility, all tied up in the richness of interpersonal closeness with patients."[27] A more recent event is the Johnson & Johnson Discover Nursing Campaign with much the same purpose.[28]

Obviously, there is no one profile of the modern nurse, particularly in these dynamic times. However, the information obtained from these various studies tells us a great deal about the practitioners of nursing. Resources being allocated to improve the image of nursing have already demonstrated that with work, the image can be changed to one that is more positive and realistic than it has been in the past.

THE REALITY: FACTS, FIGURES, GUESSES

The information we have about the *real* nurse can also cause confusion. Demographic data, such as numbers, age, marital status, and employment, are usually acquired by taking a sample and then projecting to the total number. By the time that these and other facts are published, they may be somewhat outdated. However, by comparing them with earlier data, a trend or a change can be detected. Exhibit 4.6 shows some of the latest information available on nurses. Some of the interesting trends in the employed population over the last years are a slow increase in the number of men and nonwhite nurses, and nurses as a group are getting older. A dramatic drop in the number of nurses with a diploma as the highest credential and an increase in those with associate and baccalaureate degrees reflects educational trends. Hospitals have consistently employed the largest number of nurses, but the percentage is slowly declining. Even though the percentage of NPs and clinical specialists has remained quite small, this category was not even listed before the 1977 surveys.

A NURSING PROFILE

The most current, comprehensive demographic data about nurses is contained in the *National Sample Survey of Registered Nurses,* conducted every four years by the Division of Nursing of the Department of Health and Human Services. The most recent was published in 2000. Exhibit 4.6 summarizes data from the 2000 survey and includes comparisons with 1980, 1988, 1992, and 1996 information. There are easily discernible trends. In March 2000, an estimated 2,696,540 individuals were licensed to practice nursing in this country, 63 percent more than in 1980. This produced a ratio of 782 registered nurses for every 100,000 in population.[29] Though there was a 5.4 percent increase in the total registered nurse population between 1996 and 2000, it was the lowest gain in all of the previous national surveys. The highest increase was between 1992 and 1996, by an estimated 14.2 percent. In 2000, 18.3 percent of RNs reported not being employed in nursing, the most since 20 percent in 1988. Still, almost 82 percent of nurses continued to nurse. No survey has been completed for 2004. The data below is the latest available.

The predominant setting for the employment of nurses continued to be the hospital, but the decline in workforce concentration in this market continued, from 66.5 percent of employed RNs in 1992 to 59.1 percent in 2000. It is interesting to speculate whether this decline is due to fewer hospital beds (1.0 million in 1983 to less than 700,000 in 2000),[30] occupancy rates (73.6 percent in 1983 and 46.3 percent in 2000),[31] or the tendency in some places to substitute nurses aides for RNs as a cost-cutting strategy. The current eagerness in many hospitals to rebuild their nursing staffs could make these numbers look very different in the future.

The health care settings which showed the greatest increase in RN employment were noninstitutional. RN employment in ambulatory and public/community health practice areas has increased almost 100 percent since 1980. It is difficult to determine the exact nature of these numbers since the Division of Nursing has changed these categories in the latest reports. Public/community health settings now include state and local health departments, visiting nursing services, community

Exhibit 4.6 Who Are the Nurses?

	2000	1996	1992	1988	1980
Total RN population employed in nursing[a]	2.7 million 81.7% (about 23.2% part-time)	2.5million 82.7% (about 23.7% part-time)	2.2 million 82.7% (about 25.7% part-time)	2.0 million 80.0% (about 26% part-time)	1.7 million 76.6% (about 24.6% part-time)
Sex					
Female	94.6%	95.1%	96.0%	96.6%	96.1%
Male	5.4%	4.9%	4.0%	3.3%	3.0%
Ethnic-racial background					
White/non-Hispanic	86.6%	89.7%	91.1%	91.7%	90.4%
Black	4.9%	4.2%	4.0%	3.6%	4.3%
Asian/Pacific Islander	3.7%	3.4%	3.4%	2.3%	2.4%
Hispanic	2.0%	1.6%	1.4%	1.3%	1.4%
American Indian/ Alaskan native	0.5%	0.5%	0.4%	0.4%	0.28%
Age					
Under 25	2.5%	2.3%	2.1%	3.9%	9.6%
25–34	15.8%	18.3%	23.6%	29.8%	36.2%
35–44	30.6%	34.4%	34.7%	29.5%	23.3%
45–54	29.9%	25.1%	20.6%	19.1%	17.2%
55–64	14.6%	13.7%	12.7%	12.3%	15.7%
65 or over	5.7%	5.7%	5.6%	5.0%	4.5%
Marital status					
Married	71.5%	72.3%	71.5%	70.6%	70.6%
Divorced/separated/ widowed	17.9%	17.6%	16.5%	15.4%	13.8%
Never married	9.9%	9.8%	11.1%	13.0%	14.8%
Places of employment					
Hospital	59.1%	60.1%	66.5%	67.9%	65.6%
Nursing home	6.9%	8.1%	7.0%	6.6%	8.0%
Community health	12.8%	13.1%	9.7%	6.8%	6.6%
Physician's office/ ambulatory care	9.5%	8.5%	7.8%	7.7%	5.7%[b]
Nursing education	2.1%	2.3%	2.0%	1.8%	3.7%
Student health service	4.7%	3.0%	2.7%	2.9%	3.5%
Occupational health	2.1%	1.0%	1.9%	1.3%	2.3%
Private duty		N/A	0.6%	1.2%	1.6%
Public/community health (includes occupational and school health)	18.2%				
Other	3.6%	3.4%	3.0%	3.6%	1.7%
Type of position					
Staff nurse	60.0%	61.9%	61.6%	66.9%	65.0%
Head nurse/supervisor	8.4%	10.3%	9.6%	10.9%	13.1%
Administration (service and education)	5.7%	5.3%	6.2%	6.6%	4.8%
Instructor	2.1%	3.5%	3.5%	3.8%	4.7%
Clinical specialist/clinician	2.0%	3.1%	1.9%	2.9%	2.1%
Nurse practitioner/midwife	3.6%	2.1%	1.4%	1.5%	1.3%
Nurse anesthetist	1.1%	1.0%	1.0%	1.0%	1.1%

Exhibit 4.6 (continued)

	2000	1996	1992	1988	1980
Nurse practitioner/clinical nurse specialist	0.54%				
Other	16.5%	10.0%	6.5%	6.6%	6.8%
Higher education					
Doctorate	10.2%	0.6%	0.5%	0.3%	0.2%
Master's		9.1%	7.5%	6.2%	5.1%
Bachelors in nursing	32.7%	28.8%	27.3%	25.1%	20.7%
Other bachelors		2.5%	2.6%	2.3%	2.6%
Diploma	22.3%	27.2%	33.7%	40.0%	50.7%
Associate degree	34.3%	31.7%	28.2%	25.2%	20.1%

[a] Data refer to employed nurses. Some figures do not total 100% because of no response and rounding of figures.
[b] Refers to physician's office only.
Source: DHHS Division of Nursing, *National Sample Survey of Registered Nurses*, 1980, 1988, 1992, 1996, 2000.

health centers, student health services, occupational health, and more. Ambulatory care settings are physician-based practices, nurse-based practices, and health maintenance organizations.

The "aging" of the RN population continues. In 2000 the average age of the RN was 45.2, as compared with 40.3 in 1988. In 1980, 52.9 percent of RNs were under the age of 40, as compared to 2000 when less than 32 percent were that age. The most significant drop was among RNs under 35, 40.5 percent in 1980 and 18.3 percent in 2000. In the under-30 category, there was a drop from 25.1 percent in 1980 to only 9.1 percent in 2000. The average age for completing a nursing program in 1985 and earlier was about 24 years old. From 1995 to 2000, the age rose to an average of 30.5 years old. That age varies by program type, with associate degree graduates averaging 33.2 years, diploma at 30.8, and baccalaureate at 27.5 years old. Contributing factors to this "aging" are the fact that associate degree graduates are generally older and an increased proportion of nurses are prepared in these programs. Further, nursing is attractive as a career to young retirees looking for a career change, individuals with prior academic degrees, and those who were licensed practical/vocational nurses (LPN/LVNs). As a class these individuals are older, and contribute to the "aging" effect.

By 1992, the majority of nurses received their basic preparation for nursing in an academic as opposed to a service setting. In the first sample survey of 1977, 75 percent of nurses were originally diploma school graduates. In 2000, only 29.6 percent came from this origin. Corresponding figures for RNs who reported completing an associate degree program increased from 11 percent of all nurses in 1977 to 40.3 percent

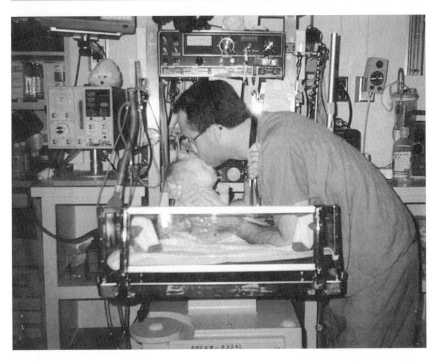

Nursing requires intellectual ability, technical competence, and the capacity to continue to care. (*Courtesy of U.S. Army Center of Military History*)

in 2000. Baccalaureate graduates increased from 17.3 percent in 1980 to 29.3 percent in 2000. In 2000, about 18.6 percent of the RN population had completed additional academic preparation beyond the entry program. Almost 24 percent of RNs originally prepared in baccalaureate programs and 15.5 percent of associate degree graduates go on for further formal education.[32]

The family status of nurses has changed very little since 1996. They are predominantly married (71.5 percent), about 17.9 percent widowed/ separated/divorced, and 9.9 percent never married. Regardless of family status or the presence or absence of children, most nurses worked. In 2003, nurses employed full-time had a mean annual wage of $52,810, with those in California, Maryland, Massachusetts, Hawaii, and New York achieving higher salaries.[33] Considering salaries in the context of the work force, the greatest economic gains for nurses come at the peak of a shortage, proving the truth of the supply and demand principle.

The numbers of nurses with master's or doctoral preparation increased to 10.2 percent in 2000. Also of note is the shifting focus of nurses with advanced degrees. The primary emphasis of the master's degree for

51.5 percent was clinical practice as opposed to 43.4 percent in 1992. Twenty-three percent focused on management in 1996 compared to 24 percent in 1992; and 20 percent on education, a change from 22.3 percent in 1992 and 41 percent in 1977. At the doctoral level, the most identified focus was education for 37.5 percent (36.8 percent in 1992) and research for 34 percent (33.5 percent in 1992).[34] The functional roles of teaching and administration/management are no longer the primary focus of graduate education. The science of nursing has developed to the point where there is growing public recognition for advanced practice. And this trend is continuing; in 2002 only 3.4 percent of the graduates from master's programs majored in education (teaching). In this same year, 53.0 percent of master's enrollees and 60.1 percent of master's graduates were NP or combined NP/CNS majors. These programs focus on preparing individuals for clinical practice and may not result in a large number of graduates pursuing doctoral education.[35] The salaries in advanced practice have outpaced teaching. Schools of medicine and law have retained faculty by basing their salaries on the market, and supplementing their earnings through faculty practice opportunities or salary adjustments. Nursing has not followed suite. This is one of the reasons that we are currently experiencing a profound shortage of nurse educators.

However, nurses are recognizing that doctoral preparation is necessary for credibility in higher education; and there is a growing market for nurse–researchers in business and industry, health care organization, and more. Our educational pathways and preferences are a sign of our maturation as a profession. A high proportion of baccalaureate graduates choose graduate education, but RN-to-baccalaureate programs suffered a sharp decline of 7.2 percent in 2000.

MINORITY GROUPS IN NURSING

Studies on the general population of nursing students and graduates are inevitably influenced by the fact that the majority of nurses are both women and white. There is increasing interest in the minority groups in nursing, such as Blacks, Native Americans, and Hispanics, but also including the male minority.

Nursing recruitment for all ethnic minorities has gradually become more successful, stimulated particularly by federal grants available since 1965. However, despite these efforts, and although there has been an increase in the *numbers* of ethnic minorities, their *proportion* among employed RNs has not shown remarkable gain (see Exhibit 4.6). White/non-Hispanics were 86.6 percent of the RN population in 2000. There is an observable increase in the minority presence in basic nursing education programs over the past few years. Minority enrollment accounted for 26.7 percent of students in 2003, and 22.4 percent of the graduates in that same year.[36] There are many perceived and real financial and cultural barriers that impede recruitment and retention of minority students to nursing. One of the most serious may be the shortage of role models among faculty and leaders in nursing service for minority students to emulate. Minorities only account for 10 percent of the faculty in colleges of nursing.[37]

There are serious implications here for a nursing workforce that must be prepared to minister to a population in which the minority presence is currently 25 percent and rapidly growing.[38] It also perpetuates a vicious circle. Minority presence among graduate students in nursing is less than in baccalaureate programs at 11.7 percent, with the difference being especially pronounced for Blacks at 5.8 percent.[39]

Men have been neglected as potential sources of nurse power, although male nurses have existed almost as long as female nurses in the United States. By 1910, about 7 percent of all student and graduate nurses were men, but in succeeding years the percentage declined, until by 1940 it had dropped to 2 percent. Most men were graduates of hospital schools connected with mental institutions; not many schools (for men) were affiliated with general hospitals, and few coeducational ones existed (see Chapter 3). By 1960, male nurses (not including students) comprised 0.91 percent of the nursing workforce. The current 5.4 percent reflects a significant increase in the number of male nurses in the workplace. In 2003, men represented 10.7 percent of enrollments in all basic RN programs, and 9.8 percent of graduates, with associate degree programs attracting a slightly greater number of men.[40] This trend has been attributed to a variety of circumstances, including the general economic recession, employment opportunities in nursing, and the good salary gains achieved during the period of the nursing shortage.

Men in allied health roles or with other health care experience represent a major recruitment pool for nursing. They should not be expected to choose traditional male specialties, such as emergency, anesthesia, or intensive care, but should be urged to consider a whole range of career choices. They should be supported in career mapping to build a future in the profession.

When looking at the issues regarding the role of minorities in nursing, it is important to remember that cultural differences stem from a myriad of components in all our backgrounds—gender, religion, ethnicity, and even geography. The same insensitivity that thwarts our attempts to increase the ethnic, racial, gender, and religious diversity among the ranks of nurses hampers our ability to minister to those who are different from ourselves. Thus, it is important to be aware of and sensitive to minority issues in nursing but not to give them greater weight than the human issues that affect all people and are the mainstay of nursing care.

KEY POINTS

1. The basic criteria of professionalism include the qualities of autonomy, altruism, a defined body of knowledge, research, career commitment, social value, and ethics.
2. Nursing is defined in many ways, but the concept of caring for the individual as a whole is generally consistent.
3. Basic nursing functions include interviewing, examining, evaluating, treating, referring, collaborating, and caring for persons during their periods of dependence.
4. The nursing process and classification systems for nursing diagnosis, interventions, and outcomes are a way of organizing data for nursing care.
5. The emphasis of nursing on holistic man is evident in the work of nursing theorists beginning with Florence Nightingale.
6. The public see nurses as vital for their safety and advocacy in the health care delivery system, and a resource for curtailing escalating cost.
7. The image of nursing in the media is often distorted, but the public may also form a more lasting image, whether positive or negative, through direct contact.
8. Each nurse must take some responsibility for creating a true, positive image of nursing and challenging dysfunctional stereotypes.
9. Changes in the growing RN population include an older average age for working nurses and a higher level of education.
10. Since nursing is a large profession made up of a diverse population, information about the background and attitudes of subgroups, as well as of the majority, helps nurses understand one another better.

STUDY QUESTIONS

1. Detail your personal beliefs about the nursing metaparadigm: man, health, society, and nursing.
2. How relevant to modern times are the traditional qualities associated with professions?
3. Describe how well nursing meets the criteria necessary to be considered a profession.

4. Predict future changes in the National Sample Survey of Registered Nurses, and justify your predictions.
5. What is the usefulness of the classification systems for Nursing Diagnosis, Nursing Interventions, and Nursing Outcomes?
6. Give a specific example of how you can apply nursing theory to practice.

REFERENCES

1. Flexner A. Is social work a profession? *Proceedings of the National Conference of Charities and Correction.* New York: New York School of Philanthropy, 1915.
2. Pavalko R. *Sociology of Occupations and Professions.* Itasco, IL: Peacock, 1971.
3. Levenstein A. A road to professional growth. *Nurs Mgmt* 15:7, 1985.
4. Truog R, et al. The problem with futility. *New Engl J Med* 12:326, 1992.
5. *Nursing's Social Policy Statement*, 2d ed. Washington, DC: American Nurses Publishing, 2003.
6. Caplow T. *The Sociology of Work.* Minneapolis, MN: University of Minnesota Press, 1954.
7. Pearson L. Seventeenth annual legislative update: How each state stands on legislative issues affecting advanced nursing practice. *Nurse Pract* 30(1): 10–22, 2005.
8. ANA disturbed by Supreme Court decision on nurses as supervisors. *News Release.* Washington, DC: ANA, May 24, 1994.
9. Ford L. The nurse practitioner question. *Am J Nurs* 74:2188, December, 1974.
10. *Nursing's Social Policy Statement*, p 2.
11. Ibid.
12. *Nursing: Scope and Standards of Practice.* Washington, DC: American Nurses Association, 2004.
13. Orlando IJ. *The Dynamic Nurse–Patient Relationship: Functions, Process and Principles.* New York: J.P. Putnam's Sons, 1961.
14. Carpenito LJ. *Nursing Diagnosis: Application to Clinical Practice*, 9th ed. Philadelphia: J.B. Lippincott, 2003.
15. *Nursing Diagnosis: Definitions and Classification 2005–2006.* Philadelphia: NANDA, 2004.
16. Dochterman J, Bulechek G. (Eds.): *Nursing Interventions Classification (NIC)*, 4th ed. St. Louis: Mosby, 2004.
17. Moorhead S, Johnson M, Maas M. (Eds.): *Nursing Outcomes Classification (NOC)*, 3d ed. St. Louis: Mosby, 2004.
18. NANDA International. President's Report, December 20, 2004: http://www.nanda.org/html/news.html. Retrieved March 4, 2005.
19. Shindul-Rothschild J, et al. 10 keys to quality care. *Am J Nurs* 97:35–43, November 1997.
20. Joel L. *Kelly's Dimensions of Professional Nursing*, 9th ed. New York: McGraw-Hill, 2003.

21. *Nursing and the Quality of Patient Care: 1996 Survey.* Princeton, NJ: Princeton Survey Research Associates, 1996.
22. Knight K. Nurses score high on a public scale. *Nursing Spectrum*, September 20, 1999, p NJ4.
23. The Gallup Organization. Nurses top list in honesty and ethics poll, December 7, 2004: http://www.gallup.com/poll/content/login.aspx?ci= 14236. Retrieved March 2, 2005.
24. Gordon S. *Nursing Against the Odds.* Ithaca, NY: Cornell University Press, 2005.
25. Gordon S. *Life Support.* Boston: Little, Brown, 1997.
26. Sigma Theta Tau International. *The Woodhull Study on Nursing and the Media: Health's Invisible Partner.* Indianapolis, IN: Center for Nursing Press, 1998.
27. Joel L. NCNIP/Advertising Council campaign challenges resistant stereo-types. *Am J Nurs* 22:13, February 1990; *Am J Nurs* 97:7, May 1997.
28. Johnson & Johnson. Discover Nursing Campaign: http://www. discovernursing.com. Retrieved March 2, 2005.
29. USDHHS Division of Nursing. *National Sample Survey of Registered Nurses: Preliminary Findings.* Washington, DC: The Division, February 2001.
30. *Managed Care Digest Series 2000: Institutional Highlights Digest.* Kansas City, MO: Aventis Pharmaceuticals, 2000, p 8.
31. Ibid.
32. USDHHS Division of Nursing, op cit.
33. U.S. Bureau of Labor Statistics: http://bls.gov. Retrieved March 1, 2005.
34. USDHHS Division of Nursing, op cit.
35. Berlin LE, Stennett J, Bednash GD. *2002–2003 Enrollment and Graduations in Baccalaureate and Graduate Programs in Nursing.* Washington, DC: American Association of Colleges of Nursing, 2003.
36. National League for Nursing. *Nursing Data Review, Academic Year 2003.* Vol. 1: *Contemporary RN Nursing Education.* New York: The League, 2004.
37. A Report of the Sullivan Commission on Diversity in the Healthcare Workforce. *Missing Persons: Minorities in the Health Professions.* Washington, DC: The Commission, 2004.
38. Ibid.
39. NLN Center for Research in Nursing Education and Community Health. *Trends in Contemporary RN Nursing Education.* New York: The League, 1997.
40. NLN, ibid, 2004.

Updates can be found at

 http:/www.JoelTheNursingExperience.com

HELPFUL WEBSITES FOR PART 2

American Nurses Association: http://www.nursingworld.org

American Association of Colleges of Nursing: http://aacn.nche.edu
American Cancer Society: http://www.cancer.org
Children's Defense Fund: http://www.childrensdefense.org
Chronicle of Higher Education: http://chronicle.com
Information Please (repository of general information):
    http://www.infoplease.com
International Council of Nurses: http://cn.ch
Lippincott Publishers, Nursing Center: http://www.nursingcenter.com
National Center for Health Statistics: http://www.cdc.gov/nchs
National League for Nursing: http://www.nln.org
Elder Care Issues: http://www.elderweb.com
Nursing Spectrum: http://www.nursingspectrum.com
U.S. Bureau of the Census: http://www.census.gov
U.S. Bureau of Labor Statistics: http://bls.gov
U.S. Department of Education, Educational Research and Improvement Center
    (ERIC): http://www.ed.gov
U.S. Department of Health and Human Services: gateway to consumer
    information on health and health services: http://www.healthfinder.gov
U.S. Department of Health and Human Services, Healthy People: www.cdc.gov/
    nchs/about/otheract/hp2000/2000
University of Iowa, Center for Nursing Classifications. Nursing Outcomes
    Classification: http://www.nursing.uiowa.edu/noc
University of Iowa, Center for Nursing Classifications. Nursing Intervention
    Classification: http://www.nursing.uiowa.edu/nic

PART 3

NURSING PRACTICE

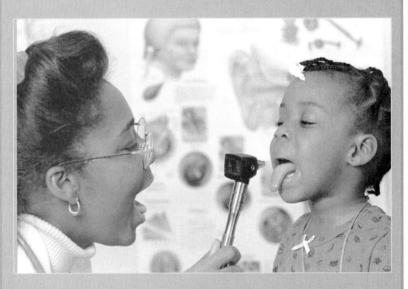

Nurses are uniquely suited to primary care. (*Courtesy of the Visiting Nurse Association of Central Jersey, Red Bank, New Jersey*)

Chapter 5

Education and Research for Practice

OBJECTIVES

After studying this chapter, you will be able to:

1. *Identify four ways in which nursing education programs are alike.*
2. *Compare the major types of education programs leading to RN licensure.*
3. *Explain briefly the various alternatives for RNs seeking a baccalaureate.*
4. *Describe briefly two trends or issues in nursing education and how they may affect future education.*
5. *Present the key points in landmark actions related to entry into practice.*
6. *Discuss the controversies surrounding continuing education.*
7. *Define nursing research.*
8. *Identify the problems in putting nursing research into practice.*

Unlike most professions, nursing has a variety of programs for entry into the profession (also called *basic, preservice,* or *generic* education). This situation confuses the public, some nurses, and employers. The three major educational routes that lead to RN licensure are the diploma programs operated by hospitals, the baccalaureate degree programs offered by four-year colleges and universities, and the associate degree (AD) programs usually offered by junior (or community) colleges. An option for second-degree students who are interested in nursing has become a fast-track to complete the baccalaureate and to progress directly to the master's degree and specialization.

Although at one time diploma schools educated the largest number of nurses (there were more than 1100 such programs in the early 1900s), they have experienced a dramatic decline with the movement of nursing into higher education. In 2003, only 69 programs awarded the diploma, 846 the associate degree, and 529 the baccalaureate for a total of 1444 basic nursing education programs.[1]

Sixty percent of all new RNs are graduates of associate degree programs. In 2000, of 71,000 candidates for RN licensure, 59.6 percent were associate degree graduates.[2] After five straight years of decline, 2003 shows that entry-level nursing school enrollments are up 10.4 percent, and graduations increased by 5.2 percent.[3] Enrollments in graduate and higher degree programs in nursing were managing to hang on at current levels with master's degree programs down 0.1 percent and doctoral and doctoral programs up 1.5 percent from 2000 to 2001. There was a significant increase in postdoctoral programs.[4] The pattern, then, has been an increase in all collegiate programs and the virtual elimination of diploma programs. The domination by AD graduates has contributed to the aging of the RN workforce.

This chapter gives an overview of the various educational programs in nursing, educational innovation including distance education, continuing education, research, and related issues and trends.

PROGRAM COMMONALITIES

There are certain similarities that all basic nursing programs share, in part because all are affected by the same societal changes:

1. Nursing education is becoming more expensive, and financial support is less available for schools and students. Both state and federal governments have been tightening the financial reins on programs. Tuition seldom covers the cost of education, but, even so, it has been rising consistently. The monies available to students are more usually loans as opposed to grants and scholarships. Also, the federal government has become more demanding in pursuing the payback of loans, with colleges/universities being penalized if a large amount of default is associated with their students.

2. The student population is more heterogeneous. Though there are still students of the traditional college age, a growing number are older. It is not unusual to have a grandparent in a class as more mature individuals look for a new or better career. Many students

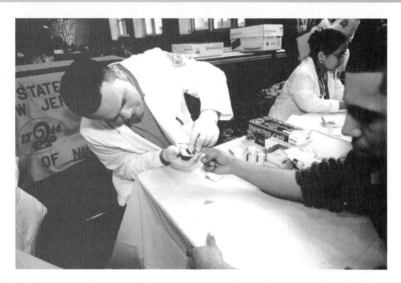

Health fairs provide an excellent opportunity for students to refine their practice skills. (*Courtesy of Rutgers–The State University of New Jersey, College of Nursing, Newark*)

bring other academic credentials, and previous success in fields that are both related or unrelated to nursing. All programs are including more men, by a small but definite percentage. Overall the percentage of minority students has not increased, although the profession as a whole sees the recruitment of minority students and the development of minority leadership in nursing as a priority.

3. Educational programs are generally more flexible. The admission of a very mixed and older student body, including aides, licensed practical nurses (LPNs), and RNs seeking advanced education, has required a second look at proficiency and equivalency testing, self-paced learning, new techniques in teaching, distance technology, and the external degree program. Programs must be geared to the unique educational needs of the adult learner, and faculty must be sensitive to their special needs and life circumstances, and the approaches to learning which suit them best.

4. The nursing community has a history of supporting upward mobility through education. Though it is still true that the shortest distance between two points is a straight line, many find it impossible to take that route. The classic example are those students who begin as an LPN/licensed vocational nurse (LVN), move on to the AD, sit for the RN licensing exam, and subsequently complete a baccalaureate in nursing. Programs can be found that will recognize the earlier educational experience and give credit toward the next credential.

5. State approval is required and national accreditation is available for all basic programs. Every school of professional nursing which prepares for entry into practice, as well as practical nurse programs, must meet the standards of the legally constituted body authorized to regulate nursing education and practice within that state. These agencies are usually called *state boards of nursing* or some similar title. Without the approval of these boards, the graduates of the school would not be eligible to take the licensing examination. In addition, most schools of nursing seek accreditation by the National League for Nursing Accrediting Commission (NLNAC) or the Commission on Collegiate Nursing Education (CCNE). Accreditation is a voluntary matter, not required by law. Increasing numbers of schools seek it, however, because it represents a nationally determined standard of excellence. The absence of accreditation may affect a school's eligibility for outside funding or impede the graduates' entrance into BSN or graduate programs or their ability to obtain grants and loans.

6. Faculty and clinical facilities are scarce resources. Faculty with the recommended doctoral degree for baccalaureate and graduate programs and the master's degree for other programs are in scarce supply. Clinical facilities are at a premium. Most schools use a variety of experiences, and in some geographical areas several schools may be using the same clinical areas for student experience. In rural areas, distance, small hospitals, and the absence of a variety of placements are problems. It is important to search out placements that support quality nursing practice, and to choose experiences which are representative of today's health care settings. The hospital is only one among many settings for nursing practice. Any educational program without a generous exposure to community practice and home care, and long-term care in varied forms, is suspect. How adequately are students being prepared for their life's work? Though community experiences may be difficult to identify, suitable options have to be sought.

7. There is a slow but perceptible trend toward involving students in curriculum development, policymaking, and program evaluation. Consumerism, accreditation criteria, and the maturity of students are making some inroads on faculty and administrative control of schools.

8. All nursing students have learning experiences in clinical settings. Somewhere a myth arose that only practical nurse and diploma students gave "real" patient care in their educational programs; that AD students barely saw patients; and that baccalaureate students rarely focused on "doing." In fact, the time spent in the clinical area differs among programs within a particular credential as much

as it does among various types of programs. In all good programs, students care for patients in order to gain skill and apply theoretical content. There should also be experiences in caring for larger numbers of patients. This opportunity can diffuse some of the inevitable "reality shock" that comes with graduation and your first job.

THE NURSING ASSISTANT

It has been traditional that nurses are helped in their work by individuals called nursing assistants, orderlies, nurses' aides, attendants, or more recently, unlicensed assistive personnel (UAPs). This category of workers has received added attention lately because of their increased presence in hospitals, often for the purpose of reducing the numbers of RNs needed to give care. The result has sometimes been an adversarial relationship between RNs and management with UAPs caught in the middle.

This group of care-givers was traditionally prepared through on-the-job training. In 1987, the dissatisfaction with the quality of care in this nation's nursing homes resulted in a series of amendments to the Omnibus Budget Reconciliation Act. One of these amendments required that nursing aides in facilities qualifying for Medicare reimbursement be certified, and that certification be based on 75 hours of instruction including an examination to verify competency in both theory and practice. Though this process is handled by the state, there are specific federal guidelines. Many states have requirements that exceed those of Medicare. By 1990, all nursing assistants in long-term care facilities were required either to have had a competency evaluation or to have completed an approved course. In each state the certification is awarded by a different administrative agency, but for the most part it is the Board of Nursing, Department of Health and Human Services, or the Department of Health. Long-term care aides were singled out for this degree of scrutiny because of the vulnerability of the population they serve, the frail elderly, and the token amount of supervision from the RN. In some ways, this was to compensate for unsuccessful legislative attempts to increase the numbers of RNs required in nursing homes.

There are similar certification requirements for home health aides, although the evaluation requirements seem to be less stringent. To some degree there is the assumption that the home-bound are more in control because they are candidates for community living. The skeptic would say they can be even more isolated and potentially open to abuse and victimization. Though the incidents of unloving care are few, they do exist.

Though the functions of nurses' aides are governed by state law and there is a great deal of inconsistency, some comments are possible.

Nurses' aides are generally responsible (under the direction and supervision of the RN) to maintain a safe environment, perform basic nursing skills, grooming, and helping with feeding, elimination, and mobilization. The most important thing for the RN to remember is that the aide functions under the RN's license. It is the RN who supervises and determines the appropriate utilization of any unlicensed worker involved in direct patient care. The basic education course for this assisting role may be given by a health care facility, high school, vocational/technical school, community college, or a privately owned program which may be run for profit and guarantee no employment. Nursing home aides and in some states home-care aides must have completed an approved program.

Many schools of practical nursing will award some credit for a formal nursing assistant course, thereby creating the first rung in a career ladder. Certification of assistive personnel has never been an issue for hospitals, where the assumption has been that patient contact is more limited and the RN presence is intense enough to honor the true meaning of delegation and supervision. This has not always been true in recent years. Since the salaries of professional nurses have increased and, in the wake of the recent nursing shortage, considerable hospital restructuring has occurred, UAPs have been used more extensively in hospitals, and there are often no consistent criteria for training or responsibilities. Issues of competence, motivation, security, and supervision have been raised. Staff nurses say they need more "help," yet UAPs often generate fear, distrust, and a perception of inadequate preparation. Nursing must move to clarify these issues and institute solutions.

PROGRAMS FOR PRACTICAL NURSES

Professional nurses work closely with practical nurses (PNs) in many practice settings. Both PN education and licensure are different from those of RNs, but because of changes in health care, an increasing number of PNs have been entering RN programs at either a beginning or an advanced level.

PNs (called *vocational nurses* in Texas and California) fall into three general groups: (1) those with experience but no formal education who have taken state-approved courses to qualify them to take state board examinations and become licensed; (2) those who have been licensed through a grandfather clause; and (3) those who have graduated from approved schools of practical nursing and, by passing state board examinations, have become licensed in the state or states in which they practice. There are also a few PNs who were enrolled in RN programs and were permitted by their state law to take the PN examination after a

certain number of courses. The large majority of LPNs/LVNs are licensed by examination (NCLEX-PN). Although LPNs in the first and second categories can be legally employed, employers with a choice usually prefer graduates from an approved school who have been licensed by examination. (A grandfather clause is a legal device that allows persons who can show evidence that they have been practicing in a field to attain or maintain licensure even though the requirements have been changed and made more stringent.)

Formal PN education actually came later than that of the trained nurse. Although many women who nursed family and friends in the last 100 years were probably considered a type of PN, the first formal training programs were started by the Brooklyn, New York, YMCA in 1893. The three-month course taught home care of chronic invalids, the elderly, and children. Included were cooking, care of the house, dietetics, simple science, and simple nursing procedures. The program's success inspired similar courses in other states, but the first school was not organized until 1897. By 1945 there were only 36 schools, and only a few states had any kind of legislation regulating PN practice. After World War II, the nursing shortage and considerable federal funding for vocational education set the stage for extraordinary expansion. Most of the early postwar programs, of about one year's duration, were in public schools, with practical experiences supervised by graduate nurses in cooperating hospitals. Generally, no tuition was charged, although exploitative trade schools often charged much and gave little. By the 1950s there was more pressure for regulation, with states gradually requiring licensure.

LPN education takes place primarily in vocational/technical schools and community colleges, with fewer programs offered in secondary schools and hospitals, and is commonly 12 months in length. Most programs are publicly funded. Interestingly, tuition at community colleges is about the same per year for LPN and ADN programs. In 1984, "concern for job safety" due to the layoffs that followed diagnosis-related groups (DRGs) prompted the National Federation of Licensed Practical Nurses (NFLPN) House of Delegates to endorse expansion of the PN curriculum to at least 18 months. An implementation date of 10 years was set, but no real action followed. In 1986, North Dakota changed its educational requirement for LPN licensure to a two-year community college program.

Not all LPNs or LPN faculty agreed with this decision. However, some programs began planning to phase into an AD level. Already existing are PN programs that are the first year of a two-year AD program. A student may exit at the end of the year, become licensed and work, or become licensed and not work and continue into the second year and eventually become eligible for the RN licensure examination (NCLEX-RN). Some RN programs, particularly for the AD, give partial or total credit for the

PN program (often only if the PN has also passed the licensing examination). PNs aspire to become RNs, and most frequently use the route of the AD. This observation, combined with the fact that minority students are more likely to choose an LPN program than an RN program, may predict a more diverse RN workforce in the future. A concerted effort has also been made to upgrade nurses' aides, home health aides, and other paraprofessional health care workers to LPN status through career ladders.

Legitimate PN programs must be approved by the appropriate state nursing authority and may also be accredited, usually by the NLNAC; then the student is eligible to take the licensing examination (NCLEX-PN) to become an LPN or LVN. The licensing law is now mandatory in all states.

Today, LPN programs are distributed throughout the nation, although most are in the South (45 percent) and fewest in the West (15 percent). The number of programs and number of admissions have fluctuated, depending on the availability of RNs, and the extent to which the LPN can be substituted for the more costly RN. In 1992, as a direct response to the industry shortage of RNs, there was more than a 4 percent increase in LPN school enrollment, which reversed with the end of that shortage.[5] LPN programs have declined from a peak of 1319 in 1982 to a current 1107 which are state approved, but very few pursue accreditation. In 1996, of 1132 PN educational programs, only 216 were accredited.[6]

PN programs emphasize technical skills and direct patient care, but a (usually) simple background of the physical and social sciences is often integrated into the program. Clinical experience is provided in one or more hospitals and other agencies. The number of skills that are taught increases each year, probably because of employers' demands. The National League for Nursing (NLN) has published statements on LPN entry-level competencies.

The major employment site for LPNs has shifted again and again, based on the availability and salary expectations of the RN. During the years when RN salaries were significantly depressed and hospitals were proud to claim an all-RN staff, the presence of the LPN in hospitals declined. During the RN shortage of the late 1980s, LPNs were again hired for hospital practice. Within these same years, the American Nurses Association tirelessly lobbied for the 24-hour presence of an RN in nursing homes. As a governmental compromise to the economically strained nursing home industry and given the perceived shortage of RNs, the modifier *registered* was changed to *licensed*, allowing the hiring of either LPNs or RNs. Based on this event, LPNs have become the dominant licensed presence in nursing homes, and their competency statements speak to a continuing accountability for care delegated to unlicensed health care providers.

Studies on the role activities of the LPN show a great deal of state-to-state inconsistency. There is also a tendency for LPNs to expand their practice once they become experienced. This is accomplished through a sequence of events: an educational program appropriate to the activity, supervised practice, documented competency, continued supervision, and appeal to the state board of nursing for an interpretation which makes the activity allowable. However, despite the fact that many of these activities have become a usual part of LPN practice, they are not included in the basic education. This may be due to the political need to avoid lengthening the educational program. LPNs report administering IV medications, starting IVs, hemodialysis monitoring, pronouncing death, inserting GI tubes, ventilator care, central line management, management of total parenteral nutrition (TPN), as some examples. These situations are of great concern to the RN, who is not only legally responsible but bound by a code of ethics.

DIPLOMA PROGRAMS

The diploma or hospital school of nursing was the first type of nursing school in this country. Before the opening of the first hospital schools in the late 1800s, there was no formal preparation for nursing. However, after Florence Nightingale established the first school of nursing at St. Thomas's Hospital, England, in 1860, the idea spread quickly to the United States.

Hospitals, of course, welcomed the idea of training schools because, in the early years, such schools represented a low-cost supply of nursing resources. With some outstanding exceptions, the education offered was largely of the apprenticeship type; there was some theory and formal classroom work, but for the most part students learned by doing, providing the majority of the nursing care for the hospitals' patients in the process.

Gradually these conditions improved, faculty were better educated, and students had more classroom teaching. Yet, even as late as the 1950s, many classes were taught by doctors, and the focus was on giving care in the hospital, with the how sometimes more important than the why. When sciences were taught by a nearby college, courses were designed especially for nurses, often at a lower level than for other students. The student was typically a white, single, 18-year-old female who had to live in the dormitory. Breaking rules about curfew, smoking, drinking, and especially marrying meant dismissal, no matter how excellent the student.

This is no longer true. Today, in order to meet standards set in each state for operation of a nursing school and to prepare students to pass the licensing examinations, diploma schools must offer their students a truly educational program, not just an apprenticeship. Hospitals conducting such schools employ a full-time nurse faculty, offer students a balanced mixture of coursework (in nursing and related subjects in the physical and social sciences) and supervised practice, and look to their graduate nursing staff, not their students, to provide the nursing service needed by patients. The educational program has been generally three years in length, although most diploma schools have now adopted a shortened program. Upon satisfactory completion of the program, the student is awarded a diploma by the school. Competencies of the graduate focus on direct patient care, and practice within prescribed and predictable situations.

This diploma, it should be understood, is not an academic degree. Because most hospitals operating schools of nursing are not chartered to grant degrees, no academic (college) credit is routinely given for courses taught by the school's faculty. (Exceptions are some external degree programs and some nonnursing baccalaureate programs that offer "blanket credit" to RNs. The latter type of degree may be a problem when seeking graduate education in nursing.) For this and economic and educational reasons, large numbers of diploma schools enter into cooperative relations with colleges or universities for educational courses and/or services. It is not uncommon for diploma students to take regular physical and social science courses and, occasionally, liberal arts courses at a college. If these courses are part of the general offerings of the college, college credit is granted. Credit is usually transferable if the nursing student decides to transfer to a college or continue toward the baccalaureate degree. If the course is tailored to nursing only, it may not be transferable to satisfy baccalaureate requirements, but may have to be counted as an elective.

The primary clinical facility is the hospital, although the school may contract with other hospitals or agencies for additional educational experiences. Advocates of diploma education usually say that early and substantial experiences with patients seem to foster a strong identification with nursing, particularly hospital nursing, and thus graduates are expected to adjust to the graduate role without difficulty.

Hospital schools provide other necessary educational resources, facilities, and services to students and faculty, such as libraries, classrooms, audiovisual materials, and practice laboratories. When it was taken for granted that students would be housed, good schools had dormitory and recreational space, as well as educational facilities. Such housing has now become optional to the student, and if used must be paid for and may also be used by others educated in or involved with the hospital.

The perceptible shift away from diploma school preparation for nursing can be explained (in an oversimplified way) by three factors:

1. The expense of maintaining a school is substantial, and that cost has often been absorbed by patients and their insurers. This practice has become unacceptable, resulting in inadequate funding, and difficulty maintaining standards, including attracting qualified faculty.
2. Increasing numbers of high school graduates are seeking some kind of collegiate education with the assurance that credits earned will be accepted for transfer.
3. The nursing profession is becoming ever more committed to the belief that preparation for nursing, as for other professions, should take place in institutions of higher education.

The vast majority of current diploma programs are NLN accredited, and many of the schools that dissolved or were "phased into" AD or baccalaureate programs were also accredited. Strong, vital schools were encouraged to seek degree-granting status where state laws allowed. Other hospital schools moved to enter into a formal relationship with collegiate institutions.

Although hospitals are less likely to operate schools, they continue as the clinical laboratories for nursing education programs. In the communities where new AD or baccalaureate programs are opening, there is often planning for the new programs to evolve as diploma programs close—a phasing-in process. This cooperation enables prospective candidates for the diploma program to be directed to the new program, qualified diploma faculty to be employed by the college, and arrangements made to use space in the hospital previously occupied by the diploma school. Cooperative planning provides for continuity in the output of nurses to meet the needs of the community.

ASSOCIATE DEGREE PROGRAMS

A relative newcomer to the scene of nursing education is the associate degree (AD) program, usually offered by a junior or community college and two years in length. This program prepares graduates for the RN licensing examination. This type of program, offered in a college setting but not leading to a baccalaureate degree, was not even envisioned by nursing educators of the late nineteenth and early twentieth centuries.

The AD program is the first nursing education program to be developed under a systematic plan and with carefully controlled experimentation. In 1951, Mildred Montag published her doctoral dissertation describing a nursing technician able to perform nursing functions described as considerably more prescribed and narrower in scope than those of the professional nurse and broader than those of the PN.[7] This nurse was intended to be a bedside nurse who was not burdened with administrative responsibilities. Experience with the Nurse Cadet Corps during World War II supported the concept of providing a shortened nursing program. The emerging community college was seen as a suitable setting for this education since it would place nursing education in the mainstream of education, and the burden of cost would be on the public in general rather than on the patients, as was the case with diploma programs. An AD in nursing would be awarded at the end of two years. As originally conceived, the program was considered to be complete in itself or terminal, rather than a step toward the baccalaureate.

A five-year project to test this idea of the AD nurse was initiated in 1952, with seven junior colleges and a diploma school participating. The results of the project showed that AD nursing graduates could carry on the intended nursing functions, that the program could be suitably set up in junior colleges with the use of clinical facilities in the community at no charge, and that the program attracted students. The success of the experiment plus the rapid growth of community colleges combined to give impetus to these new programs.

The entire concept of the AD nursing program as terminal has changed over the last 25 years. Obviously, no educational program should be terminal in the sense that graduates cannot continue their education toward another degree. Trends have continued toward enhancing articulation opportunities for AD-RNs into baccalaureate nursing programs. However, the AD nurse need not continue formal education to hold a valuable place in the health care system.

The practice of the AD graduate has often been called technical, as differentiated from professional. Whether the term *technical* will continue to be used is not clear. The concept of a technical worker, honored in other fields, has not been fully accepted in nursing, possibly because it is considered a step down from the *professional* label that has been attached to all nurses through licensing definitions and common usage over the years. Montag predicted the difficulty which would be associated with choosing an appropriate term for this new type of nurse.[8] The use of the term *technical* was rejected by the NLN Council of Associate Degree Programs in a 1976 action and the term *associate degree nurse* (AD nurse) was suggested. Yet, neither has this term been commonly used.

More important than the name are the role and functions of the AD nurse. Because of nursing shortages, as well as lack of understanding of

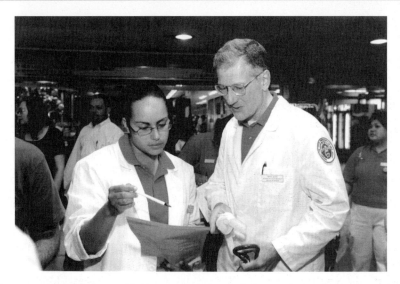

The nursing student quickly learns that the artfulness of practice is a cognitive artfulness. (*Courtesy of Rutgers–The State University of New Jersey, College of Nursing, Newark*)

the abilities and preparation of AD nurses, a tendency to use the diploma nurse of previous years as a standard, and general traditionalized concepts of nursing roles, employers have often not assigned AD nurses in the manner that best suits their preparation. Like nurses throughout the centuries, AD nurses have been placed quickly in team leader and charge nurse roles, positions in which they were not intended to function.

The NLN has published a role and competencies statement for AD nurses, which provides guidelines for identifying their expected level of practice at graduation and six months later. The document is very comprehensive. The introduction notes that AD education has as its goal to prepare RNs to provide direct client care. The competency statements are distinguished by what they do not say. They do not mention leadership, community health practice, or evaluation of research findings for their applicability to practice.[9]

Over the years, as Montag predicted, the AD course of studies has varied and changed. For instance, when college policies permit, there is a tendency to put a heavier emphasis and more time on the nursing subjects and clinical experiences, sometimes through the addition of summer sessions. Some programs are also adding team leadership and managerial principles because their graduates are put in positions requiring these skills. Today, most AD programs are between 18 and 24 months in length, but some require that all science and general education courses be completed before the nursing program is begun, which may lengthen the program considerably. It should be possible to complete degree requirements in four semesters of full-time study.

There has been some complaint that AD nurses are not proficient in certain technical skills and require too much orientation to the responsibilities of a staff nurse. AD educators believe that the need for additional clinical experiences is not suggested more frequently than for graduates of other programs. It is unrealistic for employers to expect new graduates to function as seasoned practitioners. Almost everyone agrees that AD graduates have a good grasp of basic nursing theory, have inquiring minds, and are self-directed in finding out what they don't know. It is also generally agreed that a good orientation program is the key to the satisfactory adjustment of any new graduate to the work setting.

AD programs are the fastest-growing segment of nursing education for a variety of reasons. Clearly, the availability of AD programs in a community; the generally low cost; the fact that this is usually the shortest way to RN licensure; the increasing possibilities of educational career ladders; and the reality that most employers do not differentiate much in salaries for RNs with different kinds of education, are all important factors. AD programs are distributed throughout the United States, with most in the Midwest and the South. The makeup of AD students (and graduates) is distinctly different from that of the other programs. There are a larger number of Hispanics in two-year institutions as opposed to Asian–Americans and Blacks, who gravitate to baccalaureate programs. AD students are also more likely to be older, married with children, and working part-time. There is some indication that they are more likely to continue to work in the community where they went to school. AD programs have been attracting second-career students and second-degree students, perhaps, in part, because of the brevity of the program. The perceived brevity of the program may be misleading, as many baccalaureate programs offer "fast-track" opportunities, especially designed for the second-degree student. The result can be a bachelor's degree for the same amount of time invested. The long-term implications of all these factors for nursing in general are discussed later.

BACCALAUREATE NURSING PROGRAMS

The first baccalaureate program in nursing was established in 1909 under the aegis of the University of Minnesota, through the efforts of Dr. Richard Olding Beard. Since then, these programs have become an increasingly important part of nursing education and have grown steadily in numbers.

The baccalaureate graduate obtains both a college education with a bachelor's degree and preparation for licensure and practice as a registered professional nurse. The baccalaureate degree program includes courses in general education and the liberal arts, the sciences germane to and related to nursing, and nursing. In most programs, courses in the nursing major are concentrated in the upper division, the last two years of the program. As in the other nursing programs, the baccalaureate program has both theoretical content and clinical experience.

The most notable differences between baccalaureate education and the other basic nursing programs are related to the extent of liberal education, depth in the natural and behavioral sciences, development of intellectual skills, and the addition of community health practice, leadership experiences, and teaching and management concepts, although some of the other programs do include a limited amount of such content. Baccalaureate nurses have the opportunity for a diverse education, and almost all programs allow free electives in the humanities and the sciences, as well as nursing courses. Nursing majors meet the same admission requirements and are held to the same academic standards as all other students. The nursing program is an integral part of the senior college or university as a whole and is usually four years in length. The baccalaureate in nursing degree is the gateway to graduate study.

Although technical skills are essential to nursing, learning activities that assist students to develop skills in recognizing and solving problems, applying general principles to particular situations, and establishing a basis for making sound clinical judgments are emphasized. This enables the nurse to function when a familiar situation takes an unexpected turn or when it is necessary to deal with an unfamiliar situation. The unique artfulness of the baccalaureate nurse is cognitive.

Like other nurse educators, those in baccalaureate programs constantly review (and often revise) their nursing curriculum, but they have given relatively little attention to the liberal arts component, even though this part of the program is essential in setting the baccalaureate nurse apart. In 1986, an interdisciplinary "Panel for Essentials of College and University Education for Professional Nursing" reported the recommendations of its two-year study to the American Association of Colleges of Nursing (AACN), its sponsor. The report had two components, one related to nursing knowledge and the other to liberal education. The panel members noted that a liberally educated person can responsibly challenge the status quo and anticipate and adapt to change. Their recommendations were that the education of the professional include (among other things) the ability to write and speak effectively, think analytically, understand a second language and multicultural traditions, interpret qualitative data, use computers, and appreciate the social role of the fine and performing arts.[10] Finally, they noted that nursing faculty are responsible for integrating knowledge from the liberal arts and sciences into professional nursing education and practice. "Liberally educated nurses make informed and responsible ethical choices and help shape the future of society as well as the nursing profession."[11] Amazingly, the report did not serve as a catalyst for change.

Most BSN graduates select hospitals as their first place of employment but then often turn to community health nursing. Those hospitals that have primary nursing, which gives nurses individual responsibility for a group of patients, seem most likely to attract and retain baccalaureate nurses. Graduates with long-term plans for teaching, management, or clinical specialization continue into graduate study.

A baccalaureate in nursing offers many career opportunities, a fact that is widely acknowledged. Equally important is the fact that in the last 10 years, when nursing has been under particular scrutiny, many reports and studies have agreed that what is required to meet the nursing needs in today's complex health care environment is more baccalaureate nurses. A recent report by the National Advisory Council on Nurse Education and Practice, an advisory body to the federal Division of Nursing, urged that at least two-thirds of the basic nurse workforce hold baccalaureate or higher degrees in nursing by 2010. Presently, only about 43 percent do.[12] Many hospitals have established "BSN-preferred" policies for new hires. For example, the Veterans Administration, the nation's largest employer of registered nurses, has established the baccalaureate degree as the minimum preparation its nurses must have for promotion beyond entry-level positions beginning this year, 2005. However, the baccalaureate program is usually more expensive for students than other basic programs. This is a serious problem, as funding cuts lessen student aid.

A major phenomenon in baccalaureate nursing is the many RNs entering these programs. In part, this is because nurses are eager to advance in their careers and see more options available with a baccalaureate degree. Since employers are aware of this and look for ways to keep their nurses, many offer tuition reimbursement as a fringe benefit. When this is added to the new flexibility offered RNs by baccalaureate educators, nurses find it less difficult to go to school, work, and maintain family responsibilities (although it is never easy). Many programs are designed especially for returning RNs. Other RN–BS tracks exist within regular baccalaureate programs, with the nurses main-streamed into the basic curriculum. In most baccalaureate programs, RNs receive credit and/or advanced standing for their previous nursing education through challenge examinations, or articulation agreements, often statewide. Frequently, courses and clinical experiences are individualized to meet the RNs' needs and goals. The degree, however, is the same for basic and RN students. More than 600 RN to BSN programs are available nationwide, including 169 programs offered in a more intense, accelerated format. Program length varies between one and two years depending upon the school's requirements, program type, and the student's previous academic achievement. Enrollment in RN to BSN programs is increasing in response to calls for a more highly educated nursing workforce. From 2002 to 2003, enrollments increased by 8.1 percent, the first such increase in RN to BSN programs in six years.[13] There are also 137 programs available nationwide to transition RNs with diplomas and associate degrees to the master's degree level (MSN, MS or Master of Science in Nursing degree). These programs prepare nurses to assume positions requiring graduate preparation, including the advanced practice roles. The number of RN to MSN programs has doubled within the past 10 years, from 70 programs in 1994 to 137 programs today. According to AACN's 2003 survey of nursing schools, 23 new RN to MSN programs are in the planning stages.[14] These programs prepare nurses to assume positions requiring graduate preparation, including the advanced practice roles.

Another noticeable trend is the increase of entry-level students who already have a baccalaureate or advanced degree in fields other than nursing. Most of these students will receive a second baccalaureate, although some may be enrolled in entry-level masters or the professional nursing doctorate program. Depending on how many previous courses can be credited toward the BSN, their program may consist primarily of upper-division major nursing courses. Some baccalaureate programs have been especially designed for these students. Actually, such programs may not take much more time for completion than an AD program. Often these second-careerists do not realize, or are not told, that they will need a nursing baccalaureate for career advancement, regardless of their nonnursing degrees. The other option which has become very popular with these students is an accelerated BS–MS program in which they acquire a nursing baccalaureate on the way to a nursing master's degree. These programs are described next.

OTHER PROGRAMS LEADING TO RN LICENSURE

There are educational programs which grant a master's degree in nursing as the basic (entry) educational credential. A variation on this theme is the accelerated masters for students with a nonnursing bachelor's degree. The bachelor of science in nursing is completed as an interim step, and the student moves on to specialty preparation at the master's level. A student may sit for the licensing exam after completion of the baccalaureate degree, depending on state law, and then continue directly to the master's degree.

The first program for a professional doctorate (ND) for college graduates was established at Case-Western Reserve in 1979. It was designed for "liberally educated men and women who are gifted intellectually, willing to invest themselves in a rigorous, demanding, rewarding program of study, and committed to a sustained professional career."[15] As described, the program should be located only in universities with health science centers preparing several types of health professionals. Because such universities also offer advanced graduate education, ND students are prepared in an academic climate of scholarship and research. Faculty are prepared at the highest level of scholarship, with some engaged in teaching and research and others, jointly appointed, master's prepared clinicians engaged in clinical practice, teaching, and some aspect of research. The curriculum prepares the ND graduates to become proficient in the delivery of primary, episodic, and long-term nursing care, and to evaluate their own practices and the practice of those who may assist them in giving care. Graduates of this program would continue study in a clinical specialization and/or a functional area such as teaching, management, or clinical practice. As is true of medical students, whose professional degree is a doctorate, they may also obtain a master's or PhD concurrently with the first doctorate. This innovative approach, seen as a major step toward the emergence of nursing as a full-fledged profession, has now been adopted by several other universities, but many questions are still raised as to the functions, role, and job market for graduates and the best organizational structure for the program. This program may just be an interim step in our development.

GRADUATE EDUCATION

THE MASTER'S DEGREE

In 2000, about 10.2 percent of the nurse population had at least a master's degree. Today, the purpose of master's level education is to prepare professional nursing leaders in the areas of advanced practice, teaching, and management. Nurses with these special skills and knowledge are desperately required now and will be for the foreseeable future. Only about 15.8 percent and 13.4 percent of students in master's study indicate an interest in administration or education respectively; whereas over 50 percent are committed to clinical practice.[16] This represents a significant change from another era when graduate education was dominated by preparation for teaching and management/administration. In many ways the pendulum may have swung too far, given the crisis proportions of faculty shortages.

Graduate programs in nursing vary in admission requirements, organization of curriculum, length of program, and costs. Admission usually requires RN licensure, graduation from an approved (or accredited) baccalaureate program, a satisfactory grade point average, achievement on selected standardized tests, and sometimes nursing experience. Part-time study is available in most programs, but often certain courses must be taken in sequence, requiring at least some full-time study. The motivation for part-time study is often economic. Being in demand, the RN can arrange work hours that accommodate an academic schedule, and earn much more than graduate assistantships or federal traineeships would provide.

Not all graduate programs offer all possible majors. The degrees granted are usually the MS (Master of Science with a nursing major), MSN (Master of Science in Nursing), MEd (Master of Education with a major in nursing), MA (Master of Arts with a major in nursing), MNSc (Master of Nursing Science), MN (Master in Nursing), or MPH (Master in Public Health with a nursing major). The differences are sometimes obscure. More important than the letters is the assurance that the program will provide the content and developmental experiences to achieve master's level competencies in your chosen role, and the hours of practice that will allow you to sit for national certification. Both the NLN and AACN have authored competency statements. In *Essentials of Master's Education for Advanced Practice Nursing*, the AACN identifies the content areas for the general core competencies that every graduate of a master's degree program in nursing is expected to demonstrate, and additional content for the advanced practice core competencies which are then supplemented by the specialty content. Specialty content is the product of a consensus-building process involving the appropriate specialty association(s). The general core competencies are organized under seven content areas, and the advanced practice competencies under three content areas.[17] The reader is referred to Exhibit 5.1, which contains the organizing model.

Most master's programs offer study of a clinical area, such as medical–surgical nursing, maternal–child nursing, community health nursing, or psychiatric nursing, including cognates in the specialty, supportive natural and/or behavioral sciences, and supervised clinical experience. The depth of clinical study varies in relation to the functional role selected: teaching, management, or advanced clinical practice. A practicum (planned, guided learning experiences that allow a student to function within the role) is usual for the functional role as well as the area of clinical specialization, and most often they are combined. Practice varies from program to program, from one or more days a week for a semester to almost a year's full-time residency. Acquisition of research methods is also considered essential. In general, master's education in nursing includes introduction to research methods. Debate continues around whether a thesis or independent study project should be a degree requirement. As the terminal degree became the doctorate, the credits for the master's have decreased, and many programs have eliminated the thesis, choosing to reserve any independent research experience for the dissertation. Contrary to this trend, the AACN recommends some type of a capstone experience which allows integration of learning in the master's program. One example of a capstone according to the AACN definition is a thesis or research project,[18] though other options may also be appropriate.

The latest opportunity in master's study is the clinical nurse leader (CNL). Observing the complexity in health care, the AACN and a host of allied academic and practice partners have proposed the preparation of a generalist clinician at the master's degree level. Admission requirements differ from school to school, but generally expect a baccalaureate degree either in nursing or in a nonnursing area. Some programs require that the candidate be an RN, others prepare for entry into practice and licensure within the CNL course of study. The CNL would oversee the care coordination of a distinct group of patients in addition to providing direct patient care in complex situations.[19] The need for this caliber of clinician is reinforced by Aiken's research, which confirms that patient mortality rates are significantly improved when care is provided by health care teams with higher percentages of nurses prepared in baccalaureate and graduate degree programs.[20] Currently

---

Exhibit 5.1 Content Areas for Core Competencies of Master's Graduates in Nursing

Content Areas of Core Competencies for All Master's Graduates

    Research
    Policy, organization, and financing of health care
    Ethics
    Professional role development
    Theoretical foundations of nursing practice
    Human diversity and social issues
    Health promotion and disease prevention

Content Areas for Advanced Practice Core Competencies

    Advanced health/physical assessment
    Advanced physiology and pathophysiology
    Advanced pharmacology

Source: AACN. *The Essentials of Master's Education for Advanced Practice Nursing.* Washington, DC: The Association, 1996.

77 education-practice partnerships have registered interest in piloting a CNL program, and 12 universities have established a CNL course of studies.[21] The credentialing of the CNL, whether the workplace is ready to assimilate this new role, and the manner in which the CNL will work with the advanced practice nurse are just some of the questions still to be answered. The reader is urged to seek more information on this evolving program through the AACN website, www.aacn.nche.edu/CNL.

DOCTORAL EDUCATION

The first American nurse to earn a doctorate received her PhD in psychology and counseling in 1927, although the first doctoral program for nurses opened at Teachers College, Columbia University, in 1924, offering the EdD in nursing which is still its hallmark. Until 1946, when two of the 46 colleges and universities offering advanced programs in nursing also initiated doctoral education for nurses, nurses who wanted doctoral studies had to attend programs outside of nursing, or Teachers College. By 1969, some 25 different doctoral degrees were being awarded to nurses, including the Doctor of Nursing Science (DNS or DNSc), Doctor of Nursing Education (DNEd), and Doctor of Public Health Nursing (DPHN), as well as Doctor of Philosophy (PhD) and Doctor of Education (EdD).

Although many nurses are still enrolled in nonnursing doctoral programs, the choice has become the doctoral degree in nursing. The PhD is the most prestigious and appropriate for anyone making an educational decision today. Sometimes the university denies nursing this option because of the notion that nursing science is not advanced enough; therefore, the school chooses a DNS or DNSc instead. What's the difference? Theoretically the PhD is a research degree that prepares scholars for research and the development of theory. The professional doctorate (DNS, DNSc, DSN, EdD, DPH) is an advanced practice degree with an emphasis on functional role, be it clinical practice, education, or the executive role. Research is an inherent part of the program, but the goal of that research is to bridge the gap between theory, research, and practice. The PhD is interested in the creation of knowledge for its own sake; the professional doctorate searches out new answers for their practical use, most notably to improve the human condition. By 2002, some 81 different post-entry doctoral programs awarded degrees in nursing, including one offering the Doctor of Nursing Practice (DNP), seven the Doctor of Nursing Science (DNS or DNSc), four the Doctor of Science (DNS), sixty-nine the Doctor of Philosophy (PhD), and one the Doctor of Education (EdD). The most recent addition is the practice-oriented doctorate (DrNP or DNP) which would provide a specialty area and preparation for advanced practice.[22] This credential, the DNP, is in many ways a complement to the CNL master's preparation mentioned earlier in this chapter. It could also be conceived as the next step in academic preparation for current APNs.

The point has already been made for the urgent need to expand our pool of doctorally prepared nurses. The reasons are many: to expand the science, to secure our status in higher education, to bring the credibility of the degree to nursing service, and to establish an active research presence in our practice sites.

OPEN CURRICULUM PRACTICES

It has already been documented in this chapter that the new order of education demands responsible flexibility: the flexibility to allow students to enter and exit a course of studies, and to try self-pacing and independent study where it suits their personal needs (as a class these techniques have been called the "open curriculum"). Other ways of providing flexibility and convenience in education are through "summer and weekend colleges," and the use of distancing technology to bring instruction to students in inaccessible locations. This radical restructuring of education is part of a larger social upheaval. Consumers of every service and product are questioning why there can only be one way of doing things. The once impossible has been made possible through nursing faculty who are sensitive to the needs of students struggling for upward mobility through education. However, sympathy is worthless unless it makes things happen. There were educators willing to risk their reputations on innovative curriculum design, and others who worked with them to perfect systems of evaluation. Without credibility in evaluation, flexibility may be seen as little more than a "quick trick" to increase enrollment. In fact, most innovation and flexibility demands students who are highly motivated and self-directed. The terms attrition and retention take on new meaning, and cannot be measures of success in the traditional sense.

One of the most innovative and pioneering variations on the "open curriculum" is the external degree, or "virtual" university. This is independent study validated by testing, an approach long used in other countries (as early as 1836). In the United States, Excelsior College of Albany, New York (formerly Regents College), pioneered this approach for nursing. Excelsior shares many goals and activities with conventional campus-based programs. However, it differs significantly in the ways students learn and the methods used to recognize and credential that learning. Rather than providing classroom instruction, Excelsior provides the focus for learning through its degree requirements and related study materials. It provides a comprehensive system of objective assessment of college-level knowledge and skills, transfer credits from regionally accredited colleges, proficiency examinations, nursing performance examinations, and other specialized evaluation procedures. Excelsior grants credits whenever college-level knowledge is validated through the use of faculty-approved, objective, academic assessment methods.

Since 1972, Excelsior has developed associate, baccalaureate, and master's degree programs in nursing through grants and federal funds. All degrees are NLN accredited. ADN graduates, who are primarily LPNs, are eligible for licensure in 48 states; since 1975 the pass rate on licensure examinations has averaged 94 percent, with scores typically higher than those of the New York State and national averages. The graduate degree is a master of science in nursing administration with a concentration in nursing informatics.

In March 2005, there were more than 17,000 students enrolled at Excelsior, about 16,000 in the ADN, 1242 in the BSN program, and 319 in the master's program. Retention of students in the program continues to be a problem. Overall, about 25 percent of Excelsior students withdraw over time.[23]

Nearly 80 percent of the BSN candidates are RNs from diploma or AD programs, with an average of 10 years' experience in nursing, and an average age of 40. Many BSN students have baccalaureate, master's, or doctoral degrees in other fields. Approximately 75 percent of the graduates state intentions of continuing with graduate school.

The performance examinations are conducted by some 250 nurse faculty members, all of whom have completed the extensive training developed and administered by Excelsior. These performance examinations are administered on weekends throughout the year at the national network of Regional Performance Assessment Centers created and established by Excelsior. The written nursing examinations are administered by computer at some 160 locations throughout the country and at embassies and military bases throughout the world. Further information may be obtained by consulting their website: http://www.excelsior.edu.

Excelsior is no longer the only "external degree" option. Several others exist and can be identified through the National League for Nursing, the American Association of Colleges of Nursing, or the Internet.

DISTANCE EDUCATION

Distance education is as old as correspondence courses, but has taken on a new meaning with the consumer outcry for easy access to education, the knowledge explosion, and technology which makes it possible to transcend time and distance. It is both an instrument of social change and a response to that change. Distance education involves the geographical separation of learner and instructor, the use of technology for communication which allows us to transcend both time and distance, the capacity for bi-directional communication, and sometimes the absence of a peer group.

Distance education involves both synchronous and asynchronous technology. Synchronous allows the students and instructor to be together in "real time," while asynchronous allows the scheduling of course responsibilities according to your personal preference. Synchronous technologies include ITV (interactive television), chat rooms, and teleconferencing. Some asynchronous approaches are threaded discussions (students placing responses to a discussion topic on an Internet site, but not simultaneously), the Internet, e-mail queries of instructor and transmission of assignments, accessing course materials, and testing using a course-specific website, videotapes, faxes, and computer disks, as well as textbooks and study guides.

The distance experience is strange and uncomfortable for many students, but makes it possible to offer smaller, more specialized courses, and convenience. No difference has been found in student achievement when compared with the traditional classroom experience.[24]

In choosing a "distance" course, it is important to be an informed consumer. Inquiry about some of the following points would be wise:

- Has the instructor taught by "distance" before? (The learning curve is often steep for faculty.)
- What are the variety of teaching/learning strategies used? (Variety and a combination of synchronous/asynchronous techniques make for quality.)
- How quickly can you expect to obtain feedback from your instructors when you direct a question to them? (Immediate gratification is one positive of distance.)
- How many students are there in a course, and how many sites are connected electronically with what number of students at each site (for ITV)? (It is often possible to create your own peer group.)
- In the case of ITV, will there be a technician and/or a facilitator at each site? (Equipment failure can be a big problem, and an academic presence of some type is common in many "distance" courses.)
- What equipment do I need to participate, and if I do not personally own appropriate equipment how can I participate? (Equipment is often available to you through public libraries, elementary and secondary schools, your workplace.)

Distance education is here is stay. Many colleges of nursing offer complete degree programs using a combination of distance techniques and modalities. One of the largest distance learning student bodies in the world is part of UNISA, the University of South Africa, with more than 200,000 people enrolled worldwide in 2000.[25]

CONTINUING EDUCATION

Professional practitioners of any kind must continue to learn because they are accountable to the public for minimum safe practice. This commitment is impossible without lifelong learning and updating. For nurses, specifically, continuing education (CE) is needed to keep abreast of changes in nursing roles and functions, maintain practice competency, and modify attitudes and understanding. (It is commonly accepted that the half-life of knowledge today is about five years, and less in the sciences.)

In the 1970s, a number of states enacted legislation requiring evidence of CE for relicensure of nurses (and of certain other professional and

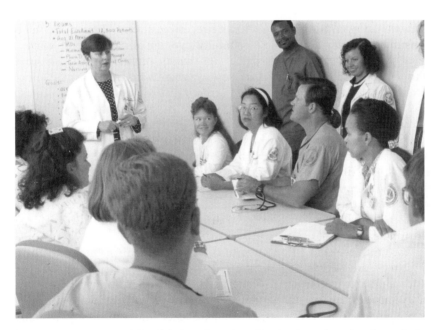

A career in nursing assumes life-long learning. Continuing education through the workplace agency is a valuable benefit. (*Courtesy of the U.S. Department of Veterans Affairs*)

Exhibit 5.2 States/Territories with Mandatory Continuing Education for Relicensure, 2003

Alabama	Mississippi
Arkansas	Nebraska
Alaska	Nevada
California	New Hampshire
Delaware	New Mexico
District of Columbia	North Mariana Islands
Florida	Ohio
Iowa	Puerto Rico
Kansas	Rhode Island
Kentucky	Texas
Louisiana	U.S. Virgin Islands
Massachusetts	Utah
Michigan	West Virginia
Minnesota	Wyoming

Source: *Journal of Continuing Education*: http://www.slackinc.com/jcen

occupational groups). According to a recent survey, 28 state and territorial boards of nursing now have continuing education requirements for renewal of licenses for the RN and LPN/LVN (see Exhibit 5.2), and 42 state boards of nursing now have continuing education requirements for reentry into active practice.[26] Additionally, all states currently recognize advanced practice in nursing, and most make that legal recognition of an individual contingent on national certification which entails continuing education for recertification.[27] The requirements for renewal of the RN license generally average about 10 to 15 contact hours annually. The requirements for reentry into RN practice vary widely from as little as 20 hours over two years to as much as a 300-hour approved nurse refresher course. Formalized programs are given under the auspices of educational institutions, professional organizations, and commercial for-profit groups. Most of these providers have been accredited by either the American Nurses Credentialing Center (ANCC), a national accrediting and certifying board for nursing, or the state board of nursing, so that their programs will be acknowledged as legitimate sources of CE. Most programs use the contact hour, which is nationally accepted as the unit of measurement for all kinds of CE programs. A contact hour is the measure of 50 minutes of an approved, organized learning experience.

More nurses seem to be attending formal programs. How much CE improves practice is still debated; however, many impact evaluation studies appear to confirm that there is benefit, albeit inconsistent. It has been shown that the motivation of the learner and the opportunity to apply what is learned are key factors. Opportunities and funds to attend programs are often part of collective bargaining agreements. However, nurses, if they consider themselves professionals, should be prepared to pay for their own CE.

Is CE readily available to most nurses? Despite some justifiable complaints that formal face-to-face and/or distance learning are not available in all geographical areas, there are many ways for nurses to continue professional development independently or through independent study. Examples of self-directed learning activities include self-guided, focused reading, independent learning projects, individual scientific research, informal investigation of a specific nursing problem, correspondence courses, self-contained learning packages using various media, directed reading, computer-assisted instruction, programmed instruction, study tours, and group work projects. Some nursing journals have developed self-learning programs that include official credit hours, for a minimal fee and completion of the evaluation process. There are also other innovative ways in which nurses are offered learning opportunities, such as through television, telephone systems, satellites, and other forms of telecommunication, as well as increased regional programs by nursing organizations. One of the richest sources of CE is the Internet. Some of the best Internet locations are used as references throughout this book and are listed at the end of each part. The opportunities for CE in nursing are considerably greater than they were some years ago.

TRENDS AND ISSUES IN EDUCATION

THE 100-YEAR DEBATE: EDUCATION FOR ENTRY INTO PRACTICE

Of all the issues that create heated debate within nursing (and outside), the one that causes the strongest reactions is also the oldest. The question of how nurses should be educated to enter the nursing field, often abbreviated as "entry into practice," has been going on for almost 100 years. With the first training programs, hospital based and controlled, there were early concerns about the need to move away from the apprenticeship model. These programs had never been totally like the Nightingale model. Nightingale, for instance, advocated a better-prepared, career-oriented nurse, as well as a bedside nurse. The first baccalaureate program in 1909 added liberal arts and a degree to the nurses' education, but not much, if any, change in the nursing part of the curriculum. Nevertheless, there were now two kinds of programs. With the initiation of the AD program, there were three that produced the vast majority of nurses; and a generic master's was already in existence.

What is wrong with having choices? Confusion results from several distinctly different ways of educating nurses, which presumably produce different outcomes, yet all graduates still take the same licensing examination and have the same title, RN. They may then hold the same kinds of jobs with the same expectations, the same responsibilities, and often the same salary. If so, what justification is there for three major educational programs, not to mention the generic master's and doctorate?

In the late 1950s and early 1960s, both ANA and NLN made a variety of statements that focused primarily on the baccalaureate as the necessary educational degree for professional nursing. Since an important function of ANA is that of setting standards and policies for the nursing profession, it was the ANA that made the definitive statement in 1965. A strong recommendation by the Committee on Education resulted in the ANA position that nursing education should take place within the general educational system. Reaction to the "position paper" was decidedly mixed. (This is actually correctly titled "Educational Preparation for Nurse Practitioners and Assistants to Nurses—A Position Paper.") Although the concept underlying the paper had been enunciated by leaders in nursing since the profession's inception, reiterated through the years, and accepted as a goal by the 1960 ANA House of Delegates, many nurses misunderstood the paper's intent and considered it a threat. Probably the greatest area of misinterpretation lay in the separation of nursing education and practice into professional, technical, and assisting components. Minimum preparation for professional nursing practice was designated at the baccalaureate level, technical nursing practice at the AD level, and education for assistants in health service occupations was to be given in short, intensive preservice programs in vocational education settings rather than in on-the-job training. An obvious omission in the position paper was the place of diploma and PN education. A large number of hospital-based diploma graduates, students, faculty, and hospital administrators were angered by this. A major source of resentment was that the term *professional nurse* was to be reserved for the baccalaureate graduate.

Even in this period of confusion, it was recognized that the largest system of nursing education at the time, the hospital school, could not be overlooked or eliminated by the writing of a position paper. Later, both the ANA and the NLN prepared statements that advocated careful community planning for phasing diploma programs into institutions of higher learning. It was also pointed out that as PN programs improved and increased their course content, their length would be close to that of the AD program, making the programs competitive and the continuation of both irrational. Nevertheless, the storm has raged for 40 years, although repeated attempts have been made to clarify the content and intent of the position paper. ANA suffered a membership loss due to the alienation of many diploma nurses. As expected, social and economic trends have gradually brought about many of the changes suggested by the position paper.

In 1976, the New York State Nurses' Association's voting body overwhelmingly approved introduction of a "1985 Proposal" in the 1977 New York State legislative session. Although variations of the proposal evolved over the next few years, the basic purpose of the legislation was to establish licensure for two kinds of nursing. The professional nurse would require a baccalaureate degree, and the other, whose title changed with various objections, would require an AD. The target date for full implementation was 1985; currently licensed nurses would be covered by the traditional grandfather clause, which would allow them to retain their current title and status (RN). The bill did not pass but was consistently reintroduced during each legislative session. The 1985 Proposal became both a term symbolizing legal recognition of baccalaureate education as the entry requirement for entry into *professional* nursing and a rallying point for nurses who opposed this change. There was, and continues to be, considerable opposition from some diploma and AD nurses and faculty, some hospital administrators, and some physicians. Nevertheless, an increasing number of state nurses' organizations voted at their conventions to work toward the goal of baccalaureate education for professional nursing.

The NLN has played an interesting role in the entry into practice debate. In 1979, it supported all pathways (baccalaureate, associate, diploma, and practical nursing). Given the structure of the NLN and its historic position as the accrediting body for each level of nursing education, this statement is understandable. In 1982, however, the board of directors endorsed the baccalaureate degree as the criterion for professional practice. This position was affirmed when the voting body met in June 1983. (See the convention reports published in *Nursing Outlook* in the odd years during that period.)

Later affirmations by the NLN board that called for two separate licensing exams infuriated the AD programs and community college presidents, who threatened to pull out of NLN agency membership.[28] There was a demand for clarification and objections that this action downgraded AD nurses for the sake of elevating BSN nurses. (From all this agitation came a number of organizations whose purpose was basically to support AD nursing and to protect AD nurses and programs from ANA and NLN actions they saw as detrimental.) The LPNs were not happy either. An interesting nonaction occurred at the next NLN convention, where the issue was tabled indefinitely, but publicly.

Entry into practice and its possible corollary, changes in nurse licensure, continue to be major issues in nursing. Most nursing organizations, at the state and national level, have taken a stand supporting baccalaureate education as the appropriate education for the "professional" nurse. After that, there is still disagreement as to whether the "other" nurse would be the AD nurse with separate licensing and if the PN would remain the same. Some think that AD education should be required for the practical nurse, leaving only two levels of nursing. Because this means a major change in nurse licensure, which is always a political as well as legal issue, only one state has taken that big step. The North Dakota Board of Nursing changed its administrative rules so that since 1987 the baccalaureate degree is the required educational credential for those wishing to take the RN licensure exam, and for practical nursing it is an AD. Although there was a legal attempt by several hospitals to prevent this from happening, the North Dakota attorney general ruled that this decision was within the purview of the board. No other states were successful in their plans for legislation to move the "entry" debate, probably because of a more pressing issue, the nursing shortage. Opponents seized on the shortage to maintain that this was not the time to make such changes because all types of nursing education programs were needed. Even when reputable studies (see Appendix 1) recognized the need for baccalaureate nurses, the approach suggested was often to encourage educational mobility. This refers to articulation of diploma and AD programs with those awarding baccalaureate or higher degrees, as well as more high-quality and flexible on- and off-campus programs for RNs to attain their baccalaureate.

In the long debate about the nature of education for practice, it is not surprising that there are those who think that the system should stay as it is; some who believe the AD nurse should progress to the baccalaureate degree in a time-limited period defined by the law; others who opt for changing the baccalaureate nurse's title and license to set them apart; a few who are anticipating the time when a professional doctorate in nursing practice, like the MD and DDS of physicians and dentists, will be the standard for entry into practice; and still others who see certification with the requirement of a baccalaureate degree as the additional credential to distinguish professional nursing.

Some natural fears of nonbaccalaureate nurses are to be expected—that they will lose status and job opportunities and that those who desire baccalaureate education will find it too expensive, unavailable, or rigidly repetitive. As to the first, there is, and already has been, some selectivity; in the latter, there has been significant progress in making RN/BSN programs accessible, affordable, and challenging. These issues will not be quickly resolved, but inevitable societal and professional changes, such as the decrease in diploma schools, the increasing complexity of health care, and the expectations of professional practice (nursing is the only health profession for which entry is less than a baccalaureate) will be major factors in the final outcome.

Because nursing loses power every time we battle internally, it is essential that nurses work together toward a satisfactory conclusion of the entry issue, one that includes appreciation and respect for all competent nurses and focuses on providing the best possible nursing care to the public. In the meantime, there has been a quiet revolution, one that may end the recurrence of the entry into practice issue that has followed nursing throughout its history. Although many RNs are not convinced that baccalaureate education necessarily means professionalism, others are and back to school they go.

NURSING RESEARCH

One essential quality of a profession is the constantly evolving nature of practice based on scientific inquiry, and the assumption that practice will be evidence-based. This standard of evidence-based practice includes research utilization as one of its components and not as a synonym. RNs, regardless of their basic program, are oriented to research during the educational experience; and research is no longer an unfamiliar presence in clinical sites.

DEFINING TERMS

Schlotfeldt's definition of the term *research* is classic: all systematic inquiry designed for the purpose of advancing knowledge.[29] Notter made a useful comparison between problem solving related to patient care (sometimes also described as the *nursing process*) and scientific inquiries.[30] Both go through such steps as (1) identifying a problem, (2) analyzing its various aspects, (3) collecting facts or data, (4) determining action on the basis of analysis of the data, and (5) evaluating the result. These steps may be relatively simple or very complex; they may involve laboratory equipment, human experimentation, or neither. Research may be designated as *basic*, the establishment of new knowledge or theory that is not immediately applicable, or *applied*, the attempt to solve a practical problem. Either way, the same steps are taken. Simply put, the questions to be studied through the research process arise from practice and the ultimate aim is to enhance our understanding of that practice so as to offer better service to the public.

Research may then be further characterized as quantitative or qualitative. *Quantitative* research is the more objective and uses data-gathering techniques that can be replicated and verified by others. It produces information that can be counted or measured using standardized instruments. The approach is deductive: identifying the question of interest, and reviewing the literature to determine what has been done in order to identify a conceptual framework or organizational structure for ideas on which to base the study. *Qualitative* is the more subjective, and focuses on questions that cannot be answered by quantitative designs. It is particularly useful in understanding perceptions and feelings, and answering the question "why?" Its approach is inductive, proceeding from the careful analysis of individual situations in order to evolve a conceptual structure to explain the phenomenon of interest.

There are also the broad categories of design: experimental and nonexperimental. If the research influences the subjects in any way, the research is *experimental*; if not, it is *nonexperimental*. There are numerous types of design in each of these categories, but the basic difference is whether the researcher manipulates or influences the subjects.

RESEARCH UTILIZATION

A more frustrating issue is the utilization of nursing research. After all, no matter how critical the findings of research studies may seem, if they are not tested in practice over a period of time, in a variety of settings, the results might still be questioned. If they are not used at all, practice may change, but it will not change as a result of research. The first step is communication, especially from researcher to practitioner. In the last few years, means of reporting research have increased considerably, with many more publications and conferences sponsored by organizations, universities, the government, and others, and the Internet offers ready access to many research products.

Nevertheless, putting research into practice has made slow progress. Most nurses giving direct patient care do not read research journals or have contact with nurse researchers. Obstacles most frequently reported by them in relation to using research findings are reading and understanding the report, relevance of findings for practical situations, inability to find research findings, suggestions too costly or time-consuming to implement, resistance to change in the workplace, and lack of worthwhile rewards for using nursing research.

Some clear trends are now emerging that may turn this situation around. First, researchers are beginning to realize that they have a responsibility for translating the research into terms and concepts understandable to the staff nurse, and presenting their research results in places other than research conferences. Also, nursing research is being done in clinical sites, with nurse researchers and staff working together. Having organized research programs in a significant number of clinical

Exhibit 5.3 Examples of Nursing Research Products with Significant Cost and Quality Implications for Practice

- Shorter hospital stays and earlier discharge for low-birthweight babies with home follow-up by APNs.
- Improved ability of nursing home residents to manage their daily activities without assistance.
- Reduction of urinary incontinence in older women through exercises and training.
- Identification of patients who are most at risk for pressure ulcers.
- Reduction of high blood pressure in young black men.
- Reduction of the number of low-birthweight babies and expensive hospital stays.
- Use of physical contact between mother and baby to benefit temperature, breathing, and sleep of premature babies.
- Identifying pain-reducing drugs that work better for women. (U.S. pain costs are $100 billion a year.)
- Improved condition of Latinos with arthritis and diabetes.
- Teaching children how to prevent and manage their asthma symptoms.
- Improved measurement techniques for the determination of obesity in children.
- Reduction of the use of restraints in the institutionalized elderly.
- Comprehensive discharge planning and follow-up programs for elderly patients with complex medical-surgical conditions using visits and telephone contact by advanced practice nurses.
- Monitoring vital signs for early detection and treatment of sepsis.
- Enhancing adherence to diabetes self-management behaviors.
- Improving the quality of life and reducing the care costs for Alzheimer's disease patients by using exercise and special monitoring.
- Use of saline flush to maintain patency of peripheral intravenous locks.

settings will take time, but the advances that have been made are impressive. Exhibit 5.3 presents some research products with obvious cost and quality implications for practice.

THE NATIONAL INSTITUTE FOR NURSING RESEARCH

One dramatic acknowledgment is that, in 1986, a National Center for Nursing Research (NCNR) was established at the National Institutes of Health (NIH). Congress not only overrode a presidential veto (and NIH objections), but key senators on both sides of the aisle spoke to the value of nursing research and the need for a visible national center. The Secretary of DHHS announced the establishment of the NCNR

> for the purpose of conducting a program of grants and awards supporting nursing research and research training related to patient care, the promotion of health, the prevention of disease, and the mitigation of the effects of acute and chronic illnesses and disabilities. In support of studies on nursing interventions, procedures, delivery methods and ethics of patient care, the NCNR programs are expected to complement other biomedical research

programs that are primarily concerned with the causes and treatment of disease.[31]

The NCNR was awarded the full status of an institute in 1992, becoming the National Institute for Nursing Research (NINR).

The NINR supports research, research training, and career development in health promotion and disease prevention, acute and chronic illness, and nursing systems, which include such areas as innovative approaches to delivery of quality nursing services, strategies to improve patient outcomes, interventions to ensure availability of resources, and bioethics research, a special initiative. A number of research training awards exist for beginning and advanced nurse researchers through individual and institutional predoctoral, postdoctoral, and senior fellowships. The research initiatives considered for 2007 include:[32]

- Physical activity and comorbidity in mobility-limiting disorders.
- Reducing health disparities among children.
- Transitions in the pediatric cancer trajectory.
- Biotechnology in self-management and informal care-giving.
- Multicultural issues in HIV research.
- Opportunities for research in environmental health.

RESPONDING TO AN INEVITABLE FUTURE

The recurrent problems and issues of the profession should not distract us from taking charge of our future. It is time to read the cues in the environment, and take decisive action around our educational and research agendas.

- Demand that you be prepared to function in a community-based, community-focused health care system that demands continuity and integration of services.
- Expect from the outset that you must be accountable for your practice, including cost and quality implications.
- Look for experiences to prepare for practice in a multicultural society; realistically this may be no more than becoming aware of one's own biases and accepting others as they are, including their personal definition of health and wellness.
- Look for true interdisciplinary education in the form of required courses and joint practice experiences.
- Empower consumers, making consumers the gatekeepers for their own health.
- Realize that you can never learn everything, so make content process. Focus on critical thinking, evidence-based practice,

collaboration, shared decision making, a social epidemiological viewpoint, and analyses at the systems and aggregate level.

○ Identify the databases that hold the information you need and be sure you know how to access them.

○ Remember it will be a luxury to be just responsible for your practice; you must have the skills to delegate and to evaluate the performance of assistive personnel.

○ Demand faculty-to-student relationships that are more egalitarian and characterized by cooperation and community building. After all, it is the people that make the difference.

○ Inquire whether faculty are equipped to teach for a community-focused health care system.

○ Expect employers to be involved in the work of curriculum design, so that nursing education is truly preparing individuals suited to the realities of practice.

○ Look for recruitment and retention efforts to target individuals of diverse racial, cultural, and ethnic backgrounds, especially faculty and graduate students.

○ Shift the emphasis for research toward studies concerned with health promotion and disease prevention at the aggregate and community level.

○ Seek more balance between the traditional definitions of scholarship and the "scholarship of application," so that you can use these products in your daily practice.

○ Look to your faculty to be actively involved in the job placement of their graduates, so that you can claim your place in new employment markets.

KEY POINTS

1. Nursing education programs share certain concerns: escalating cost, recruitment challenges, a change in student mix, scarce faculty and clinical facilities, consumer demands for flexibility in education, and more.

2. Nursing education programs differ in many ways, particularly in the expected competencies of their graduates.

3. RNs seeking baccalaureate education have many more choices than they did a generation ago, including self-directed learning activities and external degrees.

4. Educational programs preparing for entry into nursing practice must reflect health care as it is delivered in the twenty-first century.

5. Continuing education is an ethical and professional responsibility, whether or not it is legally required.
6. Issues about education for entry into practice focus on whether baccalaureate education should be required for the professional nurse and AD education for a technical or associate nurse, how and when this should be accomplished, and whether it should be legally required.
7. Beginning with the ANA's position paper on education in 1965, the actions of the various nursing organizations have tended to support baccalaureate education for professional nursing.
8. Nursing research is a systematic inquiry into questions and problems arising from the practice of nursing.
9. Problems of translating the findings of nursing research into action are related to the lack of knowledge about nursing research held by many practicing nurses.
10. Nurse researchers have made significant improvements in health care possible.

STUDY QUESTIONS

1. How did you decide what nursing education program to choose, and what advice would you give to someone else confronted with the same decision?
2. What is your proposed resolution to the education for entry-into-practice debate?
3. How would job descriptions for a baccalaureate prepared nurse and an associate degree nurse differ?
4. Form an opinion about mandatory continuing education for relicensure, and state your rationale.
5. Review the articles in five or six recent issues of *Nursing Research*. Give your opinion on the value and relevance of these studies to nursing.

REFERENCES

1. National League for Nursing. *Nursing Data Review, Academic Year 2003*. Vol. 1: *Contemporary RN Nursing Education*. New York: The League, 2004.
2. American Association of Community Colleges: http://www.aacc.nche.edu. Retrieved July 10, 2002.
3. National League for Nursing, op cit.
4. American Association of Colleges of Nursing. Enrollments Rise at U.S. Nursing Colleges and Universities Ending a Six-Year Period of Decline: http://www.aacn.nche.edu/Media/NewsReleases/enr101.htm. Retrieved July 20, 2002.

5. National League for Nursing. *Nursing Data Review*. New York: The League, 1994.
6. NLN Center for Research in Nursing Education and Community Health. *Nursing Datasource*, Vol. II. New York: The League, 1997.
7. Montag M. *The Education of Nursing Technicians*. New York: Putnam, 1951, p 70.
8. Ibid, p 13.
9. National League for Nursing. *Educational Competencies for Graduates of Associate Degree Nursing Programs*. Boston: Jones and Bartlett, 2000.
10. American Association of Colleges of Nursing. *Essentials of College and University Education for Professional Nursing*. Washington, DC: The Association, 1986, p 4.
11. Ibid, p 5.
12. American Association of Colleges of Nursing. Fact Sheet: The Impact of Education on Nursing Practice. http://www.aacn.nche.edu/edimpact/index.htm. Retrieved March 1, 2005.
13. American Association of Colleges of Nursing. Degree Completion Programs for Registered Nurses: RN to Master's and RN to Baccalaureate Programs, October 2004: http://www.aacn.nche.edu/Media/FactSheets/DegreeCompletionProg.htm. Retrieved March 1, 2005.
14. Ibid.
15. Schlotfeldt R. The professional doctorate: Rationale and characteristics. *Nurs Outlook* 26:309, May 1978.
16. DHHS Division of Nursing. *National Sample Survey of Registered Nurses: Preliminary Findings*. Washington, DC: The Division, February 2001.
17. American Association of Colleges of Nursing. *The Essentials of Master's Education for Advanced Practice Nursing*. Washington, DC: AACN, 1996.
18. Ibid.
19. American Association of Colleges of Nursing. The Clinical Nurse Leader: http://www.aacn.nche.edu/Media/FactSheets/CNLFactSheet.htm. Retrieved July 13, 2005.
20. Aiken LH, et al. Educational levels of hospital nurses and surgical patient mortality. *JAMA* 290:1617–1623, September 24, 2003.
21. AACN, Clinical Nurse Leader, op cit.
22. American Association of Colleges of Nursing. AACN Position Statement on the Practice Doctorate in Nursing, October 2004: http://www.aacn.nche.edy/DNP. Retrieved February 12, 2005.
23. Interview. Todd Thomas, Director, Institutional Research, Excelsior College, Albany, NY, March 10, 2005.
24. Distance learning is changing and challenging nursing education. *Issue Bulletin*. Washington, DC: AACN, January 2000.
25. The Distance Educator: http://www.distance-educator.com. Retrieved March 2, 2005.
26. State and Certifying Boards/Associations: CE and Competency Requirements. *Journal of Continuing Education in Nursing*, January/February 2004: http://www.slackinc.com/allied/jcen/2003ce.htm. Retrieved March 1, 2005.
27. Ibid.
28. Two-year colleges prepare for battle over nursing programs. *Chr Higher Ed* 2, April 23, 1986.

29. Schlotfeldt R. Research in nursing and research training for nurses: Retrospect and prospect. *Nurs Res* 24:177, May–June 1975.
30. Notter, L. *Essentials of Nursing Research*, 2d ed. New York: Springer, 1978, pp 20–23
31. Merritt D. The National Center for Nursing Research. *Image* 18:84–85, Fall 1986.
32. National Institute of Nursing Research, January 25, 2005: http://ninr.nih.gov/ninr/about/adv-council.html. Retrieved March 8, 2005.

Updates can be found at

 http://www.JoelTheNursingExperience.com

Chapter 6

Career Opportunities

OBJECTIVES

After studying this chapter, you will be able to:

1. *Discuss the dynamics which create periodic nursing shortages and surpluses.*
2. *List the basic competencies most employers expect the new graduate to have.*
3. *Identify job opportunities available in the first years after graduation.*
4. *Recognize the types of positions that require advanced study.*

A TIME OF UNLIMITED OPPORTUNITIES

One of the most exciting aspects of nursing is the variety of career opportunities available. Nurses, as generalists or specialists, work in almost every place where health care is given, and new roles and positions seem to arise yearly. In part, this is in response to external social and scientific changes—for instance, shifts in the makeup of the population, new demands for health care, discovery of new treatments for disease conditions, recognition of health hazards, and health care legislation. In part, these roles for nurses have emerged because nurses saw a gap in health care and stepped in (nurse practitioner, nurse epidemiologist) or simply formalized a role that they had always filled (nurse thanatologist).

Usually, further education is required to practice competently in specialized areas, which are expected to grow. There is a distinction that must be made here between practice in a specialized area, and practice as a specialist. They are different, the former deriving more from experience and informal and continuing education, and the latter assuming a master's degree in advanced practice with a defined clinical area of study. Both are necessary. Specialized practice will vary to some extent according to the site of practice and the level and degree of specialization that is necessary in that site. For instance, in a small community hospital, a nurse may work comfortably on a maternity unit, giving care to both mothers and babies; in a tertiary care setting, perinatal nurse specialists, psychiatric nurse specialists, and nurses specializing in the care of high-risk mothers may work together; in a neighborhood health center, the nurse–midwife may assume complete care of a normal mother and work with both the pediatric nurse practitioner (NP) and hospital nurses.

In addition, nurses hold many positions indirectly related to traditional patient care as consultants, administrators, teachers, editors, writers, executive directors of professional organizations or state boards, lobbyists, health planners, utilization review coordinators, risk management specialists, epidemiologists, sex educators, case managers, and even anatomic artists, and legislators.

There are few careers that can offer the diversity of nursing. Almost always, a switch to a different kind of practice or a different setting means building on your basic nursing and experience, learning some new theory, and adjusting to new practice rights and responsibilities. Even if you stay in the same job, there are opportunities to try new techniques or broaden your responsibilities. The frequent crises in health care delivery present unlimited opportunities for nurses to show what they can do. With all these choices, it is difficult to find any one way to present areas of practice. In this chapter, the approach used is first to describe positions and the responsibilities and conditions of employment for each of the types of positions that a nurse can hold at graduation or shortly afterward. (You may wish to refer to Chapter 3, to review the settings in which health care is given, and Chapter 4, to see where nurses work.) An overview of other nursing opportunities is then given. Exhibit 6.1 describes some of the positions that require advanced education and experience. Further information is available from the specialty nursing organizations, educational programs, and career articles published in various nursing journals, some of which are listed in the Bibliography, as well as in Chapter 15 of Joel, *Kelly's Dimensions of Professional Nursing*, 9th edition (New York: McGraw-Hill, 2003). The obstacles to advanced practice are discussed in detail in *Dimensions*.

In discussing conditions of employment, specific salaries are usually not given or are presented as a range or average because there are dramatic geographic variations (highest in the West, lowest in the North Central and Southern states, but rising in the Sunbelt) and according to whether they are urban, rural, or suburban. Listings of current salaries are reported periodically in many nursing journals, federal statistics, ANA reports, and Appendix 2 of this text.

NURSING: SHORTAGES AND SURPLUS

Throughout the history of nursing there have been repeated shortages and, though less frequently, surpluses. Controversy has raged over the causes of these shortages, with less curiosity about how to deal with the periods of oversupply. One major incident of oversupply occurred during the Great Depression, when families could not afford private duty nurses and hospital nursing was done primarily by students. Another, more recent episode, had a short life: the prospective payment system described in Chapter 3 panicked hospitals, and as they closed units and sometimes laid off nurses there was a talk of a nurse oversupply. This panic lasted for about a year, because it was soon clear that, under the new system, even more nurses were needed to care for the very ill patients. Therefore, in 1986, as one nursing journal talked of layoffs another reported a surfacing shortage. Hospital admissions were rebounding, patient acuity was increasing, alternative health care facilities that required nurses were expanding, and new nonnursing opportunities were opening up for nurses. More nurses were choosing to work part-time and nursing enrollments were sagging. When these factors showed no signs of changing, the situation suddenly became a crisis. How do you define a crisis in what has always been a recurring nursing shortage? Probably not only when nurses and hospitals see a problem, but also when it becomes headline news in the *New York Times*, *Time* magazine, and the *Wall Street Journal*. This scenario has been repeated on numerous occasions.

DYNAMICS OF THE CYCLE

Nurse shortages have always been a response to either public need (as in wartime) or an economic expedient. The relatively low salaries of nurses and their readiness to take on a broad range of responsibilities have continually made them an excellent value. Regardless of the cause, each shortage has prompted organized nursing to rise to the occasion, producing ever greater numbers, but the demand has never been satisfied. Instead demand increases salaries and eventually economic conditions force more restraint in how and when the professional nurse is used. An oversupply follows, and history repeats itself.

The profession's reaction to every shortage in memory has been to respond blindly to external pressures, devising solutions with little thought about the long-term consequences. Nurses were the logical choice to provide continuity and caring as hospitals became commonplace for care of the sick. Inadequate numbers of nurses for both home care (which was the more usual site for the sick) and hospitals inspired the establishment of diploma schools. In another example, nurses for World War I were drawn from the ranks of college-educated women and received further concentrated education for nursing at the Vassar Camp, a program that, if protected and strengthened, would have allowed nursing to resolve its perpetual struggle for educational parity with more established professions. However, nonnurse influentials terminated the Vassar project once wartime need was past. World War II saw the licensed practical nurse proposed as a solution to home-front shortages, and the Cadet Corps, which became the prototype for associate degree education.

THE SHORTAGE

The nursing community had done its work well and without question. By 1988, RN employment was at an all-time high. There was one employed nurse for every 142 Americans, most of whom were well and self-sufficient.[1] Nursing services were being offered in more varied and diverse settings, yet nursing salaries had experienced little consistent growth over the years. Nurses willingly expanded and contracted their work, responding to the need of their patients and their employers. Nurses were the ultimate multipurpose worker, easily taking on the work of a variety of other providers. It became the mark of status in hospitals to boast of an all-RN staff. This theory of economic advantage is one explanation for the shortage that should allow us to have more control in future cycles.

The shortage of the late 1980s did provide us with some new challenges and opportunities. Organized nursing was moved to a spirit of solidarity when, in 1988, the American Medical Association (AMA) proposed the creation of a new caregiver, the registered care technologist (RCT), to supplement hospital nurses. Hospitals were the hardest hit by the shortage. In some situations 22 percent of nursing positions were vacant (5 percent is considered full employment). The RCT was to follow the orders of the physician but be supervised by the nurse.[2] The proposal was illogical and insulting, and moved nursing to a unity and assertiveness that has since come to characterize its management of issues.

The shortage of the 1980s can be traced to several unique situations. In fact, in some ways it really was a different shortage, a point well established by the Secretary's Commission on Nursing.[3] An insatiable demand stemming (at least in part) from a more intensely ill hospital patient, the fact that nurses are the most versatile health care workers (and perhaps the most dedicated and docile), and increasing demands for nursing services in what had been secondary markets (home care, nursing homes, ambulatory care) set the stage. A general disenchantment among women with nursing as a career choice (about 90 percent of nurses are women) resulted in enrollment declines of more than 28 and 19 percent in baccalaureate and associate degree programs, respectively.[4] So, the demand was high and the future was bleak.

The National Commission on Nursing Implementation Project (NCNIP) (see Appendix 1), jointly sponsored by the leadership of organized nursing and nonnursing groups, spearheaded a major public relations campaign directed at selecting nursing as a career. This initiative, conducted with the Ad Council (counterpart to legal aid, provides pro bono marketing services for essential, though needy, causes), in combination with a general economic recession in this country (nurses could always find work), resulted in a dramatic increase in applicants to educational programs. It was this renewed interest in nursing that put the "aging" of the field into high gear. Nursing became a preferred choice for the mature learner, such as those making midlife and later life career changes.

During this nursing shortage, nursing spoke out boldly and detailed what had to be done to recruit and retain nurses. Nurses needed fair wages and attractive benefits, emancipation from the nonnursing duties that kept nurses from their patients, status and prestige, and the opportunity to build a career.

Salary gains were noteworthy through 1991, although, when adjusted for inflation, increases only amounted to 3 percent per year.[5] In 1988, the American Organization of Nurse Executives (AONE) proposed a 100 percent differential between starting salary and the most experienced individual in a job classification. The growing salary range is particularly important. Salary compression, and the fact that in the late 1980s staff nurses received no increments for experience and additionally would reach their maximum earning capacity in about five years, made it impossible to realize much economic advancement over a lifetime of work. It should also be noted that there are very real salary variations between practice sites and employers; nursing homes pay 15 percent less than hospitals, with government salaries lagging behind the private sector.

The health care industry (especially hospitals and nursing homes where the shortage was greatest) have taken additional steps to resolve their shortage problem. An increasing number recruited nurses abroad, hired contract or "traveling" nurses, employed nurses from supplementary staffing agencies (creating problems of quality and continuity of care), or formed their own pool of nurses who worked per diem. Benefits were commonly withheld from per diem or part-time workers.

Particularly interesting was the variety of techniques used to attract and retain nurses. Among the benefits were flexible benefits (giving choices); dental, vision, and malpractice insurance; reimbursement for unused sick time; added vacation days (one hospital offered a nine-month year); free educational seminars; added conference days; child care programs; subsidized housing; a sabbatical after a number of years of service; differentials for shift, weekends, education, and certification; longevity bonuses; paid parking; purchasing discounts; health and fitness center discounts; nonmandatory float policies and frequent-floater bonuses; even maid service and a food purchasing cooperative.

Although hospital administrators have been advised for decades, through many studies on nursing, on what it takes to retain nurses, the advice seemed to fall on deaf ears all too often. By 1990, with a drastic shortage at hand, there was at least some greater inclination to listen. Once salaries, and often benefits, were competitive in most hospitals in a particular commuting area, attention had to turn to improving the environment and the conditions of work where nurses practice. Some changes were elementary and cost little but had been largely ignored, including better communication with access to administrators, attitude surveys, open forums, nurse-relations programs, newsletters, physician–nurse liaison committees, nurse-recognition and nursing image days, positive stories about nurses and advertisements praising nurses in local newspapers, employee-of-the-month programs, appreciation of nurses by physicians, directors' letters of commendation, and anniversary and recognition teas or receptions. There were also reward systems, including clinical ladders, clinical excellence-in-nursing awards, promotions from within, and liberal transfer policies.

Most important, the value of the nurse and the nurse's work was demonstrated by involving nurses in various types of planning, shared governance, and nurse empowerment. In many facilities, nurses determined their own schedules, regulated their own staffing needs, and were accountable for their own productivity. Employing assistive personnel placed under the control of nursing to do the fetching, carrying, transporting, message-taking, and other nonnursing tasks often left to nurses was a good use of resources.[6]

Another important recruiting and retention factor was flexibility in scheduling. Some innovations were weekend 12-hour days for a full week's salary, 12-hour shifts and shorter work-weeks, and top pay for unpopular shifts. Some of these longer shifts have since been questioned and eliminated, because they exist for the convenience of the nurse and possibly to the detriment of the patient. There are also signs of better interprofessional relationships between nursing and medicine. Many physicians recognized the need for more collegial relationships and worked in their own settings toward this goal. The lack of such relationships is considered one aspect of nurses' dissatisfaction.

Clearly, the hospital shortage received most of the publicity, but other areas of nursing such as home care also dealt with shortages. These agencies tried to match the salary and benefit packages of hospitals, as well as many of the communication and service approaches. One practice area of particular concern continues to be long-term care (LTC). Because of fiscal constraints, poor image, and the fact that the federal government mandates only a token RN presence, nurses have been less attracted to nursing homes.

SURPLUS MOVES IN TO TAKE ITS PLACE

However, our success in managing the shortage of the late 1980s and early 1990s provided no consolation as a surplus moved in quickly to take its place. Nursing enrollments had rebounded due to vigorous and sophisticated recruitment, and a greater number of nurses were working than ever before. But change moved too quickly, and the solutions we created to ease the pain of the shortage were used to our disadvantage.[7]

Organized nursing proposed that one way to assure more hours at the bedside was to unburden nurses of those tedious nonclinical duties which could just as capably be done by someone else; but growing economic pressure in the health care industry opened the door to a much broader interpretation, and these cheaper workers were substituted for the RN in direct care. In 1996, over 60 percent of respondents to the largest ever survey of the nursing community claimed that within the past year they had personally observed a reduction in the number of RNs giving direct care, and almost half reported the substitution of part-timers and agency personnel for RNs in permanent full-time positions.[8]

Other surveys reported the reduction in service or staff in areas such as housekeeping (mentioned by 40 percent of respondents), clerical (40 percent), supplies (31 percent), laboratory services (28 percent), and pharmacy (24 percent). As support services are cut back, more work inevitably falls on the shoulders of nurses, and it is probably that general usefulness and cooperative nature that has made our frequent under-utilization so acceptable to the industry. In instances more than

70 percent of the RN's time may have been consumed in support activities and nonnursing functions.[9]

Meanwhile, there had been almost 30 percent increase in hospital-based RNs alone between about 1986 and 1996,[10] but as statistics will show, the numbers are misleading and deserve some explanation. So where have all the nurses gone? The versatility of nurses has not gone unnoticed, and they have become the preferred choice for a broad spectrum of nonclinical roles: risk management, infection control, utilization review, case management, discharge planning, and so on. They are not necessarily in direct care, nor visible to the staff nurse, but they are there. Clinically, nurses have been dispersed to new areas, with a 70 percent increase of RNs in hospital outpatient areas between 1988 and 1992. In 1996, almost 15 percent of all hospital RNs were in emergency rooms, and primary care and specialty clinics. Factor in the higher acuity (sicker patients, more technology, more to be done for patients in the fewer days that they are allowed for care) and there has been 20 percent growth in the complexity of hospital inpatients.[11]

So, in the span of less than 20 years, we have run the gamut of a violent shortage, a more painful surplus, and are in the midst of another shortage in 2005. The rhetoric is familiar, we are saying that this shortage is different, but for once it is. The aging nurse workforce, the general labor scarcity in ancillary professions and support staff, and the global nature of this shortage are new factors, but just the beginning. Public opinion has been a major factor in today's shortage/surplus cycle. Consumers have conveyed the message that they want a nurse, and in an era of competition, the health care industry has responded. Americans have not just bought a media message; the complexity and instability of health care warrant rich staffing. The increased acuity and complexity of our patients does not only need more nurses, they need more sophisticated nurses; they must be experienced and highly skilled for today's practice. If much of our workforce is the older nurse, many of who have long histories in the profession and are expert, our practice environments will have to be redesigned to accommodate them. There is growing proof that the shortage of nurses in America's health care industry is putting patients at risk.[12]

WHAT EMPLOYERS EXPECT FROM A NEW GRADUATE

Although there is growing disagreement over what positions new graduates are qualified to accept, there is very little confusion over what employers expect from a new graduate. It used to be expected that the first job would be as a staff nurse in a hospital. New graduates were a little nervous over their competence, especially in the technical skills, and the employer began to provide many opportunities to perfect techniques. In 2003, a National Council of State Boards of Nursing (NCSBN) survey showed that almost 70 percent of employers offered preceptorships that lasted an average of 6.7 weeks. These preceptorships were most common in hospitals (80.9 percent) and home health agencies (72.9 percent). Thirty-six percent of new graduates reported that their employers customized these activities to their individual needs. A standardized approach was much more common in long-term care facilities, as was an orientation program of about 3 weeks as opposed to a preceptorship experience.[13]

Internships and residencies are another type of first experience, and though they may come in many forms, basically the new nurse is gradually oriented to all aspects of nursing care, with partial assignments, good supervision, and the opportunity to get experience in specific tasks as well as in overall care of patients. While this relieves some of the pressure of feeling less than competent in what might be an understaffed, busy practice setting, the price is a lower salary for that period and the possibility that not all the teaching promised will be delivered.

It is evident that nurses become specialized very quickly after graduation. The American Nurses Credentialing Center (ANCC) first-level certifications for competence in specialized areas of practice are testimony to this fact and are discussed in Chapter 11. In short order after graduation, the scientific knowledge erodes which allowed safe practice in a variety of areas, and you become most capable in the practice area where you have chosen to start your career. This being the case, there is good reason to select the patient population or practice setting which most interests you from the very beginning. This is also a good argument for *cross-training* in the workplace. Cross-training assumes an opportunity to build practice competency with more than one patient/client population. The challenge becomes to maintain those skills over time. It is in the best interest of the employer to provide appropriate experiences.

Given that some of the issues surrounding competence and entry into the job market have been identified, it remains to describe what competence means to the new graduate and the employer. What is expected of you as a beginning staff nurse? You will find statements on activities in Chapter 4. Most of these were identified through the opinion of experts. The most valid statements on the expected competencies of the new graduate come from the "role delineation" studies and other surveys conducted periodically by the NCSBN as the basis for developing the licensing exam (NCLEX-RN). A random sample of newly licensed registered nurses are surveyed within 6 months to one year of graduation to determine what activities are most important and most prevalent in their current practice settings. Respondents reported spending one-third of their working hours doing some variety of paperwork. In 2003, skill sets of major importance in their current practice setting were: critical thinking/clinical decision making, medication administration skills, psychomotor skills, and therapeutic relationship skills.[14] A similar study completed in 1993 provides more descriptive information.[15] At that time the newly licensed RN was expected to:

1. Practice safely and protect themselves and the patient:
   - use universal precautions;
   - perform cardiopulmonary resuscitation and the Heimlich maneuver;
   - recognize medical emergencies and intervene (embolus, hemorrhage, insulin shock, etc.) until a more qualified provider arrives;
   - monitor changes in the patient's condition and safety of equipment.

2. Coordinate care and supervise assistive personnel.

3. Communicate effectively:
   - help patient and family understand care and expected outcomes;
   - provide culturally competent care;
   - document accurately, completely, and in a timely fashion.

4. Be proficient in basic technical skills (no further clarification offered, specific skills depend on clinical focus).

5. Complete work assignment within the time frame of the shift (the best response to the question: how fast do I have to be?).

The similarities and differences are obvious, and may be due to the research methodology or changes in practice over time.

HOSPITAL PATIENT CARE POSITIONS

The basic requirement for a staff position is graduation from an approved school of nursing and nursing licensure or eligibility for licensure. The new graduate may be designated as a graduate nurse (GN) and must take and pass the licensure examinations within a specific period. Sometimes a lesser salary is offered until the RN is acquired, and the new graduate may be limited to a general nursing unit, that is, not the coronary care unit or another that requires an investment of extensive additional education. Nevertheless, in the hospital, the variety of experiences is endless.

In some cases, hospital nurses will be required to rotate shifts; in most cases, they will be expected to work holidays. It is possible to work part-time in most hospitals. Usually there are salary differentials for working evenings and nights. In recent years, flexible hours and shifts have become popular. The amount of practice autonomy varies considerably. Opportunities for promotion may be through clinical advancement or movement into managerial roles.

Positions described in hospital nursing include all those in which the employing agency is a hospital, whether private or voluntary, general or special, and whatever the size. The one element all hospitals have in common is that they are in existence primarily to take care of patients. The greatest differences from an employment point of view are types of responsibility, advancement opportunities, and salaries.

Hospitals may differ in size, location, ownership, and kinds of patients, but in addition, there are a variety of other characteristics that are important in predicting the quality of a hospital as a workplace. Some of these qualities were described in the magnet hospital study of the early 1980s; our observations have become more sensitive in the intervening years (see Appendix 1). The organization that attracts and retains nurses values the service they bring to patients and expects them to be responsible for their own practice. This sentiment can be detected by the presence of a peer review system, and the fact that peer appraisals are taken seriously in promotion and retention decisions. In some situations this respect results in the decentralization of managerial functions to the unit level. Simply put, autonomy and intrapreneurship are not only tolerated but also encouraged. Staff nurses are treated as professionals, responsible for both their practice and the environment in which they practice. Nurses find this respect in hospitals that provide the mechanisms for career advancement: career ladders, opportunity for internal promotion, financial assistance for both formal and informal education, and flexible work scheduling for personal needs, including the pursuit of educational goals. Beyond a fair compensation and benefit package, the greatest satisfiers to staff nurses are quality of care issues: support personnel to relieve RNs of nonnursing duties and participation in decisions about staffing and patient care policies. Nurses see themselves as part of a health care team, and expect to be treated with the respect accorded to other provider professionals. They see their own status determined to a large extent by the status and respect accorded to the chief nurse executive (CNE). In other words, they value strong central leadership with optimum individual practice autonomy.

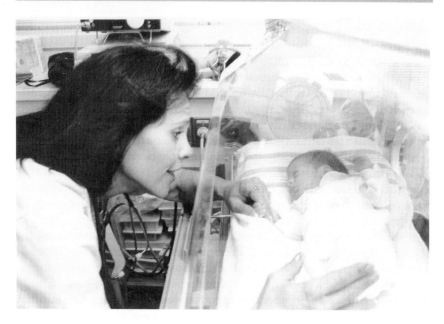

Caring for infants and children has its very special rewards. (*Courtesy of the Valley Hospital, Ridgewood, New Jersey*)

Nurses want to participate in decisions about the environment in which care is given, systems of nursing care, and one's personal practice. How each of these relates to the other two, and the nature of governance and control, is of special interest and will differ from setting to setting. Some models may be based on a system of *participatory management*, others may claim *shared governance*. The terminology may be overlapping, but it is agreed that significant participation of the staff nurse in decision making is important, with a free flow of information in all directions. Nurses must be offered not just participation but ownership in the organization. In all these models, nurses have not only autonomy but also the corollary responsibility. For instance, in one model, which the participants called *collaborative governance*, day-to-day decision making took place at the unit level. The process required special education for the head nurse, renamed the clinical manager, consisting of topics such as in budgeting, team building, performance evaluation, counseling, and so on. In other examples of participatory management, all decision making is centralized, staff nurses and managers come together to develop policy and decide on aspects of operations, each holding an equal amount of authority (put simply, perhaps too simply). Although not all hospitals require participation of this intensity or share authority to this extent, nurses weighing employment options need to consider the environment in which they would be most comfortable. Some people prefer a more traditional relationship and structure. The mode of governance will affect the nurse's job responsibilities, and is not restricted to hospitals, but is also found in other sites for care, such as community health and nursing homes. To understand the intricate tapestry that is nursing, students will have to read carefully and make quantum leaps in their thinking from time to time.

Many hospitals still have fewer than 100 beds, so there may be relatively little separation of specialties, with the exception of obstetrics, pediatrics, and psychiatry. However, when there is a declining census, hospitals in the same geographical area are beginning to cooperate by sharing their facilities: one may have the only pediatrics unit, another the only cardiac surgery. Therefore, the staff nurse may still become specialized. Positions in the emergency room and the outpatient department, operating room, rehabilitation unit, or intensive care unit (ICU) may require specialized training, but programs such as an outpatient surgery or "overnight" unit, or home care services, present challenges in nursing without necessarily mandating more formalized education.

In most hospitals, the range of experiences is endless. Larger hospitals and those in medical centers may offer a greater variety of specialties, exotic surgery, and rare treatments, as well as the advantages of being in the center of hospital, medical, and nursing research. Smaller hospitals may be less impersonal, located in the nurse's own community, and provide the opportunity to be a generalist on smaller patient units. Also, the smaller nonteaching hospital may offer many more opportunities in skills, whereas in a teaching center those "hands on" experiences are often reserved for medical students. A nurse is usually hired for a particular specialty unit (except for very small hospitals), but it is not uncommon to be asked to "float"—replace a nurse on any unit. Floating should not extend to units that require special knowledge and skill unless the nurse is "cross-trained"—preparing a nurse for practice competence in two or more specialty areas. There should be clarity on the floating issue before you accept a position. In some hospitals, there are "float pools" or resource teams—highly skilled nurses who never have a regular unit, and are compensated for this role.

Depending on the policies a hospital has regarding promotion, a nurse could become a head nurse without further education, but not without experience. *Head nurses* are in charge of the clinical nursing units of a hospital, including the operating room, outpatient department, and emergency room. They may also be called, more recently, *nursing coordinators* or *clinical coordinators*. Head nurses are accountable to the next higher person in the organizational hierarchy, usually the supervisor, or, in a smaller hospital, the assistant director of nursing or the director. The head-nurse position is the first management position most nurses achieve (or perhaps that of assistant head nurse, who may share some of the head-nurse functions and substitute for the head nurse in his or her absence).

It is the head nurse's job to manage the operations and nursing care in a relatively small area of the hospital, ensuring its quality. This may or may not include supervision of ward clerks in their clerical activities. With the trend toward decentralization of nursing authority, the head nurse is expected to give more attention to acting as a consultant and teacher for staff, to following the clinical progress of the patients, and to maintaining communication with physicians and other health personnel. In most instances, the head nurse works only the day shift, but may alternate on weekends and holidays with the assistant head nurse.

There are a number of other employment opportunities for nurses in hospitals, although they may have only an indirect relationship to traditional nursing care, and are often in a department other than nursing service. Nurses on the intravenous (IV) team are specially trained, and responsible for all the IV infusions given to patients (outside of the operating room and delivery room). They usually bring the appropriate solution to the patient, add ordered drugs, and start and/or restart the IV infusion. In some institutions they are also permitted to start a blood transfusion.

The nurse–epidemiologist or infection control nurse focuses on surveillance, education, and research. The surveillance aspect is designed for the reporting of infections and the establishment, over a period of time, of expected levels of infections for various areas. Patients with infections are checked to see whether the infection was acquired after admission. Reports are used for epidemiologic research, and the staff are educated in the prevention of infection. Nurses have also been trained as epidemiologists in public health agencies, where they perform similar but broader duties that involve the total community. Another challenging role is that of ombudsman, or patient advocate, in which a nurse acts as an intermediary between the patient and the hospital in an attempt to prevent or resolve problems of the patient related to the hospital or hospitalization.

Another role may be in quality assurance (QA), with a variety of titles. Although these persons may have a medical records background, most are nurses. The primary function of QA practitioners is to assess and evaluate indicators of the outcomes of care. The position arose from the increasing requirements of the Joint Commission on the Accreditation of Health Care Organizations (JCAHO), as well as demands on the part of payers and consumers for accountability. Their numbers are estimated to be in the low thousands. QA work includes but goes beyond the boundaries of nursing. Working with the professional staff, they determine the indicators to be studied, gather and analyze data, disseminate results, and recommend corrective action. Individuals in these roles may report to a variety of areas in the organization: the CNE, director of medical records or finance, or the chief operating officer (COO) as examples.

It has also become common for nurses to assume roles in utilization review (UR) and in coordination of community health or community education. UR is the internal monitor to determine whether patients are being admitted and discharged appropriately and whether resources are used properly during the period of hospitalization. It is a role that is imperative to the fiscal integrity of the institution. The community health coordinator may direct the program for outpatient teaching and participate in educating the community to the needs and contributions of the hospital.

STANDARDS OF CLINICAL NURSING PRACTICE

To help attain the goal of quality in nursing practice, in 2004 the ANA revised the *Standards of Clinical Nursing Practice*. These are general

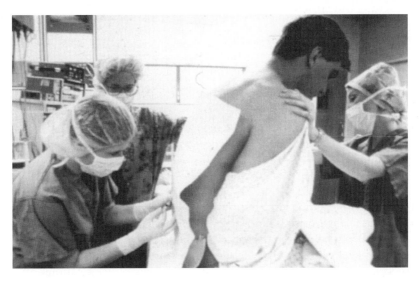

Nurse anesthetists are among the highest paid advanced practice nurses. (*Courtesy of the American Association of Nurse Anesthetists [AANA]*)

standards; they apply to all RNs engaged in clinical practice, regardless of specialty, practice setting, or educational preparation, and serve as the framework for specialty standards. These standards consist of *Standards of Care* (patient centered) and *Standards of Professional Performance* (provider centered).[16] Each standard is accompanied by measurement criteria to allow a determination on competence. Assessment is the first standard under "Standards of Care" and is included here as an example. Exhibit 6.2 presents a list of ANA practice standards and the year each was published.

Standard I: Assessment

The nurse collects Client Health Data

Measurement Criteria

1. The priority of data collection is determined by the client's immediate condition or needs.
2. Pertinent data are collected using appropriate assessment techniques.
3. Data collection involves the client, significant others, and health care providers when appropriate.
4. The data collection process is systematic and ongoing.
5. Relevant data are documented in a retrievable form.

Standards should remain stable over time. Criteria must reflect current practice, and so will change with advances in knowledge, practice, and technology.

Literally hundreds of specific nursing tasks are involved in meeting these standards, some of which can be carried out by less prepared workers. It is the degree of nursing judgment needed, as well as knowledge and technical expertise, that determines who can best help any patient.

ASSIGNMENTS FOR DELIVERING CARE

Three basic methods of assignment for delivering day-to-day care to patients in the hospital (and perhaps nursing homes and other inpatient facilities) are functional, team, and case. In *functional nursing*, the emphasis is on the task; jobs are grouped for expediency and supposedly to save time. For instance, one nurse might give all medications, another all treatments; aides might give all the baths. Obviously, the care of the patient is fragmented, and the nurse may lose the sense of "real" nursing.

Nevertheless, this approach is used in many facilities, especially on shifts that are understaffed. The work gets done; there may be limited nurse or patient satisfaction.

Team nursing presumes a group of nursing personnel, usually RNs, LPNs, and aides, working together to meet patient needs. It became popular after World War II, when the shortage of nurses was acute. For team leader, a baccalaureate degree had been suggested by the Surgeon General's Consultant Group on Nursing as early as 1963, but there are often not enough baccalaureate graduates to fill these positions. Other team members are under the direction of the team leader, who assigns them to certain duties or patients, according to their knowledge or skill. The team leader has the major responsibility for planning care and coordinating all activities, acting as a resource person to the team (though not always prepared to do so). Often, the team leader is the only nurse directly relating to the physician, and, too often, actual patient contact is infrequent or sporadic. The original concept of the team has been diluted. Planning and evaluation are seldom a team effort; conferences to discuss patient needs are irregular; and too frequently, the team leader has a mostly functional role, doing treatments and giving medications in an endless cycle. Nevertheless, the professional nurse should expect to be part of a nursing team, or, more likely, leader of this team, because most hospitals utilize some version of team nursing, at least to the extent that the RN supervises and directs other nursing personnel in patient care. Another noteworthy variation of team nursing is Manthey's "Partners in Practice," which matches different skill mixes of professional, technical, and assistive nursing personnel on a permanent basis to work in an arm's length relationship.[17]

Primary nursing was instituted in the 1970s and is a somewhat confusing designation for the *case method*, in which total care of the patient is assigned to one nurse. A major difference between primary nursing and other methods of assignment is the accountability of the nurse. The patient has a primary nurse, just as she or he has a primary physician. A nurse is a *primary nurse* when responsible for the care of certain patients throughout their stay and an *associate nurse* when caring for the patients while the primary nurse is off duty. Ideally the primary nurse is responsible for a group of patients 24 hours a day, even though an associate nurse may assist or take over on other shifts. The primary nurse is in direct contact with the patient, family/significant others, and members of the health team, and plans cooperatively with them for total care and continuity. The head nurse then is chiefly in an administrative role. Almost always the primary nurse is an RN. Sometimes the nursing team involved in primary nursing consists of all RNs, with the exception of aides who are generally limited to "hotel service," dietary tasks, and transportation. There is almost unanimous agreement that the primary

Exhibit 6.1 Positions in Nursing Requiring Advanced Preparation

Position	Qualifications[a]	Practice setting	Responsibilities	Working conditions
Clinical Nurse Specialist (CNS): Psychiatric/mental health, medical/surgical, community health, perinatal, oncology, geriatric, pediatric, and a limitless number of other highly specialized areas.	Master's degree in clinical specialty with functional preparation as a CNS; certification for advanced practice to comply with state and federal law.	Usually hospitals; increasing number in CH/PH; also ambulatory care; private practice; nursing homes.	Direct care of selected patients in specialty; nursing staff development; consultation with nursing and other health professionals; identification of populations at risk; sometimes research; may include middle management functions. Focus on systems of care as a whole as well as care of individual patients. A heavily "mediated" role (often works through other people rather than personal "laying on of hands"). Prescriptive authority in many states.	Salary usually middle manager level. Hours may be flexible. Benefits depend on setting. If position includes management, may be structured into 8-hour shifts; hours may be long. Sometimes called at home. If self-employed, must arrange own benefits.
Nurse Practitioner (NP): Clinical practice focus is broadly defined when compared to the CNS, family practice, adult and women's health, psychiatric NP, school and college health practice, geriatrics, pediatrics, to name a few. Recently you will see the acute care NP, in many ways to fill a gap created by disappearing medical residency programs.	Dramatic shift to exclusive master's preparation over the past 30 years; many NPs still currently only hold certificate preparation; certification expected to comply with state and federal law.	Community and ambulatory settings; private practice; joint practice with physicians; growing presence in nursing homes and in hospitals.	NPs assume some functions which were once the exclusive domain of the physician; prepared chiefly for the primary care role (first and continuing contact for patient in the delivery system), though the acute care NP challenges this assumption; concerned with health promotion, disease prevention, diagnosis and treatment of minor acute illness, and management of chronic disease. Focus is overwhelmingly on the one-to-one relationship with individual clients. Prescriptive authority of some form in every state and territory.	Salary and benefits may be negotiable, but generally about some as for CNS. Hours may be flexible, depending on setting. Need for significant malpractice insurance.

	Education	Setting	Responsibilities	Salary/Conditions
Nurse anesthetist (CRNA)	Graduation from an accredited master's program in nurse anesthesia; national certification; there are clinical nursing doctorate programs in anesthesia.	Operating and delivery rooms in hospitals, surgicenters, emergency rooms, some doctor's offices.	Pre- and postanesthesia care, administration of anesthetic agents, resuscitation services, pain management, respiratory care, establishment of arterial lines. Practice in all but one state without anesthesiologist supervision. Medicare reimbursement dependent on anesthesiologist except where state waiver has been secured.	Salary among the highest in nursing; not usually under the nursing department; day into early evening hours with frequent call; need for substantial malpractice insurance coverage.
Nurse-Midwife (CNM)	Accredited nurse—midwifery programs vary from 8 months to 2 years; a growing trend toward master's preparation; certification required.	95 percent of CNMs attend births in hospitals. 11 percent in freestanding birth centers, and 4 percent in the home. Pre- and postnatal care in ambulatory sites including clinics, physician's offices, and so on.	Require formal collaborative arrangement with an obstetrician to provide consultation and management of high-risk patients; practice includes prenatal care, labor and delivery, immediate care of newborn, postpartum, family planning, and well-woman care.	Significant malpractice insurance requirements; hours may be erratic depending on patient needs.
School or college health nurse (student health service)	Usually baccalaureate/ master's (same as for teachers) preparation; frequently require special courses and certification as designated by state regulations; may be a school NP with a master's degree and certification.	Any type of school, public or private, kindergarten through high school; also colleges, universities.	Vary with requirements of board of education; may be first-aid-type care with some health teaching; routine screening for visual and hearing problems; record keeping. For NPs, same as NP responsibilities.	Depends on types of schools—salary/benefits (health plans, retirement). Could be same as for teachers; salary often lower without master's degree or at least postbaccalaureate credits. Same holidays and vacations as teachers. Usually work only days except in higher education.

(continued)

Exhibit 6.1 (continued)

Position	Qualifications[a]	Practice setting	Responsibilities	Working conditions
Nursing faculty (formal academic setting)	Depends on educational program. Baccalaureate for LPN to doctorate for universities. Nursing degree (BSN and/or MSN) preferred, sometimes legally required. Usually require experience, sometimes specialization.	Trade schools, hospitals, junior colleges, colleges, universities.	Develop and carry out curriculum; prepare for and teach courses in classroom, laboratory, and clinical settings; recruit, select, promote, counsel, and evaluate students; develop special projects; work on committees to meet needs of program and/or students; may be expected to do research, write, and be involved in nursing and community activities, especially in colleges and universities; may be expected to hold joint positions in the clinical setting, especially in higher education; also involved in campus activities.	In higher education, salaries vary according to rank (instructor to professor), education (doctoral/nondoctoral), and whether a 10-month or calendar year contract is given. Hours flexible; may have evening classes; may do much work at home; may work during academic year only; may become tenured if criteria are met (emphasize scholarship, particularly research).
In-service education (staff educator)	From simply good clinical experience to a master's, the latter especially for a department director.	Hospitals, nursing homes, public health/community health.	Sees to orientation and ongoing education of nursing staff as related to competencies and work role. May require similar preparation to nursing faculty for teaching classes.	May have salary and benefits somewhat in range of middle management if director; teachers usually receive less. Most programs given during the day, but may also include evenings and nights for other shifts.

Title	Education	Settings	Responsibilities	Salary/Benefits
Nurse executive/nurse administrator; director of nursing; vice president for nursing; assistant administrator	Preferred: baccalaureate in nursing with master's or doctorate in nursing administration. Other degrees in administration, business also acceptable. In smaller settings, baccalaureate and experience. For nursing home, varies from job experience and RN only to master's degree.	Any place that nursing services are given. Most employed in hospitals, nursing homes, public health/community health agencies (PH/CH). Some corporate positions with responsibilities for nursing in several settings.	Varies with size of operation. May not include day-to-day operations. Planning, organizing, controlling, evaluating nursing services; includes personnel management, labor relations, budget, working with other administrators and public. May be limited to nursing department or include other departments. Should be part of the top management team.	Negotiable salary and benefits; flexible hours (may be long). Lowest salaries/benefits usually in nursing homes.
Middle management; supervisor; clinical coordinator—various titles	Nursing baccalaureate and master's preferred with clinical and/or administrative focus/experience. Still some acceptance of no degree (especially in nursing homes) with good clinical and/or head nurse track record.	Usually hospitals, PH/CH. In nursing homes, may be the only nurse at night.	Participate in nursing policymaking and problem solving; supervising and evaluating delivery of nursing care; collaborating with other departments; coordinating staff activities, possible scheduling of staff; recruiting, selecting, evaluating personnel; sometimes facilitating research; coordinating student learning experiences.	Salary should be higher than that of staff nurse but isn't always if nurses are unionized. May have same benefits as staff nurses plus additional managerial perks such as meeting expenses.
Nurse researcher	Usually a doctorate; sometimes advanced research training and experience.	Any health care setting; universities; private research groups; government agencies.	Develop and carry out research; assist others in applying research findings; train nurses in research.	Negotiable salary, except for government positions where salaries are established according to a set schedule. Hours flexible.

°All require current licensure and, generally, experience in nursing.

Exhibit 6.2 ANA Nursing Practice Standards and Year Initially Published/Revised

Nursing Practice (1973)
Psychiatric–Mental Health Nursing (1973, 1994, 2000)
Medical Surgical Nursing (1974)
Orthopedic Nursing (1975)
Neuroscience Nursing (2002) (Neurological and Neurosurgical Nursing 1977)
Urological Nursing (1977)
Pediatric Oncology Nursing (1978, 2000)
Cancer Nursing (1979)
Cardiovascular Nursing (1981)
Perioperative Nursing (1981)
Rheumatology Nursing (1983)
Maternal–Child Nursing (1983)
Child and Adolescent Psychiatric–Mental Health Nursing (1985)
Practice in Correctional Facilities (1985, 1995)
Rehabilitation Nursing (1986)
College Health Nursing (1986, 1997)
Community Health Nursing (1986)
Home Health Nursing (1986, 1999)
Gerontological Nursing (1987, 1995, 2001)
Hospice and Palliative Care (2002) (Hospice Nursing 1987)
Oncology Nursing (1987)
Primary Health Care Nurse Practitioner (1987)
Addictions Nursing (1988, 2004)
Organized Nursing Services (1988)
Clinical Nursing Practice (1991, 1998, 2004)
Cardiac Rehabilitation Nursing (1993)
Nursing Professional Development: Continuing Education and Staff Development (1994)
Nursing Informatics (1994)
Respiratory Nursing (1994)
Otorhinolaryngology Clinical Nursing (1994)
Acute Care Nurse Practitioner (1995)
Pediatric Clinical Nursing (1996, 2003)
Oncology Nursing (1996)
Nurse Administrators (1996, 2004)
Advanced Practice Registered Nursing (1996)
Forensic Nursing (1997)
Diabetes Nursing (1998, 2003)
Parish Nursing (1998)
Genetics Clinical Nursing (1998)
Intellectual and Developmental Disabilities Nursing (2004) (Developmental Disabilities
    and/or Mental Retardation Nursing 1998)
Home Health Nursing Practice (1999)
Public Health Nursing Practice (1999)
Nursing Informatics (2001)
School Nursing Practice (2001, 2005)
Vascular Nursing (2004)
Neonatal Nursing (2004)
Faith Community Nursing (2005)
Pain Management Nursing (2005)
Plastic Surgery Nursing (2005)

nursing model is the most satisfying to patients, families, physicians, and nurses, and that care is of high quality.

However, each method of assignment has its strong points and liabilities. Functional assignment may be the most administratively efficient because of its division of labor according to specific tasks, but almost no one says that either patient or nurse finds it preferable to others. Team nursing, when done according to the original concept, may be satisfying to the team who can give their attention to a small group of patients and also develop an esprit de corps that compensates for the time expended in conferencing and work coordination. It is often seen as expensive because of the need for this additional time spent. Primary nursing, considered the most "professional" of assignments, also has its detractors; additional stress, role overload, and role ambiguity are cited.

Functional, team, and case methods (primary) are distinguished from one another by the extent to which they allow continuity of the provider of care, the use of assistants to the RN and the roles these assistants assume, the degree to which activities as compared with the complexity of the clinical situation drive decisions on the assignment of personnel, and the autonomy or decentralization of authority and accountability. Given these basic categories, there are endless variations on each theme. New graduates should be aware of some of these variable models and of their own comfort zone in practice.

ASSISTANTS TO THE NURSE

Another reality of nursing is the significant presence of assistive personnel, both those who provide environmental support and others who have some role in patient care. The work of environmental support personnel may include stocking supplies and checking equipment, transporting patients and equipment, cleaning patient units, checking the work of other departments, and moving furniture. It has been recommended that these people be carefully trained and oriented to their responsibilities. In the best of situations, they are accountable to the head nurse and under the organizational control of the nursing department.

Environmental support staff must be distinguished from unlicensed assistive personnel (UAP) who are trained to assist the RN in providing care, and are often referred to as "nurse extenders." *Delegation* is essential to the RN/UAP relationship. In delegating, an RN transfers the responsibility for task performance from themselves to another person, but the *accountability* both for the process and the outcome of the task remains with the RN. A further distinction is made between direct delegation where there is verbal direction concerning a specific situation, and indirect delegation which involves an approved list of activities or allowable tasks which are sanctioned by the organization. While indirect delegation may offer some consistency, it can never substitute for or supersede the independent judgment of the RN.[18] It is rare for RNs to be responsible solely for themselves, and in fact most professionals accomplish a lot of their work through others. Students should be prepared for this reality within their educational program. The ANA cautions that risk exists:[19]

- When the RN knowingly delegates a nursing care task to a UAP that only a licensed nurse can perform, or when the delegation is contrary to law or involves a substantial risk of harm to a person or client.
- When the RN fails to exercise adequate supervision of the UAPs to whom patient care tasks have been delegated.
- When the RN knowingly delegates a patient care task to a UAP who has not had the appropriate training or orientation.

The issue of UAPs and the RN is honeycombed with legal and ethical dilemmas. Can the RN plead ignorance of the extent of the UAP's preparation when a mistake is made and the patient is harmed? How adequate is the degree of supervision provided to assistive personnel in nursing homes? Will the requirement of certifying home health aides and nursing home assistants legitimize their work to the extent that they will eventually become independent of RN supervision? Since these two categories of "nurse extenders" have very little direct supervision and care for the most compromised of our public, how is safety to be assured?

DIFFERENTIATED PRACTICE/THE CLINICAL LADDER

Because the expected competencies of the various kinds of nursing education programs differ, theoretically the responsibilities of each type of nurse should also differ in the staff nurse position. Unfortunately, the tendency is often to assign all nurses to the same kinds of tasks and responsibilities, so that differences are not consistently maximized.

In an informal way, differentiating among nurses based on their competence has existed for many years. Some feel that education is the best basis for such practice distinctions, others say that the model should be built on levels of demonstrated competence, that is, the clinical ladder approach. Still others combine the two.

There are many variations of a *clinical career ladder*.[20] Most organizations use a committee composed of the CNE, other representatives of management, and staff nurses to develop and implement a career-ladder plan, but other approaches are also used. Criteria are set, usually

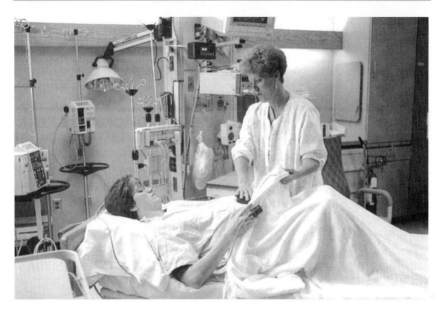

Today's labor and delivery nurses find themselves caring for more and more women with serious medical problems. (*Courtesy of Magee-Women's Hospital, Pittsburgh*)

including educational levels, experience, clinical competencies, certification, continuing education, peer and supervisory evaluation, and seniority. Positions are categorized as I, II, III, and so on, based on these criteria. It is important that moving up the ladder not be a form of tokenism and that there be added rights and responsibilities as one progresses. In some settings, added expectations are in areas such as patient and family education, leadership and coordination, and research. In another, reaching the role expectations and competencies of primary nursing is the second level, and the nurse may choose to stay there. Both lateral and vertical mobility should be possible, allowing one to progress yet stay at the bedside or move into a managerial role. A ladder should allow for a change in patient population and in job pressures and expectations. In other words, a nurse may move to another type of nursing, if qualified. Some nurses may choose realignment (downward mobility), perhaps as they choose to go to school. The guiding principle is for nurses to plan and develop their own careers. Through self-assessment, the first step, nurses identify their knowledge, skills, values, and interests in the context of the practice setting, and additionally what rewards are important to them. Salary changes accompany each change in levels.

In preparing for the review that determines one's readiness to progress, the nurse usually prepares a portfolio that contains information demonstrating ability to meet the performance criteria of a particular level of nursing practice. Information may include a case study, a patient-teaching tool, a discharge plan, a nursing database, or other evidence of the nurse's abilities as well as evidence of educational advancement (formal course work or continuing education). The review process should be objective and involve both peers and administrators. If it is determined that the nurse does not meet the criteria, she or he should have a clear idea of what areas of behavior or practice need to be strengthened. Because both increased salary and prestige are at stake, career ladders must be carefully developed, managed, and explained.

Not everyone likes the clinical career ladder. Some nurses find it time-consuming to develop a portfolio, even with help; some do not want peer evaluation. Others think it really doesn't measure "a good nurse." Still others simply don't care and want to stay where they are. However, if their salaries "top out," nurses may prefer to "ladder" instead of "level."

SUPPLEMENTAL STAFFING AGENCIES

An employment option is to be placed in a position through a supplemental staffing agency sometimes called a temporary nursing service (TNS). Nurses most commonly using TNSs are some new graduates, nurses enrolled in advanced educational programs, nurses with small children who cannot work full time or all shifts, or nurses who simply prefer the flexibility. The TNS will pay them a salary for the hours worked, with the usual legal deductions, after billing the institution or the patient or client using the worker's services. There are some TNSs who treat the nurse as an independent contractor as opposed to an employee. The distinction is important since you are responsible for your own social security and tax payments as an independent. You also forfeit protections that are legally guaranteed to employees. There are local and national agencies, and selecting a reputable one is extremely important. Job assignments may be made an hour or a week ahead, but the nurse is not obligated to take it; however, no agency is interested in a no-show. As well as a great deal of flexibility and variety, there are also disadvantages, even with a good TNS: no job security, sometimes only the minimum rate paid by the area hospitals with no increases, and of course the constant reorientation to new nursing units and patients, even to new hospitals, although some nurses limit themselves to one particular hospital. The fact that "agency nurses" are sometimes looked down on by regular staff as incompetent (although they may simply be unfamiliar with that hospital's procedure) also creates problems for these nurses.

A variation of temporary nursing is the "travel" nurse, who accepts short-term contracts directly with a hospital anywhere in the country and sometimes abroad. Arrangements are made through an agency. The hospital usually gives only the benefits required by law, but pays for the nurse's travel and sometimes arranges for or provides housing. The nurse must get a temporary license in each state where employed. Although the variety is exciting for many nurses, the place of work is seldom ideal, as there usually is a problem—strikes, extreme short-staffing, or other poor practice conditions. Because TNSs are widely used during a nursing shortage, some states have put regulations in effect, both setting standards and limiting what can be charged. Nursing homes that use TNSs have been particularly concerned by what they consider outrageous costs.

NURSING IN EXTENDED AND LONG-TERM CARE FACILITIES

The distinction between skilled and intermediate beds in nursing homes has been largely abandoned. All of today's nursing home residents are frail and seriously compromised in their self-care. Instead, the most important distinction is the payer source, mostly Medicaid, and to a lesser extent Medicare and personal pay. Medicare recipients are confined for a limited period on the assumption that their conditions are transient and there will be positive progress. In contrast, Medicaid funds long-term continuing care. The difference in reimbursement rates between the former and the latter are considerable. Residents of these facilities are not only the elderly, but include people of many ages and stages of disability, including those with neurological problems, victims of trauma, multiple sclerosis, and so on. More RNs are working in nursing homes today, although the majority of caregivers are practical nurses and certified nursing assistants (CNA).

Nurses may have positions in nursing homes similar to those in hospitals, with the additional role of facility administrator being assumed by some nurses. In this case, the nurse must be certified for the position, and although the individual's knowledge of nursing may be extremely helpful in understanding the need for quality care, being a nurse is not a requirement for certification.

The director of nursing, who has the same kinds of responsibilities as any other director of nursing, is sometimes expected to act as the administrator's assistant. In small nursing homes, the director might assume both roles. Because most facilities are for-profit, the financial management is extremely important. The administrative nurse should be well prepared in managerial skills; unfortunately, that is rare.

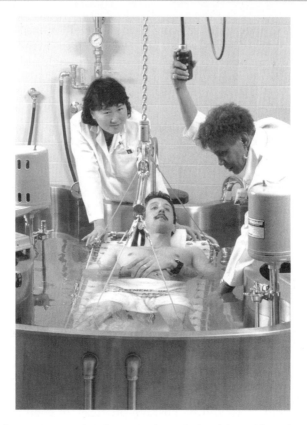

Nursing in long-term care involves ongoing relationships with patients and often responsibility for total care. (*Courtesy of the U.S. Department of Veterans Affairs*)

In most nursing homes the pace is slower and the pressure less than in other settings for care. Nurses interested in nursing home care enjoy the opportunity to know the patient better in the relatively long-term stay and to help the patient maintain or attain the best possible health status. This is not the area of practice for someone impatient for quick results. Both rehabilitative and geriatric nursing require a larger amount of patience and understanding. In rehabilitation, nurses work closely as a team with related health disciplines—occupational therapy, physical therapy, speech therapy, and others. In geriatric nursing, the nurse works to a great extent with nonprofessional nursing personnel and acts as team leader, teacher, and supervisor. It may well be that there is only one licensed nurse in a nursing home per shift, with practical nurses as charge nurses and aides giving much of the day-to-day care.

Because the patients are relatively helpless and often have no family or friends who check on them, the nurse must, in a real sense, be a patient advocate. Physicians make infrequent visits and in some cases, where there are limited or no rehabilitative services, the nurse is the only professional with long-term patient contact.

For this reason, geriatric nurse practitioners (GNPs) are considered a tremendous asset in nursing homes. The GNP is responsible for assessing patients and evaluating their progress, performing certain diagnostic procedures, and interpreting the results. She or he diagnoses and treats minor acute illness and monitors and manages chronic conditions, as well as promoting health and preventing disease. Additional important functions are assessing personal and family relationships, patient and staff relationships, and life situations that may affect the patient's health status. In some nursing homes, the GNP is on 24-hour call.

Requirements for employment are similar to those in hospitals for like positions, although often the need for a degree is not emphasized. Conditions of employment and salaries have improved, but are not as good as those in hospitals. Because, under Medicare, orientation and subsequent in-service education are mandatory, the nurse has an excellent opportunity to learn about long-term nursing care and the concepts and techniques of geriatric nursing. Because the increase of older people is one of the trends in society, geriatric care is being given greater attention, and workshops, courses, and programs are available in the field. With an aging population, there are also likely to be good job opportunities for some time to come.

SUBACUTE CARE

Both hospitals and nursing homes have been recently aggressive in establishing "subacute" care units. Subacute care is for the patient who needs more clinical sophistication and professional monitoring than is possible in a nursing home, but less than is routine in a hospital. Though the rationale may be clinically sound, the motivation is often more economic than altruistic. Beds are better filled than standing empty. Both hospitals and nursing homes are vying for these programs. In reality, they can best service different constituencies. The nursing home has a natural capability for rehabilitation and restoration; the hospital is equipped to handle the step down from acute illness.

The premier provider in a "subacute" service is nursing. The jeopardy is that this service sector will become medicalized, and that nursing will be construed as basic, but not the essential ingredient in clinical success. Should we fail in building our case, subacute care will only provide a ready occasion to cut cost by reducing the presence of professional nurses and substituting assistive personnel who will be presented as adequate to the challenge. Requirements for employment are similar to those for staff nurses in hospitals or nursing homes.

PUBLIC HEALTH/COMMUNITY HEALTH NURSING

Public health nursing (PHN) synthesizes the knowledge from the nursing and public health sciences to promote and preserve the health of individuals, families, and communities. This area of specialization is population focused, community is client, and the provision of personal health services is only important as they benefit the community as a whole. The goal is to improve the health of the community by identifying subgroups (aggregates) within the population that are high risk for illness, disability, or premature death; directing resources toward these groups; and monitoring the adequacy of the response to these efforts. Home care is also a part of the community health agenda, recognizing that outreach to the sick and vulnerable in their homes is a community responsibility. Home care is not just a service to the acutely and chronically ill brought into the home as an option to the hospital. The setting creates new rights and responsibilities for both the nurse and the patient.

ANA has revised standards for community health, public health, and home health nursing practice. The standards for public health and community health nursing practice have been consolidated given their mutual focus on populations, and home health practice has been recognized as a distinctive area of personal care services.

Today, public health nurses (PHNs) practice in many settings. Most are employed by agencies that may carry the title of public health, community health, home health, or visiting nurse. They may be official—governmental and tax supported (e.g., a city or county health department); nonofficial or voluntary—agencies supported to a great extent by community funds (e.g., visiting nurse or home health service); or proprietary—for profit. These agencies range in size and services from small, employing only one or two PHNs, to very large, employing a sizable staff of professional nurses, other health professionals, practical nurses, and home health aides and homemakers.

PHN employment opportunities are not limited, however, to these agencies. Nurses may also be employed by hospitals to conduct home-care programs or to serve as liaison between the hospital and the community. They may work with other organizations, private and governmental, in need of the kinds of services the PHN is prepared to provide in schools, outpatient clinics, community health centers, walk-in clinics for drug addiction and sexually transmitted diseases (STD), migrant labor camps, and rural areas.

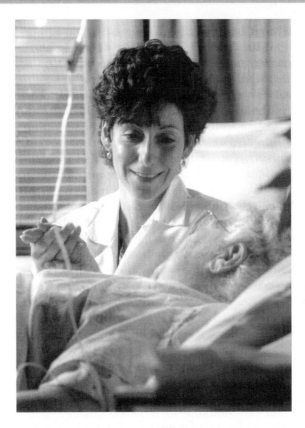

Subacute care services are being established in many hospitals and nursing homes. (*Courtesy of the U.S. Department of Veterans Affairs*)

Visiting nurses, or home health nurses, regardless of their place of employment, also carry out these functions and may, in addition, give physical care and treatments. With the advent of much earlier discharge from hospitals, patients are quite a bit sicker when they go home, and these nurses are required to know how to care for the acutely ill. If the nurse assessment indicates that such care does not require professional nurse services, home health aides/homemakers may be assigned to a patient/family, with nurse supervision and reassessment. Visiting nurses have also set up clinics that they visit periodically in senior citizen centers or apartments, as well as in the single-room occupancy (SRO) boarding homes commonly used for welfare clients in large cities. There are also many liaison roles with hospitals, HMOs, clinics, geriatric units, and various residences for the long-term disabled and mentally ill or retarded, primarily to assist in admission and discharge planning, as well as coordinating continuing patient care.

Besides state licensure, and for some agencies, prior nursing experience, one major qualification for PHN work is ideally graduation from a baccalaureate nursing program. Many graduates of these schools go on to earn a master's degree and are thus prepared educationally for a lifetime career in this field. Because of the shortage of nurses with the prescribed PHN preparation at the present time, however, graduates of diploma and AD programs can and do find positions in this field, working at the beginning level and under supervision. In some areas they work only in clinics. Some employers encourage nurses to work toward a baccalaureate degree by providing tuition or scholarship grants.

In 2000, 18.2 percent or 402,282 RNs worked in community and public health settings, including state or local health departments, community-based home health agencies, various types of community health centers, student health services, and occupational health services. Over 44 percent of nurses employed in community and public health settings have a baccalaureate or higher degree.[21]

In the past, PHNs enjoyed standard daytime hours, with most working Monday through Friday. However, with the move toward more care in the community on a 24-hour basis, PHNs are expected to rotate shifts and work weekends, much the same as nurses employed in institutions.

A unique and distinct aspect of PHN practice is the self-sufficiency and autonomy required when working in a setting "without walls." You have to know a lot, be clinically versatile, a critical thinker, have a quick mind, and be willing to confront your own biases.

Nurses in community practice have to relinquish the implied authority of hospital practice. Control is in the hands of the patient who will decline or grant access to his home. Anticipating this, nurses should have the personality attributes that allow them to deal successfully with such situations. Even if the setting is a clinic, there is no force that can make a client come or return or, for that matter, follow any prescribed regimen.

Many studies have documented the need for public health nurses to use interventions with clients and families that are specific to ethnic, cultural, and social values. Families may reject health teaching if it is perceived to be judgmental or prejudicial on the part of the health care provider.

Professional nurses who select PHN as a career need outstanding ability to adjust to many types of environments with a variety of living conditions, from the well-to-do in a high-rise apartment house to the most poverty-stricken in a ghetto or rural area, and to appreciate a wide range of interests, attitudes, educational backgrounds, and cultural differences. They must be able to accept these variations, to understand the differences, to communicate well so as to avoid misunderstandings and misinterpretations, and to be able to give equally good nursing care in every situation. PHNs in any position must use excellent judgment and are expected to use their own initiative. They have the opportunity to work with persons in other disciplines and other social agencies to help provide needed services to the clients, services that may include financial counseling, legal aid, housing problems, family planning, marital counseling, and school difficulties. In some instances, PHNs are not only case finders, but also case coordinators—patient advocates in every sense.

OFFICE NURSING

Office nurses are employed by physicians or dentists to see that their patients receive the nursing they need, usually in the office. Office nurses may give all of this care or assign certain duties to other personnel who work under their direction and supervision. If working for several doctors or dentists in a group practice, the nurse may supervise a staff of several employees. Nurses may be employed in a one-doctor general practitioner's office, which requires general skills, or they may be employed in a specialist's office, which requires special skills. For instance, surgeons may employ nurses who can also act as scrub nurses in surgery done at the hospital or assist them in office surgery.

What the office nurse does in terms of nursing will depend largely upon the employer's type of practice, daily schedule of appointments, and attitude about nurses' scope of practice. Tasks may be as routine as giving medications, chaperoning physical examinations, preparing equipment, and seeing that the patients' records are completed and filed at the end of the day. Better utilization would include observation, communication, teaching, and coordination with community health agencies. A few nurses make hospital patient rounds with or without the physician. Unfortunately, in too many instances the employer expects the nurse to be hostess, secretary, bookkeeper, errand girl, housekeeper, purchasing agent, public relations expert, and laboratory technician as well, work that in today's complex environment require a host of specialized talents. One of the most far-reaching effects on office nursing is the presence of the NP, who is often part of the physician's private practice and assumes much responsibility for patient care.

Most office nurses do have considerable experience. Salaries and working conditions in this field are, generally speaking, both flexible and variable, representing private arrangements between the individual office nurse and the employer. Office nurses sometimes say they are willing to make some sacrifices in salary because the hours or responsibilities of office nursing fit their tastes or general life situation.

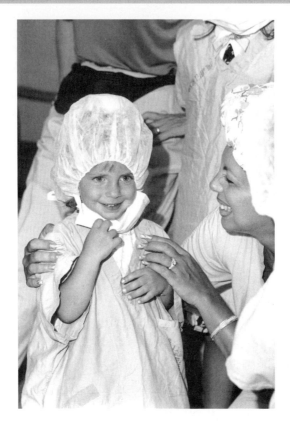

There are many novel practice opportunities such as this nurse who is conducting a hospital preadmission orientation for a child. (*Courtesy of the Valley Hospital, Ridgewood, New Jersey*)

Both salary and fringe benefits are likely to be lower than those for the hospital staff nurse. However, most office nurses seem to enjoy a friendly and congenial relationship with their employing physician or physicians and usually succeed in negotiating mutually satisfactory working conditions and salary. They appear to stay in the job longer than most nurses, an average of nine years.

CASE MANAGEMENT

The *case manager* role has surfaced with prominence in recent years as the health care delivery system is confronted with rising cost and increasingly complex patients. The case manager is discussed here as opposed to the nursing roles requiring advanced preparation in Exhibit 6.1, because there is no consensus as to the necessary qualifications for this area of practice. The title of case manager or nursing case manager is used haphazardly for anyone who coordinates care or services. In the proper use of the term, case managers should be used very judiciously for only the most costly and complex clinical situations.[22]

Case management may occur telephonically, or through paper trails or the physical presence of the client. Case managers may be employed by third-party payers (managed care systems or insurers), a health care facility, or the patient themselves (independent case managers). Regardless of who pays for the service, the manager's primary allegiance should be to the client. Case management should access the client to both the clinical sophistication and business acumen to make informed and personally acceptable decisions about the management of their health care regimen within the resources available to them. Case managers can expertly build the case for the conversion of benefits included in a policy or managed care agreement into other services which may be more suited to the client's needs and lifestyle. Where case managers are employed by the payer, they can approve such exceptions. Case managers coordinate, integrate, and negotiate all services on behalf of their clients. They challenge providers to consider options where treatment is ineffective. They advocate for the client in every sense of the word. Assignment of a case manager is an option for a patient to accept or reject, except in situations of worker's compensation, where the service is mandatory.

Although you need not be a nurse to be a case manager, 85 percent are. Because case managers are only necessary in the most complex cases, many believe that this role should be an integral part of master's preparation for advanced practice. This is not currently the case, with nurses of many skill levels filling this role.

OCCUPATIONAL HEALTH NURSING

The occupational health nurse (OHN), then called the industrial nurse, reportedly began in 1888 with services provided by Betty Moulder to a group of coal miners in Drifton, Pennsylvania. In 1895, the Vermont Marble Company hired Ada Mayo Stewart to care for ill and injured workers and their families. She is generally credited with being the first industrial nurse, as much has been reported about her activities.

Two department stores were the next to provide similar health services for their employees: the John Wanamaker Company of New York in 1897 and the Frederick Loeser Department Store in Brooklyn in 1899. Early in the 1900s more and more industries on both the east and west coasts recognized the economic value of keeping employees healthy and established similar health services. Adding impetus to the trend was the enactment of workers' compensation laws (beginning in 1911), which emphasized accident prevention to employees on the job, and provided for disability compensation for work-related injured or ill workers and encouraged immediate and expert attention to injuries received at work. This development brought more industrial nurses into the work sites.

For many years nurses employed in these positions called themselves industrial nurses. In 1958, however, the industrial nurses within ANA voted to call their field occupational health nursing, which reflected the broader and changing scope of practice within the specialty. Other organizations also adopted the newer term, including the American Association of Occupational Health Nurses (AAOHN). A key factor in the changes in OHN was the enactment in 1970 of the Occupational Safety and Health Act. That act created the National Institute for Occupational Safety and Health (NIOSH) to provide education to occupational health and safety professionals through the establishment of Educational Resource Centers (now called Education and Research Centers) and to research occupational health problems and recommend health and safety standards.

The Occupational Safety and Health Administration (OSHA) was also established to guarantee a "safe and healthful workplace." OSHA inspects the nation's workplaces for health and safety hazards, but its effectiveness has been blunted by lack of funds and the resistance of some employers, who have sometimes sued and won to limit the access of OSHA's inspectors. Nevertheless, unions, environmentalists, and other interested citizens have pressed for more action.

Guided by an ethical framework made explicit in the AAOHN Code of Ethics, occupational health nurses encourage and enable individuals to make informed decisions about health care concerns. Confidentiality of health information is integral and central to the practice base. Occupational health nurses are advocates for workers, fostering equitable and quality health care services and safe and healthy work environments.[23]

The OHN may work in a multidisciplinary setting or multinurse unit; however, more than 60 percent of OHNs work alone. Physicians are often employed on a contractual basis and provide medical services as needed, but in most cases the OHN nurse is the manager of the unit.

Whether this nurse functions in a sophisticated manner in the delivery of health care depends on his or her education and experience, and the policies of the employer. As a nurse practitioner or clinical nurse specialist, the nurse gives primary care and makes a diagnosis. She or he assesses the worker's condition through health histories, observation, physical examination, and other selected diagnostic measures; reviews and interprets findings to differentiate the normal from the abnormal; selects and carries out the appropriate action and referral as necessary; and counsels and teaches. The practitioner must also be concerned with the physical and psychosocial phenomena of the workers and their families, their working environment, community, and even recreation.

When the nurse does not function in an expanded role, standing orders or directions prepared and signed by the medical director give the necessary authority to care for conditions that develop while the employee is on the job. In a more conservative environment, where a nurse does not have specialized preparation, activities may be limited. However, these usually include first aid or emergency treatment, assisting the physician, carrying out certain diagnostic tests, and keeping health records. The ability to take and recognize abnormalities in electrocardiograms and to do eye screening, audiometric testing, and certain laboratory tests and x-rays is also important. In addition, the nurse must be vitally concerned with the safety of the employees and often conducts worksite tours with management and the safety engineer to help plan a practical safety program.

The scope of the OHN's practice has broadened considerably. More emphasis is being placed on health promotion activities to keep the worker well. There is an increased emphasis on worker health problems that may or may not be directly caused by the job but affect worker performance—alcoholism, emotional problems, stress, drug addiction, and family relations. In many cases, the nurse may be involved in developing employee assistance programs and in counseling and therapy.

Graduation from a state-approved school of professional nursing and current state registration are basic requirements for OHN. More employers are requiring a college degree and many find a graduate degree desirable. A career OHN may seek certification by the American Board for Occupational Health Nurses, an independent nursing specialty board authorized to certify qualified OHNs.

Salaries and fringe benefits vary according to the size of the industry or business and its location. The usual company benefits include vacations, sick leave, pensions, and insurance. Working hours are those of the workers; thus, in an industry with work shifts around the clock, nurses are usually there also. Although some industries carry professional liability insurance that supposedly covers the OHN, it may not apply in all cases of possible litigation. It is advisable, therefore, for the nurses to carry their own professional liability insurance.

PRIVATE DUTY NURSING

For many years, private duty nursing was second only to hospital nursing in its attraction for professional nurses, but each year has seen a decrease in the total number of nurses in this field of practice, particularly younger nurses.

Private duty nurses are independent practitioners in almost complete control of where they will work, when they will work, the types of patients they will care for, and when they will take vacation or days off. They are limited in what they can charge for services only by the prevailing fee in their community, which is not legally binding.

Private duty nurses make their availability for service known through a nurses' registry, an employment agency, local hospitals, and personal contacts with other nurses, doctors, and members of the community. Individual nurses may build up a list of "clients" composed of families and doctors who always try to engage them whenever they need private duty nurses. Some work only as specialists.

A private duty nurse is usually employed (by the patient or family) to nurse one patient in the hospital or home. Wherever they are, the nurse is responsible for the patient's care while with him or her. When the nurse leaves for any length of time, arrangements must be made for care in the interim. This is also done if the nurse wishes a day or so off after being with a patient continuously for a number of weeks.

Most patients requesting private duty nurses are quite ill, or at least require a great deal of care physically and/or mentally. Some examples may be individuals who have undergone serious surgery or patients with strokes, cancer, and burns. Moreover, there is always a percentage of patients who can afford three nurses around the clock and who simply wish to have someone constantly at hand. These patients may not be in critical condition but require an enormous amount of individualized care. Free from the pressures of time and heavy patient care loads that often harass the staff nurse, private duty nurses have the opportunity to give truly comprehensive professional care to their patients, with limited concern for hospital routines.

For success in private duty nursing and greatest job satisfaction, the private duty nurse must have a genuine liking for people and must be able to adjust well to a wide variety of personalities, establishing and maintaining warm yet professional relationships with both patients and their families, no matter how long a case may last. This nurse must enjoy giving direct comprehensive nursing care to one patient. Naturally, it is necessary to be currently licensed in the state where the nurse practices, with the exception of times when patient and nurse may be traveling and

of age, have earned a qualifying degree from an accredited program, and must also meet medical, security, and licensure requirements.

The Commissioned Corps is a personnel system composed entirely of health professionals; it is an all-officer corps. It is also one of the seven uniformed services of the United States including the Air Force, Army, Navy, Marine Corps, Coast Guard, and the Commissioned Corps of the National Oceanic and Atmospheric Administration. In the event of a national emergency or war, the President may, by issuing an executive order, declare the PHS Commissioned Corps a military service. Pay, allowances, and other privileges are comparable with those of officers in the armed services. Rank appointments are made depending on the nurse's length of training and experience.

The PHS offers excellent opportunities for students in baccalaureate nursing programs for periods of 31 to 120 days through the Commissioned Officer Student Training and Extern Program (COSTEP) and Senior COSTEP Program. Both programs are highly competitive and based upon the needs of PHS agencies. (At this time the program has been severely curtailed by budget restraints.) COSTEP allows students to serve in assignments at any time during the year; however, the majority of students are hired for the summer months.

In Senior COSTEP, students are assisted financially during their final year of school in return for an agreement to work for PHS after graduation. The student is appointed as an active-duty PHS officer during the senior year and receives monthly pay and allowances as an ensign (01) grade officer. Additional support, in the form of tuition and fees, *may* be paid by a supporting agency or program of the PHS. Following graduation, the student agrees to work for the agency or program that provided the financial support for twice the amount of time supported.

As mentioned earlier, most of the clinical positions are in the IHS and NIH Clinical Center. Almost half of all the 5000 PHS nurses work for IHS. IHS is responsible for providing comprehensive care to over 1 million American Indians and Alaska Natives, in hospitals, health centers, and clinics across the United States. Most of the facilities are located west of the Mississippi. The NIH Clinical Center, in Bethesda, MD, is a world center for biomedical research. Approximately 900 nurses conduct research, help design experimental treatments, monitor patient responses, analyze data, and educate patients and families. The other PHS agencies employ nurses, though opportunities are more limited than with IHS and NIH.

The National Health Service Corps (NHSC) was originally authorized in 1970 to recruit health care personnel to urban and rural communities that have critical health manpower shortages. NHSC funds are offered to primary health care professionals for service in community-based systems of care throughout the United States and its territories.

The graduate will receive a specified amount for each year, up to three years, of service in a shortage area. The funds are given after graduation.

DEPARTMENT OF VETERANS AFFAIRS NURSING SERVICE

The Department of Veterans Affairs (VA) was established in 1930 as a civilian agency of the federal government. Its purpose is to administer national programs that provide benefits for veterans of this country's armed forces. In 1989 the agency was elevated to cabinet status. The VA operates the nation's largest organized health care system, composed of 172 hospitals, over 200 outpatient clinics, more than 100 nursing home care units, and 26 domiciliaries. More than 1.3 million veterans receive inpatient and outpatient care through the VA system yearly. The Veterans Health Services and Research Administration employs more than 35,000 professional nurses.

To accomplish its objective of providing high-quality health care, the VA has developed extensive programs in research and education. A majority of VA medical centers are affiliated with medical schools, schools of nursing, and other health-related schools in a network of health care facilities that cover the entire country. Individual hospitals range in size from approximately 110 to 1400 beds, most of which provide care for patients with medical, surgical, and psychiatric diagnoses. A few hospitals are predominantly for the care of patients with psychiatric diagnoses. Many VA health care facilities have outpatient clinics and extended-care facilities, such as nursing home care units.

VA medical centers are administered through the Veterans Health Administration, headed by the Under Secretary for Health. The Nursing Service functions within this agency under the leadership of an Assistant Chief Medical Director for Nursing Programs.

The VA has established the baccalaureate degree as the minimum preparation its nurses must have for promotion beyond the entry-level beginning in 2005, and has committed $50 million over a five-year period to help VA nurses obtain baccalaureate or higher nursing degrees.[27] To qualify for an appointment in the VA, a nurse must be a U.S. citizen, a graduate of a state-approved school of professional nursing, currently registered to practice, and meet required physical standards. Graduates from a professional school of nursing may be appointed pending passing of state board examinations.

Nurses employed in VA are covered by a locality pay system (LPS). The LPS is designed to ensure that VA nurses are paid competitive rates within local labor markets. As such, salary ranges vary according to facility location. There are several levels of salary grades for VA nurses.

Qualification standards relating to education, experience, and competencies are specified for appointment or promotion to each grade. The VA salary system recognizes excellence in clinical practice, administration, research, and education. Nurses, including those giving direct patient care, receive salaries commensurate with their qualifications and contributions. A Nurse Professional Standards Board reviews performance and recommends promotion or special salary advancement according to established criteria. A nurse appointed to one VA medical center may transfer to another with continuity of benefits and without loss of salary.

Personnel policies in the VA include a variety of health and life insurance options (partially paid for by the federal government), retirement plans, and liberal annual and sick leave benefits, tuition reimbursement, uniform allowance, annual physical examination, and a smoke-free workplace.

The VA Nursing Service emphasizes continued learning and advanced education. There is a Nursing Career Development Program to provide opportunities within the system. Nurse researchers are employed in some VA medical centers and in the national office. NPs and CNSs function in specific units, clinics, or satellite facilities.

ARMED SERVICES

Despite similarities, there are specific differences among the Army, Navy, and the Air Force Nurse Corps. All the armed services have a reserve corps of nurses to provide additional nurses to care for members of the services and their families in time of war or other national emergencies. Nurses may join the reserve without having joined the regular service; requirements are similar. A certain amount of continued training (which is paid) is required. There are opportunities for promotion, continuing education, and fringe benefits such as low-cost insurance, retirement pay, and discounted on-post shopping. More information is available from the reserve recruiter of the particular service. In the services, nurses have the economic, social, and health benefits of all officers, as well as the opportunity for personal travel. After discharge or retirement, veterans' benefits are available.

In all the armed services, nurses are commissioned at an officer rank and may advance to a top rank. The basic requirement for a commission are similar: physically qualified, licensed, U.S. citizen (usually), and educationally qualified. All nurse corps officers in the U.S. Army, U.S. Navy, and U.S. Air Force are required to hold a baccalaureate degree to practice as an active duty Registered Nurse.[28]

OTHER CAREER OPPORTUNITIES

It would probably be impossible, or at least extraordinarily lengthy, to give information about every career possibility available for nurses. A list of specific positions directly related to nursing, not even including clinical specialization or subspecialization, runs into the hundreds when the diverse settings in which nursing is practiced are considered. Overall, these are clinical nursing, administration/management, education, or research (or a combination of all), but the specific setting brings its own particular challenges. Each may require knowledge of another culture and the physical and psychosocial needs of these people, such as nursing in an Indian reservation, or a new orientation to practice such as working in an HMO, or in juvenile court, or the prison system, or even camp nursing. Almost all types of nursing are practiced in international settings for WHO, the Peace Corps, or Project Hope—not easy jobs, but rewarding and often exciting. Some require a baccalaureate.

In some cases, specialization or subspecialization, usually demanding additional education and training, becomes a new career path. There are any number of these, and as each becomes recognized as a distinct subspecialty, involved nurses tend to form a new organization or a subgroup within the ANA or some related organization to develop standards of practice. Recent interest in such areas as women's health care, men's health care, family planning, thanatology, and sex education have brought an interdisciplinary context that gives additional dimension to our practice.

When nurses assume positions such as editors of nursing journals or nursing editors in publishing companies, they not only draw on their nursing background but must also learn about the publishing field and acquire the necessary skills. In the same way, nurses employed as lobbyists, labor relations specialists, executive directors or staff of nursing associations, nurse consultants for drug or supply companies, or administrative consulting firms and staff for legislators or governmental committees, all use their nursing but must learn from other disciplines not related to nursing and develop new role concepts.

As health care and nursing expand, some nurses will develop positions undreamed of. It seems safe to say that opportunities and challenges in nursing today are practically limitless.

KEY POINTS

1. Nursing has been plagued by cyclical shortages and surpluses.

2. Because of social and economic factors that can create rapid and unexpected demands in health care, it is difficult to predict the number of nurses that would provide a balance of supply and demand.
3. Nursing positions are available or can be developed in every setting where health care is given.
4. There is a clear picture of the behaviors that employers expect of the new graduate.
5. There continues to be disagreement as to whether differentiated practice should be built on competence or education.
6. Staff nurses need participation in clinical decision making and a free flow of information about the issues.
7. Standards of practice and the accompanying measurement criteria allow a determination on competence of nursing care, and competence in the professional role.
8. Three basic models for assignment of patient care exist: functional, team, and case method, and subsequent endless variations.
9. It has become rare for nurses only to be responsible for themselves; they accomplish much of their work through others.
10. There are a number of employment opportunities for nurses, and they are often in a department other than nursing service.
11. There is no consensus as to whether or not the case management role is reserved for the advanced practice nurse.
12. Perhaps the oldest entrepreneurial role is the private duty nurse.

STUDY QUESTIONS

1. Interview an advanced practice nurse. Who and what does (s)he see as the major facilitators and impediments to her/his work?
2. What do you see as the solution to the cyclical shortage/surplus of nurses?
3. What should an employer expect from a new graduate?
4. Identify the ideal position for yourself after graduation and why?
5. What are the benefits and liabilities of employing nurses from a temporary nursing service?
6. Give several intrapreneurial examples of nursing practice.

REFERENCES

1. Aiken L. Charting the future of hospital nursing. In Lee PR, Estes CL (Eds.): *The Nation's Health,* 4th ed. Boston: Jones & Bartlett, 1994, pp 177–187.

2. Leavitt JK, Herbert-Davis M. Collective strategies for action. In: Mason DJ, et al (Eds.): *Policy and Politics for Nurses*, 2d ed. Philadelphia: W.B. Saunders, 1993, pp 166–183.
3. *Secretary's Commission on Nursing: Final Report*, Vol. I. Washington, DC: Government Printing Office, 1988.
4. McKibbon RC, Boston C. An overview: Characteristic impact and solutions. Monograph 1 in *The Nursing Shortage: Opportunities and Solutions*. Chicago: American Hospital Association/American Nurses Association, 1990.
5. Buerhaus P. Is another shortage looming? *Nurs Outlook* 46:102–108, May–June 1998.
6. Joiner G, Wessman J. Expanding shared governance beyond practice issues. *Recruit Restruct Rep* 10: 4–7, November–December 1997.
7. Grando V. Making do with fewer nurses in the United States, 1945–1965. *Image* 30:147–149, Second Quarter 1998.
8. Shindul-Rothschild J, et al. Where have all the nurses gone? *Am J Nurs* 96:25–39, November 1996.
9. Aiken L, Salmon M. Health care workforce priorities: What nursing should do now. In Harrington C, Estes C (Eds.): *Health Policy and Nursing*, 2d ed. Sudbury, MA: Jones & Bartlett, 1997, p 174.
10. Joel L. Setting the record straight on hospital RNs. *Am J Nurs* 96:7, September 1996.
11. Aiken and Salmon, loc cit.
12. White S, Hewes C. Interview with a quality leader: Linda Aiken on the healthcare industry and workplace issues. *J Healthc Qual* 25(3):21–23, May–June 2003.
13. Smith J, Crawford L. *Report of Findings from the 2003 Employers Survey*. Chicago: NCSBN, 2004.
14. Smith J, Crawford L. *Report of Findings from the Practice and Professional Issues Survey*. Chicago: NCSBN, 2004.
15. Chornick N, et al. *Job Analysis of Newly Licensed, Entry-Level Registered Nurses*. Chicago: National Council of State Boards of Nursing, 1993.
16. American Nurses Association. *Nursing Scope and Standards of Practice*, 3d ed. Washington, DC: ANA, 2003.
17. Manthey M. Nursing's message to the world: An interview with Barbara Blakeney. *Creat Nurs* 9(3):4–8, 2003.
18. *Registered Professional Nurses and Unlicensed Assistive Personnel*, 2d ed. Washington, DC: ANA, 1996.
19. Ibid, p 10.
20. Taylor N. Magnet Conference attracts hundreds of nurse leaders. *Nurs Mgmt* 35(12):22, December 2004.
21. National Sample Survey of Registered Nurses: http://bhpr.hrse.gov/healthworkforce/rnsurvey/rnss1.htm. Retrieved March 10, 2005.
22. Cohen E, Cesta T. *Nursing Case Management*. St. Louis: Mosby, 2001.
23. *Standards of Occupational Health Nursing*. Atlanta, GA: American Association of Occupational Health Nursing, 1994.
24. Aydelotte M, et al. *Nurses in Private Practice*. Kansas City, MO: ANA, 1988, pp 19–20.
25. Pinchot G. *Intrapreneuring*. New York: Harper & Row, 1985.

26. Ibid.
27. American Association of Colleges of Nursing. The Impact of Education on Nursing Practice: http://www.aacn.nche.educ/Media/FactSheets/ImpactEdNP.htm. Retrieved July 13, 2005.
28. Ibid.

Updates can be found at

 http://www.JoelTheNursingExperience.com

Chapter 7

Leadership for an Era of Change

OBJECTIVES

After studying this chapter you will be able to:

1. Define autonomy and describe how a nurse functions autonomously in patient care.
2. Discuss three theories of leadership.
3. Compare two different approaches to leadership.
4. Identify five sources of power.
5. Recognize those conditions that make change most acceptable.
6. Describe how mentorship works.
7. Identify the relationship of nursing to feminism now and in the future.
8. Describe how nurses can prepare to influence health policy in their community.
9. Explain how you can market a positive nursing image.

Why bother to concern yourself with issues of power, autonomy, and influence? Maybe you don't care whether nursing is considered a profession. Maybe, right now, you plan to do your nursing job, do it well, and not get involved in issues of politics and power. Leave that to those who enjoy it. It's not as easy as that. "Right now" will become the future, and unless you're unlike most people you'll want a part in deciding the future. Chances are that you will be in the workforce for as long as 45 years. (Even if you started your nursing program late in life, you

294

probably expect to work for at least 15 or 20 years.) Chances are also that you will be an employee most of that time, with all the constraints a bureaucracy can put on you. Without doubt you're going to want, at the least, some say about how you do your job, how best to care for your patients or clients. You won't be alone. Every survey and study done about nurses' job satisfaction comes up with autonomy as a major factor, and with autonomy, there is accountability—to the public.

If nurses do have the ability and responsibility to control their practice so that they can give the best possible care, then they have to use their knowledge, talents, and numbers to influence health care, either directly through personal leadership, or through leaders they choose. They need to develop collegial relations that provide a support system; they need to help one another. Too often nurses have discovered this too late and have had to scramble to catch up in a health care system where the power figures started their influence training early. As a nurse, you can't divorce yourself from what your profession is; its influence or lack thereof will affect your working life in every way. A strong profession can make your practice more rewarding. Whether or not you choose to be an activist now or see that role only as part of the dim future, it's not too early to know where nursing is in the power game and who the players are.

NURSING AUTONOMY

Professional *autonomy* has been defined as the right of self-determination and governance without external control. Identified as components of autonomy are control of the profession's education, legal recognition (licensure), and a code of ethics that persuades the public to grant autonomy. A distinction has been made between *job content* autonomy, the freedom to determine the methods and procedures to be used to deal with a given problem, and *job context* autonomy, the freedom to name and define the boundaries of the problem, the role relationships with other providers, and the price to be paid for our service. The keys to autonomy as applied to nursing are that no other profession or administrative force can control nursing practice, and that the nurse has freedom of action in making judgments in patient care within the scope of nursing practice as defined by the profession.

The issue of nursing's autonomy as a profession was discussed in Chapter 4. By admission, nursing does not have full autonomy, but we have made significant progress. Current restrictions on autonomy are experienced in both one's personal practice and with the discipline as a whole. The common practice for government to consult with the AMA on health care legislation has often been presented as proof of the autonomy of American medicine. We can debate whether the interpretation is correct; but given that it is, American nursing has moved closer to that standard through the American Nurses Association's prominence on Capitol Hill.

There are other indicators of progress toward autonomy for nurses. *Shared governance* models that bring staff nurses and nursing service managers together to achieve consensus on clinical management, *peer review* as a mechanism in retention and promotion, *nursing staff organizations*, and the right to *professional staff privileges* when JCAHO or Medicare guidelines are applied as they are written, are all intermediate steps toward full autonomy.

Most nurses do not identify with the issues of autonomy as they are played out in the profession. They are more concerned with their personal practice; but nurses have gravitated toward roles that hold the promise of autonomy. For the staff nurse this has been primary nursing. Primary nursing in its distinguishing features holds promise of autonomy but will depend on how these qualities are played out given the presence of an administrative hierarchy. It is consistently agreed that the primary nurse:[1]

- Is responsible for comprehensive and continuous care of the patient from admission to discharge.
- Makes independent decisions that need not be ratified by any other provider.
- Consults with patients and their support systems to allow informed and acceptable decisions.
- Accesses others to the information they need to participate intelligently in care of the patient.
- Decides how nursing care will be delivered, and communicates this to those who will share in implementing the plan.
- Participates in a communication triad with the physician and patient.
- Participates as an equal and fully accountable member of the health care team.
- Has ready access to peer support and participates in peer review.
- Incorporates consultation, continuing education, and research into their practice.

Issues of autonomy may be particularly frustrating when the professional is an employee. The nature of these conflicts surfaced in a U.S. Supreme Court decision of May 1994. The decision places in question the distinction between those actions that an employed professional initiates as part of their autonomous practice in contrast to those that are initiated on behalf of the employer. The distinction is important and will be questioned more as professionals are less frequently entrepreneurs.

A LEADER AMONG LEADERS

Leadership is "every nurse's domain." Leadership is about influencing the behavior of others. Registered nurses influence the behavior of their patients, provide leadership to the nursing care team, and are often called as individuals to be the leader among leaders as the professions speaks out on behalf of the public welfare.

LEADERSHIP: A HISTORICAL PERSPECTIVE

Successful leadership depends on the artful blending of four forces: the leader, the followers (for without followers there are no leaders), the immediate organization, and the environment or context within which the goal is to be accomplished (see Exhibit 7.1). Early writings on

Exhibit 7.1 The Interplay of Forces in Leadership

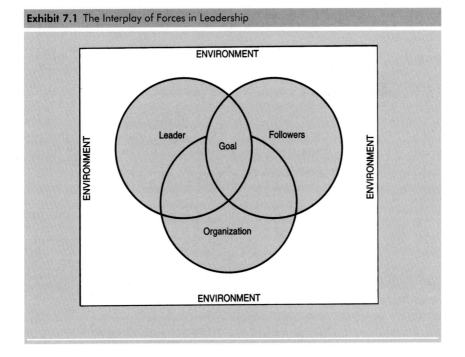

leadership focus on the style and theoretical orientation of the leader. It was assumed that there was a basic instability in human relations and that leaders must control the behavior of their followers to ensure the desired results. Freedom and independence were only metered out to followers once they had proved their motivation, readiness, capability, and so on. Regardless of the labels, the qualities of control of behavior and freedom continue to be central to the process of leadership.

Aspiring leaders have been encouraged to select an approach most suitable to themselves or the situation at hand. Finding no suitable match, one could always create an eclectic style, borrowing from a variety of orientations. The best advice is that there must be a good fit between a situation, the qualities of the leader, and the traits of the followers.[2] There is no one combination that is right all of the time, and many combinations are possible. Leadership theories help us to see the options:

- *The great man theory:* As old as Aristotle, this tells us that some are born to lead and others are born to be led. Confusion exists here over which traits are necessary to acquire leadership and which are needed to maintain it. Personality is not viewed as an integrated whole, and the impact of environmental and situational factors, including followers, is ignored. A better interpretation would be that one may be born to a position, but that does not guarantee that it could have ever been achieved or will be maintained.

- *Charismatic theory:* The ability to lead is dependent on an emotional commitment from followers. Followers feel secure in the presence of the leader, which is particularly helpful when sacrifices that could only be expected based on personal loyalties are asked of followers. Many of our most successful revolutionary leaders have been described as charismatic. Note that the allegiance is to a specific person. Removal of that person can often result in loss of progress, unless there has been a planned strategy to transfer leadership to a new personality.

- *Trait theory.* Personality studies abound. The traits of successful leaders closely approximate those observed in successful executives (see Chapter 15). They are described as endowed with vision, motivating followers to buy into that vision, sharing just enough of their vision to motivate people without overwhelming them, and distinguishing their relationships with humanism. They live with human respect and expect no less from their followers.[3] Other traits associated with leadership include: intelligence, emotional maturity, creativity and ability to see novel solutions for problems, possessing initiative, listening carefully, ability to derive meaning from even clouded communications, skilled at persuasion, a good judge of people, social, and socially adaptable.

- *Situational theories.* Leadership depends on the situation. Who will be the most successful leader at any one point in time is relative, depending on the best match with the circumstances: amount of pressure, task at hand, technical demands, closeness of the working relationship, and on and on.

- *Contingency theory.* This school of thought is situational and prescriptive. It involves a three-dimensional model that aims to create the best fit between leader–follower relations, the task at hand, and the resources or support that can be accessed by the leader due to their position or status. In other words, there is no one leadership style that is suited to every situation.

- *Path–goal theory.* The leader structures work for subordinates and removes obstacles so that they can be successful. Caring and consideration is added to the leadership prescription based on the needs of the group. These qualities have been singled out in many surveys on leadership.

- *Life cycle theory.* The most appropriate leadership style is based on the maturity of the followers. With growing maturity there is less need for structure, and greater need for the leader to assume an active role in the work at hand, and focus on relationships.

- *Behaviorists.* Leaders have styles that place them on a continuum from *bureaucratic* to *autocratic* to *participatory* to *consultative* to *democratic* and finally to *laissez-faire.* The distinguishing qualities are whether followers need to be motivated by internal or external forces and how much of a role followers actually have in decision making. Further, does communication flow from the top down, or take some other route; and is criticism overt, covert, punitive or constructive? Each style depicts the degree of control exerted by the leader with a complementary restriction on the freedom allowed subordinates. Maximum control by the leader and maximum freedom by the followers are mutually exclusive. The ultimate external "locus of control" is the bureaucrat who neither follows self nor followers, but defers to organizational policies.[4] Democratic leadership assumes that some degree of autonomy (the ability to act without permission) has been voluntarily relinquished by all participants for the common good. Laissez-faire does not assume that the followers are directionless, but that they need to be left alone to decide how to complete their own work.

- *Dual factor theory.* Satisfaction and dissatisfaction are not presented as direct opposites, but as separate entities. An increase in satisfaction is brought about by attention to the humanistic aspects of leadership. The removal of the dissatisfying elements does not necessarily result in satisfaction. These principles were widely applied to nursing during the last shortage.[5]

CONTEMPORARY LEADERSHIP

Contemporary approaches to leadership build on many traditional theories, but evolve into something different that better fits the tempo and values of life in this new century. The leader and followers are fused into a whole that is greater than the sum of its parts. The process is to break down old hierarchies and build commitment around a shared vision. The leader may facilitate and support, but only lead at the pleasure of the followers. Disequilibrium is not something to avoid, but inevitable and sometimes the stimulus for action. Networking outside of the group is seen positively. Stability comes from the human relationships. This represents the converse of earlier models, where the presumed instability was in the human relationships.

A body of knowledge has taken shape around the dynamics of this *transformational leadership*. Earlier work, which was primarily *transactional*, assumed that differences between leader and follower were sure to be an obstacle and demanded attention in planning and execution. In a transformational context, these concerns are not primary; rather the goal is for the leader and the followers to evolve toward a shared agenda. All parties grow and develop through the process. History does not repeat itself, but patterns recur as cyclical events that challenge any leader to be self-sufficient. See Exhibit 7.2 for a comparison of transactional and transformational leadership.

Transformational leadership focuses on creating the social architecture to sustain a vision, and the attitudes and behaviors that allow progress in these uncertain times. This brand of leadership builds on organizational trust first, because of the organization's likelihood of greater permanence, and then on leaders with positive self-regard and a capacity for humanism. The trick is to bridge the gap between transactional and transformational leadership. The insights generated by the transactional school of thinking are not to be dismissed but should be enhanced with new assumptions and ways of operating.

The literature supports an additional variation on leadership, perhaps best suited where both the environment and the organization are unstable (a very likely picture in the health care industry today). The dynamics here may require a very narrowly defined goal and a very special group of participants. A collegial style is proposed as the natural complement for leadership. In this context, leadership is relative and functional only once it is legitimized by the group. In other words, the claim to leadership must

Exhibit 7.2 Qualities of Transactional and Transformational Leadership

Quality	Transactional	Transformational
General orientation	Technical	Philosophical
Assumptions	Instability in human relations; stability in the environment and organizations	Instability in the environment; stability in human relations and relative stability in organizations
Response to goal	Reactive	Proactive, visionary
Plan for action	Predetermined by vision of the leader	Creation of shared vision
Prevailing focus	Content	Process
Roles	Division of labor	Group unified by goal; roles emerge over time and in response to work plan
Group dynamics	Competitive	Collaborative
Emotions	Work to distance feelings	Accept and recognize feelings and work them through
Cognitive qualities	Rational, objective, strive to decrease complexity and ambiguity	Acknowledge complexity and ambiguity; value intuition
Decision making	Directive	Participative
Governance	Managerial	Self-governance
Human relations	Work to ensure stability	Assume and exploit stability
Leadership style	Command/control	Facilitate/protect/empower
Distribution of power	Centralized	Decentralized
Structure	Hierarchy	Networking

be achieved. Collegial leaders are catalytic, not merely consultative or facilitative. They do not build teams but integrate the assets of the group. Although the "buck" does stop somewhere, leadership is shared, as is the responsibility and recognition for success. Communication is authentic and genuine, with emphasis on precision in communicating the message, whatever the form may be. Supervision and motivational techniques are nonexistent because these qualities reside in the individual.[6] Shared vision, responsibility, and accountability are more than rhetoric. The narrowly defined goal is another concession to today's instability. Once the work of the group is done, the participants disband. This is called *ad hocracy*. It removes the pressure of long-term commitment from the participants and recognizes that each challenge is new and different.

PERSPECTIVES ON POWER

Leadership involves power, the power to move people to a desired effect, the power to secure and retain resources. The first step toward personal empowerment (the ability to act) is to recognize that you have power.

Power may be associated with your position, awarded by a system, given to the leader by the followers, or shared with the followers by the leader. Most basically, power is the by-product of a social relationship, and is given or it does not exist. Individuals derive their power from specific sources, and then use that power according to their personal power orientation. A typology of sources of power, deriving from the work of many authors, is presented here:

- *Coercive power*—real or perceived fear of one person by another.
- *Reward power*—perception of the potential for rewards or favors by honoring the wishes of a powerful person.
- *Legitimate power*—derives from an organizational position rather than personal qualities.
- *Expert power*—knowledge, special talents, or skills held by the person.
- *Referent power*—power flowing from admiration, or charisma, usually rooted in similar backgrounds or some other mutual identification.
- *Information power*—exclusive access to information needed by others.
- *Connection power*—privileged connections with powerful individuals or organizations.
- *Collective power*—ability to mobilize a critical mass or a system on your behalf.

We often infer that people who claim to have power actually do, but when studied more carefully, they have no claim or legitimacy. Additionally, power invariably fills any vacuum. People generally want peace and order. In situations of stress or chaos, someone will come forward and will be given the power to restore order.

One's power orientation indicates how an individual perceives or values power. Is power an essential part of one's identity, even if it is never used constructively? "He could do so much good if he only wanted to." Is power interpreted as the exclusive possession, something that is not shared? "You never quite feel that she is telling you everything." One's power orientation may be seen exclusively or in combination as:

- *Good*—power as natural and desirable and used in an open and honest manner. Would probably build on expert, reward, and legitimate power sources.
- *Resource dependent*—power depending on possession of things, including information, property, wealth. Associated with withholding patterns in the information power source. Greatly diminished in a computer age and the growing presence of transformational leadership.

- *Instinctive drive*—power as a personality attribute, and usually associated with referent power.
- *Charisma*—influence over people through personal magnetism. Power often given to people who are ill-prepared or even destructive, and could stifle the growth of those who do the giving.
- *Political*—drawing heavily on referent, connection, and collective sources, power is linked to an ability to negotiate the system.
- *Control and autonomy*—the power broker always calls the shots operating from a base of coercion, information, and connection.

The power sources of individuals in combination with their power orientation allows prediction on how they will function and provides you with a model to identify your own *capacity* and *style*. It can also provide direction for what people expect before they will give power.

Power and influence are sometimes equated, because both affect or change the behavior of others; however, when they are separated, it is on the theory that power is the potential that must be tapped and converted to the dynamic thrust of influence. Almost all authorities agree that a person or group must be valued on some level in order to

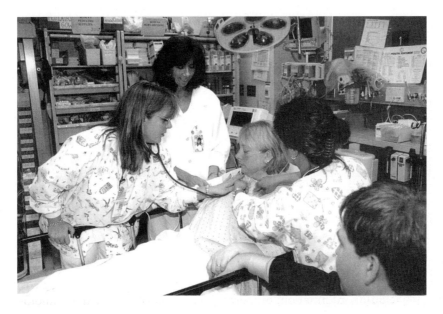

The power for nurses is in their practice, which allows them to make a rich contribution to interdisciplinary patient care. (*Courtesy of Hackensack University Medical Center, Hackensack, New Jersey*)

have power or influence, again reinforcing the interpersonal dimension of the concept.

Does nursing have power? Considering these concepts, it is clear that nursing has the *potential* for power with its overwhelming numbers, its special knowledge and skill, and its place in the public trust. Nursing leaders also have power of various kinds, including positional power in high government policy-making positions; but what of nurses as individuals? They are still complaining of lack of power on the job—the lack of autonomy and of involvement in budget setting and in policy making. Yet nurses do not seem to mobilize their constituency, or capitalize on their position at the center of health care information networks. Is it a historical pattern of obedience to authority, which has been transmitted by education and practice? Is it their social, cultural, or economic background? Is it because, according to personality tests, nurses have a low power motive? Is it that they think they do not have what it takes to be powerful and influential—for whatever reason? Groups or individuals "choose" to obey for a number of reasons: habit, fear of sanctions, moral obligation, self-interest, psychological identification with someone in charge, indifference, and lack of self-confidence. No doubt there are nurses who fall into one or more of these categories.

However, those who maintain that lack of self-confidence is the root cause for nurses' apparent lack of interest in gaining power should remember that "both the powerful and the powerless tend to take existing social systems for granted and rarely recognize that it is not *talent*, but rather laws, customs, policies and institutions that, in reality, keep the powerless . . . powerless."[7]

THE CONSTANCY OF CHANGE

Change will be your constant companion throughout the course of life. You will be able to feel it, see it, smell it, hear it, and taste it. You have a responsibility to change with the times, and to move the whole of nursing to action if you see indifference and too much comfort with the status quo. Your practice must change, as must the systems that support that practice. Patients must be helped to adjust to change, or to change so that they can adjust. Whether it is changing the health care practices of the newly diagnosed diabetic, or the body image of the traumatic amputee, a transition from team to primary nursing, or the decentralization of all management decisions to the unit level, the theoretical constructs and strategies are much the same.

Change is any significant departure from the status quo. Change may be planned or accidental. Planned change is a deliberate, conscious effort intended to improve a situation and make those improvements acceptable to the parties involved. In comparison, accidental change is a shift that occurs to maintain balance between a system and its environment. Planned change allows a degree of control, whereas accidental change happens despite us, and we are more or less swept along. Another way of describing change is as first-order and second-order. First-order change may happen, but the larger system remains unaltered (accommodation). In second-order change, the system itself changes (assimilation).[8] One common example may be the requirement to maintain current care plans on every patient, but are those plans merely tokenism (first-order), or do they become an essential tool in the operation of the unit, including staffing (second-order)?

CLASSICAL THEORIES OF CHANGE

Lewin's theory of change is probably the basis for the adaptations of most other theorists.[9] He identifies three basic stages: *unfreezing,* in which the motivation to create change occurs; *moving,* the actual changing, when new responses are developed and initiated; and *refreezing,* in which the change is integrated and stabilized. A further notion is that in all changes there are *driving forces* that facilitate action and *restraining forces* that impede it. Each must be identified—the first so that they can be capitalized on, and the second so that they can be avoided or modified.

Lippitt's theory includes seven phases within Lewin's stages, a delineation that is useful in thinking through action and introduces the role of the change agent, the architect of the change process:[10]

Unfreezing:
- Diagnosis of the problem.
- Assessment of the motivation and capacity for change.
- Assessment of the change agent's motivation and resources.

Moving:
- Selecting progressive change objectives.
- Choosing the appropriate role of the change agent.

Refreezing:
- Maintenance of the change once it has been started.
- Termination of a helping relationship between the change agent and the changed system.

The Lewin and Lippitt models paint a very simplistic picture of the change process. On the contrary, even the most adventuresome participants have trepidation because human nature fears the unknown. Perlman and Takacs, building on Lewin and Lippitt's work, identified ten behaviors or emotional phases in the change process. They note phases of equilibrium, denial, anger, and bargaining that coexist with Lewin's unfreezing. Then chaos, depression, and resignation coincide with the moving phase. Lastly, openness (renewal), readiness (acceptance), and reemergence (empowerment) characterize refreezing.[11] The reader can observe this same linear sequence in many paradigms, including Kubler-Ross's work on the natural phenomena of dying.[12]

CONTEMPORARY THEORIES OF CHANGE: THE NON-LINEAR

In the past, change was predictable, relatively orderly, and linear, progressing in the fashion of steps and stages. Today, change is unpredictable, and though patterns may be discernible, order is rare and the dynamics are nonlinear.[13]

Systems thinking and *chaos theory* are well suited to this environment. Chaos theory tells us "...organizations can no longer rely on rules, policies, and hierarchies, or afford to be inflexible; and that small changes in the initial conditions of a system can drastically affect the long-term behavior of that system."[14] Put another way, "The richness of the interaction among parts and between the system and its environment allows the system as a whole to undergo spontaneous self-organization."[15] More simply, "out of the box" thinking is in order.

In his discussion of organizations and individuals that will survive and thrive in our age of uncertainty (and sometimes chaos) and constant change, Senge proposes the following strategies:[16]

- *The whole is greater than the sum of its parts.* You cannot think of your work in isolation. Whereas earlier studies of leadership expected only the designated leader to focus on external events, newer thinking expects that all participants will have this broadened view.
- *Look internally for solutions to problems.* It is more comfortable to blame our misfortunes on external circumstances or personalities. They are often beyond our control, so failure is less personal. From a position of strength, the first step in problem solving should be to straighten your own thinking or behavior.
- The voguish strategy is to become proactive or to *rise to address difficult issues before* we are faced with crisis management and forced into a reactive mode. All too often, we are still reacting, though at an

earlier stage in the development of the issue. In other words, *the illusion of taking charge* is just that, an illusion.

- We are hampered by our preoccupation with events and short-term planning. Survival in today's environment of rapid change demands a *search for themes, and the identification of trends over time*. Dig under events for the real theme. The consumer demand for "final directives" is more than that; it is the public outcry for more personal control over decisions about their health.

- *We tend to adjust to a bad situation* and learn to live with it, focusing on the reality of the moment. Seeing threats for what they are requires us to slow down, compare situations across time, and attempt to forecast. Neither do we deserve kudos for tolerating an intolerable situation.

- Even given the rapid pace of change, it is *difficult or impossible today to learn from your mistakes*. Decisions made at one time and place will impact people and events in a distant time and place, often generations away. The best hedge against doing harm is to ensure that *leadership for the far-reaching issues is a blend of people from many perspectives*.

- The traditional image of *the team is useless for today's problems*. Over time most teams invest more effort maintaining their image of cohesiveness than participating in the process of change. Better suited to the times is a model where everyone has something to contribute and no proposal is dismissed. This decidedly transformational style is inconsistent with the inevitable hierarchy in transactional models. The role of the leader evolves into one of developing people, actually instigating openness and honesty while removing the threat of reprisals. The leader often assumes the position of consultant on process and facilitator, as opposed to expert and controller—a very difficult transition for those socialized into the traditional mode of leadership.

MAKING CHANGE ACCEPTABLE

The test will be in the day-to-day arduous process of implementing change. A review of the numerous change strategies and tactics reported in the literature urges the following conditions to make change more acceptable:

- Ensure that the need for change is justified, even if there is not agreement. This requires total honesty, exquisite communication, and sensitivity to the cues that you have heard. Change for the sake of change is never justified.

- Try to safeguard the future security of those who are involved in change.
- Diffuse anxiety by having those involved create the vision for change.
- It is helpful to work from a previously established set of impersonal principles.
- Change is best received when it follows other successes rather than failures.
- It is better to space events so that there is adjustment to one change before another is introduced.
- People new to the organization react to change more comfortably than people with longevity in the system targeted for change (vested interest).
- Try to guarantee that there will be personal benefits to those who participate. Things should be better, not worse, after the fact.
- Establish a venturesome environment by making change and improvement a priority.
- Choose a change agent with psychological sensitivity to serve as a bridge to other participants.
- Focus attention on the future, not the past.
- Allow for failure. Nothing is forever. Be ready to compromise once everyone is clear on the things that are nonnegotiable.
- Provide assurance of administrative support and freedom to act without the constant need for approvals.
- Encourage open expression of concerns.
- Avoid experimentation and never withhold information; be sure people see "the big picture" and know what they are doing.
- Remember, the change agent is the architect of change and participates with the intent of disengaging when the process is complete.

OBSTACLES TO THE EXERCISE OF POWER

Based on our analysis of autonomy, leadership, power and change, it becomes obvious that the single most important ingredient to advancement of the profession and protection of the public welfare is power and its conversion into strategic influence. The fact that nursing is a "sleeping giant" holds little comfort when the health care delivery system grows in instability and decisions are made which promise a less than preferred future for nurses and nursing. Though there are many situations that have minimized the influence of nursing, there are just a few which have persisted over the years and deserve special consideration.

NURSING AND FEMINISM

A point frequently made, when it is asked why nurses, with so much potential for influence, do not seem to be able to or want to use it, is that nursing is still 94.6 percent a woman's profession, and, even with changing legislation and attitudes, women as a whole are still subject to discrimination and harassment and often victims of female socialization.

For many years, most women nurses looked at nursing as a useful way to earn a living until they were married, a job to which they could return if circumstances required. Most nurses did marry and most married nurses did drop out to raise families, working only part-time, if at all. Unmarried female nurses (like male nurses) were more inclined to stay in nursing but, unlike men, frequently did not plot an orderly path to positions of authority and influence. This is similar to the career patterns of other women. In business, most women have traditionally been in their thirties or forties before they realized that they either wanted to or would be forced to continue working, and by then they were often frozen in dead-end, low-prestige (but productive) jobs. When they decided to compete for power positions in management, they were up against an "old boy" network that prevented or deterred their progress. Moreover, they had to overcome their own reluctance to be aggressive and to reject traditional female social goals.

Has the women's movement had an impact on this situation? As noted in Chapter 3, despite many obstacles still in the path of women on the way up (and even of those who aren't interested in this path), the women's movement has had a tremendous influence in improving many aspects of women's lives. Yet, nurses have had an uneasy relationship with feminists as a group, in part because many feminists have incorrect knowledge about nursing and were more interested early on in encouraging women to move into the powerful male bastions of law, medicine, and business. On the other hand, many of the issues concerning nurses such as comparable worth and child care are also feminist issues.

Feminism can be defined as a world view that values women and confronts systematic injustices based on gender. There are a number of feminist theories and ideologies, but none are anti-male, they are simply opposed to the male-defined systems and ideologies that oppress women. These feminists point out that, even now, women believe that they must choose between the male-defined feminine role and the more interesting male role. Overall, they feel that nursing, with its largely female component, follows oppressed group behavior and also tries to emulate what they see as powerful, that is, male.

Nursing tends to identify with the oppressor (administration? medicine?) and is sometimes self-aggressive. An example of this self-aggression is given in relation to the long-standing entry-into-practice battle. It is pointed out that the debate is largely taking place on the professional organization level, to which most nurses do not belong, ignoring the fears of those without a baccalaureate and the means or motivation to get one. The fact that nurses blame themselves and each other for failure to solve the complex dilemmas of the profession is seen as another form of antifeminist self-aggression.[17]

The winds of change blow constantly. As we move into the new millennium, there is a decided change in the feminist perspective. Feminists today choose a more low-key and gentler approach to their issues. They emphasize the differences between men and women as opposed to their similarities. This shift in ideology comes on the scene as nursing is more influenced to define its own uniqueness as caring. The emergent "soft feminism" is comfortable and persuasive to nursing. You could well see these constituencies converge on the issue of women's health.

PHYSICIAN–NURSE RELATIONSHIPS

Physician–nurse relationships are a large, if not major, factor in nurse autonomy. There is necessarily a fine line between overstating and understating the problems, or, as some would have it, between paranoia and servility. Physicians' recognition of nurses as co-professionals and colleagues has been present almost since the beginning of nursing, but a hard core of physicians who see and prefer a nurse-handmaiden role, although less common than even a decade ago, still exists.

Some physicians and, to some extent, a part of organized medicine seem to have limited, stereotypical images of nurses and resist nurse autonomy—either because they honestly doubt nurses' ability to cope with certain problems (bolstered, unfortunately, by the behavior of some nurses they work with) or because they are threatened by the expansion of nursing roles. The latter is demonstrated by the periodic action of certain medical societies and boards to restrict expanded nursing practice by lobbying against the expanded definitions of practice in nurse practice acts, by opposing reimbursement for nursing services unless there is physician supervision, or by using their power to limit nursing practice in a particular community or health care setting.

The reasons for problems in nurse–physician relationships have been examined repeatedly. One reason given is that physician education tends to impress on the medical student a captain-of-the-ship mentality and a need for both omniscience and omnipotence (Aesculapian authority), whereas nursing education often does not develop nurses as independent and fearless thinkers. This is also seen as one cause of the doctor–nurse game in which the nurse must communicate information and advice to the physician without seeming to do so, and the physician acts on it without acknowledging the source.

Other reasons include the different socioeconomic and educational status of doctors and nurses; the physicians' lack of accurate knowledge about nursing education and practice, and vice versa, which enables them to work side by side without really understanding each other or communicating adequately; different orientations to practice; nurses' lack of control over their practice, particularly in hospitals; and physicians' exploitation of nurses.

With more nurses looking toward advanced practice, the fact that many physicians surveyed do not seem comfortable with having nurses carry out responsibilities that were traditionally medicine has caused considerable misunderstanding. This is particularly true when nurses feel that they must prove themselves to be accepted in new roles and that a "role challenge" has been thrown out by physicians.

On the other hand, an increasing number of physicians encourage and promote nurse–physician collegial relationships and see them as inevitable and necessary for good health care. Joint practice and other collaboration, both at the unit level and in various manifestations of physician–advanced nursing practice, are evidence of this cooperation.

That doctors and nurses are willing to work together—that is, to collaborate—has a more serious meaning than symbolism. Over the years, impressive amounts of data have been gathered to show that nurse–physician collaboration has a significant outcome for patient well-being. The critical attributes of collaboration are shared planning and decision making, joint problem solving and goal setting, and genuine and open responsibility and accountability to one another and to the patient.

In a number of studies, it has been shown that this kind of collaboration had positive results by improving the conditions of geriatric patients in several settings, including lowering mortality; lowering costs; increasing patient satisfaction; improving professional nurse–physician relationships; decreasing the hospital stay of patients; and, most dramatic, being the key factor in the life or death of ICU patients.[18]

Does the doctor–nurse game still exist? Stein is convinced that there have been major changes in the decades since his first observations. He admits that in some places the game still functions as described in 1967, but he predicts that the changes visible elsewhere will spread. One factor is that "the image of nurses as handmaidens is giving way to that of specialty-trained and certified advanced practitioners with independent duties and responsibilities to their patients."[19] Physicians depend on this special expertise. Interdisciplinary models have also been shown to improve care in specialty areas. Stein adds that the many other influential roles nurses take in utilization review and quality assurance may threaten doctors' authority in clinical decision making. In explaining how and why the physician–nurse interaction has changed, he stresses the nurses' goal of becoming autonomous practitioners, changes such as the civil rights and women's movements and the nursing shortage, nurses' education in terms of both content and socialization of nursing students to relate to physicians differently than in the past, and the improved environment of some hospitals.[20]

Is Stein too optimistic? Given his caveat that the doctor–nurse game still exists and realizing that everything takes time, probably not. In recent years, there have been many more reports of health care settings where the new interdependent mode prevails.[21] Resolving this overall issue is a part of the challenge that both medicine and nursing must face.

NURSES AS EMPLOYEES IN A BUREAUCRACY

Nursing leadership has frequently blamed the employee status of nurses for our lack of empowerment. Even more telling is the fact that nursing has been buried in a department within the institutional hierarchy. Most decisions occurred at the top of the bureaucracy and few if any choices filtered down to those who gave the direct care. If, in the course of implementing those decisions, the nurse's ethics were challenged or professional goals for the patient jeopardized, any assertive action on the nurse's behalf may have resulted in the loss of a job. The rights of nurses as employees are discussed more fully in Chapter 15.

Though in many places the oppression of nurses has not changed considerably, the world of health care has changed around us. We are moving toward an era where most provider professionals will be employees in some fashion. This fact has created legal sensitivity to the fact that there are those things we do as employees, and there are other areas of accountability to the public that cannot be compromised by the demands of any employer. Relevant court decisions and public policy that recognize these distinctions enable us to speak out.

Neither has the organizational structure of health care institutions remained the same after some very tumultuous years of nursing shortage and surplus and the increased needs of patients. There is a new appreciation of long-term employees, and dollars once invested in recruitment are redirected to retention. As part of this changed philosophy, a series of studies and programs were initiated which explored the disillusionment of new graduates with their work, and the qualities of hospitals that were successful in recruiting and retaining the best and the brightest nurses. One significant factor was the powerful positioning of the chief nurse executive in the executive structure of the organization. Not that this realignment has occurred everywhere, but it has been frequent enough to allow nursing to surface as an institutional force, and the most successful nurse executives have rejected the idea that shared power is loss of power. Sharing power with staff as experts in what they do actually enhances the positions of all the shareholders.

The new century has brought a different era in the battle between nurses and the bureaucracy. The salary gains made by nurses and institutional pressures to cut costs (mostly hospital costs) have initiated restructuring and reorganization. It has become common practice to reduce the number of professional nurses on staff, substitute unlicensed assistive personnel, meet patient care needs through part-time and agency nurses, or any combination of the above. Possessed with a new militancy, nurses have taken their case to the courts, pushed their issues in public policy, and brought their concerns to the consumer. All of these strategies intend to build new sources of power.

STRATEGIES FOR ACTION

The "sleeping giant" that is nursing has begun to awaken. It is evident in the increased status of nursing and in the expansion of nursing practice to every possible setting. It is probably a healthy sign that so many nurses are saying, "But compared to what we can do and should do, it's not enough." And they're right. The major problems within nursing are caused by the lack of cohesiveness, the lack of agreement on professional goals, the lack of planned leadership development, the diversity of nurses in background, education, and position, the lack of internal support systems, and the divisiveness of nursing subcultures, all coping with a rapidly changing society. If nursing is to have the full autonomy of a profession, there must be unity of purpose and action on major issues. Leadership is vital, but grassroots nurses must be a part of the final decision, or goal achievement will continue to be an uphill struggle. Therefore, strategies (and they are not all inclusive) are suggested in the following sections that are the responsibility not just of nursing leaders but of all nurses.

MENTORS, NETWORKS, COLLEGIALITY: THE GREAT POTENTIAL

The term *mentoring* is usually defined as a formal or informal relationship between an established older person and a younger one, wherein the older guides, counsels, and critiques the younger, teaching him or her (the protégé) survival and advancement in a particular field. This is best described as a specific point on a *patron system,* a continuum of advisory support relationships that make access to positions of leadership, authority, or power easier.

At the far end of the continuum is the *mentor,* a very powerful, influential individual. Here, the relationship is the most intense (and perhaps the most stressful). A mentor supports a protégé's dreams and helps him or her to make them a reality. The mentor is a protector and supporter who provides the extra confidence needed to take on new responsibilities, new tests of competence, and new positions. Emphasis on competence is of paramount importance; the mentor teaches, supports, advises, and criticizes.

Protégés are carefully selected. True, someone who wants another for a mentor can bring himself or herself to that person's attention, but the protégé must be seen as worthy. One group of executives cited certain qualities that they looked for in potential protégés: has depth, integrity, a curious mind, good interpersonal skills; wants to impress; has an extra dose of commitment; has a capacity to care; can communicate; can understand ideas; can identify problems and help find solutions; ambitious; hard working; willing to do things beyond the call of duty; someone looking for new avenues and new challenges; someone dedicated to a purpose; and always—someone who would be a good representative of the profession. Usually the individual is also expected to be well groomed and dress appropriately.

Interest in mentoring in nursing has been rising in terms of preparation for scholarliness, development of minority nurses, and leadership in general. However, although almost everyone says that being mentored is a key to success, even quick success, others disagree. After all, there are not enough true mentors for every ambitious person, and many succeed with no mentor at all.

There is now much literature on mentoring in business and education, and a growing body of knowledge in regard to the development of today's nursing leaders. In Vance's study, 83 percent of the nursing leaders surveyed reported having mentors, and 93 percent were mentors to others.[22] The mentors were primarily women nurse educators (teachers) or teacher colleagues, advisors, and educational administrators. A more extensive study of 500 women graduates of doctoral programs also showed the importance of mentoring. Those mentored attributed much of their success to their mentors, and those not mentored expressed deprivation. The mentored were slightly more satisfied and productive in their work than were the nonmentored. With the exception of a very few of the subjects, the mentors and protégés parted amicably and have continued to be friends.[23]

A 1995 study focused on mentoring in the career development of hospital staff nurses.[24] Regardless of their age or experience in nursing, mentorship seemed to continue to be an important resource in their professional lives. Although the term mentoring was loosely defined, participants agreed that what they had experienced was a dynamic, interactive process in which influentials had moved them toward crucial career decisions or adjustments. The most influential patrons or mentors to the hospital staff nurse were select peers and nurse managers. Staff nurse peers enabled development of their clinical problem solving, and nurse managers helped with career advancement opportunities.

The *sponsor*—a strong patron, but less powerful than a mentor in shaping or promoting the protégé's career—is seen as next in the patron continuum, followed by the *guide*, less able than either of the other two to serve as benefactor or champion, but capable of providing invaluable intelligence and explaining the system, the shortcuts, and the pitfalls. (Any of these can also act as role models, although role models may also be more distant figures that are admired.) At the beginning of the continuum are the *peer pals*, peers who help each other to succeed and progress. The first step is seen as being more like the feminist concept of women helping women, less intense and exclusionary, and therefore more democratic, by allowing access to a large number of professionals.

Peer pals can create their own networks. There is a male corollary—the "good old boy" networks—which, through an informal system of relationships, provide advice, information, guidance, contact, protection, and any other support that helps a member of the group, an insider, to achieve his goals, goals obviously not in conflict with those of the group. The good old boys frequently share the same educational, cultural, or geographical background, but whatever the basis of their commonalities, mutual support is the name of the game. It could be group pressure; it could be a word to the right person at the right time; it could be simply access to information sources, but it exists. You can count on it; you can take risks; you won't be alone. (And you don't necessarily have to like each other or agree on everything.) Could this work for nurses? Why not? What is needed is a network that promotes support *of* nurses *for* nurses, men or women. A network that provides backup for the risk takers until all can become risk takers for a purpose. A network that shows unified strength on issues that can be generally agreed upon, so that the profession as well as the individual practitioner can put into practice the principles of care to which both voice commitment. A network that avoids destructive competition and instead develops new leaders at all levels through peer pals, mentors, and role models. A network that encourages differences of opinion but provides an atmosphere for reasonable compromise. In essence, a network that develops and uses the essential abilities of nurses to share, to trust, to depend on one another.

Because networking is "in" and is sometimes seen as what one writer called a "quick fix for moving up," and because it is also new to many women, it is being abused by some. Besides the warnings noted above, networkers are advised to observe both common and uncommon courtesies: do not make excessive requests; be appreciative; be sensitive to your contacts' situation; and be helpful to others.

There are already formal nurse networks in operation, often initiated by a nursing organization or subgroup made up of nurses with common interests, clinical or otherwise. The participants help each other make contacts when they relocate, or they supply needed information or suggest someone else who would know. They alert one another to job opportunities and suggest their colleagues for appointments, presentations, or awards. They give visibility to nurses and boost and praise one another, instead of being unnecessarily critical.

Could this also be called collegiality? In a sense, yes. A *colleague* is usually defined as an associate, particularly in a profession. In a thesaurus, we also find ally, aide, collaborator, helper, partner, peer, friend, cooperator, coworker, cohelper, fellow worker, teammate, or even right-hand man ("person" to comply with today's unisex requirements), and buddy. The implications are great. Colleagues may be called upon confidently for advice and assistance, and will give it. Colleagues share knowledge with one another, together rounding out the necessary information to improve patient care. Colleagues challenge one another to think in new ways and to try new ideas. Colleagues encourage risk taking when the situation requires daring. Colleagues provide a support system when the risk taker needs it. Colleagues are equal, yet different— that is, they may have varying educational preparation, experience, and positions, perhaps even belong to another profession, but when they work together for a particular purpose, that work is bettered by their cooperation.

POLITICAL ACTION

Politics may be defined as the art or science of influencing policy. There is a legitimate tendency to think of politics in the context of government, but affecting policy and operations at the institutional level is often just as important in the work life of a nurse. The term *in-house politics* has been used to describe the power nurses can have if they can determine policies and procedures that affect daily practice. An example is a policy stating that nurses may (or should or must) develop and implement teaching plans for patients or arrange for referrals to the visiting nurse, all of which have been blocked by physicians or administrators in some hospitals.

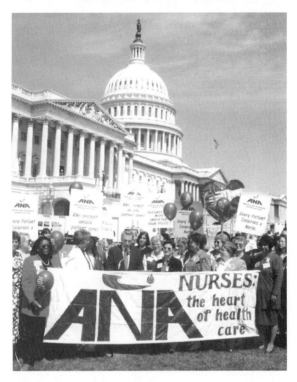

Nurses are exceptionally effective political reformers. Here nurses demonstrate for patient safety on the grounds of the U.S. Capitol. (*Courtesy of the American Nurses Association, MATTOX Commercial Photography*)

It is vital that nurses participate actively in the agencies or community groups where decisions are being made, such as local or state planning agencies. The strategy used to gain input may vary. A basic principle is applicable: before, during, and after gaining entrée, nurses must show that they are knowledgeable, that they have something to offer, and that they can put it all together into an action package. There are many places to start, for most community groups are looking for members who work and are willing to hold office (for example, church groups, charity groups, and PTAs). These activities may be seen as (1) a way of getting experience on boards, using parliamentary procedure to advantage, politicking, gaining some sophistication in influencing decisions, and (2) being visible to other groups and the public. Many community groups interlock, and by being active in some, nurses come into contact with others. However, participating nurses must be capable; there is nothing worse than having an incompetent as the first nurse on a major board or committee. That could do the profession more damage than having a nonnurse, for it appears that nurses still have to be better than those already in power to gain initial respect.

Another aspect to consider and use is the potential economic power of nurses. A nurse executive who controls a multimillion-dollar budget wields power in determining how that money is spent. This kind of status enables these nurses to move in power circles where they can cultivate individuals who influence public and private decision making. Community nurses are particularly good resources, because most make strong community contacts. Today, the participation of the consumer in health care decisions is increasing. An activated consumer who supports nursing has impact on local decision making, as well as on state and national legislation. A legislator is more inclined to hear the consumer who presumably is a neutral participant, as opposed to an obvious interest group; but nursing must sell that consumer the profession's point of view, and must balance consumer needs and nursing goals.

Although it is often through the influence of consumer groups and the community's traditional power figures that nurses get on decision-making committees, boards, and similar groups, after that, they are on their own and must be prepared, perceptive, articulate, and under control. In meetings and at coffee breaks, the politicking and the formation of coalitions may well influence which way a decision goes. Nurses who have not learned to play that game had better take lessons: using role play, assertiveness training, group therapy, group process, speech lessons—whatever is necessary.

On the level of governmental politics, nurses not only can and have influenced such issues as Social Security, quality assurance, patients' rights, and care of the long-term patient, but also have a vital interest in such issues as reimbursement for nursing services, use of technology, children's services, nurse licensure, funds for nursing education, and a national health plan. The specifics of the legislative process and political action in the governmental arena are described in Chapter 10. However, in addition, there is no reason that nurses should not run for office. They are intelligent, well educated, and know a lot about human relations. Those who have won office are not only effective, but often offer extraordinary insight into health issues. Some have been responsible for major legislative breakthroughs for nursing and health care. This is equally true of the dynamic group of nurses in regulatory agencies and congressional offices.

Regardless of the setting, there are some basic guidelines for effective political action. The first is to know the social and technical aspects of professional practice; second, to know the current professional issues and the implications for various alternative actions; third, to be aware of emerging social and political issues and trends that will affect health care and nursing; fourth, to learn others' points of view (those of potential supporters or opponents) and come to terms with what policy changes are possible, as well as desirable; and fifth, to seek allies who can espouse or at least see the desirability of a particular course of action.

PROFESSIONAL UNITY, PROFESSIONAL PRIDE

It is a political fact that the most powerful groups are those that are united. Almost always this means that an organization speaks for that group, and that is one of the purposes of a professional organization. Nursing has many organizations representing various interest groups (see Chapter 13). At times they cooperate, but too often they are at odds or simply act separately. Fortunately, more serious efforts are being made by most groups to form coalitions in relation to important issues for nurses. This trend may or may not overcome the fact that only about 10 percent of nurses belong to the largest nursing organization, ANA. Yet almost everyone agrees that support of the professional organization, where unity and a resolution of internal problems must occur, is crucial if nursing is to be an autonomous, influential power group.

Unity is hard to achieve, however, if you're not proud of yourself and your profession and what it stands for; if you're embarrassed by nursing's image or if, worse yet, you believe it. Because then, nurses are not a group with whom you want to be identified. Unity is not important because it doesn't seem worth the effort. The feeling of powerlessness is a comfort, in a sense, because it excuses you from taking action. That action *can* be taken is illustrated in the preceding pages. To look at the image of nursing is to see what you want to see. A nurse is not one kind of person, good or bad, handmaiden or entrepreneur. Nursing, like its components, has various images at various times. When you see that reflection, it should be what you want nursing to be.

A small point—or, perhaps, a large one: the fashionable image might be woman as slob, but nurse as slob is not attractive. Thirty years ago, how to dress was taught in nursing schools. A sloppy uniform was cause for a reprimand. The same was true for the RN. Then that was no longer considered appropriate; the modern student knew how to dress and behave in a socially correct manner without needing lessons. Are the results evident today? But perhaps we've come full circle. The business literature aimed at men and women is full of advice on "dressing for success," and now it might be nursing's turn. What is nursing's image when a patient is cared for by an unkempt nurse in nondescript clothes with long hair sweeping across the patient's body? Yes, the public does notice. One individual being treated in a college health clinic reported, "I wondered who that person was in blue jeans and a top like men's underwear." A noted editor said at a meeting, "If you nurses are so worried about your image, you'd better clean up your nurses." Not you? Then perhaps a little peer pressure would help—a little direct or indirect action. Personal image and nonverbal behavior do convey a message—possibly a message of "no pride, no interest." Now, both nurses and their employees are taking a second look at this state of affairs and making changes. So are students. A positive image creates power. Who better than the nurses can shape that image?

It is time to look at what nursing has accomplished and is continuing to accomplish. It is a career of unlimited opportunities. It has produced documented evidence that its practitioners make major contributions to health care, and they are reaping some recognition and rewards; but there is unfinished business. Power and autonomy do not come to the spineless, the indifferent or downtrodden, or those who think they are.

Everyone has his or her own concerns, but individuals acting in isolation are vulnerable. In this era of social revolution, ever more individuals are uniting to secure their legitimate rights and privileges. Why would nursing want less? As Edith Draper, one of nursing's leaders, said in 1893, "To advance, we must unite."

KEY POINTS

1. Practice autonomy is one of the most crucial qualities of a profession.
2. To lead others to personally meaningful change will be a constant requirement of your practice.
3. Without followers, there are no leaders.
4. The most logical view of leadership for today assumes general instability, and requires that the leader and followers fuse their strengths and move toward a shared agenda.
5. Power is the by-product of social relationships, and is given or it does not exist.
6. Nursing has the potential for power in its overwhelming numbers, its special knowledge and skills, and its place in the public trust.
7. Planned change allows us a degree of control.
8. Because of their central position in systems of care, nurses often find themselves in the role of "change agent."
9. Nurses who are women must overcome some of the stereotypes of what women can and cannot do.
10. Most nurses are employees, which creates sensitivity to the fact that there are those things we do as employees, and other areas of responsibility to the public which cannot be compromised by the demands of any employer.
11. The most influential mentors to hospital staff nurses are peers and nurse managers.

12. Physician–nurse relationships can be problems or assets, depending on how the two professions understand each other and whether each sees the other as rival or colleague.
13. Networking is an effective way to broaden professional opportunities.
14. Nurses can have a strong impact on health policymaking by their effective participation in community groups.
15. Nurses who have pride in nursing, themselves and one another, can move nursing forward toward a preferred future.

STUDY QUESTIONS

1. Give an example of an instance in which you and your employer would have a difference of opinion concerning the clinical management of a patient, and how it could be resolved.
2. In deciding on the political agenda for the state nurses association, there are a number of issues. Decide which agenda items are best handled by the state association alone and which could be better handled jointly with other associations: drug coverage for Medicare recipients, expanded prescriptive authority for nurse practitioners, health care benefits for children under six, needle-stick protection for staff nurses?
3. Identify how you would go about selecting a mentor, and why.
4. How will the changing nature of feminism impact nursing?
5. Without followers, there is no leader. Called to lead, how would you generate the followers?
6. How would you go about influencing others to participate in a change that was necessary but predicted some personal hardship for every participant?

REFERENCES

1. Webb C, Pontin D. Introducing primary nursing: Nurses' opinions. *J Clin Nurs* 5:351–358, November 1996.
2. Spreitzer G, Perttula K. *Leadership*. Hoboken, NJ: Wiley, 2004.
3. Dunham J, Fisher E. Nurse executive profile of excellent nursing leadership. In Brown B (Ed.): *Dynamics of Administration*. Gaithersburg, MD: Aspen, 1994.
4. Sullivan E, Decker P. *Effective Leadership and Management in Nursing*, 4th ed. Menlo Park, CA: Addison-Wesley, 2000.
5. Herzberg F. *Work and the Nature of Man*. Cleveland: World, 1966.
6. Porter-O'Grady T. A different age for leadership, Part 2: New rules, new roles. *J Nurs Admin* 33(3):173–178, 2003.
7. Sweeney S. Traditions, transitions and transformations of power in nursing. In McCloskey JC, Grace HK (Eds.): *Current Issues in Nursing*, 3d ed. St. Louis: Mosby, 1990, pp 460–464.

8. Watzlawick P, et al. *Change.* New York: Norton, 1974.
9. Lewin K. *Field Theory in Social Science.* New York: Harper & Row, 1951.
10. Lippitt R, et al. *The Dynamics of Planned Change.* New York: Harcourt & Brace, 1958.
11. Perlman D, Takacs G. The ten stages of change. *Nurs Mgmt* 27(4):33–38, 1990.
12. Kubler-Ross E. *On Death and Dying.* New York: Scribner, 1969.
13. Wagner C, Huber D. Catastrophe and nursing turnover: Nonlinear models. *J Nurs Admin* 33(9):486–492, 2003.
14. Ibid.
15. McDaniel R. Strategic leadership: A view from quantum and chaos theories. In: Duncan W, Ginter P, Swayne L (Eds.): *Handbook of Health Care Management.* Oxford, UK: Basil Blackwell, 1998, pp 356–377.
16. Senge P. *The Fifth Discipline.* New York: Doubleday, 1990.
17. Shea, CA. Feminism. In McCloskey JC, Grace HK (Eds.): *Current Issues in Nursing*, 4th ed. St. Louis: Mosby, 1994, pp 572–579.
18. Coombs M, Ersser S. Medical hegemony in decision making: A barrier to interdisciplinary working in intensive care. *J Adv Nurs* 46(30):245–252, 2004.
19. Stein L, et al. The doctor–nurse game revisited. *New Engl J Med* 322:547, February 22, 1990.
20. Ibid.
21. Davidhizar R, Dowd S. The doctor–nurse relationship. *J Pract Nurs* 53(4):9–12, Winter 2003.
22. Vance C. Mentorship. *Ann Rev Nurs Res* 9:175–200, 1991.
23. Spengler C. Mentor–Protégé Relationships: A Study of Career Development Among Female Nurse Doctorates. Unpublished PhD dissertation. University of Missouri–Columbia, 1982.
24. Angelini DJ. Mentoring in the career development of hospital staff nurses: Models and strategies. *J Prof Nurs* 11:89–97, March–April 1995.

Updates can be found at

    http://www.JoelTheNursingExperience.com

HELPFUL WEBSITES FOR PART 3

American Academy of Nurse Practitioners: http://www.aanp.org
American Association of Colleges of Nursing: http://nche.aacn.edu
American Association of Occupational Health Nurses: http://www.aaohn.org
American Association of Retired Persons: http://www.aarp.org
American College of Nurse Practitioners: http://www.nurse.org/acnp
American Hospital Association: http://www.aha.org
American Medical Association: http://www.ama-assn.org
American Nurses Association: http://www.nursingworld.org
Case Management Society of America: http://www.cmsa.org
Center for Health Care Strategies: http://www.chcs.org

National Association for Practical Nurse Education and Service:
    http://www.napnes.org
National Center for Continuing Education: http://nursece.com
National Council of State Boards of Nursing: http://www.ncsbn.org
National Institute of Nursing Research: http://www.nih.gov/ninr
National League for Nursing: http://www.nln.org
National Organization for Associate Degree Nursing: http://www.noadn.org
National Student Nurses Association: http://www.nsna.org
New York State External Degree Program: http://www.regents.com
The Nurse Practitioner (Journal): http://www.springnet.com/np

PART 4

NURSING ETHICS AND LAW

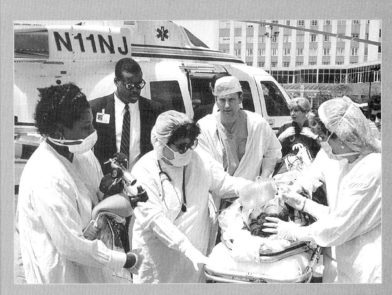

Complex high-tech care has created new issues in the areas of ethics and patient's rights. (*Courtesy of Saint Barnabas Hospital, West Orange, New Jersey*)

Chapter 8

Ethical Issues in Nursing and Health Care

OBJECTIVES

After studying this chapter, you will be able to:

1. *Differentiate between morality and ethics.*
2. *Recognize the kinds of ethical dilemmas nurses and others face in health care.*
3. *List factors that create these dilemmas.*
4. *List factors that influence the way you react to ethical problems.*
5. *Develop a way of assessing and dealing with ethical concerns.*
6. *Apply the ANA Code of Ethics for Nurses to your professional life.*
7. *Identify principles that underlie DNR procedures.*
8. *Recognize some of the major issues related to end-of-life decisions.*
9. *Understand the issue of access to care.*
10. *Identify actions you can take in relation to colleagues who are impaired by substance abuse.*

Most people who decide to enter nursing are aware that there are times when they will be dealing with life and death. If they think about it to any extent, they probably assume that they would do their best to help the patient to live or keep him or her comfortable until death. Asked whether they expected to have a conflict with the law or with other colleagues or even a conflict within themselves at such a time, they would probably react with astonishment. How could this happen? If you asked whether they expected to have any trouble behaving ethically in these situations, the reply might well be, "Why would I?"

Is that the way you felt? Is that the way you feel now? It is quite possible that the shock of dealing with ethical questions is not as great now as it might have been even a few years ago. Movies, plays, television, books, magazines, and even newspaper reports are beginning to recognize that the ethical dilemmas in health care faced every day by those in the field must also be faced by the public.

WHAT CREATES ETHICAL DILEMMAS?

Why are things different now? One simple answer is that it is a much more complex world, with many conflicting pressures on both consumers and providers. For instance:

- Technology in the form of transplants, artificial parts, and machinery, as well as new drugs, can keep alive young and old patients who would once have died, *but* the cost of surviving after such intervention may be so high financially that either the government must pay for both the treatment and lifelong care, or only the rich can afford it. An average family would become impoverished. In some cases, the public pays to keep alive a nonfunctioning human being and then has to deny resources to someone with the possibility of a productive life. Also, people's notions are changing about whether the quality of life made possible by technology, or its sanctity, is most important.
- New knowledge and techniques involving alteration of genes in a human being, and the ability to identify genes causing serious disorders, now exist, *but* this also raises questions of commercialization, cost, safety, and confidentiality.
- People are recognizing their right to make decisions about their medical treatment even if the decision would lead to death; *but* even though family and significant others agree with the individual, his or her wish may be thwarted after the individual becomes technically "incompetent," because the health professionals and/or institutions are afraid of lawsuits, and the law does not always clearly define how or whether such wishes can be carried out.
- The law does cover certain rights, such as abortion; *but* groups with their own religious or moral agendas try to prevent people from exercising those rights.

○   In general, the public accepts the idea that everyone has a right to health care; *but* there are limited resources and no one wants to pay for the reality of equal access.

These situations may not only create conflict between professionals and family but also pit colleague against colleague, health professional against administration, family against courts, lawyer against lawyer, church against individuals, and any variation of these. Yet, almost everyone wants to do what is right. What is "right"? It is not easy to decide. Look at these not uncommon ethical dilemmas:

○   A fragile man in his eighties, riddled with cancer, is admitted to the hospital. When his heart stops, he is resuscitated and awakens with tubes in every orifice. He begs to be allowed to die but is repeatedly resuscitated.

○   The nurse prepares a patient for surgery accepting the physician's statement that the patient was given an adequate explanation. No explanation was given to the patient.

○   A 26-year-old quadriplegic woman with cerebral palsy has herself admitted to a hospital and then asks to be kept comfortable, but allowed to die by starvation because she finds life unbearable. The hospital force-feeds her.

○   An 85-year-old man with many illnesses has been fasting in a nursing home to hasten his death. His daughter supports his decision, and he dies in a few days.

○   A retarded boy refuses kidney dialysis because he is afraid. Effort is made to relieve his anxiety rather than moving others on the hospital's waiting list forward into therapy.

○   A 70-year-old man suffered a stroke and his mental capacity seemed to fluctuate between competence and confusion. He was kept in constant restraint since earlier in his hospital stay when he had fallen. His family supported the decision, but the patient was violently opposed to this as an indignity. The patient was told that the restraint was for his "own good" and that he had no choice in the matter as long as his condition remained unchanged.

○   A baby is born with Down's syndrome and various other congenital defects, one of which requires immediate surgery in order to save the infant's life. The parents refuse permission because they believe that the child, if she survives, will not have a reasonable quality of life and they will not be able to care for her.

○   Another baby with similar defects undergoes surgery, but the mother, an unwed teenager, cannot keep the child. It is in a public institution, requiring total care for all of its five years of life.

- A depressed patient admitted to a mental hospital refuses electro-shock therapy after several treatments because he thinks it will kill him even though he is improving with treatment. He cannot care for himself at home, and his wife cannot manage his erratic behavior. He is committed, under the state's laws, given the treatment, and recovers.

- A 17-year-old high school girl goes to the school nurse. She is pregnant and requests information about abortion. The nurse is strongly opposed to abortion on religious grounds. She does not feel able to deal objectively with the situation and refers the girl to a colleague for information.

- Two men on the same hospital unit have a cardiac arrest within several minutes of each other. The first to arrest is an alcoholic street person with various other conditions; the other is a businessman with a wife and four children. There is one cardiopulmonary resuscitation cart. The resident says, "First come, first served" and resuscitates the alcoholic; the businessman dies.

- A young couple with two boys decide that they can afford only one more child and want a girl. If amniocentesis indicates a boy, the mother wants an abortion.

- After genetic screening, a couple has been advised that they are carriers of a hereditary disease. Two of their teenage children have it, and one does not. When the mother becomes pregnant again, the fetus tests positive for the condition; she decides on an abortion, but both parents decide not to "spoil the children's lives" by telling them they may later manifest the disease or carry the gene that might condemn their children to that disease.

- A patient about to undergo surgery clearly does not understand the risks or the available alternatives. The nurse tells the physician, who explains that the explanation was given, but that patients seldom understand these explanations, and that the patient should be prepared for surgery.

- A patient with cancer is on an experimental drug. Although hospital policy states that the physician must get an informed consent before the drug is administered, the patient's very prestigious physician calls in and tells the nurse to start the drug because it is important to begin at once; he will be in later to get the consent. When the nurse hesitates, her supervisor tells her to go ahead.

- A colleague in the OR confesses to his friend that he has AIDS and that he is afraid to let management know. The nurse friend is concerned because the individual assists in surgery every day.

- An older respected physician in a renowned hospital has been making mistakes in surgery. The residents have been able to catch and/or repair them thus far, but the scrub nurse thinks that he ought to be prevented from operating. No physician will report him officially.

○ A 16-year-old male client brought into the emergency room with a gunshot wound to the head is declared dead. His driver's license identified him as an organ donor, but hospital staff are unable to locate his family for permission to take his organs. Another client in the same hospital will die within 24 hours without a heart transplant. The tissue of both clients match sufficiently for a transplant.

If you were the nurse involved in any of these situations, what would you do? How would you react? Whose rights are or might be violated? The patient's? The family's? The nurse's? The doctor's? Society's? Nobody's? How much would you be affected by your own moral beliefs? If your action was contrary to what the hospital administrators, the physicians involved, or even some of your colleagues thought best (for whatever reason), would you be willing to face the consequences? What if your concept of "right" collided with a legal ruling?

All of these cases cited are real, but not always made public. A nurse somewhere faced each of these difficult situations (and probably others)

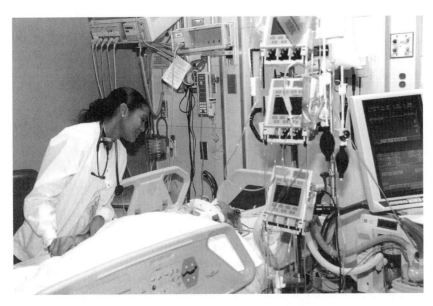

What has become the new standard of care may present significant ethical dilemmas. (*Courtesy of Hackensack University Medical Center, Hackensack, New Jersey*)

and had to make the decision to act or not to act. How that decision was arrived at is the essence of ethics.

Almost every day, some situation that has presented an ethical dilemma to family, friends, health care professionals, and health care institutions is reported in the media. One such case that recently received more than its share of attention involved Terri Schiavo of Florida. Being in a persistent vegetative state (PVS) for over a decade, the question was whether nutrition and hydration should be terminated, allowing Ms. Schiavo to die peacefully.[1] In this situation, the bitter feud between her husband (the surrogate) and her parents turned what should have been an unofficial voluntary decision into a lengthy and public legal battle. The aftermath of this case may be tinkering with the legal system over what should be a private matter, decided according to the ethical beliefs of the family and the quiet cooperation of health professionals. Once, these issues would not have come up at all. People got sick and died, probably at home. Grossly malformed infants were quietly allowed to die. There was no technology to keep these people alive, and except in very rare circumstances, available life-prolonging techniques were not used. Dying was a natural act—sad, perhaps, but inevitable.

Another result of the increasing concern about ethics in health care by both the health professions and the public is legal action. Such actions range from court decisions to legislation on both the state and federal level. Sometimes the trail from ethical problem to legal action is very clear. Unfortunately, what becomes law is not always seen as ethical by individuals and groups, and this creates problems for both practitioners and the public. The reality is that resolving ethical concerns is not easy and probably never will be. Sometimes it is also difficult to disentangle just how and where law and ethics interact. To attempt as rational an approach as possible, this chapter will focus primarily on ethical theories and principles, codes of ethics, approaches to ethical decision making, and the most common ethical situations you will meet in your practice. These include end-of-life care, assisted suicide, access to care issues, and the nurse's role as patient advocate. Ethical issues that have seen considerable legal action are discussed in Chapter 9.

As you read the sections on morality and the various theories of ethics, as well as the nursing code of ethics, consider the ethical problems given as examples and note how your decisions depend on your ethical or, perhaps, moral beliefs. Even if you are not in a position to make a direct decision, inevitably you will be in an environment where such dilemmas will continue to occur, and you will have to come to some understanding about how you can deal with them, directly or indirectly. There is no such thing as "no decision."

FACTORS THAT INFLUENCE ETHICAL DECISION MAKING

MORALS AND ETHICS

There is a tendency to use the words *moral* and *ethical* interchangeably in the literature of health professions. However, in the last few years, the need to differentiate between the two terms has become more evident. Morality is generally defined as behavior according to custom or tradition, instilled early in life, and in accordance with a group's norms. Moral behavior is often derived from religious beliefs, though social influence plays a significant role. Ethics, by contrast, is the free, rational assessment of a course of actions in relation to principles. To be ethical a person must take the additional step of exercising critical, rational judgment in decisions. Ethics is what ought to be. People can be moral, but must aspire to be ethical. Bioethics is the application of ethical theories and principles to situations in health care. Laws are rules of social conduct made by man to protect society, and these laws are based on concerns about fairness and justice.

Kohlberg, structuring a theory of moral development, used the term *stages* for individual phases of moral thinking:[2]

- Preconventional reasoning—right or wrong depending on authority out of the desire to avoid punishment (the mother, the law, the boss, and so on).
- Conventional reasoning—right or wrong from the family or group out of a desire to maintain existing social relationships. Success, in a conventional sense, based on who those groups are.
- Postconventional reasoning—right or wrong based on objective thinking, universal principles, which supersede the authority of groups.

Although his theory is still widely used when discussing moral development, there is some disagreement with this approach, most particularly because he only had male subjects. Although the term moral is used in this analysis, the postconventional level displays ethical thinking as explained by Krowczyk and Kudzma:[3]

> At this stage, morality is based on decisions of conscience, made in accordance with self-chosen principles of justice, which are comprehensive, universal, and consistent. These principles are abstract and ethical, rather than concrete moral rules.

Gilligan was particularly disturbed that Kohlberg did not acknowledge the concerns and experience of women in moral development. She carried out a study designed to clarify the nature of women's moral judgment as they faced the moral dilemma of whether to continue or abort a pregnancy. Results showed that women's moral judgment differs from that of men. For women, the worst problem was defined in terms of exercising care and avoiding hurt. The infliction of hurt was seen as selfish and immoral.[4] Chally describes a woman's moral development proceeding "... from initial concern for survival, to focus on goodness, to a principled understanding of care."[5]

Noddings' model, building on the work of Gilligan, is more recent, and has been given considerable attention in nursing. She centers her ideas on the value of care and caring, stressing that caring is a relationship, not a unilateral activity. "The choice to enter a relationship as one caring ... is grounded in a vision that we hold of our best selves," our "ethical ideal."[6] Caring has been getting increased attention as a "value" on which nursing practice is based—a moral-ethical concept. It cannot be said to be only feminine, since men in nursing (and other fields) certainly embrace this concept as much or as little as women in the "caring professions."[7]

The whole issue of ethics versus morals may seem to be purely philosophical; however, given the differentiation described, individuals often struggle with what may be a conflict between ethical behavior and personal religious beliefs.

ETHICAL THINKING

All ethical dilemmas are not solvable, but they are resolvable. Even where the choice is between two equally undesirable alternatives, taking no action may be worse than making a choice. With this in mind, there are three levels of decision making in solving ethical problems: (1) the immediate level, in which there is no time for reflection (the two men in cardiac arrest); (2) the intermediate level, in which there is some time for explanation and reflection (the woman with the metastatic cancer); and (3) the deliberate level, in which there is enough time to get information and to think and consult in order to make a rational decision (the parents with the hereditary disease). The deliberate level of decision making is probably the most common.

Nurses involved in decision making need all the help they can get, since even the ethical problems that seem most easily resolved seldom are. The examples given earlier are indicative of the difficulties. There are a number of aids available. From a practical point of view, the guidance of an ethics consultant or ethics committee can help nurses think out the alternatives, along with others involved. A decision-making model also helps clarify thinking. The nursing code of ethics and its interpretative statements put the focus on the nurse's responsibility. Ethical theories and principles provide an overall background. There are many detailed descriptions of these approaches in the nursing and health care literature—ethics books and articles by the hundreds, some more readable than others. Interested nurses may find it useful to assemble an ethical library to which current articles can be added. The principles do remain the same, but discussions of new problems and approaches (and there is always something new) can make a nurse more secure in decision making.

FRAMEWORKS/PRINCIPLES FOR DECISION MAKING

There are a number of frameworks or systems on which ethical decisions may be based. Those that are most relevant to ethical decisions in health care are utilitarianism and deontology.

The framework of *deontology* (formalism, duty-based ethics) asserts that the rightness or wrongness of human actions is considered separately from consequences of that action. Decisions are based on fundamental principles that are absolute and imperative. This standard does not change as the situation changes.

Utilitarianism is also called situational ethics. It is based on two underlying principles: "The greatest good and the least amount of harm for the greatest number of people," and "The end justifies the means." Utilitarian rules assume that they contribute to the common good and are not arbitrary, yet rules will change according to the circumstances surrounding the decision to be made. In other words, the situation determines whether the act is right or wrong.

In addition to these frameworks that are used for our ethical decisions, there are basic principles that seem to recur and give meaning to a particular situation. In fact, at the heart of the ethical dilemma is often a conflict between two or more of these basic principles. Understanding what principle is operative and how it relates in the client's situation is the beginning of resolving the dilemma. These principles are defined below:

- *Autonomy* is the responsibility placed on the health care professional to accept the uniqueness of the person. It is recognition of the fact that a person's purposes cannot be abridged because they do not agree with a certain social norm or clash with our own. Patients have a right to self-determination; to make health care decisions for themselves. There are times when a health care professional must act for a patient, but in these emergency situations, the patient has tacitly agreed to limited intervention.
- *Justice* is the obligation to be fair to all people; to treat each equally regardless of race, sex, marital status, medical diagnosis, social

standing, economic level, religious belief, or sexual preference. Another interpretation takes this a step further to define justice as equal rights for everyone and the greatest benefit given to the least advantaged. With this latter reasoning, people would be preferentially treated according to their need. This expanded definition is *distributive justice.*

- *Freedom* derives directly from the standard of autonomy. A patient does not have to deliver the agency of his will to the doctor/nurse. Freedom not only recognizes an individual's right to be told about what will happen to him, but to consent.
- *Veracity* means truthfulness; to allow yourself to know the true nature of your patient; to be confronted with true ideas and to have freedom to choose to deal with them; to tell and be told the truth. The restriction would be when the telling of truth would harm the patient
- *Privacy* involves the right to be protected against intrusive contact from others.
- *Confidentiality* is the obligation to hold certain information as privileged. This is not to be confused with the legal standard of privileged information, and there will be times when the law would have us break confidentiality.
- *Beneficence* speaks to the quality of interaction with the patient; the constant attitude of doing good toward those under our care; not demeaning the human status of your patients by violating their rights.
- *Nonmaleficence* is the reverse of beneficence. It instructs us to protect from harm those who cannot protect themselves (justified paternalism). From another perspective, it tells us to do no harm to our patients, either intentionally or unintentionally.
- *Fidelity* is faithfulness or loyalty to responsibility accepted as part of the practice of nursing. It is the basis for accountability.

These theories/principles, which have been presented very briefly, and others, are often complex and sometimes appear more philosophical than practical. However, they provide a beginning for ethical decision making.

CODES OF ETHICS

Another guide to ethical behavior is a professional code of ethics. In the last several years, ethical behavior has been increasingly a topic of discussion in almost every field—business, politics, law, and, perhaps most of all, health. Codes of ethics, by whatever name, have been common in professions for some time. It is generally conceded that medicine was the first profession in the United States to adopt a code of ethics, but law, pharmacy, and veterinary medicine were also early comers. However, in the last decade or so, an interesting phenomenon has occurred: ethics has become fashionable, and codes have been newly adopted by organizations representing business and industry.

A code of ethics is considered an essential characteristic of a profession, providing one means whereby professional standards may be established, maintained, and improved. It indicates the profession's acceptance of the trust and responsibility with which society has invested it.

The professional association first adopted a "Code for Nurses" in 1950, with the latest revision to come before the ANA House of Delegates in 2001. This document is periodically revised and interpreted to reflect current practice. There are those who support short and succinct statements in the code, with interpretative statements and guidelines that elaborate on meaning. Others prefer more detailed documents, which warrant frequent revision. The ANA 2001 Code of Ethics for Nurses is presented in Exhibit 8.1.

Exhibit 8.1 American Nurses Association Code of Ethics for Nurses (2001)

The ANA House of Delegates approved these nine provisions of the new Code of Ethics for Nurses at its June 30, 2001, meeting in Washington, DC.

1. The nurse, in all professional relationships, practices with compassion and respect for the inherent dignity, worth and uniqueness of every individual, unrestricted by considerations of social or economic status, personal attributes, or the nature of health problems.
2. The nurse's primary commitment is to the patient, whether an individual, family, group, or community.
3. The nurse promotes, advocates for, and strives to protect the health, safety, and rights of the patient.
4. The nurse is responsible and accountable for individual nursing practice and determines the appropriate delegation of tasks consistent with the nurse's obligation to provide optimum patient care.
5. The nurse owes the same duties to self as to others, including the responsibility to preserve integrity and safety, to maintain competence, and to continue personal and professional growth.
6. The nurse participates in establishing, maintaining, and improving healthcare environments and conditions of employment conducive to the provision of quality health care and consistent with the values of the profession through individual and collective action.
7. The nurse participates in the advancement of the profession through contributions to practice, education, administration, and knowledge development.
8. The nurse collaborates with other health professionals and the public in promoting community, national, and international efforts to meet health needs.
9. The profession of nursing, as represented by associations and their members, is responsible for articulating nursing values, for maintaining the integrity of the profession and its practice, and for shaping social policy.

Source: American Nurses Association, *Code of Ethics for Nurses with Interpretative Statements,* Silver Spring, MD: American Nurses Publishing, 2001.

The 2001 revision of the Code is accompanied by Interpretative Statements that present under each statement in the Code a specific clinical or professional situation that is of relevance. The following list includes some of the situations that are explicated to infuse the Code with meaning for contemporary practice:[8]

1. The right to self-determination.
2. Primacy of the patient's interests.
3. Confidentiality.
4. Protecting participants in research.
5. Addressing the impaired nurse.
6. Delegating nursing activities.
7. Moral self-respect.
8. Environmental influences on ethical obligations.
9. Responsibility to the public.
10. Intraprofessional integrity.

Since the mid-1980s many additional position statements for implementing the Code have come from ANA. These are regularly reviewed and updated and some of particular interest are listed in Exhibit 8.2. The Code as well as the complete content of these statements can be accessed through the ANA website at http://www.nursingworld.org.

The International Council of Nurses (ICN) also has authored a code of ethics. The latest version was presented in 2000 (see Exhibit 8.3). There are striking contrasts with earlier versions. Over the years, language has appeared that makes explicit the nurse's responsibility and accountability for nursing care, and statements have been deleted that ignored the nurse's judgment and showed a dependency on physicians that nurses worldwide no longer see as appropriate.

Exhibit 8.2 American Nurses Association Position Statements on Ethics and Human Rights

- Human Cloning by Means of Blastomere Splitting and Nuclear Transplantation
- Privacy and Confidentiality
- Assisted Suicide
- Nurses' Participation in Capital Punishment
- Promotion of Comfort and Relief of Pain in Dying Patients
- Cultural Diversity in Nursing Practice
- Discrimination and Racism in Health Care
- Nursing Care and Do-Not-Resuscitate (DNR) Decisions
- Active Euthanasia
- Foregoing Nutrition and Hydration
- Nursing and the Patient Self-Determination Acts
- Risk Versus Responsibility in Providing Nursing Care
- Reduction of Patient Restraint and Seclusion in Health Care Settings

Exhibit 8.3 International Council of Nurses' Code of Ethics for Nurses (2000)

PREAMBLE

Nurses have four fundamental responsibilities: to promote health, to prevent illness, to restore health, and to alleviate suffering. The need for nursing is universal.

Inherent in nursing is respect for human rights, including the right to life, to dignity, and to be treated with respect.

Nursing care is unrestricted by considerations of age, color, creed, culture, disability or illness, gender, nationality, politics, race, or social status.

Nurses render health services to the individual, the family, and the community and coordinate their services with those of related groups.

THE ICN CODE

The ICN Code of Ethics of Nurses has four principal elements that outline the standards of ethical conduct.

Elements of the Code

1. Nurses and people

   The nurse's primary professional responsibility is to people requiring nursing care.

   In providing care, the nurse promotes an environment in which the human rights, values, customs, and spiritual beliefs of the individual, family, and community are respected.

   The nurse ensures that the individual receives sufficient information on which to base consent for care and related treatment.

   The nurse holds in confidence personal information and uses judgment in sharing this information.

   The nurse shares with society the responsibility for initiating and supporting actions to meet the health and social needs of the public, in particular those of vulnerable populations.

   The nurse also shares responsibility to sustain and protect the natural environment from depletion, pollution, degradation, and destruction.

2. Nurses and practice

   The nurse carries personal responsibility and accountability for nursing practice, and for maintaining competence by continued learning.

   The nurse maintains a standard of personal health care such that the ability to provide care is not compromised.

   The nurse uses judgment regarding individual competence when accepting and delegating responsibility.

   The nurse at all times maintains standards of personal conduct which reflect well on the profession and enhance public confidence.

   The nurse, in providing care, ensures that use of technology and scientific advances are compatible with the safety, dignity, and rights of people.

3. Nurses and the Profession

   The nurse assumes the major role in determining and implementing acceptable standards of clinical nursing practice, management, research, and education.

   The nurse is active in developing a core of research-based professional knowledge.

   The nurse, acting through the professional organization, participates in creating and maintaining equitable social and economic working conditions in nursing.

4. Nurses and Co-workers

   The nurse sustains a cooperative relationship with co-workers in nursing and other fields.

   The nurse takes appropriate action to safeguard individuals when their care is endangered by a co-worker or any other person.

   The ICN Code of Ethics for Nurses is a guide for action based on social values and needs. It will have meaning only as a living document if applied to the realities of nursing and health care in a changing society.

Source: Reprinted with permission of the International Council of Nurses, Geneva.

USING THE ANA CODE

The ANA Code of Ethics, like other professional codes, has no legal force, as opposed to the licensure laws, enforced by state boards of nursing (not the nurses' associations). However, the requirements of the Code often exceed, but are never less than, the requirements of the law. Violations of the Code should be reported to constituent associations of ANA, which may reprimand, censure, suspend, or expel members. Most constituent member associations (CMAs) have a procedure for considering reported violations that also gives the accused due process. Even if the nurse is not a CMA member, an ethical violation, at the least, results in the loss of respect of colleagues and the public, which is a serious sanction. All nurses should be familiar with the profession's ethical code. It is a professional obligation to uphold and abide by the code and ensure that nursing colleagues do likewise.

Implementation of the code is at two levels. The nurse may be involved in resolving ethical issues on a broad policy level, participating with a group of professional peers in the work of formulating or interpreting the code. However, the more common situation is ethical decision making in daily practice, on a one-to-one basis, on issues that are probably not a matter of life and death but must be resolved on the spot. The Code, and particularly its interpretations, are useful as a guideline here, but more than likely in specific incidents, personal reactions will be both intellectual and emotional and strongly influenced by the nurse's own cultural background, education, and experience.

GUIDELINES FOR ETHICAL DECISION MAKING

How can you tell if you are facing an ethical issue? Some ethicists maintain that all decisions made with, for, or about patients or clients or other human beings have an ethical dimension. Theoretically, then, there are ethical decisions that do not create a problem. Everyone involved may agree on an action; however, in reality, it could still be considered unethical by someone's standards. What creates most crises is the ethical dilemma—a situation involving a choice between equally satisfactory (good) or unsatisfactory (bad) alternatives or a problem that seems to have no acceptable solution; and a true dilemma is relatively rare because, if there is adequate information and time, there are clear guidelines for action. Though a dilemma may not be solvable, it is resolvable. Even when there is no right or wrong between two *equally* unfavorable actions, taking no action may be even worse than making the choice.

admissions consent has already been ruled to be almost completely worthless for anything other than avoiding battery complaints, because it does not designate the nature of the treatment to be given. What has emerged are forms that contain all the required elements for the informed consent process, usually individualized by the physician of each patient and often in an appropriate foreign language. Although many people think of informed consent only in terms of hospitalization, there are already some court cases that indicate that the concept embraces the continuum of health care, such as a clinic or doctor's office. An interesting aspect of one of these cases was that the physician was held to have breached his duty by failing to inform the patient of the risk of not consenting to a diagnostic procedure, in this case a Pap smear. The patient died of advanced cervical cancer.

THE NURSE'S ROLE IN INFORMED CONSENT

What is the nurse's role in informed consent? To provide or add information before or after the doctor's explanation has been given? To refer the patient to the doctor? To avoid any participation? The advice given varies. Some suggest that getting involved in informed consent is

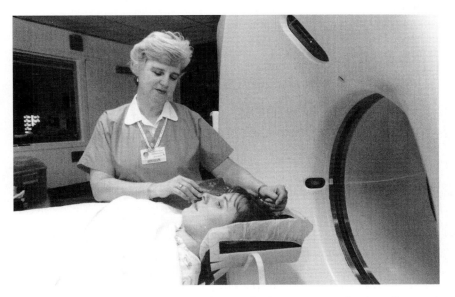

Ultimately it is the patient's right to choose whether or not to submit to diagnostic and therapeutic procedures. (*Courtesy of the Valley Hospital, Ridgewood, New Jersey*)

simply not the nurse's business and is best left to the doctor; others consider it a professional responsibility.

It is generally agreed that nurses do not have the primary responsibility for getting informed consent. However, they do have the responsibility to collaborate with the primary provider, who is more than likely the physician or the advanced practice nurse. Though a nurse may witness the signing of the informed consent form, they are not responsible for explaining the treatment. Neither is the nurse responsible for determining whether the primary provider has truly explained the treatment, risks, benefits, and alternatives. One nurse attorney offers the following statement: "Professional nurses are responsible for determining that the elements of valid consent are in place, providing feedback if the patient wishes to change consent, and communicating the patient's need for further information to the primary provider."[10] Even this straightforward answer is full of uncertainties. The question asked by most nurses is how much can be told, especially if the physician chooses not to reveal further information. Patients' questions may range over a variety of topics, including what you are doing to the patient and your qualifications (if so, answer honestly), to interpretation of what the doctor said (explain in lay terms), to "What's wrong with me?" (first find out what the patient knows, and urge them to speak to their primary), or "Is my doctor any good?" (tell patients that they have a right to ask their doctor for his or her qualifications and experience or to get a second opinion).

A variety of other opinions are offered, but a point that is always made is that the patient's lack of information should always be discussed with the doctor and, if there is no response, with administrative superiors. There is nothing wrong with questioning the patient to see what he or she really understands and clarifying points, providing that you know what you are talking about. If you decide to give further information, it should be totally accurate and carefully recorded, and the fact that it was given should be shared with the physician and others. The nurse should be careful not to give new information that might contradict or conflict with information already given by the physician, thus interfering in the physician–patient relationship. Nurses have found ways to make the patient aware of knowledge gaps so that they ask the right questions, but it is unfortunate that many are still employed in situations in which it could be detrimental to them to be the patient's advocate.

Of course, if the patient is coaxed or coerced into signing without adequate explanation, the consent is invalid. Moreover, if the patient withdraws consent, even verbally, the nurse is responsible for reporting this and ensuring that the patient is not treated. This is a legal responsibility not only to the patient but also to the hospital, which can be held liable. In one case, a competent patient refused intubation and, although persuaded by nurses to agree, the delay caused her to die from lack of oxygen. The family sued for wrongful death and won initially, but on appeal, a court held that if a competent patient had refused treatment, the physician could not be held responsible for her death.

Hospitals are beginning to use a clerk to witness the consent form, after the physician provides an explanation, on the theory that only the signature is being witnessed, not the accuracy or depth of the explanation. Other hospitals ask the physician to bring another physician, presumably to validate the explanation. Where nurses still witness the form, it should be clear *what* they are witnessing—the signature or the explanation. Hospital policy can clarify this situation. Usually, nurses' chances of liability in such acts are considered to be minimal.

The nurse's specific responsibility is to explain nursing care, including the whys and hows. An interesting idea to think about is whether you should tell patients about the risks of the *nursing* procedures you do, even though this is not a legal requirement. (Nor does it prevent you from doing so.) The answer seems to be maybe, but carefully.

THE RIGHT TO DIE

Perhaps because improved technology has succeeded in artificially maintaining both respiratory and cardiac functions when a person can no longer do so, the definition of *clinical death* as the irrevocable cessation of heartbeat and breathing is no longer pertinent. In 1968, faculty of the Harvard Medical School identified certain characteristics of a permanently nonfunctioning brain. In the years since, all states have passed legislation using variations of those criteria to define *brain death*. Translated into statutory language, the concept is typically expressed as follows:[11]

> An individual who has sustained either (1) irreversible cessation of circulatory and respiratory functions, or (2) irreversible cessation of all functions of the entire brain, including the brain stem, is dead. A determination of death must be made in accordance with accepted medical standards.

Experts say that the use of the term "brain death" has been unfortunate. It has perpetuated the mistaken notion that there are two *kinds* of death, brain death and real death. The more accurate term and the one less likely to confuse both professionals and the general public is "death as determined by neurological criteria." Such semantic precision is important. Almost 35 years after the concept was developed, otherwise careful nurses and physicians still betray their confusion by such inappropriate behavior as labeling as "brain dead" patients who are comatose or by hesitating to remove life support from patients who are certifiably dead.

The determination of death by neurological criteria is a common diagnosis only in specialized units, particularly trauma centers. In such settings, staff members are clear that "dead is dead." They recognize that the diagnosis, though painstaking and time-consuming, is rarely difficult. They speak to family members in terms of "death" as they continue to test for signs of brain stem responsiveness. Finally, when they are convinced that death has occurred, they turn off the ventilator rather than asking family permission to do so. Thus, "brain death" illustrates a general truth: there is nothing so practical as a clear concept and nothing so mischievous as a confused concept. For instance, in 1994, at the hospital's expense, the family of a brain-dead teenager took her home on life support, in the determined belief that she was alive. In a time of talk about rationing, stated some ethicists, it was appalling that a dead person continues to be treated, and doctors cannot discontinue life support. Whether the hospital feared prolonged litigation and thought that sending her home was less costly in the long run is unknown.

The popular label of "right to die" has been applied to a long series of famous court cases in which patients and, more often, their surrogates have fought to have life-sustaining treatment discontinued. The label is misleading because, strictly speaking, there is no "right to die." The rights to which these patients and their families have actually appealed are either (1) the right to freedom from undue state interference, often called the right to privacy, and (2) the right to self-determination. The first of these rights involves an appeal to constitutional guarantees. The second is based in our long tradition of common law.

Most of the "right to die" cases have been heard exclusively in state courts because they have not entailed legal questions appropriate to federal judicial review. Hence, it is not surprising that different states have evolved different standards. A review of selected "landmark" cases will illustrate the point.

In the Saikewicz case, the high court in Massachusetts upheld a decision not to give a severely retarded 67-year-old more chemotherapy that would be unpleasant for the sake of a short extended life span. (He died a month later of pneumonia.) That court ruled that such decisions on behalf of incompetent patients should be made only with explicit permission of the courts. A very different procedure was established by the New Jersey Supreme Court in the Quinlan case. In this case, a 22-year-old woman received severe and irreversible brain damage that reduced her to a persistent vegetative state (PVS). Her father petitioned the court to be made her guardian with the intention of having all extraordinary medical procedures sustaining her life removed. The court ruled that the father could be the guardian and have the life support systems discontinued with the concurrence of her family, the attending physicians, who might be chosen by the father, and the hospital ethics committee. (After disconnection of the respirator, Karen Quinlan continued to live another ten years, sustained by fluids and other maintenance measures, in a nursing home.) In a long series of subsequent cases the New Jersey Supreme Court has held to its initial stance that such decisions belong in the traditional control of family and primary caregivers. However, courts in some other jurisdictions have continued to insist on a role for judicial review.

One might suppose that nonemergency cases involving competent patients would be clearer. In such cases, there can be no question about whether the elements of informed consent have been satisfied. When someone wants to discontinue kidney dialysis today because the quality of life is unacceptable, there is relatively little objection. That may be because the patient is ambulatory and may simply choose not to come back for treatment. Yet when a competent 77-year-old California man with multiple serious ailments, but not at the point of dying, wanted the right to have his respirator turned off because *he* found the quality of life unbearable, neither the hospital, nor the doctors, nor the court would allow him to do so, and no other hospital or doctor would accept him. (He had signed a living will and other documents.) His arms were restrained to prevent any action on his part; the hospital said he continued to "live a useful life." His medical and hospital expenses were by then almost \$500,000.[12] William Bartling died the day before the state appeals court heard his case. Six weeks later the court ruled that he did have the constitutional right to refuse medical treatment, including the respirator. The family sued the hospital.

Also in California, a 26-year-old woman almost totally paralyzed from cerebral palsy found the quality of her life intolerable and had herself admitted to a hospital and asked the staff to keep her comfortable and pain-free, but to let her starve herself to death. They refused, and a court supported that decision. She was described by psychiatrists as "mentally stable," not clinically depressed. She finally signed herself out to a nursing home in Mexico, but found that she would have been force-fed there also and consented to eat. Later that year Elizabeth Bouvia returned to California and again appeared in court because doctors in the facility in which she was now a patient cut down her medication for pain. The court supported her.[13] Ironically (or, perhaps, understandably from a psychosocial point of view), the patient ceased her efforts as soon as her right to do so had been affirmed by the court.

In New Jersey, a lower court agreed to removal of a nasogastric tube on an 84-year-old incompetent (but not brain-dead) woman, Ms. Conroy, at the request of her nephew. The case was appealed, but the patient died before a final appellate decision was reached. In the Conroy decision, the New Jersey Supreme Court ruled that termination of any medical treatment, including artificial feeding, on incompetent patients is lawful as long as certain procedures are followed. (Ms. Conroy had indicated, but not in writing, that she would not have wanted to live under those conditions.) The decision came too late for Ms. Conroy, who died with the feeding tube in place. This case was considered different because the person was in a nursing home, but Annas maintains that the distinction should not have been made. Another problem with the final decision was that, although the court articulated the right of competent adults to refuse treatment, it failed to provide any way to allow proxies to exercise the right on behalf of incompetent patients.[14]

This was demonstrated again in the similar Hilda Peters case in New Jersey, this time in part because the ombudsman mandated by the Quinlan decision forbade the removal of her feeding tubes even though the man with whom she lived had her medical power of attorney and there was verbal (not written) evidence that she, too, would not have wanted to survive in this condition. The ombudsman said that he did not want to rule in this way because he believed Peters would not want to live, but that he had a legal obligation to do so because a 1985 ruling by the Supreme Court said that a feeding tube could be removed only if the patient were expected to die within a year. (Expected by whom?) However, in 1987, the New Jersey Supreme Court made three rulings, for Peters and two others, that were expected to influence other states. The court said, first of all, that these life-or-death decisions should be made not by a court, but personally or through a surrogate. The rulings also provided immunity from civil and criminal liability for those making such decisions "in good faith."

It is interesting to note that the New Jersey court decided that the care setting *did* matter. Because Ms. Conroy was in a nursing home, rather than in a hospital, the court modified its principle of leaving such decisions entirely in local hands. Citing a history of rights abuses in nursing homes and noting that nursing homes are less open to multidisciplinary scrutiny by highly trained professionals, the court insisted on review by the independent state office of the ombudsman before any withholding or withdrawing of life-sustaining treatment. This outside review applies only to elderly persons institutionalized in nursing homes and psychiatric hospitals and is justified wholly in terms of their perceived special vulnerability.

In the years since the Conroy decision, nursing homes have increasingly come under scrutiny. In most states, regulatory oversight has been extended and, in some ways, improved. The efforts of professional organizations and the further development of geriatric specialization in medicine, nursing, and social work are having a general, if unevenly distributed, effect. Even ethics committees are becoming more common in nursing homes.

Such legal processes can take a long time. The Paul Brophy case in Massachusetts is an example.[15] It took two years and the refusal of the U.S. Supreme Court to review the case (which would have taken even longer) before, after many contrary rulings, his wife, a nurse, could have him transferred to a hospital that was willing to do what he would have wished and removed his feeding tube. He died eight days later, kept comfortable but not fed, and cared for by his wife.

People like Mrs. Brophy and the parents of Karen Ann Quinlan, though motivated by the plight of their own family member, have ended up by doing a service to the entire community. These cases are called "landmark" because the decisions had implications far beyond the persons whose names they bear. These cases are also detailed here to show the movement we have experienced in the last 20 years, although there is inevitable periodic backsliding. Most often these cases were prompted when physicians or an institution refused to allow treatment to be discontinued.

As noted in Chapter 8, the idea of having a loved one die of thirst or starvation, as the pro-life group describes it (although there is little evidence that a PVS patient has such sensations), is naturally repugnant to families, and the pressures on them are great. Some advocates with a religious affiliation are strongly opposed to removal of food and hydration, although others are not. Physicians and nurses are likewise divided in their feelings, and are often confused as to whether their discipline and the public consider such removal unethical. Nurses have occasionally criticized families contemplating removal of life support (especially artificial feeding) and in some cases have reported them to authorities or alerted right-to-life organizations. Others have stated the opposite point of view. In all such cases, the nurses are the ones in intimate contact with the patient; if the decision is to let the patient die, it is their responsibility to keep the patient as comfortable as possible.

Because of the confusion, it may be helpful to cite, specifically, the AMA or ANA statements on the issue. In 1986, the AMA Council of Ethical and Judicial Affairs issued a statement on "Withholding or Withdrawing Life Prolonging Medical Treatment," declaring that "life-prolonging medical treatment and artificially or technologically supplied respiration, including nutrition and hydration, may be withheld from a patient in an irreversible coma even when death is not imminent."[16] In 1992, the ANA Board of Directors adopted a "Position Statement on Forgoing Artificial Nutrition and Hydration." This policy is in essential agreement with that of the AMA and the Hastings Center's "Guidelines on the Termination of Life-Sustaining Treatment." Its central assertion is: "Like all other intervention, artificially provided hydration and nutrition may or may not be justified."[17] Thus, the ANA has distinguished tube feeding from assisting dependent people with feeding by mouth, an ancient and continuing form of care that is always obligatory.

It was inevitable that, given the controversy on these issues and the fact that there may be several hundred thousand PVS patients, a case would eventually reach the U.S. Supreme Court, probably as a privacy (Fourth Amendment) issue. The first right-to-die case to go before the Court was that of Nancy Cruzan, a 32-year-old woman who was injured in an auto accident in 1983 and was eventually determined to be in a PVS. In 1988, her case was the first in Missouri to raise the question of whether feeding tubes can be equated with other life-sustaining medical treatments and whether patients in Nancy's condition have any rights regarding their care. The parents, stating that this would have been Nancy's wish, wanted to have the implanted gastrointestinal tube removed. A probate judge ruled that they could, but was overruled by the Missouri Supreme Court, which relied on a Missouri statute requiring "clear and convincing" evidence of a patient's prior wish that life support be removed.

The U.S. Supreme Court's decision in Cruzan is complex. The court upheld the general concept, implied or asserted in so many cases from *Quinlan* onward, that there is a constitutional right to refuse life-sustaining treatment. Moreover, the court ruled that artificially delivered nutrition and hydration is not legally distinct from other kinds of medical intervention and thus may be withheld or withdrawn in the same way as other treatment. Finally, the court upheld the right of the Missouri legislature to insist on "clear and convincing" evidence of prior wishes.[18] While clearly not requiring other states to adopt such a strict standard, the court ruled that Missouri's statute does not violate the United States Constitution.

Although this decision is considered, legally, as very narrow, since it relates only to Missouri, and is considered by some as embracing form over substance, it is perhaps also indicative of the conservative bent of the Supreme Court in 1990. In his dissenting opinion, Justice William Brennan argued that the Missouri rules are out of touch with reality; that people do not write elaborate documents about how they might die and what interventions physicians might have to prolong life; and that, after all, friends and family are most likely to know what the patient would want, even without written instructions. He added that by ignoring such evidence, the Missouri procedure "transforms [incompetent] human beings into passive subjects of human technology."[19]

As for Nancy Cruzan, after a friend came forward to say that Nancy would not have wanted to be kept alive under the conditions present, the state withdrew its objections and Nancy was allowed to die, with her family at her bedside. An interesting point on this general issue is that a study of court decisions on withdrawing or withholding treatment found that they are often affected by gender. Whereas men's treatment preferences, even without a living will, were considered by judges, those of women, even with a living will, were rejected or not considered.[20] This is particularly true of pregnant women; several states limit the applicability of their advance directives during a pregnancy.[21]

ADVANCE DIRECTIVES

"Advance Directives" is the generic name embracing both instruction directives (living wills) and proxy directives (appointment of someone to act when the directive maker is incapacitated). Living wills are written documents or statements by competent persons setting forth how they wish to be cared for at the end of their lives. The beginning statement of a living will generally says that the maker is "emotionally and mentally competent" and that he or she directs the physician and other health care providers, family, friends, and any surrogate appointed by him or her to carry out the stated wishes if the maker is unable to do so. The intent is to withhold life-sustaining treatment if there is no reasonable expectation of recovery from a seriously incapacitating or fatal condition. The directive also has space for specific directions about treatments the individual may refuse, such as "electrical or mechanical resuscitation of my heart when it has stopped beating"; "nasogastric tube feedings when I am paralyzed or unable to take nourishment by mouth"; "mechanical respiration if I am no longer able to sustain my own breathing." If such a list is already present in the document, the person is directed to cross out all that do not reflect his or her wishes and/or to add others. Two witnesses sign the document; sometimes it must be notarized. Of course, the living will can be withdrawn at any time by the maker, but otherwise it stands as a clear indication of his or her wishes.

In 1977, California enacted a Natural Death Act, the first "legal" state living will. The next year, Arkansas, Idaho, Nevada, New Mexico, North Carolina, Oregon, and Texas followed with similar statutes. All states and the District of Columbia have now enacted such laws. All grant civil and criminal immunity for those carrying out living will requests.

In 1984 California enacted a law entitled the Durable Power of Attorney for Health Care, which was the first of its kind. This law allowed terminally ill patients to designate another individual to make life-or-death decisions in the event that the patient was unable to do so. The agreement conveys the authority to consent, refuse, or withdraw consent "to any care, treatment, service, or procedure to maintain, diagnose, or treat a mental or physical condition." Like living wills, durable power of attorney provisions are now recognized throughout the

Exhibit 9.1 Example of a Generic Combined Advance Directive for Health Care[a]

As a competent adult, I have the right to make decisions about my health care. If a time comes when I have been determined to be incapacitated due to a mental or physical condition, I, _____, am now declaring my wishes regarding the health care to be given. If I am diagnosed as having an irreversible or incurable disease or condition, and this has been determined to be terminal, or if I am permanently unconscious. I direct that all life-sustaining measures be withheld or discontinued even if this would hasten my death. All appropriate care necessary to provide for my personal hygiene, dignity, and alleviation of pain should be given.

Specifically, I do not want the following life sustaining measures [Example—artificially provided fluids and nutrition]:

_____

_____

I hereby designate the following individual as my health care representative [declares durable power of attorney]:

_____

                                                  (Name, address, telephone number)

If, at any time, that person is unwilling, unavailable, or unable to serve in this capacity, I designate the following person(s):

_____

             (Name, address, telephone number of one or more persons)

_____

_____

                              Signature of person making this directive

Witnesses (names, addresses)

[a] This example is presented merely to show the *type* of information in an advance directive. Each state has its own, which should be used.

United States. They are also known as "proxy directives," and the person who has been designated may variously be known as the "proxy," the "health care representative," or the "person with durable power of attorney for health care." Some forms include designation of an alternative surrogate, "should my surrogate be unwilling or unable to act in my behalf." This document must also be witnessed. Sometimes both components, will and proxy, are combined in one document. A sample generic form is shown in Exhibit 9.1.

Although probably a generic living will, that is, not the official state document, would be seen as a clear indication of a person's intent, legally the forms specific to the particular state in which the individual lives should be used. These can be obtained from the state or from the Compassion in Dying Federation at http://www.compassionindying. org/ad.php. (They also offer advice and a number of informational publications for the public and professionals.)

Federal law now requires all health care institutions receiving Medicare or Medicaid reimbursement to maintain policies and procedures regarding advance directives. The Patient Self-Determination Act (PSDA), which became effective on December 1, 1991, applies to hospitals, nursing homes, hospices, and home health agencies. It further requires that each newly enrolled patient be asked whether he or she has an advance directive. If the answer is "yes," a copy is to be placed in the patient record. If the answer is "no," the patient must be offered information about the right to execute such a document. The PSDA also requires institutions to provide education on advance directives both to staff and to the community.

Having an advance directive would seem to give a person a guarantee that his or her wishes would be carried out, but this is not necessarily so. There are a number of problems. To begin with, the vast majority of people do not have an advance directive of any kind; probably fewer than 25 percent have one. It is constantly recommended that physicians, nurses, and social workers educate patients about the need for advance directives. One study showed that even one simple educational intervention significantly increased the completion of forms for durable power of attorney.[22]

Most health institutions provide educational materials of some kind on admission, and theoretically, there is follow-through by nurses and/or social workers. Nurses cite particular problems. One is that nurses often are unsure of their prerogative to discuss advance directives with patients and family members. Some are uncomfortable in either initiating such a discussion or responding to patient or family queries, often because they lack appropriate information themselves.[23] Staff education and policies that fully inform nurses about the law and advance directives should help resolve this. Another concern is that whether or not the patient has a written directive, it is not always clear as to whether that is what he or she really wants, whether there was undue influence from someone either to consent to or forgo treatment. Additionally, patients may also change their minds, over time, about which procedures or treatments they want to sustain life. This is particularly true in these days of burgeoning technology. What was extraordinary treatment five years ago, may be quite ordinary today. The substance of advance directives should be periodically reviewed with a knowledgeable professional and verified. Neither are patients always knowledgeable about the consequences of treatment decisions before completing a written directive.

Nurses may be aware of other inaccuracies and inconsistencies in these documents because of their prolonged contact with patients. There are cases where patients have living wills but have not told anyone, including their doctors. Facilitating self-determination in relation to end-of-life decisions is emphasized by the PSDA. The well-informed nurse can help patients think through just what they do want. Furthermore, assuring nurse–physician collaboration in counseling patients would go a long way to guarantee that patients have a realistic understanding about their treatment decisions.

Because so few of the elderly have advance directives, and many decision-making dilemmas arise when their wishes and values are not documented, the barriers to such documentation were investigated in one nursing home. As is true of other patients, few physicians discuss advance directives with the elderly, in part not to provoke undue anxiety. Reasons cited by patients for not having a living will included ignorance about what it is, a notion that God, family, or doctors would decide what to do, and general fatalism. Those who did have documents often did not update them, and their verbal statement of what they wanted was sometimes different from that recorded. In one study, it was found that an additional problem is that sometimes when the elderly person is admitted to an acute care facility, the advance directives are not available.[24] (One of the things that people should know is to discuss and give copies to the health care provider, family, friends, or spiritual advisors and store the original in a safe but available place.) When they are available, they appear to influence treatment in the vast majority of cases. Why not in *all* cases was not explained, but other studies indicate that the physicians' attitudes are a major factor. Another study found that, with other factors controlled, the physicians who were more willing to withdraw life support were young, were specialists, practiced in tertiary care settings, and spent more time in clinical practice; those less willing were Catholic or Jewish. An unexpected finding was that almost half of those queried were either neutral or unwilling to withdraw life support, regardless of supportive legal actions and statements by AMA and ethicists.[25] Physicians (or nurses) who will not or cannot in good conscience honor an advanced directive should withdraw from the case, first arranging that the care is taken over by someone whose values are the same as the patient's.

The ANA position paper on the nurses' role regarding the PSDA states that the nurse should assume a major role in facilitating informed decision making by patients, including, but not limited to, advance directives. The position paper recommends that the legally mandated questions about advance directives be made a part of the nursing admission assessment.[26] In fact, this recommendation has not been implemented in most hospitals. Where it has been, nurses are obliged to learn about advance directives and about the applicable state law that applies. On the whole, nurses who are thus aware and knowledgeable feel empowered in their role as patient advocates.

Nurses also realized that it would be helpful to know whether, when a surrogate has been selected by a person, both agree on what the future patient really wants done. In one study, it was found that they did indeed have general agreement on treatment issues, with the exception of use of chemotherapy. The surrogate was more likely to have chemotherapy used. This reinforces the need for clear understanding between patient and surrogate. Actually, very few individuals may desire the standard approach to advance care planning whereby preferences for specific life-sustaining treatments are documented and these requests are strictly followed near death. Instead, patient autonomy may be better served by emphasizing discussion of process preferences and leeway in decision making.[27]

Can a third party interfere with a surrogate's decision? They have certainly done so. Usually, these are people with strong "right to life" beliefs and affiliations, and they seek court orders to act as guardians or otherwise try to stop discontinuation of treatment. Three cases illustrate the problems. The first and most recent involves Terri Schiavo, who, being in a PVS for 15 years, had her gastrostomy feedings and hydration discontinued by her husband. As her surrogate, he believed that she would not have wanted to live in her current condition. That opinion was contested by her parents, who, despite the opinion of countless experts to the contrary, believed she could be helped by various exceptional therapies. The parents were so adamant in their convictions that they fought to the highest level of the court system and appealed directly to the U.S. Congress and to the President to send the case back to the federal courts. But the courts at every level supported her husband's case and rejected requests to have her feeding tube reinserted.[28] Terri Schiavo finally died, but the episode initiated very heated public debate between pro-life and pro-choice constituencies. The majority (60 percent) of the public believes her feeding tube should have been removed.[29] A tangential, but very real outcome of the Schiavo case was the media frenzy that it evoked, and the involvement of politics and politicians with choices that should be very personal and private.

Another case is that of Sue Lawrence, who was in a PVS following brain surgery. After several years, the family realized that her situation was hopeless; family physicians and clergy agreed. Nevertheless, the nursing home wanted a court order authorizing removal of treatment and absolving the facility of any related liability. The parents petitioned the court to remove Sue's feeding tube. The court agreed, and she was transferred to a hospice where artificial nutrition and hydration were stopped. Nearly two weeks later a religiously oriented group petitioned in Superior Court to appoint an emergency guardian so that treatment could be restarted. This was done, but the guardian resigned shortly thereafter and was succeeded by an attorney affiliated with the pro-life group. Although the Indiana Supreme Court expedited a ruling supporting the family and stating that an emergency guardian should never have been appointed, their conclusion did not come down until after Sue had died, still connected to the feeding tube. The family had suffered great pain and outrage, with the only consolation being that the court's ruling would make it much less likely that other families in Indiana would suffer third-party intrusion.[30]

A final situation concerns Christine Busalacchi, who was involved in a serious auto accident and suffered extensive brain damage when she was 17. After a year of intensive therapy that could not help her, and after consultation with physicians, priests, and ethicists who affirmed the principle that when medicine has nothing further to offer a person, it is appropriate to stop therapy, her father, Peter, decided that continued treatment was keeping Christine in a condition she never would have wanted. However, Christine was in the same facility as Nancy Cruzan, and he knew that with the media attention to Nancy's case, which had not yet reached the Supreme Court level, it would be impossible to get court permission to stop treatment. His attempt to move her to a facility outside of Missouri was blocked by the rehabilitation center and the Missouri Department of Health. Even with lower court victories for Peter Busalacchi, the attorney general and governor were determined to block the transfer. Fortunately, a newly elected attorney general stopped the state's appeal; however, the judge accepted a petition for guardianship from a total stranger and granted a 10-day restraining order, which was dismissed after 10 days. Christine died shortly afterward. The father noted, "These people didn't care about Chris. They didn't want to know who she was, what she was like, or what she wanted. They cared only about what they wanted."[31]

Third-party intervention creates both emotional and financial problems. Even though the courts tend to support the family and/or surrogate eventually, the family is thrust into judicial and media spotlight during the process, which only adds to their pain in having to make difficult decisions in the first place. The best remedy to prevent interference is for people to have carefully thought-out advance directive and a designated surrogate. The other is to have legislation that clearly defines who has a legitimate interest in making treatment decisions.

When an individual has no living will and has not designated a specific surrogate, physicians have traditionally consulted the "next of kin" or close friends. With increased litigation, they are becoming more reluctant to use such an informal process, and with more third-party interference, cases often end in court. Now over 39 states and the District of Columbia have passed laws that establish a prioritized list of surrogate decision makers with the authority to make medical decisions for patients who cannot make such decisions themselves and did not or could not record their treatment preferences in advance. In all but six of those states, statutes give priority to the spouse as decision maker for an incapacitated person.[32] If the surrogate does not know what the patient would have wanted, he or she must base the decision on what he or she believes is in the patient's best interest.

RIGHTS OF THE HELPLESS

Children, the mentally ill, the mentally retarded, and certain patients in nursing homes are often seen as relatively helpless, because they have been termed legally incompetent to make decisions about their health care for many years. Often the rights overlap, as when a child or elderly person is mentally retarded.

THE MENTALLY DISABLED

For mental patients, state laws and some high court decisions have served the same purpose. Both have focused on mental patients' rights in the areas of voluntary and involuntary admissions; kind and length of restraints, including seclusion; informed consent to treatment; the rights of citizenship (voting); the right of privacy, especially in relation to records; rights in research; and, especially, the right to treatment. Although rulings have varied, the trend is toward the protection of these rights, even to the point of giving a voluntary mental patient the right to refuse psychiatric medication. In some situations, a structured internal review system in which patients can appeal treatment decisions has seemed to work. In his analysis of autonomy and the psychiatric patient, Matthews considers possible justifications for the denial of the right to refuse treatment on the part of these patients. He justifies this right, based on the right to make decisions about one's own life, however irrational, as long as they do not harm others. In light of this discussion, it is argued that mentally disordered people cannot be denied this right on grounds of their "irrationality," which is anyway a vague concept with several meanings.[33]

Court decisions have supported this decision. The landmark decision of *Wyatt v. Stickney* clearly defined the purposes of commitment to a public hospital and the constitutional right to adequate treatment. Later, an Oklahoma court's decision in *Rogers v. Okin* that gives a voluntary mental patient the right to refuse psychiatric medication created a furor. The appeals court modified the ruling, holding that voluntary patients could be forced to choose between leaving the hospital or accepting the prescribed treatment. (Or physicians could modify the treatment.) Later, a Massachusetts court ruled that an incompetent person could refuse medication if he was able to express a "sensible" opinion, unless there was a proven danger to the public. A number of states have enacted legislation protecting the right of the mentally ill to refuse medication.[34] Other rulings have determined that if the mentally incompetent cannot understand the benefits or dangers of treatment, the family must be fully informed and allowed to make the decision. However, if there is no family to make these decisions, the debate rages. Ultimately, this is a state by state issue, and practitioners should be aware of the fact.

RIGHTS OF CHILDREN AND ADOLESCENTS

It is a general rule that a parent or guardian must give consent for the medical or surgical treatment of a minor except in an emergency when it is imperative to give immediate care to save the minor's life. Legally, however, anyone who is capable of understanding what he or she is doing may give consent, because age is not an exact criterion of maturity or intelligence. Many minors are perfectly capable of deciding for themselves whether to accept or reject recommended therapy. In cases involving simple procedures, the courts have refused to invoke the rule requiring the consent of a parent or guardian for a *mature minor*. If the minor is married, a member of the armed services, or has been otherwise *emancipated* from his or her parents, there is likely to be little question legally.

States cite different ages and situations in which parental permission is needed for medical treatment. The almost universal exception is allowing minors to consent to treatment for venereal disease, drug abuse, and pregnancy-related care. Although it has been understood that health professionals have no legal obligation to report to parents that the minor has sought such treatment, a few states are beginning to add statutes that say that the minor does not need parental permission, but that parents must be notified. In 1983, the Reagan Administration issued a rule that would require parents to be notified whenever children under 18 years of age received any contraceptives from federally funded family planning clinics. After a number of court challenges, this was overruled as infringing on a woman's right to privacy. However, some states continue to set up obstacles, and nurses who counsel teenagers should check the current law.

The entire question of permission for contraception, abortion, and sterilization is in flux. The key appears to be a designation of *mature minor*; emancipated minors are treated as adults. In general, there has been a national trend toward granting minors the right to contraceptive advice and devices, but the political power of conservative groups who oppose this trend is being felt.

Since 1976, when the Supreme Court held that states may not constitutionally require the consent of a girl's parents for an abortion during the first 12 weeks of pregnancy, the reproductive rights of teenagers have been gradually eroded by state legislation and federal edicts influenced by conservatives and right-to-life groups. More than half the states have laws requiring teenagers to notify one or both parents, even if divorced, and/or to get permission from them before an abortion. Most of these laws had not been enforced on constitutional grounds. However, that picture changed when the Supreme Court heard two cases requiring parental notification. The justices ruled five to four, in June 1990, that states had a right to make such a requirement of unmarried women under 18 as long as there was an alternative of judicial by-pass (speaking to judge instead) if the law required notice to both parents. The five conservative justices did not allow for the fact that one or both parents might be abusive, alcoholic, or drug-addicted, or even that the pregnancy might be due to incest. While pro-choice forces continue to work to overturn these restrictive state laws, the more conservative Congress and Supreme Court, as well as the current political power of conservative forces, make this an uphill battle. Ironically, should the young woman decide against an abortion and elect to bear the child, she can receive care related to her pregnancy without parental consent in almost every state. An unwed mature minor may also consent to treatment of her child.

The question of whether parents may make a decision for a child, if the child's well-being is their prime consideration, has not been decided with any consistency. The legal principles involved are *parental autonomy*, a constitutionally protected right; *parens patriae*, the state's right and duty to protect the child; the *best interest doctrine*, which requires the court to determine what is best for the child, and the *substituted judgment doctrine*, in which the court determines what choice an incompetent individual would make if he or she were competent.

In 1986, two-year-old Robyn Twitchell died of a bowel obstruction because his parents, who were Christian Scientists, did not seek medical help. They believed prayer would take care of the situation. In 1990, a jury found them guilty of manslaughter and they were sentenced to probation and community service; they also had to pledge to seek medical care for their other children. Yet, other Christian Scientists have interpreted their religion's precepts differently, considering surgery a purely "mechanical" intervention, which is permitted. Understanding some of the nuances of this religion as related to health care is helpful to the nurse and other health professionals who have difficulty with the concept that illness is caused by "mental" rather than physical factors and that seeking medical care "departs from the practice of Christian Science."[35]

Several landmark cases occurred in the early 1980s. In Illinois, newborn Siamese twins joined below the waist and sharing an intestinal track and three legs were not expected to live. "Do not feed, in accordance with parents' wishes" was written on the chart. However, several nurses did feed the babies, and someone reported the situation to a government agency. A court order was obtained to gain temporary custody of the children, and a neglect petition was filed. The parents (a doctor and nurse) and the doctor were charged with attempted murder, a charge that was later dismissed. Four months later, they regained custody of the children, whose care had mounted to several hundred thousand dollars. They were also in danger of losing their licenses.[36]

In Indiana, about a year later, a Baby Doe was born with Down's syndrome and a correctable esophageal fistula. The parents refused surgery, and their decision was upheld by the courts. The child was deprived of artificial nutritional life support and died. Although similar action had been taken in other Baby Doe cases, this one came to the attention of President Reagan. It resulted in a federal regulation that threatened hospitals which neglected such children with loss of funds under Section 504 of the Rehabilitation Act of 1973 (which protects the handicapped). Large signs had to be posted alerting people to a "hot line" number to call to report such incidents. After a series of legal challenges, this regulation was ruled unconstitutional—"arbitrary and capricious," among other things. Eventually, an alternative suggestion by the American Academy of Pediatrics was agreed on: establishment of infant bio-ethics committees (IBCs) with diverse membership whose responsibility, in part, would be to advise about decisions to withhold or withdraw life-sustaining measures. This was encouraged in the "Baby Doe" law, the federal Child Abuse Amendments of 1984, which labeled withdrawal or withholding of medically indicated nutrition "child abuse." However, a regulation basically left the decision as to whether such nutrition might be "virtually futile" up to the physician.[37]

The courts have also supported refusal of treatment for infants. A child born HIV-positive with cocaine withdrawal and numerous other problems was placed under the guardianship of the Illinois Department of Children and Family Services to make decisions on the child's medical treatment. A requested DNR order eventually went to an appeals court where the child's condition was evaluated and the DNR order was supported.[38] In another case, the parents of Cody Glasner sued because Cody, one of twins delivered by cesarean section, was resuscitated, although the parents had been told he was dead *in utero*. The doctors never let the parents make any decisions about Cody's treatment. They took home a fragile baby requiring extensive medications and treatments, and they still had the other twin to care for. After 33 months, Cody died at home after the parents decided not to put him back on a ventilator. In still another, the physician father of a very premature baby with probable brain damage, who took the baby off the respirator, was prosecuted but acquitted. He and his wife had asked doctors not to resuscitate the baby at birth, but they did so anyhow.[39]

The pain—and cost—of futile medical care for babies is periodically reported in the media, as in the cases where the infant has only brainstem activity. Sometimes, as in the case of Baby K in Virginia, the court supported a mother with a firm Christian faith who insisted on further care, including tube feedings for an anencephalic baby, which the hospital considered futile and inappropriate care. This prompted a debate on costs and ethics, since the baby could never be a sentient human being and the public money spent could have provided many health care services for other children. On the other hand, physicians in one Washington state hospital considered the dialysis of another premature baby, Ryan Nguyen, futile, inappropriate, and immoral. The parents sought and obtained an emergency order from the Spokane County Superior Court requiring the hospital to give any care necessary to stabilize and maintain the child's life. Because of the media reports, physicians from another hospital offered to accept Ryan for treatment. He had surgery and recovered well, requiring no dialysis and taking food by mouth. This case led to a discussion of how the "Baby Doe" regulations did or did not serve their purpose.[40]

At the other end of the age spectrum regarding children is whether teenagers should be permitted to forgo treatment. The trend is to letting them do so under the "mature minor rule."[41] In several cases, young men with cancer had either chosen not to have additional transplants and medication (after others had failed) or to discontinue chemotherapy. Choice in Dying recommends that mature minors make their wishes known through family discussions and advance directives. This is considered particularly important for children with chronic or potentially life-threatening conditions. A few states allow emancipated minors to complete advance directives, but usually makers must be 18 or over. Four states allow parents to complete advance directives for children suffering from a terminal illness.

An interesting right-to-die situation involving a minor came to the Maine courts in 1990. Chad Swan, in a PVS and being tube-fed after an accident, developed several medical complications. With the concurrence of his physician, his family filed for a court order permitting the termination of the feeding. The court ruled that there was clear evidence, based on Chad's statements reported by his family, that he would not want to be maintained in a PVS, but the state attorney general appealed because Chad was only 17 years old. The Maine Supreme Court then expanded a previous right-to-die decision to include minors capable of making a serious decision to forgo treatment.

A basic right that children have is not to be abused. Child abuse is reportable in every state, although defined differently. Hospitals, all health professionals (including nurses), and sometimes schoolteachers, are required to report reasonable suspicion of child abuse. Failure to do so may expose the individual to civil and, perhaps, criminal charges. In most states, those reporting in good faith are rendered free from civil liability (lawsuits) for having made the report.

Nurses should ask three questions about a child's injury: Has the child suffered injury or harm? Does the injury appear nonaccidental or inconsistent with the history given? Did the parent or caretaker cause the injury or fail to prevent it? If yes, the nurse should report a case of suspected child abuse and carefully gather and report specific information.[42]

Sexual abuse is usually part of the statutory definitions of child abuse even if no physical injury has occurred. Among the specific forms of sexual assault identified are rape, incest, sodomy, lewd or lascivious acts upon a child under 14, oral copulation, penetration of a genital or anal opening by a foreign object, and child molestation.[43]

The entire issue of identification and reporting has become particularly sensitive since sexual abuse of children has become more visible, and children have died. The question has been raised as to whether it is always in the best interest of the child and family to report the situation, if changes are being made. On the other hand, health professionals, teachers, and social agencies have been sued for *not* reporting or following through on these cases. The minor's right of protection extends to her or his school where, in most states, the law stipulates what punishment a teacher can employ to maintain discipline in a classroom or school. Private schools are not always subject to the same legal restrictions as public schools in this respect.

RIGHTS OF PATIENTS IN RESEARCH

When a nurse is participating in research, at whatever level, ensuring that the rights of patients are honored is both an ethical and a legal responsibility. Nurses should know the patients' rights: self-determination to choose to participate; to have full information; to terminate participation without penalty; privacy and dignity; conservation of personal resources; freedom from arbitrary hurt and intrinsic risk of injury; as well as the special rights of minors and incompetent persons previously discussed. For instance, nurses have been ordered to begin an experimental drug knowing that the patient has not given an informed consent. The nurse is then obligated to see that the patient does have the appropriate explanation. This is one more case in which institutional policy that sets an administrative protocol for the nurse in such a situation is helpful.[44] If the nurse is the investigator, she or he must observe all the usual requirements, such as informed consent and confidentiality.

Any institution that applies for research funding from DHHS is required to have in place an Institutional Review Board (IRB). Some multidisciplinary panels are charged with protecting human subjects from both unduly dangerous procedures and from abuses of their rights. These IRBs vary widely in the rigor of their processes, despite being tightly regulated. Some IRBs subject proposals for research to very careful scrutiny; others are much less effective.

Some boards may be less protective of patients' rights than they should be, especially in the area of informed consent. There is usually no follow-up to determine whether the plans to preserve subjects' rights that are presented in the proposals are really carried through. There is also criticism about lack of consistency in proposal approval. However, the IRB is generally seen as a safeguard to patients.[45]

There is no requirement that there be nurses on these boards, even if the boards are in hospitals or other health care agencies. Nurses can bring a useful perspective and should probably propose themselves for membership where not already invited. However, they should be properly prepared and knowledgeable about research.

PATIENT RECORDS: CONFIDENTIALITY AND AVAILABILITY

There is some evidence that, in situations other than the legally required ones, confidentiality of patients' records has been frequently violated. From birth certificates to death certificates, the health and medical records of most Americans are part of a system that allowed access by insurance companies, student researchers, and governmental agencies, to name a few. It was never realistic for hospital patients to think that medical information about them would be completely confidential, even when staff followed all the basic rules about not discussing patients except in clinical situations. And confidentiality fell even more in jeopardy with the advent of computerized record-keeping, which has grown by leaps and bounds in the last decade. Being aware of this, the *Health Insurance Portability and Accountability Act* of 1996 (HIPAA) has established rules to ensure that all patient account handling, billing, and medical records are protected. But HIPAA only applies to medical records maintained by health care providers, health plans, and health clearing-houses—and only if the facility maintains and transmits records in electronic form. A great deal of health-related information exists outside of health care facilities and the files of health plans, and thus beyond the reach of HIPAA. The reader is referred to, "HIPAA Basics," www.privacyrights.org/fs/fs8a-hipaa.htm, for more comprehensive information. The extent of privacy protection given to your medical information often depends on where the records are located and the purpose for which the information was compiled. The laws that cover privacy of medical information vary by situation. And confidentiality is likely to be lost in return for insurance coverage, an employment opportunity, your application for a government benefit, or an investigation of health and safety at your work site. In short, you may have a false sense of security.

Some provisions of the HIPAA demand that patients must be able to access their records, be able to correct errors, and must be informed of how their personal information will be used. Other provisions involve confidentiality of patient information and documentation of privacy procedures. It is these requirements that have led to a

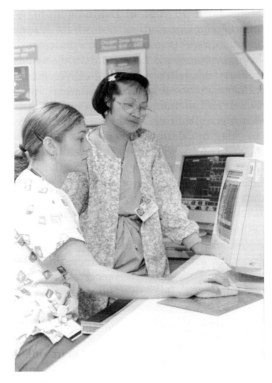

With the use of electronic patient records comes the responsibility to assure confidentiality. (*Courtesy of Robert Wood Johnson University Hospital, New Brunswick, New Jersey*)

new vigilance in record-keeping which dramatically affects the day-to-day practice of the nurse. Though passed by the Congress and signed by the President in 1996, its provisions did not become mandatory until April 2003. An orientation to HIPAA regulations is part of any workplace orientation. The important message here is that the patients' records are personal and confidential, and that this confidentiality is scrutinized intently.

Though HIPAA was passed first by the Congress, the federal Freedom of Information-Privacy Act (FOIA) was operational first. FOIA denies access to an individual's medical record without that person's consent. In addition, the Fair Health Information Act of 1994 addresses the need for federal law to protect confidential material. Still, there was consensus that these laws would not be able to protect the confidentiality of records in an electronic age. And so HIPAA took shape, with all of its provisions for security in an era of computer-based patient records.

Physicians and hospitals have historically been hostile toward the concept of sharing the record with the patient. Some attorneys serving health care facilities tend to share that feeling, often because they fear that patients may detect errors or personal comments that will result in a legal suit. (Actually, patient access has been mandated in Massachusetts since 1946 without a single reported adverse incident.) Whether or not any person involved in health care still feels that way is immaterial. Almost without exception, the patient's medical record is available to him or her on request—and sometimes without request.

It is interesting to review the literature over the last 20 years to see the changes in attitude and legislation. There were always physicians and others who saw sharing the record with the patient as not only fair, but sensible. Rather than worry that a patient would be too frightened or too stupid to understand, these practitioners had a philosophy of openness.

Choice in the matter of sharing the record has ended. Whereas it is legally recognized that the patient's record is the property of the hospital or physician (in the office), the information that the record contains is not similarly protected. Though federal laws supersede state laws in guaranteeing access to records, there are always idiosyncrasies. All states allow patients direct access to their records depending on the location of those records. In the others, individuals have a probable legal right to access without going to court.

Do you have any legal responsibility to be an intermediary? The answer is more complex than just "yes" or "no." A nurse would not generally hand a patient the chart at request. Most states, as well as health care agencies, have a protocol to be followed for access to records. This usually involves providing both privacy and an opportunity for the physician and/or another person to explain the content. However, patients often do not want to see their charts if they feel that they are being given full information and are treated decently. Nurses certainly have a role in giving that open and humane care, but if the patient does ask, they should know the specific procedure in their agencies so that they can tell those patients.

OTHER ASPECTS OF PATIENTS' RIGHTS

PRIVACY

Nurses and others who work with patients must be especially careful to avoid invading the patient's right to privacy, which is identical to that of any other person. There are a number of special concerns. Consent to treatment does not cover the use of a picture without specific permission, nor does it mean that the patient can be subjected to repeated examinations not necessary to therapy without express consent; and undue exposure during examination must also be avoided. It has been recommended that the patient should be informed as to what confidentiality can be expected both ethically and legally. If the patient is the subject of a clinical conference, identifying aspects of the patient should be disguised to maintain anonymity.

Exceptions to respect for the patient's privacy are related to legal reporting obligations. All states have laws requiring hospitals, doctors, nurses, and sometimes other health workers to report on certain kinds of situations, because the patient may be unwilling or unable to do so. Nurses often have responsibility in these matters because, although it may be the physician's legal obligation, the nurses may be the only ones actually aware of the situation. Even if such reporting is not required by a law *per se*, regulations of various state agencies may require such a report. Common reporting requirements are for communicable diseases, diseases in newborn babies, gunshot wounds, and criminal acts, including rape. As noted earlier, child abuse is always reportable, and more recently, so is spouse and elder abuse. Procedures vary greatly, but in elder abuse, in each state, the nurse is included as a reporter. In most states, the abuses covered are physical abuse, fiduciary abuse, neglect, and abandonment.[46] The nurse may be obligated to testify about otherwise confidential information in criminal and abuse cases.

As the AIDS epidemic grew, new reporting problems arose. By 1987 all states had added AIDS to the list of reportable diseases. Many, but by no means all, require reporting of AIDS carriers, that is, the reporting of positive test results for the human immunodeficiency virus (HIV). Physicians have been willing to make these reports because of the virulence of the disease and the need to maintain the best possible epidemiological records. However, the problem arises of whether to notify the family, especially a spouse or lover, of a person with AIDS. Many patients object to notification and therefore will not come for testing, creating a situation that may be even more serious. State laws vary regarding a provider's legal duty to warn potentially exposed partners, when an HIV-infected client clearly indicates that he or she will not notify their partners or make the necessary information available for health department staff to make the notification. In cases related to other infectious diseases, judges have ruled that the physician had a duty to inform the third party. Theoretically, the third party could sue the physician if infected and not warned. As a rule, this kind of reporting is a public health department's responsibility, but it has not yet been determined whether, for instance, a home health nurse with information on AIDS-related conditions has a duty to tell the family.[47]

Confidential information obtained through professional relationships is not the same as *privileged communication*, which is a legal concept providing that a physician and patient, attorney and client, and priest and penitent have a special privilege. Should any court action arise in which the person (or persons) involved is called to testify, the law (in many states) will not require that such information be divulged. Not all states acknowledge that nurses can be recipients of privileged communication, but there are specific cases in which the nurse–patient privilege has been accepted, especially in the case of advanced practice nurses.[48] Another issue is that psychiatric nurses, like other psychotherapists, have a responsibility to warn potential victims about their homicidal clients (the "Tarasoff principle," named after a case in which a psychiatrist did not do so). Other than such a situation, however, a new ruling by the Supreme Court in 1996 has recognized the therapist–patient privilege, including as "therapists" psychotherapists and other mental health professionals.[49]

ASSAULT AND BATTERY

Assault and battery, although often discussed with emphasis on the criminal interpretation, also has a patients' rights aspect that is related to everyday nursing practice, especially when dealing with certain types of patients. In many cases, where the action taken could come under this legal category, it is particularly important to chart fully and accurately. Grounds for civil action might include the following:

1. Forcing a patient to submit to a treatment for which he or she has not given consent either expressly in writing, orally, or by implication.

Whether or not a consent was signed, a patient should not be forced, for resistance implies a withdrawal of consent.

2. Forcefully handling an unconscious patient.
3. Lifting a protesting patient from the bed to a wheelchair or stretcher.
4. Threatening to strike or actually striking an unruly child or adult, except in self-defense.
5. Forcing a patient out of bed to walk postoperatively.
6. In some states, performing alcohol, blood, urine, or health tests for presumed drunken driving without consent. There are some "implied consent" statutes in motor vehicle codes that provide that a person, for the privilege of being allowed to drive, gives an implied consent to furnishing a sample of blood, urine, or breath for chemical analysis when charged with driving while intoxicated. However, if the person objects and is forced, it still might be considered battery. Several states, acknowledging this, have enacted legislation to insulate hospital employees and health professionals from liability.

As a rule, intentional torts, such as assault and battery, are not covered by malpractice insurance.

FALSE IMPRISONMENT

As the term implies, *false imprisonment* means "restraining a person's liberty without the sanction of the law, or imprisonment of a person who is later found to be innocent of the crime for which he was imprisoned." The term also applies to many procedures that actually or conceivably are performed in hospital and nursing situations *if they are performed without the consent of the patient or his or her legal representative.* In most instances, the nurse or other employee will not be held liable if it can be proved that what was done was necessary to protect others.

Among the most common nursing situations that might be considered false imprisonment are the following:

1. Restraining a patient by physical force or using appliances without written consent, especially in procedures where the use of restraints is not usually necessary. This is, or may be, a delicate situation because if you do not use a restraint, such as siderails, to protect a patient, you may be accused of negligence, and if you use them without consent, you may be accused of false imprisonment. This is a typical example of the need for prudent and reasonable action that a court of law would uphold.

2. Restraining a mentally ill patient who is dangerous neither to himself nor to others. For example, patients who wander about the hospital division making a nuisance of themselves usually cannot legally be locked in a room unless they show signs of violence. If they do, you must still be careful.

3. Using arm, leg, or body restraints to keep a patient quiet while administering an IV infusion may be considered false imprisonment. If this risk is involved—that is, if the patient objects to the treatment and refuses to consent to it—the physician should be called. Should the doctor order restraints for the patient, make sure that the order is given in writing before allowing anyone to proceed with the treatment. It is much better to assign someone to stay with the patient throughout a procedure than to use restraint without authorization.

4. Detaining an unwilling patient in the hospital. If a patient insists on going home, or a parent or guardian insists on taking a minor or other dependent person out of the hospital before his or her condition warrants it, hospital authorities cannot legally require him or her to remain. In such instances, the doctor should write an order permitting the hospital to allow the patient to go home "against advice," and the hospital's representative should see that the patient or guardian signs an official form absolving the hospital, medical staff, and nursing staff of all responsibility should the patient's early departure be detrimental to his or her health and welfare. If the patient refuses to sign, a record should be made on the chart of exactly what occurred, and an incident report probably should be filed. Take the patient to the hospital entrance in the usual manner, if possible.

5. Detaining for an unreasonable period of time a patient who is medically ready to be discharged. The delay may be due to the patient's inability to pay the bill or to an unnecessarily long wait, at his or her expense, for the delivery of an orthopedic appliance or other service. In such instances, you may or may not be directly involved, but it is always wise to know the possibility of legal developments and to exercise sound judgment in order to be completely fair to the patient and avoid trouble.

LEGAL ISSUES RELATED TO REPRODUCTION

Laws permitting abortion have varied greatly from state to state over the years. In early 1973, the Supreme Court ruled that no state can interfere with a woman's right to obtain an abortion during the first trimester (12 weeks) of pregnancy. During the second trimester, the state may interfere only to the extent of imposing regulations to safeguard the health of women seeking abortions. During the last trimester of pregnancy, a state may prohibit abortions except when the mother's life is at stake (*Doe v. Bolton* and *Roe v. Wade*).

Theoretically, all hospitals are required to perform abortions within these guidelines, and it is legal to assist with such a procedure. However, because of religious and moral reasons, some institutions are exempted from complying with the law, and individual doctors and nurses have refused to participate in abortions. Individual professionals or other health workers may make that choice, and there is legal support for them (conscience clause). This does not preclude the right of the hospital to dismiss a nurse for refusing to carry out an assigned responsibility or to transfer to another unit. There have been some suits by nurses objecting to transfer, but rulings have varied.

More than 30 years after the *Roe v. Wade* decision, opinions are still strong on abortion issues and now appear to be even more so; generally the same arguments are heard. The major related court cases have concerned legislation attempting to outlaw or limit abortion. Immediately after *Roe v. Wade*, with a liberal Supreme Court, the rulings were almost consistently directed at freedom of choice, in opposition to restrictions on abortion being enacted by the states and later by the conservative Reagan Administration. The rulings changed dramatically with appointments of conservative judges by Presidents Reagan and Bush, until there was a five-to-four conservative majority, with the only woman justice, Sandra O'Connor, considered the sometime swing vote. (However, she tended to be conservative on abortion issues.) The Clinton presidency's two liberal appointees provided more balance. But the stakes for the court and the law are even higher now than they were in 2000. The prospect of a change on the court is greater—eight of the justices are now at least 65—and the replacement of even one justice could affect the law on issues such as abortion rights, affirmative action, religion's role in government, and the division of state and federal powers, all issues around which there is great controversy among the public and divergence in thinking among members of the Court.[50]

The case *Webster v. Reproductive Health Services*, in 1989, was considered a turning point. The Supreme Court provided the states with new authority to limit a woman's right to abortion by upholding a Missouri law that banned abortions in tax-supported facilities except to save the mother's life, even if no public funds are spent; banned any public employee (doctors, nurses, others) from performing or assisting with abortions except to save a woman's life; and required testing of *any* fetus thought to be at least 20 weeks old for viability. Then, in 1990, the Court ruled constitutional the Ohio and Minnesota laws requiring parental notification by unmarried teenagers. (Whether the girl was pregnant through incest or if there were other problems to make this difficult were ignored.)

Probably of even more concern to pro-choice advocates and even others who did not necessarily support *Roe v. Wade* was the 1991 decision on *Rust v. Sullivan*. The Court ruled that federal regulations which barred employees of clinics that receive federal funding "from discussing abortion with their patients, even if the women ask for the information or if the health care provider believes that an abortion is medically necessary" were constitutional. What shocked health care professionals was not just that poor women who had no other source of family planning would be denied full information, but that physicians, nurses, and other health care workers would be forced to withhold full information from patients, which is not only an ethical but a legal problem. Part of the majority opinion written by Chief Justice William Rehnquist stated that the women's right to have an abortion was not infringed because it was her indigence, not the regulations, that prevented it. Other statements by proponents indicated that, after all, professionals did not *have* to work in such clinics if this "gag rule" bothered them. Because so many clinics depend on Title X money, some indicated that they would abide by the regulations, others that they would figure out a way around them. A number of Planned Parenthood clinics noted that they would simply have to do without federal funding. People turned to Congress for action, but late in the session, a bill invalidating the regulations was vetoed by President Bush and Congress did not override the veto. Of all the actions relating to family planning, this one probably affected nurses most, since it prevented nurses working in Title X clinics from giving their patients full and accurate information. However, in 1993, one of President Clinton's first actions was to reverse this gag rule.

The aim of many of these cases, usually brought by a state, was to force the overturn of *Roe v. Wade*. That did not quite happen, but some state legislatures passed increasingly restrictive laws (even forbidding abortion in cases of incest and rape), in part to try to force the Supreme Court to hear the cases. Governors vetoed some of these laws, but the very fact that they had gotten through two Houses was appalling to many men and women alike. After particularly restrictive laws were overturned by federal courts in Pennsylvania, Guam, Utah, and Louisiana, their advocates planned to take the cases to the Supreme Court. Because of the clear majority of conservative justices, particularly after the retirement of Justice Thurgood Marshall in 1991, an overturn of *Roe v. Wade* was predicted by some. As a matter of fact, in 1992 in *Planned Parenthood v. Casey*, the Court upheld most of the restrictions passed by the Pennsylvania legislature, and in doing so it established a new legal standard: restrictions are constitutional so long as they do not impose "undue burdens" on a woman's right to choose. However, it is important to remember that the U.S. Supreme Court rules only on issues related to the Constitution. In these cases, the Court rules that the state or another petitioner does or does not have a constitutional right to behave in a particular way. The trend now is to give states more freedom to act.

The big issue at the turn of the century is the so-called "partial-birth abortion," done in the last trimester. It represents less than 1 percent of abortions. Congress tried several times to pass a bill forbidding this procedure, but President Clinton vetoed it. Discouraged by the federal outlook, over 40 states have taken up the matter, and several have made the bans law, demonstrating the strength of the antiabortion movement. Some young women have already sought back-alley abortionists with the expected dire results. Both pro-choice and pro-life forces have concentrated their efforts on legislators and candidates to bring about state laws that support their particular point of view. The end is not in sight.

How does this affect nurses? Nurses support both sides of this issue, as was clear by the anger or joy expressed by nurses when ANA took a pro-choice stand. Regardless of their personal feelings, however, they will care for women and young girls regardless of their choices.

Ethically, nurses must give all patients good care, but who gets what care and why, as in the Webster case, may affect nurses professionally as well as personally. As citizens, nurses must stay abreast of such important issues. For instance, many pro-life groups also object to sex education and contraceptive use, yet an astounding number of teenagers get pregnant every year. What should the role of the nurse be in this situation? It is educational to see how other countries handle these issues. It is also important to see how some of these issues interrelate. For instance, groups opposed to abortion are now becoming involved in right-to-die issues.

In one case, a dying woman was forced to have a cesarean to "save" her fetus. Both died, and later the action was ruled illegal. In still another case, a woman in a coma was denied an abortion, but later, in a similar case, one was permitted—even though a right-to-life lawyer who did not even know the woman tried to become her guardian to prevent it. And what of the Baby Doe-saved children? Who will be responsible for them? Will the family be forced to care for and pay for a severely deformed child? What of all the issues related to the fetus? Will new technology that has been successful in intrauterine surgery save some of these babies? Cure them? How will new techniques of birth control, including the abortion-inducing, pill, RU 486 and the use of other new drugs or changed use of drugs already approved for other conditions that are found to induce abortions, change the family planning scene? Laws on *family planning*, in general, also vary greatly. Some laws appear to be absolute prohibitions against giving information about contraceptive materials, but courts usually allow considerable freedom. Because there are still some state limitations and because, as noted earlier, the federal government is becoming more involved, it is important to keep up to date in this area.

There are a number of other reproduction-related rights that are also important, such as sterilization, artificial insemination of various kinds, and surrogate parenthood. *Sterilization* means termination of the ability to produce offspring. Both laws and regulations have been in the process of change. Most refer to women. There seems to be little legal concern about male sterilization, *vasectomy,* which is being done with increasing frequency. The legal consequences of unsuccessful sterilization, both male and female, have resulted in suits. Called *wrongful birth,* these suits usually seek to recover the costs of raising an unplanned or unwanted child, normal or abnormal—but usually the latter. Judgments have varied but are more likely to favor the plaintiff if the child is abnormal.

Artificial insemination, the injection of seminal fluid by instrument into a female to induce pregnancy, is evolving into an acceptable medical procedure used by childless couples, although there has been some abuse reported. (Consent by the husband and wife is generally required.) When a woman, for a fee, is artificially inseminated with a man's sperm and bears a child, who is then turned over to the man and his wife, this is termed *surrogate motherhood.* It has already created some legal problems when the woman decided not to give up the child and again when neither wanted a baby born with a birth defect.

Among the most controversial legal concerns related to reproduction are *in vitro fertilization* and *surrogate embryo transfer,* each of which is intended to enhance the fertility of infertile couples. The questions are endless here: Will the government put restrictions on such techniques as embryo freezing? (There has already been a case in which frozen embryos were awarded to a woman in a divorce settlement, somewhat like a child!) What about collecting sperm from a brain-dead patient? What of the trend to (very) multiple births?

A relatively new legal aspect of human reproduction concerns the field of *genetics,* with which nurses, physicians, and lay genetic counselors must be concerned. Some of the issues have to do with human genetic disease, genetic screening, *in vitro* fertilization, and genetic databanks. In addition, legislation, such as the National Sickle Cell Anemia, Cooley's Anemia, Tay–Sachs, and Genetic Diseases Act, has encouraged or forced states to expand genetic screening to cover other disorders. Neonatal screening, for instance, will probably be expanded considerably and offers new opportunities and responsibilities for nurses. However, with what is still a relatively new science, many legal questions will arise. Confidentiality is of major importance. If a genetic disease is discovered, the counselor should not contact other relatives, even if it would benefit those relatives, without the screenee's consent. One emerging problem is *wrongful life*, which occurs when a deformed baby is born, although abortion was an option, because the physician or other counselor neglected to tell parents of the risk.

TRANSPLANTS

Since Dr. Christiaan Barnard performed the first human heart transplant in 1967, the question of tissue and organ transplants has become a point of controversy. Tissue may be obtained from living persons or a dead body. In recent years, improvement in immunosuppressive therapy has lessened the need for close tissue matches in most cases, thus permitting most transplants to shift from living donors to cadaver donors. As that shift occurred, the need to clarify "brain death" became more apparent. Thus, the rising need for cadaver organs accelerated the process of legal acknowledgment discussed previously, the development of medical standards for determination of death by neurological criteria, and the growth of a nationwide network of tissue- and organ-sharing agencies.

Although newly bereaved families from hospitals everywhere donate cadaver organs, the largest numbers come from regional trauma centers. Not only do such centers tend to concentrate those patients who are prime candidates for donation, but also it is in such centers where the staffs develop the familiarity with and expertise in recognizing potential donors and asking the next of kin for permission to harvest organs. Such hospitals are also apt to approach the determination of death by neurological criteria with relatively greater efficiency and more nearly according to established standards.

Many potential opportunities for harvesting organs are missed because physicians and nurses are reluctant to broach the subject of organ donation or even to acknowledge in a timely and forthright fashion that their patient is or may soon be "brain dead." A reluctance to be "the bearer of bad news" or a belief that grieving family members are best served by indirect communication and "maintenance of hope" is almost surely the major factor in avoidance of timely determination of death and hence of requests for donation.

Timing is everything. This often repeated statement is especially applicable here. Highly vascularized organs are lost if the blood supply is interrupted for any significant period. Meanwhile, the ethically correct and psychosocially sensitive behavior is not to ask for organ donation until after the next of kin has been told that death has apparently occurred. ("Apparently" because of the standards requiring repeat examinations and/or confirmatory tests.) Nurses and physicians with the most extensive experience in securing family consent for organ donation insist that the ethically correct and psychosocially sensitive timing is also the timing that ensures the highest yield of donation from newly bereaved family members.

Common law once prevented the decedent from donating his own body or individual organs if the next of kin objected, and statutes prohibited mutilation of bodies. However, all 50 states have adopted, in one form or another, the Uniform Anatomical Gift Act (UAGA), approved in 1968 by the National Conference of Commissioners on Uniform State Laws. The basic purposes are to permit an individual to control the disposition of his or her own body after death, to encourage such donations, to eliminate unnecessary and complicated formalities regarding the donation of human tissues and organs, to provide the necessary safeguards to protect the varied interests involved, and to define clearly the rights of the next of kin, the physician, the health care institution, and the public (as represented by the medical examiner) in relation to the dead body. As a practical matter, however, organs are ordinarily not harvested without the explicit permission of the next of kin, regardless of the decedent's prior wishes. Of course, such permission is very likely if the newly dead family member had previously expressed a desire to donate. The UAGA does grant immunity to hospitals that harvest organs after making a "good faith" effort to locate family for permission.

Since 1987, hospitals have been required to ask the next of kin of all potential donors whether or not they wished to donate. Generally, the priority order of decision making is:

- Spouse
- Adult son or daughter
- Either parent
- Adult brother or sister
- Grandparent
- Guardian of the person at the time of death
- Any other person authorized or under obligation to dispose of the body

This "required request" law has resulted in widespread changes in hospital policies and stimulated some staff education. Most importantly, it resulted in designation of a person or set of persons who could be called when a prospective donor is identified. Such designated requesters are often both more knowledgeable about donation and more psychologically skilled than the primary physicians and nurses.

Whoever makes the request needs to take the time to give accurate information to the family, and to develop trust. Maximizing access to the patient enables them to see that their loved one is unresponsive. Frequent visits also assist the grief process. It is important to:

- Allow time for sequenced grieving.
- Provide opportunities for questions.
- Avoid use of medical jargon.
- Introduce the idea of donation and allow time for family discussion.
- Tell them that organ donation and transplant is generally approved by the major Judeo-Christian traditions.
- Explain that they may donate as many or as few organs as they wish.
- Clarify terms (if any) such as "organ" and "tissue" and their use.
- Let them know that all tissues and organs are recovered in the operating room (except corneas), and that the donor is reconstructed in such a way that traditional funeral preparations, including viewing, can be carried out.
- Have the appropriate organ donor card ready, if the family agrees.
- Give the family time to discuss the matter if members agree, then return and see if you need to clarify questions.
- Support their decision, if the family opposes the donation.

Clearly this entire process requires knowledge and finesse. However, in seeking donations, the nurse also serves on behalf of the unknown patients who receive the organs. Only a short overview is presented here, and it is well worth the effort to learn all that you can about organ transplantation.

For more than a quarter of a century, various attempts to get people to donate organs have been generally disappointing. The need for organs continues to far exceed the supply. Even now, consent rates for organ donations are not more than 50 percent, and even lower for tissues and corneas. Ten people die each day waiting for a transplant. Yet it is said that one tissue donor can provide transplantable tissue for 55 people.[51] The problem for those who seek quick solutions to the persistent shortage of organs is that the discomfort of professionals and the public is not readily addressed by legislative initiatives and institutional rule-making.

RIGHTS AND RESPONSIBILITIES OF STUDENTS

When you began your nursing program, you also in effect, if not in writing, entered into a contract with the school that does not expire until you graduate (or leave). It is understood that both students and the school will assume certain responsibilities, many of which have legal implications. The first legal commitment the school has is to fulfill the minimum requirements for curriculum, faculty, and other resources set by the state board of nursing. Although you are responsible for your own acts in a clinical setting, you are expected to be under the supervision of a qualified teacher. Having your own professional liability insurance is important.

Perhaps you want to work as an aide to earn extra money. You will have to be especially careful because you can legally function only in those capacities not restricted to licensed nursing personnel. State laws governing the practice of nursing vary widely and are subject to misinterpretation by the employing agency. Most laws classify students working part time as employees. In this capacity, if you perform tasks requiring more judgment and skill than the position for which you are employed, you are subject not only to civil suits but also to criminal charges for practicing without a license.

Undesirable student conduct may result in some discipline, including suspension or expulsion, and there has been considerable disagreement on the school's power in such circumstances. Generally, it is expected that the school's rules of conduct are made public and that the student has the right to a public hearing and due process. Legal rulings may be different when applied to private or public universities. Private universities have greater power in many ways.

Constitutional rights are most frequently cited by students in complaints: the First Amendment (freedom of speech, religion, association, expression); the Fourth Amendment (freedom from illegal search and seizure); and the Fifth and Fourteenth Amendments (due process of law). The courts recognize the student first as a citizen, so that they will consider possible infringements of these rights. Most commonly, First Amendment rights involve dress codes and personal appearance. Although schools do not possess absolute authority over students in this sense, some lower court rulings have approved the establishment of dress codes necessary for cleanliness, safety, and health.

One case concerning a student's appearance found its way to the U.S. Supreme Court in *Russell v. Salve Regina*. Sharon Russell was dismissed from her nursing program at Salve Regina College because she failed to lose weight, as she had agreed to do. Although her grades were good, her weight rose to 303 pounds and she was withdrawn from her senior year. She completed her degree elsewhere but sued for damages, partly because the faculty humiliated her about her obesity. She charged intentional infliction of emotional distress, handicap discrimination, invasion of privacy, and breach of contract. All charges were dismissed except the last. Throughout the various appeals, her award of damages was upheld. The Supreme Court heard the case on narrow procedural grounds, and the case was sent back to the First Circuit Court, and her award of damages was upheld. The question of whether obesity is legally a handicap, thus awarding a protected status, whether the way she was treated was "atrocious" in a legal sense, and whether she or the college violated a contract were points of dissension. The court did comment negatively on how the faculty treated her in relation to her obesity.[52]

Due process has been a major issue of legal contention. The rule or law must be examined for fairness and reasonableness. Are the student and faculty understanding of the rule the same? Did the student have the opportunity to know about the rule and its implications? What is the relationship between the rule and the objectives of the school? The National Student Nurses' Association (NSNA) developed grievance procedure guidelines as part of a bill of rights for students. Besides suggesting the makeup of the committee (equal representation of students and faculty) and general procedures, such points as allowing sufficient time, access to information and appropriate records, presentation of evidence, and use of witnesses were included. The usual steps in any grievance process are also followed for academic grievances: an informal process first, consisting of a written complaint and a suggested remedy by the student grievant, a written reply, a hearing with presentation of evidence on both sides, a decision by the committee within a specific time, right of appeal, and sometimes arbitration. With students, the right to continue with class work throughout the whole process is considered necessary, although in nursing, if the situation relates to a clinical problem and the safety of patients is considered a risk, further clinical experience may be put on hold until the matter is settled. At any rate a complete record of the hearing should be made.

There seem to be an increasing number of grievances filed or legal complaints made because of academic concerns, especially grades. The courts have been reluctant to enter this area of academic freedom. There has yet to be a definitive ruling on curriculum and degree requirements. Most colleges now have grievance procedures for students who think that they have received unfair grades, and these procedures must be followed first before any lawsuit can be filed. In one case a nursing student was dismissed in her second year of a community college program for "unsafe clinical behavior." After a grievance procedure, in which her dismissal was upheld, she sued, alleging bad faith on the part of the faculty. The court refused to overturn the decision. A similar case in a diploma school resulted in the same decision by another court. In still another case, a nurse who refused to take a predoctoral exam she had failed twice was terminated as a student of the university and not permitted to enter the doctoral program. She sued.

The court could find no showing of bad motive or ill will on the part of the faculty.[53]

Before the student wages an all-out battle, the situation should be considered practically. It must be proved that the grade is arbitrary, capricious, and manifestly unjust, which is generally very difficult (especially when problems have been documented). Furthermore, unless that particular grade is extremely important to a student's career, the cost and time involved are greater than even a favorable result might warrant.

Cases in which the results have been more favorable to the student are related to inadequate program advisement, and the school catalog as a written contract. A school has to deal with the nursing student according to the statements in the catalog the year she or he entered, not the later, more restrictive requirements.

Because those schools receiving federal money directly are subject to federal laws, the Americans with Disabilities Act of 1990, the Civil Rights Restoration Act of 1987, and Section 504 of the Rehabilitation Act of 1973 have created rights for students with disabilities. In one case, a prospective student with a severe hearing problem sued because she was not admitted to a community college nursing program. The court upheld the school's decision because the applicant's hearing disability made it unsafe for her to practice as a nurse. At another school, an applicant with Crohn's disease was refused because her disease process would probably cause her to miss too many classes. Although the court required the school to admit the student, the decision was later overturned on a procedural issue. In other disciplines, students have been dismissed because of contracting tuberculosis, AIDS, and other diseases; this may yet occur in nursing.[54]

Another type of student right involves school records. The types of student records kept by schools vary. They may consist of only the academic transcript, or may include extracurricular activities and problem situations, which are kept in an informal file. The enactment of the Buckley Amendment has clarified the issue of student access to records. The individual loses the right to confidentiality by waiving the right or by disclosing the information to a third person. A student's academic transcript is the most common document released, particularly to other schools and employers.

As more student activists, who are now voting citizens, request or demand certain rights as part of the academic community, more legal decisions are made, and school rules that were once ironclad have become flexible. The concept of rights need not be seen as an adversarial proceeding. Both the student and the school have a new accountability. In the long run, it might be more meaningful to look at certain student rights as freedoms and responsibilities.[55]

KEY POINTS

1. Patients are beginning to assert themselves in demanding their legal rights, and generally courts are supporting them.
2. In order to have a legal informed consent, the patient must be competent and not coerced; the process must include an explanation of the condition, the proposed treatment, alternatives, and dangers or benefits.
3. Nurses are not legally responsible for getting consents, but they should try to be sure that the patient knows what he or she consented to.
4. Court decisions, statutory and administrative law, and organizational actions seem to be favoring the patient's right to die.
5. The living will is designed to allow individuals to express to their families, health care personnel, and institutions in advance their desires about their care if they are later not able to do so.
6. Legal issues related to abortion, sterilization, family planning, and artificial insemination are becoming more complex as technology offers new options and as advocates for or against certain points of view become more aggressive.
7. The law is changing rapidly in relation to the rights of children and the mentally ill.
8. Even though an action is intended for the patients' own good, forcing them to do something can be considered assault or battery.
9. The grievance procedure is necessary in settling disputes in the educational setting.

STUDY QUESTIONS

1. How would you help a patient who is dying, and wants to convey his wishes for end-of-life care to his family?
2. What are the health care rights of an adolescent who is a Jehovah's Witness?
3. Describe the nurses' responsibility in executing an informed consent document.
4. What is the relationship between the Patient's Bill of Rights legislation and the AHA Patient's Bill of Rights.
5. The mentally ill have the right to live in the least restrictive environment possible. How do you interpret that statement, and what are some of the inherent social problems?

REFERENCES

1. President's Commission for the Study of Ethical Problems in Medicine and Biomedical and Behavioral Research. *Making Health Care Decisions.* Washington, DC: U.S. Government Printing Office, 1982.
2. Annas G. *The Rights of Patients: The Basic ACLU Guide to Patient Rights,* 2d ed. Carbondale, IL: Southern Illinois University Press, 1992, p 1.
3. President's Commission, op cit, p 1.
4. University of Washington School of Medicine. Ethics in Medicine: http:// eduserv.hscer.washington.edu/bioethics/topics/consent.htm.   Retrieved April 1, 2005.
5. Douglas H. A patient's right to truly informed consent. *Arch Surg* 135:875–876, July 2000.
6. Elger B, Harding T. Terminally ill patients and Jehovah's Witnesses: teaching acceptance of patients' refusals of vital treatments. *Med Educ* 36(5):479–488, May 2002.
7. Wolley S. Children of Jehovah's Witnesses and adolescent Jehovah's Witnesses: What are their rights? *Arch Dis Child* 90(7):715–719, July 2005.
8. University of Washington, op cit.
9. Marquis B, Huston C. *Leadership Roles and Management Functions in Nursing,* 5th ed. Philadelphia: Lippincott Williams & Wilkins, 2006.
10. Betts VT. Legal aspects of nursing. In Chitty KK (Ed.): *Professional Nursing,* 3d ed. Philadelphia: Saunders, 2001.
11. Black P. Brain death. *New Engl J Med* 229:398, August 24, 1978.
12. Annas G. Prisoner in the ICU: The tragedy of William Bartling. *Hastings Center Rep* 14:28–29, December 1984.
13. Annas G. Transferring the ethical hot potato. *Hastings Center Rep* 17:20–21, February 1987.
14. Annas G. When procedures limit rights: From Quinlan to Conroy. *Hastings Center Rep* 15:24–26, April 1985.
15. Annas G. Do feeding tubes have more rights than patients? *Hastings Center Rep* 16:26–27, February 1986.
16. American Medical Association Council on Ethical and Judicial Affairs. Opinion: withdrawing or withholding life prolonging treatment, March 15, 1986.
17. American Nurses Association. Position statement on forgoing artificial nutrition and hydration, April 2, 1992.
18. Aroskar M. The aftermath of the Cruzan decision: Dying in a twilight zone. *Nurs Outlook* 38:256–257, November–December 1990.
19. Annas G. Nancy Cruzan and the right to die. *New Engl J Med* 323:670–672, September 6, 1990.
20. Parks JA. Why gender matters to the euthanasia debate. On decisional capacity and the rejection of women's death requests. *Hastings Center Rep* 30:30–36, January–February 2000.

21. Cahill H. An Orwellian scenario: Court ordered caesarian section and women's autonomy. *Nurs Ethics* 6:494–505, November 1999.

22. Darr K. Implementing advance directives: a continuing problem for provider organizations. *Hosp Top* 77:29–32, Summer 1999.

23. Jezewski M, Brown J, Wu Y, Meeker M, Feng J, Bu X. Oncology nurses' knowledge, attitudes, and experiences regarding advance directives. *Oncol Nurs Forum* 5(2):319–327, March 2005.

24. Meisel A, Snyder L, Quill T. Seven legal barriers to end-of-life care: Myths, realities, and grains of truth. *JAMA* 284(19):2495–2501, November 15, 2000.

25. "Code" called contrary to patient's advance directives. *Nurs Law Regan Rep* 45(8):1, January 2005.

26. American Nurses Association. *Position Statement on Nursing and the Patient Self-Determination Act.* Washington, DC: The Association, November 18, 1991.

27. Hawkins NA, Ditto PH, Danks JH, Smucker WD. Micromanaging death: Process preferences, values, and goals in end-of-life medical decision making. *Gerontology* 45(1):107–117, February 2005.

28. Annas G. "Culture of life" politics at the bedside: The case of Terri Schiavo. *N Engl J Med* 352(16):1710–1715, April 21, 2005. http://content.nejm.org/cgi/content/abstract/NEJMlim050643v4. Retrieved April 25, 2005.

29. Saad L. The Schiavo Case: http://gallup.com/poll/content/login.aspx?ci=15541. Retrieved April 9, 2005.

30. Third parties—can they take away your rights? *Choices* 4:1, 4–6, Spring 1995.

31. Ibid.

32. American Bar Association. Who Gets to Decide? http://www.abanet.org/adminlaw/midyear2005/tab9.pdf. Retrieved April 7, 2005.

33. Matthews E. Autonomy and the psychiatric patient. *J Appl Philos* 17(1):59–70, 2000.

34. Curran W, Shapiro D. *Health Care Law: Forensic Science and Public Policy*, 3d ed. Boston: Little, Brown, 1991, pp 770–777.

35. Linnard-Palmer L, Kools S. Parents' refusal of medical treatment based on religious and/or cultural beliefs: the law, ethical principles, and clinical implications. *J Pediatr Nurs* 19(5):351–356, October 2004.

36. Cushing M. Do not feed. *Am J Nurs* 83:602–604, April 1983.

37. Taub S. Withholding treatment from defective newborns. *Law Med Health Care* 10:4–10, February 1982.

38. Rhodes A. Guardianship and the refusal of treatment. *Mat Child Nurs* 20:109, April 1995.

39. Minors and the right to die. *Choices* 3:1, 4–5, Winter 1994.

40. Capron A. Baby Ryan and virtual futility. *Hastings Center Rep* 25:20–21, March–April 1995.

41. Vukadinovich D. Minors' rights to consent to treatment: Navigating the complexity of State laws. *J Health Law* 37(4):667–691, Fall 2004.

42. Hornor, G. Physical abuse: Recognition and reporting. *J Pediatr Health Care* 9(1):4–11, January–February, 2005.

43. Alaggia R. Many ways of telling: expanding conceptualizations of child sexual abuse disclosure. *Child Abuse Negl* 28(11):1213–1227, November 2004.

44. Rice, B. The new rules on informed consent. *Med Econ* 77:150–152, 156–157, 161–162, June 2000.

45. Olsen DP, Mahrenholz D. IRB-identified ethical issues in nursing research. *J Prof Nurs* 16:140–148, May–June 2000.
46. Haggerty LA, Hawkins J. Informed consent and the limits of confidentiality. *West J Nurs Res* 22:508–514, June 2000.
47. University of Pennsylvania. The Duty to Warn Versus Confidentiality. January 17, 2002: http://bioethics.net. Retrieved April 9, 2005.
48. Deshefy-Longhi T, Dixon JK, Olsen D, Grey M. Privacy and confidentiality issues in primary care: Views of advanced practice nurses and their patients— an APRNet study. *Nurs Ethics* 12(1):2, June 2005.
49. Greenhouse L. Justices uphold patient privacy with therapist. *The New York Times,* June 14, 1996, pp A1, A25.
50. Biskupic J. The next president could tip the high court. *USA Today*, October 12, 2004: http://www.usatoday.com/news/politicselections/nation/president/2004–09–29-election-court-cover_x.htm. Retrieved April 10, 2005.
51. Childress J. The failure to give: Reducing barriers to organ donation. *Kennedy Inst Ethics J* 11(1):1–16, March 2001.
52. Brent N. *Nurses and the Law: A Guide to Principles and Applications*, 2d ed. Philadelphia: Saunders, 2001.
53. Ibid.
54. Keeling R. Health science students with blood-borne pathogen diseases. *J Am Coll Health* 50(3):101–104, November 2001.
55. Espeland K, Shanta L. Empowering versus enabling in academia. *J Nurs Educ* 40(8):342–346, November 2001.

Updates can be found at

 http://www.JoelTheNursingExperience.com

Chapter 10

Politics and Public Policy

OBJECTIVES

After studying this chapter, you will be able to:

1. *Define statutory law, administrative law, case law, criminal law, and civil law.*
2. *Explain how case law derives its authority.*
3. *Explain how a bill becomes a law.*
4. *List ways in which you can get information about legislation.*
5. *Describe how nurses and others can influence the legislative process.*
6. *Name and explain briefly four federal laws that have a major effect on nurses.*

Every nurse today needs to know something about law and the legislative process because there is so much in health care and nursing that is affected by law. Some federal laws influence how health care is given and how it is reimbursed. On a more personal level, other laws have to do with the rights and privileges of individuals, whether they are providers or consumers. State laws regulate our practice. Laws are implemented through the administrative process of rule making. These rules and regulations carry the weight of law and further amplify and clarify provisions of the law. Court decisions also outline certain rights, and they set precedent in cases of negligence or malpractice. Few nurses set out to break or violate anyone's rights, but there are so many complex situations in health care today that there is a tendency to feel helpless about knowing what is *legal*. Yes, you may be able to consult with your employing institution's attorney, but that isn't very practical on a day-to-day basis. Worse yet, everyone dealing with the law knows that there is no final or absolute answer—something that is quite frustrating for those who want to know exactly what they can or cannot do. Yet, there are certain principles that may serve as guidelines to avoid problems and as a basis of understanding American law and influencing it. For more details, read any nursing law book, or Chapters 17, 18, and 19 in *Kelly's Dimensions of Professional Nursing*, 9th ed. New York: McGraw-Hill, 2003.

INTRODUCTION TO LAW

As the American colonies were founded one by one, the way in which they would be governed was a primary consideration. Gradually, a system similar to that of the common law then in effect in England was adopted. However, the problems within the colonies varied so widely that each eventually developed its own procedures and laws, both common and statutory, based on its own needs.

From this evolved the concept of *states' rights*, which has played an important role in the history of the United States. The states delegate to the federal government whatever powers are specified in the U.S. Constitution, other powers are retained by the states. Any infringement of these rights, either by the federal government or by other states, is usually strongly opposed. States do adopt many of the same or similar laws as others, such as requirements for professional licensure, seat belt use, and drinking age. However, a state can retain, revise, or repeal its own laws without interference from other states or the federal government. Variance in state laws often creates a great deal of confusion and misunderstanding.

Federal law is based on the U.S. Constitution, ratified in 1789. Since then, the volume and complexity of problems facing the Congress have increased tremendously, but the Constitution always guides the actions.

The Constitution has been amended 26 times. The first ten amendments, known as the Bill of Rights, were adopted within three years of the Constitution's ratification. These amendments guarantee certain freedoms, such as freedom of speech, press, religion, assembly, and due process. They are the basis of the civil rights we hear so much about. In recent years, the Bill of Rights has had relevance to health care issues. The Fourteenth Amendment's protection of personal liberty has been used in defense of a woman's right to choose to have an abortion, and the right to assemble has allowed nurses and others to rally as an expression of concern over labor issues. It is interesting to note that the Constitution does not specify access to health care as a guaranteed right. Nor do state constitutions.

THE UNITED STATES LEGAL SYSTEM

Under the U.S. system of government, the law is carried out at a number of levels. The Constitution is the highest law of the land. Whatever the Constitution (federal law) does not spell out, the states retain for themselves (Tenth Amendment). Because they can create political subdivisions, units of local government—counties, cities, towns, townships, boroughs, and villages—all have certain legal powers within their geographical boundaries. On all levels, but most obviously on the federal and state levels, there is a separation of power: legislative, executive, and judicial. The first makes the laws, the second carries them out, and the third reviews them, a system that the founders of the United States believed would create a balance of power.

There are three basic sources of law: statutory law, administrative or regulatory law, and judicial or case law.

Statutory law refers to enactments of legislative bodies declaring, commanding, or prohibiting something. Statutes are always written, are firmly established, and can be altered only by amendment or repeal. The Nurse Education Act is one example of federal statutory law. The Social Security Act, which includes Medicare as Title XVIII and Medicaid as Title XIX, is another. Statutory laws also exist at the state level. Licensing laws for professional nurses, requiring them to be licensed before they can legally practice nursing, are examples of a state statute.

Executive, administrative, or *regulatory law* refers to the rules, regulations, and decisions of administrative bodies. In a sense, they spell out the specifics of a statutory law. For example, the DHSS Division of Nursing develops the regulations that determine the requirements for the various programs in the Nurse Education Act; the State Board of Nursing spells out the requirements for nursing programs; a city health code may adopt a patients' bill of rights as a requirement for all hospitals in the city. All have the effect of law but are more easily changed than statutory law.

Judicial law, also called *decisional, case,* or *common law,* is a body of legal principles and rules of action that derive their authority from usage and custom or from judgments and decrees of courts. Courts are agencies established by the government to decide disputes. *Superior, supreme, common pleas, district,* and *circuit courts* are various types of courts. The kind of court in which a case is brought depends on the offense or complaint.

Federal courts established in all states generally hear cases related to the Constitution. With the introduction of written decisions, one of the most important principles known in the law was born, the principle of *stare decisis*, which means to stand as decided, or "let the decision stand." Thus, if a case with similar facts has been decided finally in that particular jurisdiction, the court will probably make the same decision on a like case, citing the *precedent* of the previous case. If the precedent is out of date or not applicable, a new rule will be made.

THE LEGISLATIVE PROCESS

It is not unusual for hundreds of health-related bills to be introduced during a legislative term. If nurses want to have some control over the laws that affect their practice, it is important that they learn how to influence the legislative process. The first step is to get the necessary information, as discussed in the next section.

THE LEGISLATIVE SETTING

Even with the best intentions, no legislators can be experts on all the issues that come up. For instance, in one two-year session in Congress, 25,000 or so bills were introduced. Not all are acted on, but even reading them all is almost impossible. Therefore, all national and most state legislators have staffs of varying size, depending on seniority and other factors. Some staffs are in the capital; others are in home offices in the legislator's district in order to keep in touch with and help constituents. Some perform administrative duties, and others act as legislative aides, assistants, and/or researchers. These are individuals who summarize background material on key bills and brief the legislator on specific issues and on constituents' feedback. The legislator generally uses this information to decide how to vote. The administrative assistants share the power of the legislators, if not the glory. Committee staff do the preparatory work for items that come before committees and subcommittees, drafting bills, writing amendments to bills, arranging and preparing for public hearings, consulting with people in the areas about which the committee is concerned, providing information, and frequently writing speeches for the chairperson.

Because these assistants get information from numerous sources, it is a good idea to become acquainted with them, maintain good relations, and provide accurate, pertinent information about the issues in which you are interested. Do not ignore them; they are very influential.

A measure of the prestige a legislator has is the nature of committee appointments, where most of the preliminary action on bills occurs. Appointments are influenced or made by party leaders in the House of Representatives or the Senate (Assembly and Senate at the state level). Chairmanships of committees, extremely powerful positions, are awarded to members of the majority party, usually senior members of the House or Senate. Some committee assignments are more prestigious than others and are eagerly sought. Although there are cases in which the chairpersons of some of these committees, particularly on the national level, have remained for years, the makeup of a committee may change with each new session. It is important to know on which committee your legislators sit, because the action of committees affects the future of a bill. The same process and relationships exist, for the most part, on the state level.

HOW A BILL BECOMES A LAW

A lot of compromise goes into the legislative process, and often there is behind-the-scenes negotiating that is never seen in the open committee hearings or on the floor of the House or Senate. Nevertheless there is a formal process by which a bill becomes a law. This is presented in Exhibit 10.1. Here, the bill starts in the House, but it could just as well be in the Senate. Note particularly the steps at which you can influence the process by the various lobbying techniques described later. Some important details follow.

1. Anyone can initiate a bill. Common sources include the President and his administration; a group or organization, such as ANA; and private citizens who can convince a legislator about a need. The bill is put in the appropriate format by legal specialists.
2. One or more lawmakers sponsor the bill, with the major sponsor (the author) introducing the bill and guiding it through the legislative process. The more powerful that sponsor, the better. Bipartisan sponsorship is also desirable, because then it does not become a party issue.
3. The bill is introduced (commonly referred to as "put in the hopper") and given a number. Numbers are consecutive within each two-year session and begin with "HR" in the House or "S" in the Senate. If the bill does not become law, it can be reintroduced the following session and is given a new bill number.
4. After the bill is introduced and printed in the *Congressional Record* (*first reading*), it is assigned to one or more committees that have

responsibility for that subject. You can obtain a copy of a federal bill from your senator or representative, or from the *Congressional Record* at http://www.gpoaccess.gov/crecord/index.html. The Congressional Record includes a section-by-section analysis of the bill that is usually easier to understand than the bill itself. The text summaries and legislative status of federal bills can also be obtained at http://Thomas.Loc.gov.

5. Legislators spend a lot of time in committees. The committee chairperson is very powerful and can influence the fate of the bill by introducing it for discussion very quickly or by keeping it off the agenda for the entire session. Committees also conduct hearings, which are usually open to the public. Often nurses testify on health care issues by representing professional nursing organizations or appearing as individual witnesses. When a committee decides on a bill, it is either killed, passed as introduced, passed with amendments or as a new bill. The process of deliberating and voting on a bill is called *mark-up*.

6. If the bill is passed, the Director of the Congressional Budget Office submits an estimate of the cost of the measure, and this is included in the Committee Report.

7. The bill then goes to the full House for action on the floor (*second reading*). Visitors can watch from the gallery but may not speak during floor deliberations. If you want to know when a particular bill will be brought to the floor, it is best to contact the leadership of the appropriate house, or the sponsor of the bill. A bill is usually brought to the chamber of one house independent of events in the other.

8. At the end of floor action, the *third reading* is called for and the vote taken. Amendments added in committee or on the floor are a big factor in determining the fate of the bill. Adding amendments to a bill that seems sure to pass is a technique for putting through some action that might not succeed on its own and that may be only remotely or not at all connected to the content of the original bill. On the other hand, amendments that are totally unacceptable to the bill's sponsors may be added as a mechanism to force withdrawal or defeat of the bill. In general, amendments are introduced to strengthen, broaden, or curtail the intent of the original bill or law. If passed, they may change its character considerably. When debate is closed, the vote is taken by roll call and recorded. Passage usually requires a majority vote of the total House.

9. If the bill is passed, it goes to the Senate for a complete repetition of the process it went through in the House, and with the same opportunities to influence its passage. A bill introduced in the

Exhibit 10.1 The Legislative Process: How a Bill Becomes Law at the Federal Level

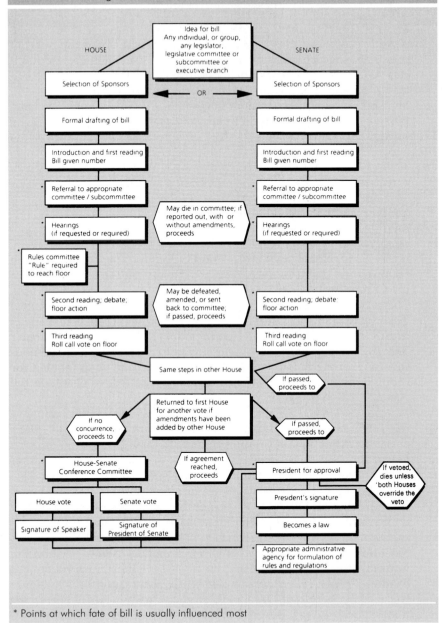

* Points at which fate of bill is usually influenced most

Senate follows the same general route, with certain procedural differences. Also, the President of the Senate is the Vice-President of the United States. Filibustering is a unique senatorial process whereby senators opposed to a motion to consider a bill may speak to it for extensive periods, thus preventing or defeating action by long delays.

10. At times, the same or a similar bill is introduced in both houses on certain important issues. If these bills are not the same when passed by each house, or if another single bill has been amended by the second house after passing the first and the first does not agree on the amendments, the bill is sent to a conference committee consisting of an equal number of members of each house. The conference committee tries to work out a compromise that will be accepted by both houses. Usually an agreement is reached.

11. After passing both houses and being signed by each presider, the bill goes to the President, who may obtain opinions from various sources. If he signs it or fails to take action within 10 days, the bill becomes law. He may also veto the bill and return it to the house of origin with his objections. A two-thirds affirmative vote in both houses for repassage is necessary to override the veto. Because voting on a veto is often along party lines, overriding a veto in both houses is difficult. However, the National Center for Nursing Research was established in 1985 through a veto override, demonstrating the political strength of nurses and others who lobbied for the bill. If the Congress adjourns before the 10 days in which the President should sign the bill, it does not become law. This is known as a *pocket veto*.

12. Another type of legislation is a resolution. Joint resolutions originating in either house are, for all practical purposes, treated as a bill but have the whereas-resolved format. They are identified as *HJ Res.* or *SJ Res.*

13. All bills that become law are assigned numbers, beginning with "PL" (Public Law, different from their original number), and then are printed and attached to the proper volume of statutes.

14. The last step is sending the new law to the appropriate administrative agency for rules to implement the law. This is another juncture at which nurses can have input. Proposed and final rules are published in the *Federal Register*, which is available at http://www.gpoaccess.gov/fr/index.html.

15. It is important to keep in mind that the federal government's fiscal year is designated by the calendar year in which it ends. Thus, the period from October 1, 2005, to September 30, 2006, is fiscal year 2006 (FY06).

INFLUENCING THE LEGISLATIVE PROCESS

There are many factors to be considered before a legislative body or even individual legislators make a final decision on how to vote on a piece of legislation. Some are probably personal—how the legislator feels about an issue. Some are internally political—support of the party leadership or a favor owed to a colleague; but likely to be the most influential is the voice of the legislator's constituency, "the folks back home." Most legislators want to be reelected to the same or a higher office. If their constituents are not pleased with them, their voting record, or their attitude, they are replaced.

Just who are these powerful constituents? Actually, they range from the ordinary householder to the powerful conglomerate, and include individuals as well as interest groups. An *interest group* is an association of people who come together to promote or protect a common cause through the political process. They represent the issues of their members and use the power of the group to influence public decisions that affect them. In recent years, nurses have become increasingly influential with their legislators. Professional organizations at all three levels of

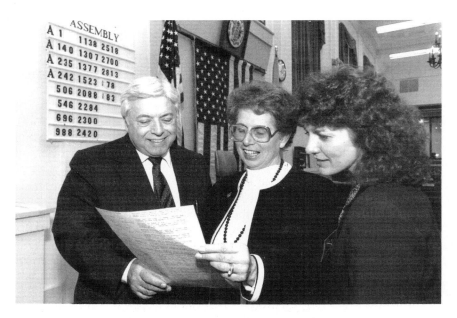

Nurses have a natural talent as legislators. Here Assemblywoman Barbara Wright (R—NJ) discusses a bill with colleagues. (*Courtesy of the New Jersey State Nurses Association*)

government, as well as individual nurses, have knowledge of the health care system and patients' needs that make them valuable resources to legislators.

One method used to influence legislation is to support a candidate, either for election or for reelection. For many decades, making political contributions has been illegal for certain groups such as ANA, and more recently, tighter constraints have been placed on contributions and spending. Because the law requires that, for some groups, campaign contributions be kept as a separate fund and that no organizational money may be used for this purpose, many groups have created separate organizations for political activity. These are known as *political action committees* (PACs). They may be located in the same office as an organization, such as ANA–PAC in ANA's Washington office, but by law their funds and activities are carefully separated from the rest of the organization's work.

Many state nurses' associations have formed state PACs based on the ANA model. They have endorsed candidates, contributed to campaigns, and encouraged fellow nurses to run for office. It is important to remember that the success of any nurse PAC depends on the input and support of individual nurses. You can always start by volunteering a small amount of time, and, in so doing, have a voice in advancing the political strength of nursing. State professional nursing organizations are a good source of information on PACs and political groups at the state level. (ANA–PAC is described in Chapter 13.)

In recent years, many political participants have criticized PACs, claiming that they make it easy for certain groups to "buy" legislators and their votes. Although it is hard to prove the exact relationship between campaign contributions and voting patterns, there is no doubt that substantial contributions help with access to public officials and create an atmosphere of familiarity. The first priority of any legislator is to get elected, and campaigning is becoming extraordinarily expensive. Recently, tighter constraints have been placed on contributions and spending. While limits are set by law on the amounts that can be given to candidates, there are ways of manipulating the system. For instance, AMA, often identified as one of the largest contributors in congressional races, has in some years contributed as much as $3 million to various campaigns.

ANA–PAC can boast of a "war chest" in excess of $1 million for every election cycle (2-year periods) since 1994. ANA–PAC is the fourth largest health care PAC in Washington, only outsized by AMA ($8 million), ADA ($6 million), and AHA ($1.5 million). It further has had the distinction of being named as the fastest-growing health care PAC in the nation. The support of nurses is an even greater asset than dollars, since where nurses believe in the candidate, they usually provide a functional grassroots network with a rich spirit of volunteerism. In 2004, ANA–PAC boasted an election success rate of 82 percent with their endorsed candidates.[1] Currently, ANA–PAC is reconsidering its strategy. Will nursing achieve more legislative support if fewer candidates are endorsed, and more funds and volunteerism are provided for a select few?

Another important, if sometimes unofficial, component of lawmaking is lobbying. *Lobbying* is generally defined as an attempt to influence a decision of a legislator or other governmental body. Since it is a type of petition for redress of grievances, lobbying is constitutionally guaranteed. Lobbying exists at several levels, from a single individual who contacts a legislator about a particular issue of personal importance, to the interest groups that carefully (and often expensively) organize systems for

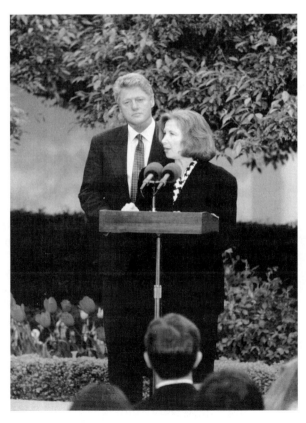

The President of ANA introduces President Bill Clinton at a Nurses' Day Reception in the Rose Garden of the White House. (*Courtesy of the American Nurses Association*)

monitoring legislation, initiating action, or blocking action on matters that concern them.

Professional lobbyists must be registered with Congress (or the Legislature in the state), and there are regulations concerning the types of organizations that may employ lobbyists. Lobbyists spend all or part of their time representing the interests of a particular group or groups. They provide information to legislators and their staffs (not necessarily objectively) and introduce resource people to them. Lobbyists are knowledgeable in the ways of legislation and are often familiar with legislators' personalities and idiosyncrasies. They keep their interest group informed about any pertinent legislation and the problems involved, and help them to take effective action.

This organized approach to lobbying, effective though it is, should not overshadow the efforts of the individual who, in effect, lobbies when contacting the appropriate legislator about an issue. Groups such as nurses have proved to be very effective in lobbying by coordinating the efforts of individuals for unified action.

NURSES AND POLITICAL ACTION

Organizations such as the ANA and various specialty groups have taken leadership roles in mobilizing nurses in grassroots lobbying. They have started educational programs and political consciousness-raising sessions, both to teach nurses techniques and strategies and to make them aware of the issues. Networks have been established which can be set in motion at a moment's notice on behalf of an issue, a candidate, or a piece of legislation. The network comprises volunteer activists with an interest in politics, experts on particular topics, or they may be drawn from a social, ethnic, or age group that is strategic.

The ANA's N-STAT program is described in Chapter 13. It is a network of trained volunteers from a variety of state and specialty organizations. Once activated, both a Leadership Team and a Rapid Response (network) are triggered. The leadership are volunteers who have already established a relationship with specific legislators. The Rapid Response creates a high volume of calls, letters, and faxes which are also focused on specific elected officials. All the activity is aimed at the grassroots, and conveys a message about support for reelection.

N-STAT is highly acclaimed for its ability to penetrate every state and district in the country. Many state nurses' associations have created similar networks for state politics. Additional participants are always welcome. However, grassroots lobbying need not occur through an organization or special interest group, it can be your personal action plan to participate more fully in government through those who represent you.

GRASSROOTS LOBBYING

There are certain ways to lobby that give a better chance of success than if you approach it with goodwill but little organization. One of the first steps is making personal contact. It is sensible to become acquainted with your legislators before a legislative crisis occurs. This gives you the advantage of having made personal contact and shown general interest, and gives the legislator or staff member the advantage of a reference point. In small communities, legislators often know many of their constituents on a first-name basis through frequent contacts at town meetings or as other opportunities arise. This personal relationship may be more difficult to manage in large areas, but the effort to meet and talk with legislators is never wasted.

Having identified and located the legislator, call for an appointment or find out when the legislator is available in his local office (or in his capital office if this is convenient for both). Before the visit, it is helpful to know the following about the legislator:

1. Geography of the legislative district and district number.
2. Present or past leadership in civic, cultural, or other community affairs.
3. Voting record on major controversial issues recently under consideration.
4. Voting record in the past on major bills of interest to nurses.
5. Subject areas of special interest, such as health, consumer affairs, and so on.
6. Political party affiliation and committee assignments.
7. Previous occupation or profession, and whether there is still some involvement.
8. Bills of major importance which have been authored or co-authored.
9. Previous contacts with nursing organizations in the area.
10. Nursing organizations' endorsements or support to opponents in past elections.

This information may be available from your nursing organization, political action groups, or literature from the legislator's office.

No one can say how such a visit should be conducted—it is obviously a matter of personal style—but generally it is wise to be dressed appropriately, to be friendly, to keep the visit short, to identify yourself as a nurse, and, depending on your level of expertise, to offer to be a resource. Comment on any of the legislator's bills or votes of which you approve. If the first visit coincides with pending health legislation, ask whether a stand has been taken and perhaps add a few pertinent comments. Probably not more than three major issues should be discussed. A *brief* written account of the key points and/or documentation of facts can be left, along with an offer to provide additional information when needed. Legislators respond best if what is discussed is within the context of what their other constituents might want. In other words, is it good for the public and not just nursing?

It is important to be prompt for the visit, but be ready to accept the fact that the legislator may be late or not able to keep the appointment. Any administrative assistant who substitutes will probably be knowledgeable and attentive, and the time will not be wasted. If distance and time make visiting difficult, a telephone call or e-mail are good approaches. The same general guidelines can be followed, and here also, making contact with the legislator's administrative assistant often serves as good a purpose as speaking to the legislator directly.

Although personal visits and calls are considered useful in trying to influence a legislator, letter writing or e-mail communication is also effective, especially if an initial introductory visit has already been made. These are also the most frequent ways to communicate. Legislators are particularly sensitive to communications from constituents. They give far less attention to correspondence from outside their state or district and are often annoyed by it. You can find a legislator's contact information at http://www.senate.gov/general/contact_information or http://www.house.gov/house/MemberWWW.shtml. Similar sites exist for state legislators. Communication received at a local office is apt to get more attention, since there is usually a larger volume of messages at the capital. Accepted ways of addressing public officials are found in Exhibit 10.2. Then, follow these guidelines:

Do:
1. Identify yourself as a nurse and a constituent.
2. Briefly renew your acquaintance, if you have met before.
3. State the specific reason for the letter.
4. Be brief and to the point.
5. Use local examples (legislators like to use these anecdotes in their speeches).
6. Give reasons for your objections or support.
7. Be sure of correct spelling and grammar and a proper format.
8. Include the bill number and title or at least its popular name, for instance, the Nurse Education Bill.

Exhibit 10.2 How to Address Public Officials

Official	Address	Official	Address
President	The President of the United States The White House Washington, DC 20500 Dear Mr. President:	Assemblywoman	The Hon. Mary Doe The State House Trenton, NJ 08625 Dear Ms. Doe:
Governor	The Hon. John Doe Executive Chamber Albany, NY 12224 Dear Governor Doe:	Mayor	The Hon. John Doe City Hall New York, NY 10007 Dear Mayor Doe:
U.S. Senator	Senator John Doe Senate Office Building Washington, DC 20510 Dear Senator Doe:	City Councilman	The Hon. John Doe City Council New York, NY 10007 Dear Mr. Doe:
Congressman	The Hon. John Doe House Office Building Washington, DC 20515 Dear Mr. Doe or Dear Congressman:	Judge	The Hon. Mary Doe (Address of Court) Dear Judge Doe:
State Senator	The Hon. John Doe Senate Chambers Albany, NY 12224 Dear Senator:	Other officials	(Not included above) The Hon. John Doe Dear Mr. Doe

Don't:
1. Be trivial
2. Be insulting, sarcastic, or threatening.
3. Use a form letter.

If speed is important, as when a vote is pending, use the telephone, a fax, or e-mail.

If you support the legislator (or any candidate), then it is politically smart to contribute to their election campaign and/or volunteer your services in the campaign. These might include house-to-house canvassing to check voter registration or to survey public support; supplying transportation to the polls; making telephone calls to stimulate registration and voting; acting as registration clerk, poll clerk or watcher, block leader, or precinct captain; raising funds; preparing mailing pieces; planning publicity; writing and distributing news releases; making speeches; answering telephones; staffing information booths; planning campaign events; or having "coffees" to meet the candidate.

Nurses who are knowledgeable about a particular issue are sometimes asked by ANA or another group to testify before a congressional committee. This requires both know-how and assurance but it can be a very interesting and satisfying experience. However, it is important to be properly prepared and do it right. (For details on how to testify, see *Kelly's Dimensions of Professional Nursing*, 9th ed. New York: McGraw-Hill, 2003, pp 414–416.)

OVERVIEW OF FEDERAL AGENCIES

The federal agencies with responsibility for health care are primarily within the Department of Health and Human Services (DHHS), although certain health-related programs are administered by other departments. An example is the Food Stamps Program, which the Department of Agriculture administers. Within DHHS, there are several major agencies: the Public Health Service (PHS), the Centers for Medicare and Medicaid Services (CMS), and the Administration for Children, Youth and Families (see Exhibit 10.3). Other divisions, such as the Administration on Aging and the Office for Civil Rights, also lie within DHHS. Most of the programs discussed in this chapter are under the auspices of the CMS or the PHS. In 1995, Congress authorized a separate Social Security Administration. Until then, the Social Security Administration was an agency within DHHS.

The Centers for Medicare and Medicaid Services (CMS) administer the Medicare and Medicaid programs. The PHS includes the Agency for Health Care Research and Quality (formerly the Agency for Health Care Policy and Research), Agency for Toxic Substances and Disease Registry, Centers for Disease Control and Prevention, Food and Drug Administration (FDA), Health Resources and Services Administration (HRSA), Indian Health Service, National Institutes of Health (NIH), and the Substance Abuse and Mental Health Services Administration (SAMHSA). The Division of Nursing within the HRSA and the National Institute of Nursing Research (NINR) at the NIH are focal points for nursing initiatives at the federal level and are discussed later in this chapter. However, nurses are involved in every agency listed, and the activities of each agency have an impact on nursing practice.

MAJOR LEGISLATION AFFECTING NURSING

Both federal and state laws have a major impact on nursing practice and education. At the state level, nurses need to know about their own

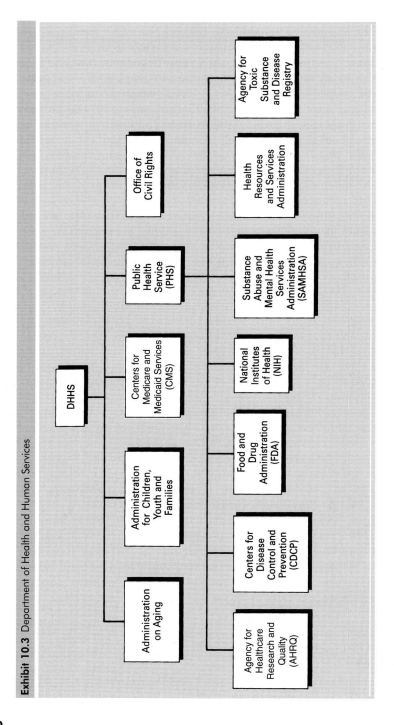

Exhibit 10.3 Department of Health and Human Services

nursing practice acts and should be acquainted with the licensure laws of other health practitioners. These are discussed in Chapter 11. Other state legislation affecting the health and welfare of nurses may be equally important, and you should keep abreast of both proposed and enacted legislation.

In this section, the focus is on federal legislation that affects the practice of nursing and the rights of nurses; occasionally, state laws that are almost universal or closely related to federal laws are included. Obviously, all health legislation fits into that category, but those laws that seem to have particular significance are highlighted here.

SOCIAL SECURITY

The Social Security Act, passed in 1935 and amended many times since, is the origin of most health and social welfare programs in this country. The act includes many titles or components, each covering a different program. The average person who talks of Social Security is most likely referring to the Old-Age, Survivors' and Disability Insurance (OASDI), which provides benefits after retirement age or in the case of total disability. Contributions to OASDI are withheld from the employee's wage, and matched by the employer. Deductions appear on the employee's paycheck under "FICA" (Federal Insurance Contributions Act). Self-employed individuals are also required to contribute. In recent years, the aging of the U.S. population has raised concerns about the solvency of the Social Security Trust Fund. In response, Congress has periodically enacted legislation to protect the program while ensuring that beneficiaries receive adequate payments. There is currently heated debate over whether to allow workers to privately invest a portion of their social security savings.

MEDICARE

Medicare, authorized under Title XVIII of the Social Security Act, is a nationwide health insurance program for the aged and certain disabled persons. In both of the two parts (A and B) of Medicare, the benefits are limited to those who are 65 years of age or older having a designated length of Medicare-covered employment, and some disabled persons under 65.

Most Americans are automatically eligible for Part A, which consists of hospital insurance (HI), upon turning 65. Others, who are disabled or in need of kidney dialysis, qualify regardless of age. Under Part A, the patient pays a small deductible (which has been increasing) for hospital care, and the federal government pays the rest. Part A also covers skilled nursing facilities, home health care, and hospice care, with certain limits in each category.

Part B of Medicare is an optional supplemental medical insurance (SMI) program available to Medicare Part A recipients upon payment of a monthly premium, which in 2005 is $78.20 monthly. Part B is financed through these premiums, along with general government funds. Ninety-six percent of Part A beneficiaries also enroll in Part B. Part B pays 80 percent of the established fee for physicians' services in excess of an annual deductible. Services covered include the physician's care in the hospital, home, or office; laboratory and other diagnostic tests; outpatient services at a hospital; therapeutic equipment such as braces; home health services; mammograms; and respite care for caretakers of homebound Medicare beneficiaries. Preventive care that the elderly often need is still unavailable under the traditional Medicare program.

The financial liabilities incurred by Medicare beneficiaries (copayments, deductibles, and uncovered services) may be paid by: the recipient themselves; a third party such as private Medigap insurance purchased by the beneficiary; or Medicaid if the person is eligible. Given the gaps in Medicare coverage, many private insurance companies sell Medigap policies to absorb the personal financial liabilities under Medicare. In 1990, Congress enacted legislation that established standards for Medigap.

Over the past decade, the federal government has promoted coordinated care and other unconventional arrangements under Medicare; one such is called Medicare Advantage. For the most part, these are prepaid, managed care plans, usually administered by health maintenance organizations or a variety of other competitive medical plans, and frequently incorporating the option of a medical savings account. Coordinated care plans may also offer benefits—such as preventive care, dental care, prescription drugs, and eyeglasses—not covered under Medicare. The managed care plan's fixed monthly premium and cost-sharing structure helps to provide predictability to beneficiaries about their out-of-pocket costs, and eliminates the need in many cases for Medigap insurance. The Medicare population has moved very slowly into these models, preferring traditional fee-for-service, regardless of its cost inefficiencies.

The Medicare program is the responsibility of CMS. CMS enters into contracts with Blue Cross–Blue Shield, commercial carriers, and group practice prepayment plans to serve as administrative agents.

Medicare Legislation

Since 1966, Congress has enacted a number of Medicare amendments aimed primarily at controlling the soaring costs of the program. There are now rigid regulations regarding the length of the institutional stay that will be reimbursed and payment for specific services. Another major concern, quality of care, has also resulted in amendments.

The most far-reaching legislative changes were the provisions of the *Tax Equity and Fiscal Responsibility Act* (TEFRA) of 1982 (PL 97–248). This legislation required the Secretary of DHHS and certain congressional committees to develop Medicare prospective payment models for hospitals, skilled nursing facilities (SNFs), and, to the extent feasible, other providers. Other cost-cutting mechanisms affecting health care facilities and providers were also included.

The work on the prospective payment mechanisms resulted in enactment of PL 98-21, variously called the *Social Security Amendments of 1983*, the *Social Security Rescue Plan,* or simply the *DRG law.* This legislation established a prospective payment system based on 467 diagnosis related groups (DRGs), categories with pretreatment diagnosis billing amounts for almost all United States hospitals reimbursed by Medicare.

What DRGs mean to a hospital is that if a patient uses more resources (days and services) than designated by the patient's DRG category, the extra costs must be absorbed. If the patient uses less, the dollar amount designated is the hospital's clear profit.

Needless to say, the DRG system had a direct effect on nursing. In some cases, hospitals desperate to cut costs chose to retain lower-paid nursing personnel, rather than RNs. Others chose to turn to all-RN staffs that could actually save money by teaching patients or by anticipating potential complications, so that the patient would be discharged before the DRG-set time. As noted in Chapter 6, the job market for nurses became tighter for a while. However, some nurses felt that this was a good time to cost out nursing services so that they could be separated from general daily charges. Others identified ways of determining patient-specific variations in nursing resource use so that these could be considered in the DRG system.[2] In general, the Medicare prospective payment system has encouraged all health care providers, including nurses, to be more aware of the cost components in health care. For nursing, this has been an advantage. Increasingly, nurse researchers have been able to document the cost effectiveness of nurse providers. Prospective payment also resulted in hospitals discharging patients "quicker and sicker." This led hospital administrators to appreciate, more than they previously did, the indispensable role that nurses have in caring for patients with higher levels of acuity in all types of health care settings.

The 1983 Medicare legislation also mandated the formation of peer review organizations (PROs) to replace the then existing professional standards review organizations (PSROs). The intent of the legislation was to establish mechanisms for quality assurance by private entities in a competitive market. PROs review only Medicare services (appropriateness of admission, discharge, and the use of resources during the episode in the delivery system). In general, each state has one PRO. However, some larger states have subcontracts with regional units. Nurses have been involved with PROs as staff and as members of PRO review boards. Consumers also play a significant role in PROs, because the 1983 law mandated that a certain proportion of the members of the PRO boards be composed of consumers. In 2001, the PROs were renamed Quality Improvement Organizations (QIOs), retaining the same mission and reporting relationships.[3]

Over the years, Congress has approved changes in the scope of services provided under Medicare. In 1990, Pap smears, mammography, and expansion of hospice benefits were added. Medicare revisions have also included reimbursement for a variety of providers once excluded from the program. Advanced practice nurses are fully reimbursable through the Medicare program. The 1989 reconciliation bill authorized nurse practitioners (NPs) and clinical nurse specialists (CNSs), working in collaboration with a physician, to certify and recertify the need for nursing home care under Medicare. A nursing home could also be paid for the services of a gerontological nurse practitioner (GNP). As a result of other policy, APNs were reimbursed when they practiced in a Federally Qualified Health Center (FQHC) or in rural or medically underserved areas.

The Physician Payment Review Commission (PPRC), which proposes policy for providers' fees, became concerned over the rising cost of Part B when compared to the better-controlled increases in Part A. A 1989 bill revamped the system of paying doctors on the basis of "customary, prevailing, and reasonable fees" and replaced it with a standard based on the total cost of the service provided, including the cost of maintaining a practice, liability insurance, and the relative value of the technical skills needed. This new methodology is based on a resource-based relative-value scale (RBRVS) that places emphasis on the service performed for a patient, instead of the traditional way of allocating fees according to the specialization of the provider. These changes in physician reimbursement under Medicare have provided incentives for expanding nonphysician and noninstitutional reimbursement, including reimbursement for nurses.

In 1991, the PPRC recommended that nonphysician practitioners (including certain nurses) under Medicare should also be paid based on a RBRVS, taking into account the differences in education and training between physicians and nonphysician providers. In January 1998, NPs and CNSs became reimbursable for services provided to Medicare recipients. The advanced practice nurse (APN) is paid approximately 80 percent of the actual charge for the service.[4]

MEDICAID

Medicaid was authorized in 1965 as Title XIX of the Social Security Act to pay for medical services on behalf of certain groups of low-income persons. It is a federal–state means-tested entitlement program, which CMS also administers. Certain groups of persons (i.e., the aged, blind, disabled, and members of families with dependent children, among others) qualify for coverage if their incomes and resources are sufficiently low. Each state designs and administers its own Medicaid program, setting eligibility and coverage standards within broad federal guidelines. As a result, substantial variation exists among the states in terms of persons covered, types and scope of benefits offered, and amount of payments for services. On average, the federal government pays 56 percent of the benefit costs and states pay the rest. Until 1986, Medicaid eligibility was tied to welfare. In that year, Medicaid was extended to include certain women and children with low incomes who were not covered by the Aid to Families with Dependent Children (AFDC) program. This change was important because state poverty levels are considerably lower than the federal poverty level and were used as AFDC eligibility criteria, thus keeping many poor women and children from receiving necessary health care. In 1997, AFDC was categorically eliminated, and Temporary Assistance to Needy Families (TANF) was established, which is discussed later under block grants.

The expansion of Medicaid in recent years has occurred incrementally, with intense deliberations at state and federal levels of government. The discussions focused on what states were required and had the option to provide under Medicaid. The changes have had a significant impact on access to and financing of health care for America's women and children. The escalating costs have caused states to cut back services. Some, such as Oregon, have set up plans that will allow more primary care and preventive services and limit more expensive services that are seen as less necessary.[5]

In 1989, nurses reached another milestone when Congress enacted legislation providing for coverage of family NP and pediatric NP services under Medicaid, as long as they are practicing within the scope of state law. Since July 1990, states have been required to cover the services of these two types of NP, regardless of whether they are under the supervision of or associated with a physician. But restrictive policies and discriminatory practices continue for APNs under Medicaid and private insurers, as well as in numerous state laws and regulations. For example, the Balanced Budget Act of 1997 encouraged states to use pediatric and family nurse practitioners, and certified nurse midwives as primary care case managers for Medicaid recipients in fee-for-service plans, but was very vague about their role in managed care, and excluded all other APNs. As Medicaid moves vigorously into managed care, this represents a barrier to the full participation of APNs.

MEDICARE AND MEDICAID IN LATER DAYS

The Medicare and Medicaid programs represent a major financial commitment and have always been shaped and reshaped as a political expedient. With increases in copayments and deductibles, older Americans are paying more out of pocket today (in dollars adjusted to a 2005 standard) than before Medicare. The prevailing technique to control Medicaid spending has been to offer a broad package of services but to pay so little to providers for delivering those services that Medicaid patients are rejected out of hand in many instances. The inappropriate use of hospital emergency rooms by the poor for primary care can be traced to the fact that other providers refuse to give care because of reimbursement that is inadequate to sustain even overhead in most cases. Hospitals cannot refuse and still qualify for federal and state monies in the form of either payment for services or programs. Financial games have allowed Medicare to survive because the poor elderly are eventually subsidized by the Medicaid program if their Medicare benefits run out. However, there are many elderly with personal resources, and they represent a large and powerful political constituency. Medicare reimbursement rates are within reason, and the requirement that providers accept the established rate as payment in full for the poor elderly is the safety net. Medicare is fully federally funded, and so federal criteria can be imposed, resulting in equity for all recipients. In contrast, the poor are often voiceless, and states must only comply with broad standards to obtain federal matching dollars. The latitude in those standards can easily create inequity.

Medicare and Medicaid are on the fast track moving toward managed care. In some situations special federal waivers are necessary, but they have been easily forthcoming, with an administration anxious to support any strategy that might reduce the likelihood of deep program cuts or tax increases. Where possible, it is advantageous that these managed care plans have a broad cross-section of members, thereby reducing the likelihood of a tiered program. It is also mandatory that, where possible, these recipients be given the opportunity to select from more than one program, introducing an element of competition. So often the Medicaid choices include facilities and providers that need patients or need beds filled, so they are willing to negotiate lower rates just to survive. These plans are offered by the same corporations that create networks (plans) for those insured through the workplace or by personal pay. Medicare recipients have more options, their numbers and dollars being higher.

The latest addition to the Medicare program is Part D, Prescription Drug Coverage. The benefit package focuses on the needs of those elderly who are the heaviest users of prescription drugs. The *Medicare Prescription Drug, Improvement, and Modernization Act* of 2003 created this benefit, which will be added to Medicare in January 2006. People with Medicare will be able to join a drug plan. All the plans will be run by private companies. These plans will offer a variety of choices for prescription drug coverage with an estimated monthly premium of $35. Once the $250 annual deductible is met, Medicare pays 75 percent of covered prescription drug costs for the next $2000. The individual is responsible for a 25 percent copayment. A beneficiary who has used $2250 in covered prescription costs is responsible for paying 100 percent of the next $2850 of covered expenses. This is referred to as the "donut hole." After a beneficiary reaches $5100 during the year, Medicare will then pay for 95 percent of any remaining covered costs for the rest of that year. This is another step in progress, but competes with state-based programs, some of which offer much more generous benefits.[6] See http://www.cms.hhs.gov/medicarereform.

BLOCK GRANTS

The block grant approach consolidates categorical programs into blocks and turns over control of money to the states, with little accounting to the federal government as to how the funds are spent. Block grants are funded through federal and state-matched funds. They shift much of the political and administrative accountability to the states, without subsequent increases in state funding, and they possibly intensify inequities among states in terms of the populations covered by the programs. The major advantage of block grants is the streamlining they provide at the federal level by consolidating programs into clusters for legislative and programmatic purposes.

In 1981, three health block grants were formed: maternal and child health, preventive services, and mental health (including alcohol and drug abuse). Congress originally designated a primary care block grant that consisted of community and migrant health center programs, but it was never officially made a block grant, and today it remains a federal program.

The Personal Responsibility and Work Opportunity Reconciliation Act of 1996 (Welfare Reform Bill) has initiated a not-so-quiet revolution in the nation's welfare programs, and there will be a direct impact on both health care and nursing. States receive a block grant for a fixed percentage of the money they spent on public assistance pre-welfare reform. This bill includes a host of initiatives which were once separately funded, such as Supplemental Security Income, nutrition programs, food stamps, Medicaid, and Temporary Assistance to Needy Families (TANF). The TANF block grant replaces AFDC which matched state funds designated for the program. State flexibility in TANF is broad, but there are some compulsory requirements to qualify: public assistance is limited to a total of 60 months; adults in families receiving assistance must work after two years; if not, community service must begin within two months of receiving benefits; unmarried minor parents must reside within an adult-supervised relationship; eligibility of aliens and naturalized immigrants for federal benefits is dramatically reduced; a parent receiving benefits must cooperate in paternity determination; and deadbeat parents will be pursued across state lines and then some to expedite child support.[7] A lot of pain and disenfranchisement of children has been predicted; others see success and a strategy similar to Roosevelt's WPA of the Depression.

HEALTH SERVICES LEGISLATION

In recent years, federal funding for AIDS has become a hot topic. One of the ongoing concerns of AIDS activists has been the lack of funding for the Ryan White Comprehensive AIDS Resource Emergency (CARE) Act, enacted in 1990 and reauthorized as amended in 1996. The bill provides for economic assistance to cities with the highest rates of AIDS to help absorb the costs of caring for people with AIDS. In addition, it established funding for community-based services to promote care for children, families, and minorities affected by the disease. The most recent amendments were applauded by AIDS advocates, and include requirements for health professions' education, and priority status for funding to programs targeted to women, infants, and children. Other new provisions are requirements for spousal notification, and voluntary testing of pregnant women and infants. Advocacy groups see the latter as the first step down a "slippery slope" to mandatory universal testing, and vigorously lobbied its exclusion from the legislation.

One of the most controversial issues pertaining to AIDS is whether the federal government should be allowed to limit immigration to this country of people who are infected with HIV. AIDS activists are against such measures, arguing that it violates human rights. Other more conservative players and government officials have taken a different stand.

They claim that AIDS is a public health threat, that neither the federal government nor the American taxpayer can afford to care for these individuals, and that lenient immigration policies with regard to HIV/AIDS increase the public's risk of transmission. This policy was enacted into law; however, the U.S. attorney general has the right to grant waivers from the exclusion. Nurses, public health professionals, and other civil rights groups continue to challenge this exclusionary policy, because HIV is not spread by casual contact, and the policy restricts the freedom of many individuals, in particular refugees seeking political asylum here.

Also in the 1980s, one of Congress's attempts to combine concerns about the cost and quality of health care was the establishment of the *Agency for Health Care Policy and Research* (AHCPR) within the PHS. The mission of the AHCPR included conducting research on the quality and effectiveness of health care services, developing practice guidelines, and assessing technology. The effectiveness initiatives are of particular importance because many policymakers look to effectiveness research as a way of controlling health care costs, empowering the consumer, reducing malpractice claims, and providing equity in treatment and care. Early in 2000, the AHCPR was refocused and renamed the Agency for Healthcare Research and Quality (AHRQ). AHRQ will serve as the government's focal point for research to enhance the quality, appropriateness, and effectiveness of health care services and access to those services. Additionally, AHRQ will form liaisons with the private sector so that the two sides do not duplicate each other's work.[8]

NURSING EDUCATION AND RESEARCH

In the 1960s, as the federal government urged the enactment of legislation to provide health care for the aged under Social Security, health facilities and personnel became matters of urgency to Washington. Ever more funds were channeled into health and education projects. At the same time, nurses were becoming more vocal, and their organizations stronger, more self-assured, and more convincing when their representatives met with legislators and appeared before legislative committees. As a result of these and other factors, several new laws were enacted in the early 1960s that supported nursing and the individual nurse.

Most significant among these was the *Nurse Training Act* of 1964 (Title VIII of the Public Health Service Act). The purpose of this law was to increase the number of nurses through financial assistance to diploma, associate degree, and baccalaureate degree nursing schools, and graduates taking advanced courses, and thus to help ensure more and better schools of nursing, more carefully selected students, a high standard of teaching, and better health care for people.

Renewal of the law has had its ups and downs over two decades, especially during the era of retrenchment in the early 1980s. However, due to the successful lobbying of nursing organizations, and individuals across the country, the program remained on the books. In 1985, federal legislation for nursing education was renamed the *Nurse Education Act* (NEA). That year was also a landmark for nurses because it marked the establishment of the National Center for Nursing Research (NCNR) at NIH. Nurses claimed victory on November 20, when the Senate voted 89 to 7 to override President Reagan's veto of the NIH bill. The House had already supported the bill in its 380 to 32 veto override the previous week. In 1993, the NCNR became the National Institute of Nursing Research (NINR). The NEA and the NINR have maintained competitive funding levels, and even grown in the toughest of economic times.

EMPLOYEE PROTECTIONS

Workers' compensation is becoming ever more important to nurses as the hazards of their work and workplace increase. These include exposure to environmental hazards, some of which are described in Chapter 15, and potentially fatal diseases such as AIDS and hepatitis B. The first such insurance to be held constitutional was the *Workmen's Compensation Act*, enacted by the state of Washington in 1911. Today, all states require

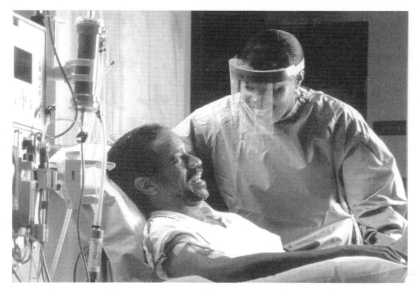

The proper use of protective gear makes a dangerous job much safer. (*Courtesy of the U.S. Department of Veterans Affairs*)

employers in industry to carry workers' compensation, but in some states, nonprofit organizations, including hospitals, are exempt. However, most nurses are covered by some version of this type of insurance. Federal employees are usually covered by the *Federal Employees' Compensation Act,* enacted in 1952.

Workers' compensation insurance, the cost of which is carried entirely by the employer, pays to employees who are injured on the job a proportion of their regular salaries for the time they are unable to work because of their injuries. If they are permanently disabled, they are entitled to additional compensation. Workers' compensation insurance laws do away with the requirement of proof that the employer was negligent or that the employee was free from contributory negligence. They also prevent court action for injuries and provide instead an administrative procedure for securing awards of compensation.

Many states have extended the coverage provided by workers' compensation laws to include occupational diseases; other states have enacted separate occupational disease acts, some of which cover all types of occupational disease; others specify which ones are covered.

The major breakthrough on the federal level was the enactment of the *Occupational Safety and Health Act* of 1970, which established administrative machinery for the development and enforcement of standards of occupational health and safety.

In recent years, health professionals and policy experts have placed growing attention on the importance of occupational health and safety, largely because of the increases in rates of many infectious diseases, such as tuberculosis, hepatitis, and HIV/AIDS. In December 1992, the *Occupational Safety and Health Administration* (OSHA) released standards on prevention of blood-borne diseases, requiring nurses and other health workers to receive protection. The standards require all employers to provide hepatitis B immunizations, as well as protective equipment and procedures, to prevent transmission of these diseases. More information on HIV/AIDS and the workplace is included in Chapter 15. In 1994, the Center for Disease Control and Prevention (CDC) issued guidelines for preventing the transmission of tuberculosis in health care facilities. OSHA has resisted requiring compliance with this standard.[9] In the summer of 1995, OSHA released a draft of voluntary guidelines on workplace violence.

Another occupational safety and health milestone occurred in May 1993, when an *Office of Occupational Health Nursing* was established at OSHA "to underscore the major role such nurses play in striving for safe and healthful workplaces." The office increased the visibility of nurses within OSHA and in related activities across the country. Despite this success, there have been some failures. The ANA has testified repeatedly before the Occupational Safety and Health Administration (OSHA) on the need for an ergonomics standard. This standard was promulgated in 2000 but repealed in March 2001 by Congress, which ordered OSHA to cease all work related to the standard. ANA continued pressing policy and lawmakers to address ergonomics hazards, and in March 2003, OSHA released nursing home guidelines for preventing musculoskeletal disorders (MSDs). According to the Bureau of Labor Statistics, nursing personnel are among the highest at risk for MSDs, with nursing aides, orderlies, and attendants ranking first (ahead of truck drivers and laborers) and RNs sixth in a list of at-risk occupations for strains and sprains. Twelve percent of nurses leave the profession annually as a result of back injuries, and more that 52 percent complain of chronic back pain.[10]

Finally, nurses have joined with others involved with occupational safety and health to push for reform of the Occupational Safety and Health Act, which has not been revised since its original enactment in 1970. One of the most important proposals for reform is to extend coverage under the law to public employees. Approximately 323,000 nurses work in national, state, or local governmental hospital settings, and they, as well as other public employees, are often exposed to blood-borne pathogens (as well as other risk factors) and are entitled to the same protection as their colleagues in the private sector.

CIVIL RIGHTS, EMPLOYMENT, AND LABOR RELATIONS

Beginning in the 1960s, a number of laws were passed to prohibit discrimination on sex as well as race, color, religion, and national origin. Many of these are particularly important to women and are referred to in Chapter 15. Some of the most important ones are discussed below.

Title VII of the *Civil Rights Act* of 1964 (Equal Employment Opportunity Law) has affected the job status of nurses because it includes a section forbidding discrimination against women in job hiring and job promotion among private employers of more than 25 persons. Executive Order No. 11246, as amended, extended the law to include federal contractors and subcontractors. Hospitals and colleges are subject to this order because of their acceptance of federal grants of various kinds.

Among other civil rights that have been given new protection are the rights of patients, children, the mentally ill, prisoners, the elderly, and the handicapped. Actions to protect these rights have come through a variety of legal means at state and national levels. Protection has increasingly been specified through regulations of various laws such as the amendments and subsequent regulations of the Social Security Act. Another is the *Rehabilitation Act* of 1973. Section 504 of that law reads, "no otherwise qualified handicapped individual in the United States shall, solely by reason of his handicap, be excluded from the participation in, be denied the benefit of, or be subjected to discrimination under any program or activity receiving federal financial assistance." The definition of *handicapped* includes drug addicts and alcoholics, as well as those having an overt physical impairment such as blindness, deafness, or paralysis of some kind. A major issue now is whether and under what circumstances AIDS patients and HIV-infected people come under this law. Some state and local jurisdictions have ruled that AIDS-related illness does come under their laws as a protected handicap. Those that do not consider communicable diseases as protected have ruled differently. In intervening years, there have been two types of renewed civil rights activity. First, the *Americans with Disabilities Act* was enacted in 1990 with the intent of barring firms from denying jobs to individuals solely on the basis of disability, as long as reasonable accommodations can be made. The legislation is aimed at protecting the nearly 43 million disabled Americans, including people infected with HIV. Discrimination is prohibited in areas such as public accommodations, transportation, and private employment. This did not prevent an applicant to a nursing school who was hearing impaired from being refused. The Supreme Court upheld the decision.

In 1991, following a veto the previous year, President Bush signed the *Civil Rights Act* of 1991. The legislation was in response to 1989 Supreme Court rulings that shifted the burden of proof from employer to employee in cases where employees experience discrimination. The 1991 bill restored the previous standard by requiring employers to prove that the hiring practice is required for the job in question. The bill pertains mostly to women and minority members who claim to have experienced discrimination in job hiring situations. Its enactment was an important step in sustaining the civil rights of all Americans.

The right to privacy also affects nurses. One of the most important federal laws in this area is the *Freedom of Information Act* (FOIA) of 1966 and the *Privacy Act* of 1974. The purpose of the FOIA is to give the public access to files maintained by the executive branch of government. Recognizing that there are valid reasons for withholding certain records, the law exempts broad categories of records from compulsory public inspection, including medical records. It also gives access to their hospital records to patients in federal hospitals.

Another step in providing access to the individual's own records was enactment of the *Family Educational Rights and Privacy Act* of 1974, also known as the *Buckley Amendment*. The basic intent of this law was to provide students, their parents, and guardians with easier access to and control over the information contained in academic records. Educational records are defined broadly and include files, documents, and other materials containing information about the student and maintained by a school. Students must be allowed to inspect these records within 45 days of their request. They need not be allowed access to confidential letters of reference preceding January 1975, records about students made by teachers and administrators for their own use and not shown to others, certain campus police records, certain parental financial records, and certain psychiatric treatment records (if not available to anyone else). Students may challenge the content, secure the correction of inaccurate information, and insert a written explanation regarding the content of their records.

The law also specifies who has access to the records (teachers, educational administrators, organizations such as testing services, state and other officials to whom certain information must be reported according to the law). Otherwise, the records cannot be released without the student's consent. The law applies to nursing education programs as well as others.

Also within the broad categories of rights are those laws related to labor relations. The first was the *National Labor Relations Act* (NLRA), one of several laws enacted to pull the country out of the Great Depression. The thesis was that labor unions could prevent employers from lowering wages, resulting in higher incomes and more spending. To achieve the growth of unions, employers had to be controlled; for instance, they could no longer legally fire employees who tried to unionize. The National Labor Relations Board (NLRB), created by law, was empowered to investigate and initiate administrative proceedings against those employers who violated the law. If these administrative actions did not curtail the illegal acts, court action followed. Only employers' violations were listed.

In 1947, the NLRA was substantially amended, and the amended law, entitled the *Labor Management Relations Act* (or *Taft–Hartley Act*), listed prohibitions for unions. Section 14(b), for instance, contained the so-called right-to-work clause, which authorized states to enact more stringent union security provisions than those contained in the federal laws.

In 1959, a third major modification was made. One of the purposes of the law, the *Labor-Management Reporting and Disclosure Act* or *Landrum–Griffin Act*, was to curb documented union abuses such as corrupt financial and election procedures. For this reason, it is sometimes called the union members' Bill of Rights. The result is a series of rights and responsibilities of members of a union or a professional organization, such as ANA, that engages in collective bargaining. Required are reporting and disclosure of certain financial transactions and administrative practices and the use of democratic election procedures. That is, every member in good standing must be able to nominate candidates and run for election and must be allowed to vote and support candidates; there must be secret ballot elections; union funds must not be used to assist the candidacy of an individual seeking union office; candidates must have access to the membership list; records of the election must be preserved for one year; and elections must be conducted according to the procedures specified in the by-laws.

Highly significant for nurses is the 1974 law that again amended the Taft–Hartley Act, PL 93–360, the *Nonprofit Health Care Amendments.* This law made private nonprofit health care facilities that had, through considerable lobbying, been excluded in the 1947 law, subject to national labor laws. These employees were now free to join or not join a union without employer retribution, a right previously denied to them unless they worked in a state that had its own law allowing them to unionize. It also created special notification procedures that must precede any strike action. The definition of *health care facility* included a broad range of acute care and community health care facilities.

In 1991 and 1994, there were Supreme Court decisions of major significance to nursing and labor representation. The 1991 ruling upheld the NLRB's rule-making which sanctioned a separate collective bargaining unit for nurses, and further found LPNs appropriately included with technical employees in the light of their skill level. In 1994, the court decided that a licensed practical nurse employed by a nursing home was a statutory supervisor because of her relationship with nurses' aides. Therefore, she was ineligible for the legal protections offered to other employees. These issues are also discussed in Chapter 15.

The inadequacies of labor law observed in the 1994 decision have been a continuing frustration to the courts, management, and the labor community. The Commission on the Future of Worker–Management Relations was created to review existing labor laws and speak on the need for corrective legislation. Observation tells us workers are different today. They want personal expression in their work, job security, and control over their day-to-day life in the workplace. In the existing economic environment, that is only possible when labor and management come together to save their industries. Commonly referred to as the *Dunlop Commission*, the panel reported in 1995 and recommended the creation of labor–management committees. (It is this provision that is suspicious, given the existing strict definitions of company-created unions.) Beyond this, the important recommendation is to narrow the definition of supervisor with the intent of protecting professionals.

The strike is the ultimate weapon in collective bargaining, and is used cautiously. The effect is weakened and retribution toward striking workers permitted when permanent striker replacements are hired. If the primary goal of collective bargaining is to level the playing field between labor and management, the strategy of permanent striker replacement frustrates that aim. In 1995, through issuance of an Executive Order, the

President barred federal contractors from hiring permanent striker replacements.[11]

Periodic shortages put nursing into a tailspin. Commissions have been created to study the problem, and nursing's organizations have come together in national recruitment efforts, and looked to enhance the pool of registered nurses through foreign recruitment and immigration. The *Immigration Nursing Relief Act* of 1990 established a five-year pilot project for use of a special work visa (H-1A) specific to foreign-educated nurses who enter the United States. Employers were required to produce assurances that no U.S. citizen was available to fill a position, and that steps were being taken to decrease dependence on foreign-educated nurses. The program sunsetted in August 1995. Another very limited temporary visa program was instituted in 2000, responding to another nursing shortage. An H-1C visa was made available to 500 nurses for work in acute care facilities in underserved areas. Foreign nurses continue to seek jobs in the United States. But immigration policies have become more demanding, since the Department of Homeland Security, strategically positioned to deal with the aftermath of 9/11, has assumed the responsibilities of the Immigration and Naturalization Service. The root causes for the instability of the nursing workforce, which have led to swings in supply and demand, must be addressed. Over-reliance on foreign-educated nurses by the health care industry serves only to postpone efforts required to address the needs of the U.S. nursing workforce.

CONSUMER PROTECTIONS

The Health Insurance Portability and Accountability Act of 1996 (HIPAA) is a piece of legislation which has prompted much overreaction in the health care community. The Act has two dimensions. Title I protects health insurance coverage for workers and their families when they change or lose their jobs. This portion has been in effect for many years. Title II, only in effect since April 2003, makes provision for the privacy and security of personal and health information through setting and enforcing standards. The standards are not so complex as would seem, and the reader is referred to Chapter 9 and the following website for more complete details: http://www.hhs.gov/ocr/hipaa.

A NATIONAL HEALTH PLAN

Our patchwork system of health care delivery and insurance has resulted in over 44 million individuals lacking health insurance, one-third of whom are children, and an equal amount with inadequate coverage.[12] Furthermore, contrary to popular belief, the majority of uninsured people are working or dependants of people who are working.

In the 1980s and 1990s, policymakers discussed various proposals to provide health coverage for the uninsured. The major obstacles to all of these proposals were that the burden of cost would fall on different shoulders, depending on the policy scheme, and that invariably the plans involved increased costs and spending. In addition, each plan targeted a different group and, unless Congress accepted some form of national health plan, there was no way to provide coverage for everyone.

Underlying all of these proposals are unanswered questions about health care as a right or a privilege. If one assumes that access to affordable health care is a right, then which level of government is responsible for it? The issue of equity needs to be addressed. Are all individuals entitled to the same level and quality of health care, regardless of their ability to pay for their care? Or can we accept a two-tiered system of care wherein those who can afford to pay more are entitled to the best quality and quantity of services their money can buy? Although the answers to these questions seem elusive, they raise important issues for nurses to consider as they become increasingly involved with the health care system.

In 1989, Congress took action to alleviate the burden of health insurance on the disabled by passing a law extending the period in which employers must let former workers who are disabled keep the group rate. The period was extended from 18 to 29 months, and the law is expected to protect the disabled, including individuals infected with HIV.

In 1990, the U.S. Bipartisan Commission on Comprehensive Health Care (renamed the Pepper Commission after its chairman, the late Congressman Claude Pepper) issued one of the most noteworthy reports. It called for extensions of job-based insurance, a national health insurance plan for those not covered by an employer, and a proposal for long-term care including a nursing home plan that was a catalyst for discussion on these issues.

In the fall of 1990, for the first time in years, the Senate Committee on Labor and Health, chaired by Senator Edward M. Kennedy, approved health reform legislation. The following year, proponents of health care reform seemed to have more support, especially as they focused on the needs of the uninsured. Legislators talked seriously about "pay or play" options, whereby employers with a minimum number of employees would have to provide health insurance ("play") or "pay" a fee that would go to a national fund to cover the costs of insuring the uninsured. By the early 1990s, most health care organizations had designed or endorsed at least one plan for health care reform. In 1991, many nursing organizations supported *Nursing's Agenda for Health Care Reform*, calling for a "basic 'core' of essential health care services to be available to everyone."

These activities were accompanied, or perhaps inspired, by two important developments that altered the political landscape. First, the business community became increasingly vocal about the financial burden of health care costs. Second, organized medicine, traditionally opposed to major social reform in medicine, shed its inhibitions and called for changes in the current health care system. With congressional leadership also pushing for health care reform and with public opinion polls pointing to the growing concern about rising health care costs, there was no doubt that health care would be a visible and determining campaign issue in 1992.

The momentum around health care reform continued well into the second year of the Clinton presidency. The best minds were brought together at the White House and the final product was the *Health Security Act* of 1993. By September 1994, health care reform was dead for the 103d Congress. The reasons for the turnabout are interesting and so predictable. Americans had become distracted from the health care agenda by more basic threats: safe streets and neighborhoods, the economy, jobs with a future, GATT and NAFTA, illegal immigrants. Most voters have access to health care, even if it is of limited and questionable value. Given that picture, there was fear of sweeping change that would in fact jeopardize one-sixth of the American economy. Incremental change—proceeding cautiously, building on successes, and allowing one step to be assimilated before another is proposed—is the preferred process, but the content was flawed too:[13]

1. Americans value freedom of choice, and the plan seemed to limit their options.
2. There is a strong distaste for the heavy hand of government.
3. A bloated federalism is particularly unacceptable.
4. Proposals that are naturally offensive to states' rights are bound to bring dissension.

Meanwhile, the Clinton Administration aroused the passion and the conscience of the nation. In the absence of national policy and perhaps because of that absence, states have begun to move forward, launching programs on behalf of the health and welfare of their citizens. It seems given that we will, over time, have universal coverage, but with a less robust benefit package than proposed by the administration. Financing will be through a combination of private and public sector resources. Managed care will dominate, but with the opportunity, for an additional cost, to select providers who are not members of the network. Indeed, the principle of reform may not be "the greatest good for the most people," but rather "a basic guaranteed standard for everyone, and the opportunity for those who are able to buy more." Prevention is guaranteed to be a driving force, as will direct access to a range of provider professionals. Care will be actively managed for some, with primary providers who will fulfill the role of gatekeeper (hopefully in a manner to help you make the best decisions on your own behalf, not to bar access to the system).

AGENCIES AND REGULATIONS

Follow-up of federal legislation requires close attention. It is not just the law itself that affects the public, but the proliferating federal regulations. Legislators have charged that regulations have been used specifically to circumvent the intent of the law; at the least, regulations often shape the legislation they are intended to carry out.

Equally important are the agencies created by the various laws, such as the FDA and Federal Trade Commission (FTC). The FTC, for instance, goes back to 1914, when the Federal Trade Commission Act was passed. It has extensive power; it can represent itself in court, enforce its own orders, and conduct its own litigation in civil courts, and it seems to have relative freedom from the executive branch of government. Its forays into the health field, with rulings on professional advertising, licensure, and other aspects of health care delivery never thought of in 1914, may indicate a direction for other administrative agencies such as FDA. On the other hand, some subjects of the FTC rulings have banded together to lobby for limitation of FTC powers. This occurred, for instance, in 1982, when attached to the FTC reauthorization bill was an amendment exempting state-licensed professionals from its jurisdiction. AMA was a major supporter; ANA was an opponent.

WHAT NEXT?

Pressure to enact legislation for the uninsured and to hold down the spiraling health care costs of this country will dominate the political scene in the next few years. These problems will be compounded by complex bio-ethical issues raised by new technologies and the need to meet all of these demands in an era of continued concerns about cost. Family concerns will also play an important role. Lawmakers will view health care policy within the context of broad social and environmental issues, both nationally and internationally. Without doubt, nurses will want to have a role in making these decisions.

KEY POINTS

1. The U.S. legal system includes statutory law, administrative law, and case law, all having specialized functions.
2. The judicial system is made up of courts at national, state, and local levels, each handling different kinds of cases, with appeals courts providing further legal review.
3. Important aspects of the legislative process include committee hearings and decisions, debate, amendments, possible conference committee agreements, final vote, administrative signature, and assignment to an administrative agency.
4. Information needed to influence legislation can be acquired from many sources, including consumer organizations, nursing organizations, governmental offices at various levels, and many publications.
5. Nurses can influence legislation in many ways by keeping legislators informed of their opinions and by supporting PACs in which they are interested.
6. Federal laws influence both the education and the practice of nurses, and have a major impact on the quality of the workplace.

STUDY QUESTIONS

1. In what political issues should nurses provide leadership?
2. How do you justify the division between federal and state powers in government?
3. What is your position on hiring foreign-educated nurses to fill positions during a shortage?
4. At what points during the legislative process is a bill most in jeopardy of being lost, and what would you do to save it?

REFERENCES

1. Dexter S, McKeon E, Whittaker S. The politics of caring. *Am J Nurs* 105(2):33, February 2005.
2. Joel L. DRGs and RIMs: Implications for nursing. *Nurs Outlook* 32:42–49, January–February 1984.
3. CMS: http://cms.hhs.gov/qio/default.asp. Retrieved April 7, 2005.

4. American College of Nurse Practitioners. Medicare Reimbursement Information and Resources: http://www.nurse.org/acnp/medicare. Retrieved April 7, 2005.
5. The Oregon Health Plan: http://www.oregon.gov/DHS/healthplan. Retrieved April 4, 2005.
6. CMS. Prescription Drug and Other Assistance Programs: http://www.medicare.gov/AssistancePrograms. Retrieved April 4, 2005.
7. Urban Institute. Welfare Reform: An Analysis of Issues: http://www.urban.org. Retrieved April 7, 2005.
8. AHRQ. Funding Opportunities: http://www.ahrq.gov/fund/funding.htm#inf. Retrieved April 7, 2005.
9. Flanagan L. *What You Need to Know About Today's Workplace*. Washington, DC: American Nurses Publishing, 1995, pp 30–35.
10. American Nurses Association. Nurses and Musculoskeletal Disorders: http://nursingworld.org/handlewithcare/background.htm. Retrieved July 13, 2005.
11. Clinton issues Executive Order on replacement workers. *Capital Update* 13:1, March 24, 1995.
12. Gralla J. U.S. Uninsured Health Care Cost Put at $125 Billion, May 11, 2004. Reuters: http://www.reuters.com. Retrieved April 3, 2005.
13. Joel LA. Health care reform: Getting it right this time. *Am J Nurs* 95:7, January 1995.

Updates can be found at

 http://www.JoelTheNursingExperience.com

Chapter 11

Health Care Credentialing and Nursing Licensure

OBJECTIVES

After studying this chapter, you will be able to:

1. Define licensure, certification, registration, and accreditation.
2. List three criticisms of licensure.
3. Describe the major controversies about institutional licensure.
4. Explain the difference between "multistate recognition" and state-to-state endorsement of licensed individuals.
5. Explain the difference between mandatory and permissive licensure.
6. Explain the meaning of a "grandfather clause."
7. List the key components of a nursing practice act.
8. List four reasons for which a license may be revoked or suspended.
9. Describe two current problems related to nursing certification.
10. Differentiate among the various ways of legalizing advanced practice.
11. Explain the meaning of "sunset legislation."
12. Identify the problems related to proving continuing competence.

For most nurses, licensure after graduation is a primary goal. For some this will be the only credential they will attain after the diploma or degree they earned from their entry-level educational program. To both the nurse and the public, being licensed is something special and important—and they are right. However, licensure is not the only credentialing mechanism in health care, nor is it (or the others) without problems. Health manpower credentialing has been criticized by consumers and the government as being one of the factors responsible for some of the serious problems in health care: fragmentation of services, accelerating costs, and poor use and distribution of health manpower.

Over the years, health manpower credentialing has been the object of considerable criticism, especially by the federal government. It has been implied that if credentialing problems were not resolved, the federal government would step in and take control away from the professions. As a result there has been both internal and external scrutiny, with minor changes that improved credentialing systems to some extent. This pressure from the federal government has almost died out, since more conservative administrations have shifted responsibility to the states. However, the issues are not resolved, and the states have responded with actions that affect every health care practitioner, including nurses. Therefore, knowing about the pros and cons of licensure and other credentialing options can help you think through some of these issues before they come to the inevitable crisis stage.

CREDENTIALING AND ITS ISSUES

INDIVIDUAL LICENSURE

Licensure is a credential awarded to an *individual* through the police power of the state. The state legislature determines what group is licensed, and with what limits. It is the responsibility of a specific part of the state government to see that the law is carried out, including punishment for its violation. Although licensure laws differ somewhat in format from state to state, the elements of each are similar. For instance, in the health professions' laws, there are sections on definition of the profession that describe broadly the scope of practice; requirements for licensure, such as education; exemptions from licensure; grounds for revocation of a license; creation of a licensing board, including members' qualifications and responsibilities; and penalties for practicing without a license.

Licensure laws are either mandatory (compulsory) or permissive (voluntary). If mandatory, the law forbids anyone to practice that profession or occupation without a license or face a fine or imprisonment.

If permissive, the law allows anyone to practice as long as they do not claim to hold the credential (such as RN).

Licensing of the health occupations was advocated in the early nineteenth century, but it was not until the early 1900s that a significant number of licensing laws were enacted. They were generally initiated by the associations of practitioners that were interested in raising standards and establishing codes for ethical behavior. Because they could not count on voluntary compliance, the associations tried to get legislation. To some critics, this movement is also seen as a way of providing members of an occupation or profession as much status, control, and compensation as the community is willing to give. It is true that as the health occupations proliferate, each group begins to organize and seek licensure.

In all of the proposals for changes in health manpower credentialing, criticism of individual licensure is implicit or explicit. Particularly in the last 15 years, the evils were cited; changes (often slow in coming) were dismissed as too little and too late. Some of the key criticisms were (and are) as follows:

1. The minimal standards of safety, theoretically guaranteed by granting the initial license, are often no longer met by some (perhaps many) practitioners because there is no organized system of monitoring continued competence. There is even the question of whether any written exam can determine safe practice in the actual work setting.

2. Specific requirements for courses, roles, and so on are rigidly specified in statutes instead of relying on administrative rule-making process. This makes timely responses to a changing environment difficult and slow. The result is that minimal standards and educational innovations in the health professions lag behind the practice realities.

3. Definitions of practice are so general that, when challenged, allocation of specific tasks may be determined by legal opinions or interpretations by lay people who cannot make an accurate judgment about what is or should be done in practice.

4. Too many licensing boards are still composed of members of that particular profession, without representation by competent lay members or allied health professions. This is seen as allowing these professionals to control the kind and number of individuals who may enter their field, with the possibility of shutting out other health workers climbing the occupational ladder and limiting the number of practitioners for economic reasons.

5. There are always some licensed practitioners who are unsafe, and even if they lose their license in one state, boards in other states may

not be routinely notified, and the individual simply crosses a state line and continues to practice.

Despite the criticism of individual licensure, it is this model that assures the allegiance of the professional to the consumer rather than to any employer. This is essential to preserve as ever more professionals become salaried employees. This issue is further discussed in Chapter 4. The fact that employers cannot force the professional to compromise their practice as defined in their practice act is a fact of law.

Of the licensed occupations, only 14 are licensed in every state (but not every territory): chiropractors, dental hygienists, dentists, nursing home administrators, optometrists, pharmacists, physical therapists, physicians (MD and DO), podiatrists, professional and practical nurses, psychologists, and veterinarians. Other practitioners find their mobility restricted as they discover that they are licensed in one state but not another. Even those licensed in all states may need to take licensing exams again when they relocate. Each state controls its own licensing exam. Nursing, with its state board examinations, now called the *National Council Licensure Examination* (NCLEX-RN), is accepted in every state. This allows for licensure by endorsement or reciprocity. That is, assuming that other criteria for licensure are met, a nurse need not take another examination when relocating from state to state.

It seems that almost all of the established or fledgling health occupations, more than 250 at the last count, consider licensing as a primary means of credentialing. This preference is largely because reimbursement for services has become associated with governmental recognition through licensure. Yet, the various weaknesses of all health occupations' licensing laws, the inconsistencies and varying standards of those seeking licensure, and the sheer numbers involved appear to be the bases for whatever enthusiasm exists for alternatives to the individual license, such as institutional licensure.

INSTITUTIONAL LICENSURE

Because so many health workers function in institutional settings, one suggested alternative to individual licensure is institutional licensure. *Institutional licensure* is a process by which a state government regulates health institutions; it has existed for more than 35 years. Usually, requirements for establishing and operating a health facility have been concerned primarily with such matters as administration, accounting requirements, equipment specifications, structural integrity, sanitation, and fire safety. In some cases, there are also minimal standards of square footage per bed and minimal nursing staff requirements. The issue in the "expanded" institutional licensure dispute is whether personnel credentialing or licensing should be part of the institution's responsibility under general guidelines of the state licensing authority.

There are various interpretations of just what institutional licensing means and how it could or should be implemented. The general idea, according to Nathan Hershey, who originated the concept, is that since health care institutions are held accountable for the actions of their employees, they should be given the responsibility of regulating them. The state licensing agency would establish certain basic standards of education and experience, but the institution would decide just what kind of position an individual could hold. An example is that of an RN returning to work after 10 or more years. Her/his RN license would not count. Instead, an aide position would be given, then an LPN position, and gradually a staff nurse level position when there was proof that skills had been regained and there was familiarity with professional and technological advances. In fact, this represents the ultimate in decentralization, allowing the organization to use personnel in varying ways, theoretically as long as safety is assured and some very broad guidelines are respected. Hershey was, then and later, rather evasive as to the place of the physician in this new credentialing picture, implying that the current practice of hospital staff review was a pioneer effort along the same lines and might as well continue to function. However, he did list as logical sites for institutional licensure organizations providing health services, such as hospitals, nursing homes, physicians' offices, clinics, and the all-inclusive "et cetera."

The advantages for the employer are obvious: potential financial savings and almost total control, including the ability to place employees where and when they would be most useful, without needing to consider individual licensing laws. For instance, an aide trained on the job might do procedures that now only RNs are permitted to do. This may or may not give the public cheaper care, but it certainly will not be better. The disadvantages for the licensed person are great. Particularly for nursing, it raises the specter of a return to the corrupted apprentice system of early hospital nursing in the United States. Probably a hospital's own personnel would be used as teacher-preceptors. Who then would do their job? How would they be compensated? How long would "students" be expected to function in their current positions with their current salaries while they "practice" the new role? And with what kind of supervision? What kind of testing programs would exist for each level? Testing by whom? With what kinds of standards? Such sliding positions might well cut personnel costs, but might they not also indenture workers instead of freeing them with new mobility?

Problems of criteria for standards are obvious. Instead of making interstate mobility easier, institutional licensure would more likely limit even interinstitutional mobility. A worker could qualify for position X in institution A, with absolutely no guarantee that this would be acceptable to institution B.

It is true that many of these practices already exist in hospitals, but it hardly seems progressive to make an unsatisfactory system legal. Expecting the state licensing agency to prevent abuse is overly optimistic. The number of inadequate and even dangerous caregiving facilities, supposedly inspected by the state but still in existence, is evidence of the problems in assuring even minimum quality. Checking who does what how well will be almost impossible, resulting in one more paper tiger— inspection by paperwork.

NURSE LICENSURE COMPACT

The licensing of nurses is a demonstration of the police power of the state, and thus handled on a state by state basis. This has become burdensome in recent years because of practice models, such as telenursing, which raise questions of practice across state lines, and the growing presence of multistate health care systems. In response to these circumstances, the National Council of State Boards of Nursing (NCSBN) developed a mutual recognition system of nurse licensure. This system is largely based on the driver's license model, requiring a *primary* license in the state of the licensee's residence. That individual could then practice in any other (*remote*) state that had enacted legislation authorizing the Nurse Licensure Compact.[1] The one-license concept could provide a number of advantages, including:

- reduces barriers to interstate practice
- improves tracking for disciplinary purposes
- promotes cost effectiveness and simplicity for the licensee
- acts as an unduplicated listing for licensed nurses
- facilitates interstate commerce

In practicing in a remote state, the licensee is subject to that state's practice laws and discipline. So, even though practice rights and responsibilities may vary state to state, this need not serve as an impediment to entering into an interstate pact. However, it is expected that the process which precedes finalization of any such agreement would promote some movement toward standardization. Since 1998, the compact has included registered nurses (RNs) and licensed practical or vocational nurses (LPN/VNs). On August 16, 2002, the NCSBN Delegate Assembly approved the adoption of model language for a licensure compact for advanced practice registered nurses (APRNs). Only those

Exhibit 11.1 Nurse Licensure Compact Implementation (as at February 9, 2005)

Compact states	Implementation date
Arizona	July 1, 2002
Arkansas	July 1, 2000
Delaware	July 1, 2000
Idaho	July 1, 2001
Iowa	July 1, 2000
Maine	July 1, 2001
Maryland	July 1, 1999
Mississippi	July 1, 2001
Nebraska	January 1, 2001
New Jersey	TBD (Signed by Governor)
New Mexico	January 1, 2004
North Carolina	July 1, 2000
North Dakota	January 1, 2004
South Dakota	January 1, 2001
Tennessee	July 1, 2003
Texas	January 1, 2000
Utah	January 1, 2000
Virginia	January 1, 2005
Wisconsin	January 1, 2000

Source: http://www.ncsbn.org/nlc/rnlpvncompact_mutual_recognition_state.asp

states that have adopted the RN and LPN/VN Nurse Licensure Compact may implement a compact for APRNs. On March 15, 2004, Utah was the first state to enter the APRN Compact.[2]

In the years since the introduction of the multistate recognition concept (nurse licensure compact), the ANA has continued to advocate for credentialing systems that best support both the needs of the consumer and the profession. The ANA had voiced concern about a loss of control over disciplinary actions, the potential loss of revenue to boards of nursing, the threat to the confidentiality of those nurses who are investigated but not necessarily charged, the erosion of states' rights, and the ability to move nurses in large numbers across state borders to dilute the effectiveness of job actions.[3] Many of these criticisms are being addressed. The reality is that multistate recognition is achieving significant success. By February 2005, 19 states had implemented the nurse licensure compact (see Exhibit 11.1 for details).

CERTIFICATION

Certification is a credential awarded to an *individual* as a mark of competence or specialization, and not just safe practice. Physicians with a general (plenary) license use certification to differentiate competency as a specialist. Traditionally, certification has been defined as a voluntary, nongovernmental credential. The agency that certifies is usually made up of experts or peers in a particular area of practice. This is no longer consistently true. Government agencies have begun to use this term more loosely in a number of situations where they either conduct the entire credentialing process or accept some private sector evidence as part of that process. We have Certified Home Health Aides (CHHAs) and Certified Nursing Assistants (CNAs) who are prepared in educational programs approved by the state, and the educational program is obligated to verify the safety of their practice. Many Boards of Nursing accept advanced practice certification as one criterion to qualify for privileges as an advanced practice nurse. In summary, neither terms nor processes are sacred or even stable today. Certifications available to nurses are included in Appendix 5.

There are additionally a range of certifications which are exclusively available to nurses with a baccalaureate degree and others that are available to any nurse. The important point is that to function as an advanced practice nurse the certification is mandatory, and the educational requirement is the master's degree. Certification may not be necessary for other nurses to practice legally, although they may be disadvantaged in the marketplace because consumers, hospitals, insurers, and managed care plans often look for certification as an assurance of quality. This private certification can be described as serving solely informational purposes, a sort of "seal of approval" from the nongovernmental board that grants it. It gives the consumer an opportunity to make more informed decisions, in that certification indicates that the practitioner has voluntarily met certain standards that other caregivers have not. Additionally, all certifiers have a recertification mechanism.

Finally, there is concern when certification is done by the professional organization that also accredits the educational program the candidate must complete in order to qualify for certification, or when the certifier also establishes the practice standards. Clearly, either situation gives the occupation inappropriate control. Professions have gradually separated these functions into independent entities. In 1991, the American Board of Nursing Specialties (ABNS) was established to set standards for the formal recognition of professional nursing specialty certification programs. Sixteen certification boards compose the membership of ABNS, collectively representing more than 50 percent of the total number of registered nurses currently certified in the United States.[4]

ACCREDITATION

Accreditation is defined as the process by which an agency or organization evaluates and recognizes an *institution* or *program* of study as meeting certain predetermined criteria or standards. Both educational programs and institutions and health care institutions often seek accreditation because it is presumably a mark of excellence, that is, it indicates that higher standards are maintained than those required by the government. Quite often, accreditation is necessary for health care facilities, as a criterion for federal reimbursement and to have medical residency programs. Educational institutions find accreditation required to receive federal or state funds for scholarships or other purposes. In these days of consumerism, accreditation is an attraction to the public.

This commentary will reveal to the reader that both accreditation and certification have begun to serve a quasi-governmental purpose. And it is those programs that are primarily described in this chapter. The Magnet status, awarded by the American Nurses Credentialing Center (ANCC), recognizes the quality of nursing service within the context of the total organization. In a more focused fashion, it serves as an accreditation vehicle. ANCC is discussed in more detail in Chapter 13.

The term accreditation is often used by state boards of nursing as they approve nursing education programs. In this instance, it does not signify a standard of excellence, but indicates that graduates have completed a program which permits them to sit for the licensing exam. This approval is mandatory. We are not speaking to this public function here, but to accreditation as a voluntary mechanism.

The major accrediting organization for diploma, associate degree, and practical nursing education programs is the NLN Accrediting Commission (NLNAC). Baccalaureate and graduate programs in nursing are accredited by both the NLNAC and the Commission on Collegiate Nursing Education (CCNE). The issues involved here relate in part to the accrediting process and in part to who should do the accrediting.

Standards are set by the profession and the degree to which a program or institution conforms with these standards is determined through the accreditation process, which includes significant consumer input. By way of example, standards for nursing practice are established by the ANA, but they are applied to the practice of an individual nurse by the American Nurses Credentialing Center (ANCC) in the process of awarding certification. It is required that the accrediting agency be autonomous and those who make credentialing decisions be free of conflict of interest and protected from any external coercion that might affect those decisions.

In most situations, the accreditor maintains a close relationship with the professional association that created it. There are philosophical and power issues: should the NLN (and NLNAC), which was given the responsibility at the reorganization of the major nursing organizations in

1952, continue to be a force in educational standard setting and accreditation in nursing? Should the American Association of Colleges of Nursing (AACN), which represents the interests of the academic deans and directors and is associated with the CCNE, become the major force? There is also the obvious matter of control and income. Considerable income is derived from activities related to accreditation: consulting, and the accreditation process itself. These resources provide attractive incentives to enter the business of accreditation or to participate in an allied association which develops standards. A final issue is the fact that the NLNAC offers a comprehensive service with all programs having the ability to seek accreditation under the same auspices. The CCNE is only interested in baccalaureate and higher degree programs, thus sacrificing this consolidation.

As noted in Chapter 3, the JCAHO accredits health care institutions and agencies. Its activities clash with nursing in at least one area. In 1965, the Community Health Accreditation Program (CHAP) was created as a joint venture between the American Public Health Association (APHA) and the National League for Nursing (NLN). These organizations brought to fruition the futuristic view that accreditation was the needed mechanism for recognizing excellence in community health practice. In 1988, CHAP became a separately incorporated, nonprofit subsidiary of the NLN. In 2001, it was spun off by the NLN and became an independent, nonprofit corporation.[5] Both groups require a self-study report and send a team for a site visit, but CHAP's visits are unannounced. CHAP, considered by many as the only consumer-oriented health care accreditation body, has an interdisciplinary board. Perhaps because of this, and its high standards, in 1992 CHAP was the first home care accrediting group to be awarded "deemed status" by DHHS. This means that instead of state surveys, CHAP has regulatory authorization to survey agencies providing home health and hospice services, to determine whether they meet the Medicare conditions for reimbursement. The JCAHO has board membership by organization, with AMA and AHA having the majority of the 21 seats, and fewer held by the American College of Physicians, the American College of Surgeons, and the American Dental Association. There are five public members. In 1992, the nursing community was awarded a seat on the JCAHO board, and traditionally one of the AHA seats is filled by a nurse. By the end of 1992, the JCAHO home health accreditation had also been awarded "deemed status" by DHHS.

Accreditation is not a simple process. Certain fees are required, and the program must complete a self-study report. If the report indicates that the criteria have been met, there is a site visit by a team of peers whose work it is to clarify, verify, and amplify the self-study and report back to the board who decides on the credential. After consideration by the board, recommendations are made to accredit for a certain period of time or not, a decision that may be appealed. (This is a very brief overview; changes in procedure are made periodically.)

Besides the criticisms of accreditation in general, another in nursing is that a university or college already goes through a regional accreditation process and that a nursing accreditation is duplicative and costly, a point that is also being made by academic administrators about other kinds of specialty accreditation.

SUNSET LAWS AND OTHER PUBLIC ACTIONS

Besides considering alternatives, improving the licensure process has become a national mandate. Although the speed of the action taken has varied from state to state, steps taken almost universally at one level or another include adding consumers and sometimes other related health professionals to each board, giving more attention to disciplinary procedures, and developing more sophisticated testing procedures. In a number of states, boards have been consolidated, sometimes under committees of lay people (or at least a majority of consumers), who make the decisions about licensing, with the individual boards acting in an advisory capacity. Although one reason given is improved efficiency, some nurses fear that this is an indirect approach to institutional licensure because these reorganizations tend to weaken nursing's control over its practice.

For some professions, improving the licensure laws to protect the public was a new experience. A motivating factor was the enactment of "sunset laws" that require the periodic reexamination of licensing agencies to determine whether particular boards or activities should be eliminated. Most of the states have now enacted such laws, a result of a lobbying campaign by Common Cause, a consumer group, to bring about legislative and executive branch oversight of regulating boards and agencies of all kinds. Common Cause identified ten principles to be followed, including a time schedule. An important component was that an evaluation was to allow for public input, as well as that of the boards and occupations involved. Consolidation and "responsible pruning" were encouraged. Although the review would be done by appropriate legislative and executive committees, safeguards were to be built in to prevent arbitrary termination of boards and agencies. These principles are generally adhered to, but states do vary in their management of sunset reviews. If a sunset law is in effect, the data and justification for existence are a joint staff–board responsibility, although the professional organizations are also usually helpful.

By 1985, most nursing boards had undergone sunset reviews, and the new or amended laws usually reflected changes in practice and the environment. Most practice acts have broadened their scope of practice, added consumers to their boards, and sometimes required evidence of current competence through various means. State boards have given increased attention to removing and/or rehabilitating incompetent nurses. Nurses in the field have continued to improve techniques of peer evaluation, implement standards of practice, and encourage voluntary continuing education (CE).

THE GRANDFATHER CLAUSE

One concern about mandatory laws is that those already practicing in the field will be abruptly removed and deprived of their livelihood. This is, however, untrue because mandatory laws are forced, for constitutional as well as political reasons, to include a grandfather clause. A *grandfather* or *waiver clause* is a standard feature when a licensure law is enacted or a current law is repealed and a new law enacted.

The grandfather clause allows persons to continue to practice the profession/occupation when new qualifications are made law. Although the concept goes back to post-Civil War days, it is also related to the Fifth and Fourteenth Amendments of the Constitution. The U.S. Supreme Court has repeatedly ruled that the license to practice a profession/occupation is a property right and that the Fourteenth Amendment extends the due process requirement to state laws. Many nurses currently licensed were protected by the grandfather clause when a new law was passed or new requirements were made, although most probably never realized it. For instance, when various states began to require psychiatric nursing as a condition of licensure, those who had not had those courses in their educational programs did not forfeit licensure.

When the grandfather clause is enacted in relation to mandatory licensure, those who can produce evidence that they practiced as, say, a PN, if applying for LPN status, must be granted a license. However, grandfathering does not guarantee employment. Thus, some employers chose not to employ "waivered" LPNs, just as they had not employed them as unlicensed practitioners.

ASSURANCES OF CONTINUED COMPETENCY

The rapidly changing scientific and technological environment has given new meaning to the image of the health care professions as dynamic. It is no longer a simple responsibility to stay on "top" of your field.

Concerns over the continuing competence of provider professionals are not new, but both licensing boards and the professions are being pressured by consumers to provide assurances about their constituencies. Continuing education, either mandatory or voluntary, has served as an interim measure, but its efficacy has been largely undemonstrated. There are other options, but they are largely talk and untested: self-assessment, readministration of a licensure exam, peer review, simulations, individual portfolios, to name a few.

This whole area has been moved center stage by pressures from the Citizen Advocacy Center (CAC).[6] The literature on the subject raises many questions. The RN goes through inherent changes from the point of new graduate to established provider of services. Where on this developmental continuum do we find the measure of competence? What is the cost of these assurances and who should bear that cost? Is competence the actual ability to perform, the cognitive artfulness, or both?

One particularly sensible suggestion is that candidates for reassessment be chosen through a random selection process, and/or that "triggers" be used to identify practitioners who merit more careful scrutiny. Such "triggers" may be recent disciplinary action, return to work after a significant hiatus, independent or isolated practice, multiple job changes over a short period, or a radical shift in a specialty area of practice. This is an area for careful thought.

NCSBN AND ANA

The National Council of State Boards of Nursing (NCSBN) and ANA represent nursing in regard to licensure. Neither has authority in this matter, but they are a significant influence in shaping the public policy agenda. The NCSBN represents the state boards of nursing and ANA represents the profession. There will be an inevitable difference of opinion between them over suggested form and language for state legislation. Definitions and models presented by the state boards will reflect nursing as it is practiced today, while the professional association is committed to presenting nursing as it should be, in the hope of moving the profession to a more ideal future. Further, the state boards have the responsibility to award credentials, and thus should be insulated from the peer group (the professional association) that sets the standard for practice. The same principles apply here as with separating certifying and accrediting bodies from their standard-setting constituencies. The NCSBN and ANA enjoy a rich liaison relationship and aim for a broad consensus on issues, realizing that they will disagree on detail. The more consistency between the policies and statements of these groups, the more the real and ideal mirror one another.

Over the years both ANA and NCSBN have provided suggested legislation/model practice acts to serve as a guide to nurses, state nurses' associations, state boards of nursing, legislators, the public, and anyone else who is interested in considering revisions to their nursing practice act. Model administrative rules usually accompany the legislative models, since the detail is worked through in regulations (administrative rules) which operationalize the law. In recent years both ANA and NCSBN have proven their sophistication, integrity, and the desire to move closer to speaking with one voice.

The emphasis on states' rights in this country makes legislative conformity difficult. For instance, in 1986, the North Dakota Board of Nursing put into effect revised administrative rules for nursing education programs. Graduates entering programs after January 1, 1987, must have completed an approved nursing program that awards the appropriate academic degree in order to be eligible for licensure. For the RN, this is the baccalaureate; for the LPN, the associate degree. The North Dakota law does not allow equivalency preparation in determining eligibility for licensure, so licensing for out-of-state graduates not fulfilling those criteria has had to be worked out.

CONTENT OF NURSING PRACTICE ACTS

Because each state law differs to a degree in its content, it is important to have available a copy of the law of the state in which you practice and, if possible, the regulations that spell out how the law is carried out. You can get these from the state board or agency in the state government that has copies of laws for distribution, and frequently they are available on-line. The language in all laws often seems stilted because the laws are written in legal terms, but the following sections can help you understand the key points.

Most nursing practice acts have basically the same major components, although not necessarily in the same order: definition of nursing, requirements for licensure, exemption from licensure, grounds for revocation of the license, provision for reciprocity (or endorsement) for persons licensed in other states, creation of a board of nursing, responsibilities of the board, and penalties for practicing without a license. Only the RN (not the LPN) licensure law or component of the nursing practice act is discussed in the following sections.

MANDATORY AND PERMISSIVE LAWS

Enactment of nurse licensure laws was one of the primary purposes of ANA at its inception (as described in Chapter 2). The first state laws were permissive. The first mandatory nursing practice act was enacted in New York in 1938, but it was not put into effect until 1947. One of the dangers of permissive licensing is that schools with poor curricula and inadequate clinical experience produce workers who can legally nurse, although they are potentially dangerous practitioners.

As of 1991, all states had mandatory licensure laws for professional and practical nurses. However, some states are loose in their interpretation of *mandatory*. States that have global exemption clauses in licensure laws stating that almost anyone can be a nurse, providing that there is some kind of supervision, are sometimes seen as permissive regardless of a mandatory clause.

DEFINITION AND SCOPE OF PRACTICE

The definition of *nursing* in the licensure law determines both the legal responsibilities and the scope of practice of nurses. Inevitably, the definition of nursing in all nursing practice acts is stated in terms that are quite broad. This is generally frustrating to nurses who turn to the definition to find out if they are practicing legally, because it does not spell out specific procedures or activities. Often such activities are not even spelled out in the regulations of the laws, and require specific interpretation by the board. A broad definition is preferable because changes in health care and nursing practice often occur more rapidly than a law can be changed, and the amending process can be long and complex. If particular activities were named, the nurse would be limited to those listed. Not only would the list be overwhelmingly long, but it is also possible that any new technique performed by a nurse would require an amendment to the law. An occasional state law does specify certain procedures but always includes the phrase "not limited to."

A practicing nurse soon finds that the nursing functions taught in an educational program may differ from those expected by an employer. The differences may be small and caused by variations in the settings of nursing care. Nursing in a medical center may require knowing more sophisticated techniques or assuming more comprehensive responsibilities in nursing care. Sometimes, whether in a large or small agency, there are procedures performed that the nurse has not learned. If the nurse has not practiced for some time, this is even more likely to happen. In other cases, the responsibilities expected in the nursing role are not in nursing care but in clerical and administrative tasks. Although this may not be desirable, it is not illegal. What concerns nurses is whether the patient-oriented care expected in the employment situation is legal or in the domain of another health profession. Many of the activities in health care overlap. A common example might be the administration of drugs, which could be done by the physician, RN, LPN, and various technicians in other hospital departments if related to a diagnostic procedure or treatment. Yet dispensing a drug from the hospital pharmacy, still done by many nursing supervisors at times when no pharmacist is on duty, is in most states a violation of the pharmacy licensing law.

Obviously, one of the greatest concerns for nurses is the possible violation of the Medical Practice Act. Nurses have gradually been performing ever more of the technical procedures that once belonged exclusively to medicine, but often these are delegated willingly by physicians. Whether nurses are always properly prepared to understand and perform them well is seldom questioned. However, as some nurses have assumed more comprehensive overall responsibilities in the care, cure, and coordination of patient care, questions have been raised by both nurses and physicians. Some are resistant to such changes; others are supportive but concerned about the legality of such acts. There are few data on nurses being disciplined for practicing medicine without a license. It should be noted that the boundaries between the professions do change over time, and that where there are questions, the board of nursing should be asked for an interpretation. An official change in public policy is not frequently needed. In the now classic DHEW report *Extending the Scope of Nursing Practice*, there is a statement that the identical act or procedure "may be the practice of medicine when carried out by a physician and the practice of nursing when carried out by the nurse."

This same report stated that there are no legal barriers to extending the scope of practice because the statutory laws governing nursing practice (the licensing laws) are broad enough to permit such extension, provided that the nurse has the proper skills and necessary knowledge of the underlying science. The report did acknowledge that at times there have been declaratory decisions of the courts about some aspect of nursing which is not included in statutes. When this happens, the profession should consider whether the statutes need to be changed.[7] That is exactly what has happened.

Governmental regulation of specialty practice has been historically opposed by leadership in both nursing and medicine. Internal regulation has been overwhelmingly favored, based on the clinical complexity of specialized practice and the fact that the science advances through research conducted in specialty areas. The reasoning continues that, for the discipline to advance and change at a pace commensurate with the science, the specialty edge must remain unencumbered by public policy and the inevitable bureaucracy it attracts.

Logical or not, it was too late for nursing to hold to this classic standard. Since almost all states already addressed advanced practice in public policy, it was a question of achieving some standardization and creating harmony between form and function. State boards of nursing held the formal authority and most were requiring a nationally recognized certification in the specialty as a minimum. They had already begun to intermingle the domains of professional and public recognition.

The latest model practice acts have achieved more consistency in language. Both versions include clear delegatory language. ANA uses bolder words about medical diagnosis and treatment, and introduces the responsibility for research. The NCSBN is clearer on the collaborative nature of the role. The title Advanced Practice Registered Nurse (APRN) is protected in both renditions. This goes beyond title protection, and verifies the existence of nurses who bring a specialized knowledge and skill to the public. Both also accept the umbrella title of APRN as inclusive of NP, CNS, CRNA, and CNM. Further, there is common agreement that detail has to exist in public policy about the rights and responsibilities of APRNs, and their educational background. Though the requirement for physician collaboration/joint practice/supervision remains in many states, it is absent in both the ANA and NCSBN model acts.[8] [The terms APRN and advanced practice nurse (APN) are used interchangeably in this book.]

Recognition of APRNs in public policy represents significant progress. The earliest approaches to formalizing the expanding role of the nurse were joint statements between nurses', medical, and hospital associations. These statements offered no legal protection, but documented mutual acceptance of an evolving pattern of practice. Lawyers found such statements helpful in mounting a defense on behalf of both nurses and physicians if their joint practices were challenged. Both ANA and NCSBN agreed that the board of nursing should be the sole authority to regulate advanced practice, but multiple board (nursing, medicine, pharmacy for the most part) involvement has resulted in some states probably finding justification in those early joint statements.

Though there has been some significant movement toward agreement about advanced practice, some disagreements continue. There was not complete comfort that the certification process as provided by professional groups guaranteed competency, and guarantees of competency became the driving force. In 1994 at their annual meeting, the NCSBN membership called to move forward and investigate the development of a national certification mechanism for NPs under its own aegis. This ignited a flurry of activity to verify the credibility of the profession's certification mechanisms. This included scrutiny of the psychometric measures of adequacy as well as reconsideration of the role of expert opinion and role delineation (examination of the actual manner in which APNs practice) studies in constructing the examinations. The expectations of NCSBN must have been adequately addressed, given that in 1995 the NCSBN membership tabled their intention to develop their own examinations for NPs in favor of working toward consensus with the major existing certifying bodies.[9] This remains an area to monitor carefully.

Despite this rather tumultuous history, the legal authority of APNs has continued to expand each year. APNs have gained tremendous legislatively sanctioned rights to diagnose, prescribe, and be reimbursed. Today, there are almost 175,000 APNs. They have title protection in every state, and in 27 states the board of nursing has the sole authority in scope of practice with no statutory or regulatory requirement for physician collaboration. In 14 states, APNs have the authority to prescribe, including controlled substances, independent of any required physician involvement in the process.[10]

Currently, the greatest differences between the ANA and NCSBN documents for model legislation are in the preferred vehicle for change. ANA relies on administrative statements for detail, while NCSBN is either silent on the vehicle or looks for codification in statutes. The ANA addresses other issues (the impaired nurse, prescriptive authority) in separate acts. ANA's caution is to avoid opening the nursing practice act wherever possible, and to keep practice act language broad, using administrative statements or rule making for amplification. The intent is both to protect the practice act and to allow easier routes for change where it is necessary.

CREATION OF A BOARD OF NURSING

The name of the state administrative agency responsible for nursing varies from state to state, as does the number of members. *Board of Nursing* is used by the NCSBN. The majority of states now have consumers or other professionals, as well as nurses, as members. These are appointed by the governor, with or without nursing input. Board size ranges from 5 to 19 appointed members, who make policy. Staff employed by the board carry out the day-to-day activities.

RESPONSIBILITIES OF THE BOARD OF NURSING

The major responsibility of a board is to see that the nursing practice act is carried out. This involves establishing rules and regulations to implement the broad terms in the law itself and setting minimum standards of practice. Usual responsibilities include approval of educational programs for nursing and development of criteria for approval (minimum standards) which address the clinical placements used for educational purposes, curriculum, faculty, and so on; evaluating the personal and educational qualifications of applicants for licensure; determining by examination applicants' competence to practice nursing; issuing licenses to qualified applicants; and disciplining those who violate the law or are found to be unfit to practice nursing, sometimes holding hearings. (Investigations and hearings are often conducted by another arm of the state government.)

Other responsibilities include developing standards for continuing competency of licensed practitioners; issuing limited licenses to those who cannot practice the full scope of nursing, perhaps owing to a handicap; interpreting the scope of practice as codified in the statutes; and developing policy for other purposes such as prescriptive authority, pronouncement of death, and so on, to the extent that the law allows. Nursing boards may hold educational programs, collect data, and cooperate in various ways with other nursing boards or the boards of other disciplines. If they operate under an overall board, certain administrative responsibilities will be carried out on a central level.

The power of the board should not be underestimated. For instance, it was simply by changing their regulations that the North Dakota Board changed requirements for RN and LPN licensure.

REQUIREMENTS FOR LICENSURE

Licensure is based on fulfilling certain requirements. The following points are usually included:

1. The applicant must have completed an educational program in a state-approved school of nursing and received a diploma or degree from that program; usually the school must send the student's transcript. Some states ask for evidence of high-school education. There is some legislative pressure that the applicant not be required to have completed the program, particularly if the uncompleted courses are in a nonnursing area such as liberal arts. Neither ANA nor NCSBN approves of this.

2. The applicant must pass an examination given by the board. This examination is currently the NCLEX-RN, developed under the direction of the NCSBN and given in every state. The examination is now offered using a computerized adaptive testing approach known as CAT.

3. Some states require evidence of good physical and mental health, but this is not recommended by either ANA or NCSBN. Actual practice varies a great deal from state to state. Handicapped students have been admitted, have graduated, and have taken state boards in some states; in others, this opportunity has been denied. Court cases can result.

4. Most states maintain a statement that the applicant must be of good moral character, as determined by the licensing board, but this, too, is impractical. The Model Act suggests terminology that refers to acts that are grounds for board disciplinary action if the nurse were licensed.

5. A fee must be paid for admission to the examination. This varies considerably among states.

6. A temporary license may be issued to a graduate of an approved program pending the results of the first licensure exam.

7. Demonstrating competence in English is required. It has been declared unconstitutional to make requirements of age, citizenship, and residence.

ENDORSEMENT/RECIPROCITY

Nurses have more mobility than any other licensed health professionals because of the use of a national standardized examination. However, there may be other requirements to fulfill for the state in which licensure is sought, and proof must be submitted that the original license is in good standing.

If all requirements are satisfactory, the nurse is granted a license without retaking the state board examination. A fee is required for this process of endorsement. Endorsement is not the same as *reciprocity*; the latter means acceptance of a licensee by one state only if the other state does likewise. This is the model of the *nurse licensure compact*, discussed earlier in this chapter. Currently, 19 states have nurse licensure compacts, which allow reciprocity, and all but one are functioning in 2005.[11]

RENEWAL OF THE LICENSE

Until the early 1970s, nursing licenses were renewed simply by sending the renewal fee when notified, usually every two years. For nurses licensed in more than one state, as long as the license was not revoked in any state, the process was the same. Usually the form asked for information about employment and the highest degree (and still does), but no attempt was made to determine if the nurse was competent. At about that time there was increased concern about the current competency of practicing health professionals, and an estimate was made that perhaps 5 percent of all health professionals were not competent for some reason. One outcome was the enactment of a mandatory continuing education requirement in a number of licensure laws; that is, a nurse's license would not be renewed unless she or he showed evidence of continuing education. A number of health disciplines have such legislation, but not all requirements are well enforced.

Forms of continuing education accepted by states include various formal academic studies in institutions of higher learning; college extension courses and studies; grand rounds in the health care setting; home study programs; in-service education; institutes; lectures; seminars; workshops; audiovisual learning systems, including educational television, audiovisual cassettes, tapes, and records with self-study packets; challenge examinations for a course or program; self-learning systems such as community service, controlled independent study, delivery of a paper, or preparation and participation in a panel; preparation and publication of articles, monographs, books, and so on; and research. The required number of hours of continuing education or continuing education contact hours varies considerably among states. *No law requires formal education directed toward advanced degrees.* In fact, although additional formal education is acceptable, the emphasis is on continuous, *updated competence in practice.* The reader is referred to Chapter 5 for an extended discussion on continuing education.

Objections to mandatory continuing education focus on the difficulty of assessing true learning; the question of whether learning can be forced (attendance does not mean retention of knowledge, change in behavior, or application of what was learned to practice); the danger of breeding mediocrity; the lack of research on the effectiveness of continuing education in relation to performance; limitation of resources, particularly in rural areas; the cost to nurses; the cost to government; the usual rigidity of governmental regulations; the problems in record keeping; and the lack of accreditation or evaluation procedures for many continuing education programs.

In 2004, 24 boards of nursing addressed maintenance of competency through mandatory continuing education.[12] Other boards no longer make it mandatory because they see a weak correlation between competency and continuing education, still others are actively exploring more creative options, and some state boards never imposed the requirement. The situation is just as tentative for other health care providers. Most state boards of nursing now have continuing education requirements for reentry into active practice. The issue is far from resolved. The trend toward mandatory continuing education has slightly accelerated, as has the demand for continued competence.

EXEMPTIONS FROM LICENSURE

This may also be called an *exception clause*. Generally exempted from RN licensure are basic students in a nursing program; anyone furnishing nursing assistance in an emergency; anyone licensed in another state and caring for a patient temporarily in the state involved; anyone employed by the U.S. government as a nurse (Veterans Administration, public health, or armed services); any legally qualified nurse recruited by the Red Cross during a disaster; anyone caring for the sick if care is performed in connection with the practice of religious tenets of any church; anyone giving incidental care in a family (home) situation; and any RN or LPN from another state engaged in consultation as long as no direct care is given.

In all these cases, the person cannot claim to be an RN of the state concerned. Over strong nursing protests, some states have also incorporated in the exemptions nursing services of attendants in state institutions, if supervised by nurses or doctors, as well as other kinds of nursing assistants under various circumstances. This, of course, weakens the mandatory aspect of the law.

GROUNDS FOR REVOCATION OF LICENSURE

The board has the right to *revoke or suspend* any nurse's license or otherwise discipline the licensee, and reinstate a license if the conditions are corrected. The reasons most commonly found in practice acts for revoking a license are acts that might directly endanger the public, such as practicing while one's ability is impaired by alcohol, drugs, or physical or mental disability; being addicted to or dependent on alcohol or other habit-forming drugs or being a habitual user of certain drugs; and practicing with incompetence or negligence or beyond the scope of practice. Other reasons are obtaining a license fraudulently; being convicted of a felony or crime involving moral turpitude or refusing to deny the charge (accepting a plea of *nolo contendere*); practicing while the license is suspended or revoked; aiding and abetting a nonlicensed person to perform activities requiring a license; and committing unprofessional conduct or immoral acts as defined by the board. The refusal to provide service to a person because of race, color, creed, or national origin has also been added in some states.

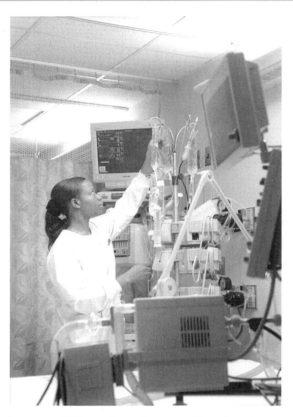

It is each nurse's responsibility to honestly assess his or her competence in clinical practice. This is what the individual license is all about. (*Courtesy of Robert Wood Johnson University Hospital, New Brunswick, New Jersey*)

The most common reasons that nurses lose their licenses are the same as those that apply to physicians—drug use, abuse, or theft. Substance abuse has become a growing concern among professionals. The exact extent of the problem is unknown, but there are a growing number of disciplinary actions involving substance abuse. Support programs have been developed by boards of nursing and state nurses' associations. Despite what has been the establishment of a substantial number of peer assistance programs, little is known about the numbers entering or leaving treatment and the degree of recidivism. Almost every state provides services for impaired nurses, but relatively few have enacted diversion legislation. The diversion concept provides the impaired nurse with immunity from disciplinary action if there has been no harm to patients, and requires voluntary entry into treatment.

The license may need to be voluntarily surrendered, but in some instances a limited license is issued after investigation of the case by the board.

As is true in obtaining or renewing licenses, a nurse can also lose his or her license because of physical or mental impairment. Legal blindness is the most common physical condition involved, but there are many exceptions, especially since the passage of the Americans with Disabilities Act (Chapter 10).

With the exception of substance abuse, it is rare that specific conditions for revocation or suspension of license are detailed in legislation or even regulations. Rather, disciplinary action may be authorized by the ubiquitous "unprofessional behavior" clause. A number of states already have regulations defining unprofessional conduct, and depending on how the licensure laws are structured, the regulations may define unprofessional behavior as it applies to all licensed health professionals (New York) or may be written into each separate law.

The courts have also played a major role in shaping interpretation. They have been opposed to trivializing unprofessional conduct and have held to the criteria of behavior that intellectually or morally creates jeopardy through practice. An example exists where the District Court in Nebraska reversed the Board of Nursing's denial of license finding that the plaintiff may be difficult to get along with and resistive to directions, but not unprofessional. Criteria used by the state of Utah date back to 1991, but remain especially clear and provide a good example:[13]

1. Failing to utilize appropriate judgment in administering safe nursing practice based on the level of nursing for which the individual is licensed.
2. Failing to exercise technical competence in carrying out nursing care.
3. Failing to follow policies or procedures defined in the practice situation to safeguard patient care.
4. Failing to safeguard the patient's dignity and right to privacy.
5. Violating the confidentiality of information or knowledge concerning the patient.
6. Verbally or physically abusing patients.
7. Performing any nursing techniques or procedures without proper education and preparation.
8. Performing procedures beyond the authorized scope of the level of nursing and/or health care for which the individual is licensed.
9. Intentional manipulation or misuse of drug supplies, narcotics, or patients' records.
10. Falsifying patients' records or intentionally charting incorrectly.
11. Appropriating medications, supplies, or personal items of the patient or agency.

12. Violating state or federal laws relative to drugs.
13. Falsifying records submitted to a government agency.
14. Intentionally committing any act that adversely affects the physical or psychosocial welfare of the patient.
15. Delegating nursing care, functions, tasks, and/or responsibilities to others contrary to the laws governing nursing and/or to the detriment of patient safety.
16. Failing to exercise appropriate supervision over persons who are authorized to practice only under the supervision of the licensed professional.
17. Leaving a nursing assignment without properly notifying appropriate personnel.
18. Failing to report, through the proper channels, facts known to the individual regarding the incompetent, unethical, or illegal practice of any licensed health care professional.

The absence of very specific language in statutes or regulations is purposeful to avoid foreclosure on unanticipated types of behavior. This problem is sometimes resolved by using the phrase "not limited to," but if the legislature has a particular concern, this may be written into the law. Some states have also adopted the ANA standards of practice as criteria for incompetence.

A particular problem in both statutory and regulating language concerns such terms as *moral, ethical, and moral turpitude*, since these can be interpreted in various ways. Model acts use phrases such as "has engaged in any act inconsistent with standards of nursing practice as defined by Board Rules and Regulations" and "a crime in any jurisdiction that relates adversely to the practice of nursing or to the ability to practice nursing."

Another issue is what a nurse should do about reporting incompetence or unprofessional conduct on the part of physicians or other health professionals. Because the nurses' code of ethics requires that she or he safeguard the patient, incompetent or unprofessional practitioners should be reported. Most surveys indicate that a large percentage of nurses would take some sort of action, usually speaking with the doctor, head nurse, or supervisor, if the patient was endangered by medical action. Few would report the physician to a peer review or licensing board. In part, this is because they fear a lawsuit. All but a few states have laws giving immunity from civil action to any person who reports to a peer review board if there is no malice, but this does not preclude being sued, even though malice is very difficult to prove. In New York, a statute was enacted requiring physicians to report other physicians' misconduct on penalty of being cited for unprofessional conduct themselves; nurses and others are also encouraged to report such misconduct. (Some have interpreted the law as requiring such reporting by all licensed professionals.) Other states have similar statutes, including states requiring nurses to report nurses. There is another problem; some nurses who have reported a physician have either been dismissed from their jobs or harassed, a situation more difficult to resolve. Whistle-blower laws can provide some protection here and are discussed in Chapter 15. A supportive working environment can also make a difference.

Although the law seems to protect the public, data show that relatively few nurses have had licenses revoked or suspended. In part, the reason is believed to be the reluctance of other nurses to report and consequently testify to these acts by their colleagues before either the nursing board or a court of law. Nursing associations and state boards are now emphasizing the responsibility of professional nurses to report incompetent practice. Most current model acts make nonreporting a disciplinary offense.

When a report is filed with the state board, charging a nurse with violation of any of the grounds of disciplinary action, he or she is entitled to certain procedural safeguards (due process). After investigation, the nurse must receive notice of the charges and be given time to prepare a defence. A hearing is set and subpoenas are issued (by the board, attorney general, or a hearing officer). The accused has the right to appear personally or be represented by counsel, who may cross-examine witnesses. If the license is revoked or suspended, it may be reissued at the discretion of the board. (Sometimes the individual is only censured or reprimanded.)

Consumers have questioned whether health care professionals are vigilant in monitoring their own against charges of incompetence and illegal behavior. To ensure the public's safety, legislation created the *National Practitioners Data Bank* (NPDB). The intent of the law is to "collect and release certain information" about the professional competence and conduct of health care practitioners. The NPDB must, by law, be consulted by any health care institution seeking to hire a new professional provider and by certifying bodies, insurance companies, and federal and state licensing agencies when they are going to certify, credential, or license a professional provider, including a nurse, for the first time. Hospitals must then recheck the data bank every two years for every provider's record. Information is required to be reported to the NPDB by these same bodies about all professional providers, including nurses, related specifically to:[14]

- Malpractice payments made by or for the nurse, including judgment, arbitration decisions, and out-of-court settlements (but not the amount spent on the defense).

○ Licensure actions such as revocation, suspension, reprimand, censure, or probation.

PENALTIES FOR PRACTICING WITHOUT A LICENSE

Penalties for practicing without a license are included in mandatory laws. Penalties vary from a minimum fine to a large fine and/or imprisonment. Usually legal action is taken. Penalties are being strengthened to deter illegal practice.

PROCEDURE FOR OBTAINING A LICENSE

Almost all new graduates of a nursing program apply for RN licensure, because it is otherwise impossible to practice. Although there is nothing to prohibit you from postponing licensure, it is generally more difficult, both psychologically and because of distancing from the educational experience, to take the state board examination (NCLEX-RN) much later.

As a rule, your school makes available all the data and even the application forms necessary for beginning the licensure procedure. Should you wish to become licensed in another state, because of planned relocation, request an application from that nursing board. Correct titles and addresses of the nursing boards of all states are found in the Career Guide of the *American Journal of Nursing*, which is published annually. The board advises you of the proper procedure, cost, and data needed.

NCLEX-RN is administered year-round using computerized adaptive testing (CAT). Applications for the examination are made to the board of nursing in the jurisdiction where you want to be licensed. You will also need to register to take the NCLEX-RN, and this process will depend on the individual state procedures. Once the licensure application has been reviewed and eligibility approved by the board of nursing, you will receive an Authorization to Test (ATT). A bulletin, *Scheduling and Taking Your NCLEX-RN*, will also be forwarded that describes the examination, procedures for making an appointment, and a list of available test center locations and telephone numbers. The NCLEX-RN is administered at *Pearson Professional Centers*. Appointments to take the exam can be made either on the Internet or by telephone. The individual candidate schedules his or her own date and time for the examination. For more information on specific candidate application procedures and requirements, contact your board of nursing.

The CAT provides for each candidate to have a unique examination because it is assembled interactively as the individual is tested.

A competence estimate based on all earlier answers is calculated by the computer as the candidate answers each question. A large question bank stores all the examination questions and classifies them by test plan area and level of difficulty. The questions are then searched and the one determined to measure the candidate most precisely in the appropriate test plan area is shown on the computer screen. This process is then repeated for each question, thus forming an examination unique to the candidate's knowledge and skills. Grades are reported simply as a pass/fail score. Both NCLEX-RN and PN are based on periodic job analyses.

The tests are the same for all nurses seeking an RN, whether graduating from a diploma, associate degree, or baccalaureate program. This has been the subject of controversy because the stated goals of all three programs are different. However, proponents of a single licensing exam state that the purpose is to determine safe and effective practice at a minimal level, and that this criterion applies equally to all levels of nurses.

Nurses who pass the licensing examination receive a certificate bearing a registration number that remains the same as long as they are registered in that state. The certificate (or registration card) will also carry the expiration date—usually one, two, or three years hence. Failure to renew promptly may mean that you must pay a special fee to be reinstated.

It is advisable to keep your registration in effect, whether actively engaged in nursing or not. The expense is nominal. All nurses continue to have the responsibility (and sometimes the legal requirement) to keep their nursing knowledge updated through continuing education.

To become licensed by endorsement, applicants must already be registered in one state, territory, or foreign country. They must apply to the state board of nursing in the new state and present credentials, as requested, to prove that they have completed preparation equal to that required. A temporary permit may be issued to allow the nurse to work until the new license is issued.

Nurses who wish to be reregistered after allowing their licenses to lapse should contact their state board for directions. An RN wishing to practice nursing in another country also needs to investigate its legal requirements for practice. Members of the armed forces or the Peace Corps, or those under the auspices of an organization such as the World Health Organization or a religious denomination, will be advised by the sponsoring group. Registration in one state is usually sufficient.

Nurses educated in other countries are expected to meet the same qualifications for licensure as graduates of schools of nursing in the United States. The procedure for obtaining a license is the same as for graduates of schools here. Additional requirements are necessary to qualify for visa status, and those will be discussed later in this chapter.

Since 1993, the United States has entered into two major trade agreements that have significant ramifications for nurses and nursing. These are the *North American Free Trade Agreement* (NAFTA) and the *General Agreement on Tariffs and Trade* (GATT). The trade pact between the United States, Canada, and Mexico (NAFTA) removes most trade barriers among these nations. This creates the world's largest free-trade zone, and permits the unencumbered movement of nurses across borders for employment opportunities given that they are qualified. ANA, partnering with the Office of the U.S. Trade Representative and a coalition of licensed professionals, worked hard to ensure state primacy and autonomy in matters related to licensing and credentialing under NAFTA. Language in the Statement of Administrative Actions clarifies that NAFTA does not permit Mexican or Canadian professionals to practice a licensed profession in the United States without meeting all applicable state licensing criteria.

THE COMMISSION ON GRADUATES OF FOREIGN NURSING SCHOOLS (CGFNS)

In the late 1960s the United States experienced an increase in nurses migrating here to practice nursing. Immigration officials were having difficulty identifying which of the nurses educated abroad, and applying for nursing occupational visas, would actually be eligible for licensure as registered nurses in the United States. At that time, only about 15 to 20 percent of the nurses educated outside the United States were passing the U.S. registered nurse licensing exam. This led the Division of Nursing to contract for two studies regarding RN licensure of foreign-educated nurses in the United States. The findings of these landmark studies on foreign nurse immigration were presented at a 1975 HEW conference attended by representatives from governmental and private organizations, including the U.S. Department of Labor, the Immigration and Naturalization Service, the ANA, and the NLN, among others.

The outgrowth of the conference was that in 1977, ANA and NLN agreed to cosponsor the establishment of an independent nonprofit organization for the purpose of developing an equitable system through which nurses educated in foreign nursing schools could gauge their chances of becoming licensed as registered nurses in the United States. Such an organization had as its mission to establish an orderly process for assessing the individual knowledge and level of preparation of each nurse applicant. These efforts would also help serve to protect the public health, by ensuring that nurses educated outside the United States meet standards that are comparable to those registered nurses educated here.

The organization created and chartered with this mission was the Commission on Graduates of Foreign Nursing Schools, or CGFNS.

Today, the Commission provides a variety of services, including the *CGFNS Certification Program* and the *Credentials Evaluation Service* (CES) for foreign-educated nurses who wish to practice in the United States. To obtain either a permanent or temporary occupational preference visa from the Department of Homeland Security, the nurse will need a CGFNS certificate or a full, unrestricted license to practice as a registered nurse in the state where they will be employed. To support these services, CGFNS is an active participant in policy discussions concerning international nursing education, licensure, and practice.

ISSUES, DEVELOPMENTS, AND PREDICTIONS

It seems that almost every month brings information about changes in nurse practice acts or challenges as to what they permit. Certification in specialty areas is growing in popularity and beginning to be recognized in the workplace, as well as by the consumer.

At the other end of the educational scale is the concern about the competence of nurses' aides. New positions are emerging for aides in hospitals and home care. As the least expensive and least prepared nursing person, the aide is still expected to detect behavioral changes that may signal a serious health problem—and is not trained to do so. Although the need for national training standards has been recognized, just who will implement them is still undecided. Some states, such as New Jersey, now regulate home health aides. How can nurses who are ultimately responsible for nurses' aides determine if they are safe and competent? Will the state boards have a role? The NCSBN has developed standards for the regulation of nurses' aides and a testing program for certification of long-term care aides as required by the government.

Equal concern can be directed at the growing responsibilities of LPNs. Many state boards are put under pressure by employers to approve procedures for LPNs that are not in their curricula, such as venipuncture. Some boards approve and demand that PN programs include these procedures in their course of study. Schools say that there is already enough to cover in one year. The impact of this problem is uncertain. Will patients be endangered? What of the responsibility of nurses who supervise LPNs? Might these new demands escalate the move toward AD education for LPNs?

On another note, nurse disciplinary problems are likely to increase. The stress of institutional staff cutbacks, caring for sicker patients with fewer people, and an uncertain job future can all be triggers for substance abuse. Support programs sponsored by the state boards and state nurses' associations were mentioned earlier. They will probably increase in number and diversity, but be evaluated as to their efficacy.

Regardless of the outcome of health care reform efforts, it is clear that there will be an increasing push for more uniform licensing standards, and removal of statutory barriers to practice. The licensure examinations are expected to continue to change. Another challenge for NCSBN is investigate the presence of item bias in NCLEX. NCLEX-RN has been criticized for not taking into consideration cultural, gender, and other factors on the part of the test-taker. With the large immigrant population, many of whom go into nursing, such things must be considered. Other issues about licensure include establishing mechanisms to ensure competence, including that of returning nurses, and developing better means of verifying credentials across state lines.

Finally, the credentialing issues in health care in general are not expected to improve greatly because they are so disorganized. More health occupations will continue to seek licensure or other legal status. All these groups will have problems similar to nursing with definition, scope, discipline, and testing methods. And what of the uncredentialed health worker? How best can we guarantee at least safe care for the public? These issues do not have simple solutions; but if someone must take the lead to initiate cooperative action, it may well be nursing.

KEY POINTS

1. There are a variety of mechanisms for credentialing nurses and other health care workers, all of which have some problems.
2. Mandatory licensure means that an individual cannot practice without a license and safeguards the public more than permissive licensure.
3. Among the criticisms of licensure are too much control by the profession or occupation, a tendency for practice requirements to be rigid and out of date, and primarily that the public has no guarantee of competence.
4. Institutional licensure, although favored by administrators for economic and other reasons, would not guarantee improved care but would limit the autonomy and mobility of nurses who now have individual licenses.
5. Nursing practice acts may vary from state to state, but they generally have the same components that define and control practice.
6. Nursing practice acts must change with the times, but the current practitioner is usually protected by a grandfather clause.

7. The most common reasons for revocation of a license are drug abuse or misuse, or other failure to meet the standards of the profession.
8. The approaches to authorizing advanced nursing practice are most commonly a combination of public/private sector partnerships.
9. Sunset legislation, which requires a review of existing laws to determine if they are fulfilling their purpose, has resulted in some good revisions of nursing practice acts.
10. A major problem with continuing education as a requirement for relicensure is that there is little evidence that it results in improved competence.
11. Many changes are occurring in the testing of individuals for nurse licensure.

STUDY QUESTIONS

1. Interview five "knowledgeable" consumers, and see what they think are the guarantees of safety and quality from their health care providers.
2. How would institutional licensure affect your professional life as a registered nurse?
3. Why do we need licensure?
4. Compare and justify some of the differences in opinion between the ANA and the NCSBN on nursing licensure.
5. The importation of nurses from foreign countries has been an ongoing solution to shortages in this country. Give your opinion on this.

REFERENCES

1. National Council of State Boards of Nursing (NCSBN). Nurse Licensure Compact: http://ncsbn.org/nlc/index.asp. Retrieved April 11, 2005.
2. Ibid.
3. American Nurses Association. Concerns Still Exist Over Nursing Licensure Compact: http://nursingworld.org/tan/99marapr/licensur.htm. Retrieved April 4, 2005.
4. American Board of Nursing Specialties: http://www.nursingcertification.org/strategic_plan.htm. Retrieved April 12, 2005.
5. Community Health Accreditation Program: http://www.chapinc.org/chap-mission.htm. Retrieved April 2, 2005.
6. Consumer Advocacy Center: Demonstrating Continued Professional Competency: A National Conference, June 2003: http://www.cacenter.org/ContCompFullFinal.pdf. Retrieved April 11, 2005.
7. The Department of Health, Education, and Welfare. *Extending the Scope of Nursing Practice*. Washington, DC: The Author, 1971.

8. NCSBN. Model Nursing Practice Act: http://www.ncsbn.org/regulation/ nursingpractice. Retrieved April 11, 2005.
9. Joel L. Advanced practice nursing in the current socio-political climate. In Stanley J: *Advanced Practice Nursing*, 2d ed. Philadelphia: F.A. Davis, 2005, pp 46–69.
10. Phillips S. A comprehensive look at the legislative issues affecting advanced nursing practice. *Nurse Pract* 30(1):14–47, January 2005.
11. NCSBN. Nurse Licensure Compact, op cit.
12. Journal of Continuing Education in Nursing. Continuing Education Requirements for Relicensure (2004): http://slackinc.com/allied/jcen/ 2004ce1.pdf. Retrieved April 9, 2005.
13. *Heinecke v. Department of Commerce, Division of Occupational and Professional Licensing*, 810 P.2d 459 (Utah App 1991).
14. Torre C. Are You Aware of Your Status with the Federally Mandated National Practitioner Data Bank, April 2004: http://www.njsna.org/ RegulaTorreUpdate/NationalPractitionerDataBank(NPDB).htm. Retrieved April 11, 2005.

Updates can be found at

 http://www.JoelTheNursingExperience.com

Chapter 12

Legal Aspects of Nursing Practice

OBJECTIVES

After studying this chapter, you will be able to:

1. Define basic legal terms.
2. Explain the elements of the standard of care as it might be applied in a court of law.
3. Give examples of legal problems nurses may encounter in caring for patients.
4. Present specific ways in which nurses may avoid malpractice suits.
5. Name three charting errors that may cause problems for the nurse in a malpractice suit.
6. Identify key points in selecting liability insurance.
7. Give examples of criminal activities for which nurses can be held responsible in their practice.
8. Explain how best to handle a situation calling for a critical incident report.
9. Explain the usual steps in a trial.
10. List the main points a nurse should know about testifying.

There are numerous ways in which nurses become involved with the law in their practice. The impact of statutory law has been previously discussed. In this chapter, other legal aspects will be considered,

475

primarily tort law involving intentional or unintentional civil wrongs. This is the kind of law that relates to the daily practice of most nurses. When cases are used to illustrate a legal principle, it is important to remember that even a landmark decision may be overturned. The law is dynamic, not rigidly fixed, and changes with changing times.

LITIGATION TRENDS IN HEALTH CARE

Part of the doctrine of common law is that anyone can sue anyone else if she or he can get a lawyer to take the case or is able to handle it personally (as is common in a small claims court). This does not necessarily mean that there is just cause or that the person suing (plaintiff) has a good chance of winning; in fact, the defendant might be protected by law from being found liable, as when someone, in good faith, reports child abuse.

Most people are reasonably decent in their dealings with others, and unless a person sustains a serious injury, they generally will not institute legal proceedings. Sometimes the cost of legal services dissuades the injured party from bringing suit. On the other hand, often the person inflicting the injury is also realistic and prefers to settle the matter out of court, knowing that it will be less costly in the long run; or insurance may pay for the damage inflicted. The parties may settle their difficulties out of court because one or the other or both wants to avoid publicity and does not want to have a court record of any kind.

Once people seemed particularly reluctant to "make trouble" for nurses, doctors, or health agencies such as certain nonprofit or voluntary hospitals, either out of respect for the services offered and/or because they presumably had so little money that it seemed unfair or pointless. The latter was probably always an inaccurate generality, but today patients and families who feel aggrieved are considerably more likely to sue any or all concerned, sometimes for enormous sums. Health care is big business. The number of claims and the monetary escalation of awards began to increase in the 1930s, declined during World War II, and then rose again, with the 1980s and 1990s seeing multimillion-dollar awards. Malpractice suits against hospitals, especially, have increased, and the doctrine of *charitable immunity,* which granted them freedom from liability, and *sovereign immunity,* which does the same for government, is gradually being wiped out in the courts.

A variety of reasons have been cited: the "litigant spirit" of the general public, what seems to be a "sue if possible; I've been injured, or I'm entitled" attitude; changing medical technology that has brought new risks, with a potential for exceptional severity of injury; sometimes high, unrealistic public expectations; the increase in specialization that has resulted in a deterioration of the physician–patient relationship; and patient resentment of depersonalized care and sometimes rude treatment in hospitals.

At the height of the malpractice crisis, a specially appointed interdisciplinary committee reported that the *prime factor in malpractice was malpractice.* However, because there are so many more medical injuries than medical claims, another major factor might be interpersonal problems between the provider and patient and frustration with the way specific complaints were handled or not handled.

When faced with a bad outcome, it has been documented that patients and family are more likely to sue if they feel that the physician was not caring and compassionate. Quality of care was not the main determinant. The main positive factors were: spending a little more time with the patient; explaining or teaching about what to expect; using some humor; encouraging patients to talk or ask questions; and checking understanding—all of which sound like rather basic considerations. These same points seem critical for nurses to consider in their practice.

However, there is also some strong evidence that people are being socialized into thinking that if something goes wrong, they should sue. One factor is seen to be the influence of the ubiquitous advertisements of attorneys on radio and television, promising legal help for a multitude of injuries and accidents. Another is explicit recommendations by other health care providers to seek legal counsel.

Most suits are settled out of court. The dramatic multimillion-dollar suits seldom result in awards anywhere near the original figure; sometimes they are not won at all, and almost always progress to the appellate level. The largest awards have the largest elements of compensation for pain and suffering, almost exclusively occurring after some negligently caused catastrophic injury, such as severe brain damage or paralysis, which obviously has an enormous effect on the victim's life. The frequent suits and large awards were part of the reason for the mid-1970s and 1980s malpractice crisis, when many physicians could not get malpractice insurance, and neither hospitals nor physicians felt that they could afford it if they could get it. In 1990, malpractice fees were being reduced; state laws limiting awards and increased caution by physicians were cited as reasons. By 1992, a study of medical malpractice cases indicated that unjustified payments were rare. Nevertheless, the issue of tort reform continues to be of major interest to Congress and state legislatures.

The vast majority of malpractice cases are against physicians or hospitals. Don't nurses get sued? Absolutely. As noted later, a good percentage of hospital and physician suits include nurses and may be based on the nurse's negligence. Because of the various legal doctrines, also explained later, the aggrieved patient has the option of suing multiple defendants. The *deep pocket* theory of naming those who can pay most has become traditional tort law strategy, as has the *fishnet theory* of suing every defendant available. Thus the likelihood of recovery from one or more defendants is greater, and a favorite defense of admitting negligence but blaming an absent party, the so-called *empty chair defense*, is defeated. Because presumably either or both the physician or the hospital has more money than the nurse, either may have to pay the award or at least more of the award, even if it is the nurse who is clearly at fault. Particularly in the case of the hospital whose liability and responsibility may be only secondary (*vicarious liability*), it may seek to recover damages from the employee primarily responsible for the loss through the process of *subrogation*, meaning that the employer can sue the employee for the amount of damages paid because of the employee's negligence.

In 1986, as the result of federal legislation, the National Practitioner Data Bank (NPDB) was established to facilitate the identification of health care practitioners who are found guilty of unprofessional conduct: malpractice claims paid, disciplinary action by a licensing board, clinical privilege suspension or revocation, or professional society censorship. In 2003, the NPDB reported that over its entire history, registered nurses (including advanced practice nurses) had only been responsible for 4512 malpractice payments, or 1.8 percent of all claims paid. Almost two-thirds (63.3 percent) of these were cases involving registered nurses, as opposed to advanced practice nurses, where almost 21 percent were associated with nurse anesthetists and 9 percent with nurse midwives. Monitoring, treatment, and medication problems characterize the situation in the majority of claims paid for registered nurses. Claims for obstetrical and surgical cases were prominent. The median and mean malpractice payment for all categories of nurses in 2003 was $132,500 and $376,140, respectively.[1]

Given these circumstances, it makes sense to know (1) the kinds of situations that lead to litigation, (2) the steps to take to avoid being sued, and (3) what to do if a patient is injured. This chapter gives an overview of the legal problems with which nurses can be involved in their practice. The major emphasis will be tort law, that is, an intentional or unintentional civil wrong. Criminal problems that may occur are reviewed more briefly.

APPLICATION OF LEGAL PRINCIPLES

The majority of incidents leading to legal action in which nurses are involved occur in an employment situation, generally the hospital or nursing home. That is to be expected because that is where most nurses work and where patients are usually sickest and most helpless. When a person is injured, the chances are that the institution will be sued, even when an employee or a physician has done the actual damage. In the case of the employee, the hospital is sued under the legal principle of *respondeat superior*: "let the master answer" or be responsible for the actions of the employees.

This does not prevent the employee from being sued, since the rule or doctrine of *personal liability* says that everyone is legally responsible for his or her acts, even though someone else may also be held legally liable, usually the institution. The latter is called *vicarious* liability, imposed without personal fault or without a causal relationship between the actions of the one held liable and the injury.

At one time, physicians were held directly responsible for any error of personnel who worked with them in a patient care situation (*borrowed servant*) on the basis of the "captain of the ship" doctrine; this has been overturned by most courts, but not all, as shown in a case described later. The institution, however, can be held accountable for physicians' acts, even if they are not employees, under the principle of *corporate negligence*. A classic example is the 1965 landmark decision of *Darling v. Charleston Community Memorial Hospital*, which has set several precedents, including opinions on staffing. Although other cases will be presented to exemplify some of these points, the *Darling* case illustrates the elements that must be present in order to have cause for action based on malpractice or negligence:[2]

- *Duty*. The nurse has assumed the responsibility for the patient's care, and must do what a reasonably prudent nurse would do in a similar situation.
- *Breach*. The nurse fails to adhere to the standard of care, for instance, inappropriate delegation or neglecting to notify the physician of a change in condition.
- *Damages*. The patient's injury is proven.
- *Causation*. The patient's injury was directly caused by the nurse's failure to meet the standard of care (proximate cause).

CASE

Darling v. Charleston Community Memorial Hospital (1965)

A minor broke his leg playing football and was taken to Charleston Community Memorial Hospital. An on-call physician set and cast his leg, and he was sent to a regular nursing unit. Nurses' notes indicate that almost immediately, the patient began to complain of pain, and his toes became swollen and dark, and later cold and insensitive. A pervasive stench permeated his hospital room. Nurses checked the leg several times a day, charted their findings, and notified the doctor who visited once but did nothing to remedy the situation. When the cast was removed three days later, the necrotic condition of the leg was obvious. After several surgical attempts to save the leg, an orthopedist was forced to amputate below the knee because of advanced gangrene. The family sued the first doctor, the hospital, and the nurses involved.

The physician settled out of court; he admitted that he had set few legs and had not looked at a book on orthopedics in 40 years. The hospital's defense was that the care provided was in accordance with the standard practice of like hospitals, that it had no control over the physician, and that it was not liable for the nurses' conduct because they were acting under the orders of the physician.

The appellate court, upholding the decision of the lower court, found that the hospital had failed in its duties to review the work of the physician or to require consultation when the patient's condition clearly indicated the necessity for such action. Additionally, the court found the hospital liable for failing to have enough specially trained nurses available to recognize the seriousness of the patient's condition and to alert the medical staff, or if they were unresponsive the hospital administration.[3]

Nursing Implications

Since Darling there have been several cases decided on the same principles. Almost every case involved a nurse who failed to provide adequate monitoring of a patient. The courts emphasized the need for sufficient numbers of nurses to monitor the patient's condition, and specially trained nurses who would recognize signs and symptoms that would require immediate medical intervention.

You must be persistent in reporting inadequate care. It is not enough to observe and record. For nurses, an additional crucial point in the decision was the newly defined duty to inform the hospital administration of any deviation from proper medical care that poses a threat to the well-being of a patient.

Two terms used here and almost inevitably in most suits are *malpractice* and *negligence*. Malpractice technically means "professional negligence." At one time nurses were only charged with negligence, but the court's view of nursing liability has changed. *Negligence* means failing to exercise the degree of care that a person of ordinary prudence would exercise under the same circumstances. Malpractice is more restricted, a specialized kind of negligence. It is the "violation of a professional duty or a failure to meet a standard of care or failure to use the skills and knowledge" that other professionals would use in similar circumstances.[4] The following cases not only illustrate incidents of negligence, but present the doctrine of *vicarious liability*. This is liability that a supervisory party, such as an employer, bears for the actionable conduct of a subordinate or associate, such as an employee. This doctrine is closely related to the concepts of *captain-of-the-ship* or *respondeat superior*.

CASE

Nelson v. Trinity Medical Center (1988)

The physician of a woman in active labor ordered assessment of fetal heart tones, an IV, and analgesia. Standing orders in that labor unit called for continuous fetal heart monitoring, but the nurse, without checking, assumed that the monitors were all in use and did not place one on the patient until an hour later. It indicated fetal distress, and despite an immediate cesarean, the infant was born with severe brain damage. According to the expert who testified, the damage was caused by placental separation, which could have been diagnosed by earlier fetal monitoring. The defendant hospital tried to invoke the captain-of-the-ship doctrine to cover the nurse's negligence. The court ruled that even though the doctor was in charge of the case, he had no direct control over what the nurse did (as opposed to an operating room situation) and that the nurse was performing a routine act. However, it was the hospital, not the nurse, who was found liable for the actions of its employee.[5]

Nursing Implications

The entire area of obstetrics is high on the list of malpractice suits. As seen here, the problem is not always that of a nurse not knowing how to handle equipment (although this also is the basis of nurse malpractice), but carelessness and false assumptions. Check whether equipment is available and working; do not guess. If it is not, notify your manager and the doctor so that other arrangements can be made. Check to see if equipment is in working order *before* it is needed. You are not at fault if equipment does not work, but it is your responsibility to report it and follow through. Again, use your nursing judgment! In this case, the nurse's neglect was considered the *proximate cause* of the child's injury.

A similar case decided in New Jersey in 2005 (*Danilczuk v. Hunterdon Medical Center*) emphasizes the jeopardy in obstetrical practice. A judge approved a $5 million settlement in a suit by parents who claimed that a labor nurse's negligence caused their child's cerebral palsy and quadriplegia. A woman was in labor when her fetal monitor showed distress caused by insufficient oxygen leading to a drop in the fetal heart rate, but the nurse on duty waited two hours before calling the obstetrician. Even though a cesarean section was performed immediately, the lack of oxygen caused severe brain damage. The child is mentally impaired, has no control over her bowels and bladder, uses a feeding tube and a tracheotomy, and will require lifetime care.[6]

The following case again illustrates negligence and the principle of vicarious liability involving the hospital and doctor.

CASE

Lewis v. Lakeland Medical Center et al. (2001)

A patient in whose body a laparotomy sponge had been left following gallbladder surgery brought suit against the surgeon, the hospital, and the nurses involved. The plaintiff asserted that the surgeon was vicariously liable for the failure of two nurses, employed by the hospital, to accurately count the number of sponges used in Lewis's gallbladder surgery. As a result a sponge was left in Lewis's abdomen and only found during a subsequent exploratory surgery for postoperative complaints. Decisions were appealed all the way to the Wisconsin Supreme Court. It was finally determined that the surgeon, who the patient had stipulated was not negligent, was not vicariously liable for the negligence of the nurses employed by the hospital. Further, the Court dismissed appeals on the grounds of either "respondeat superior" or the "captain of the ship" doctrine (not recognized in Wisconsin). Any of these arguments are severe exceptions to the basic principle that one is only responsible for his or her own acts, so courts proceed with caution when asked to impose vicarious liability or any similar doctrines on an innocent party.

The hospital settled in the early stages of the litigation, the surgeon was found not vicariously liable, and the nurses were never joined as defendants in the suit. The financial recovery against Lakeland was minimal, given that it was a county-owned facility.[7]

Nursing Implications

This Wisconsin case has several interesting points. The Court recognized that hospitals have become big business, competing with each other for health care dollars. As the role and image of the modern hospital has evolved, so too has the law with respect to the hospital's responsibility and liability toward those it serves. The issue remains whether a hospital can be held vicariously liable for the allegedly negligent acts of health care providers working either as employees or as independent contractors. Further, the issue was raised in oral argument whether the duty to put in and remove the laparotomy pads was a nondelegatable duty of the surgeon. If the duty is nondelegatable, the person is vicariously liable.[8]

Criminal negligence and *gross negligence* are sometimes used interchangeably and refer to the commission or omission of an act, lawfully or unlawfully, in which such a degree of negligence exists as may cause a serious wrong to another. Almost any act of negligence resulting in the death of a patient would be considered gross negligence. In such a situation the plaintiff may be awarded *punitive damages*, over and above the ordinary damages.

Contributory negligence is an old term that states that if you contribute to your injuries in any way, you are not entitled to any compensation.

There are only four states that still adhere to this law. The other forty-six states have done away with contributory negligence. Instead, they have some form of *comparative negligence*. In comparative negligence, the jury determines the amount of fault. For example, if a jury determines that you are entitled to $10,000 to compensate you for your injuries but also finds you 10 percent at fault, you would receive only $9000. In a contributory negligence state, in that same scenario, you would be entitled to nothing. Because comparative negligence must be proven by the defendant, as much written evidence as possible is needed. The following two cases illustrate the concept.

CASE

Naya v. Mercy Medical Center (2003)

The incident occurred at defendant's rehabilitation facility where the plaintiff, a school guidance counselor, was recovering from a stroke. Following the stroke the plaintiff was taken to a hospital where she was comatose and paralyzed on the left side. After treatment for nine days with some improvement, including the regaining of consciousness, the plaintiff was brought to the rehabilitation portion of the hospital, where she was assessed as to her status and needs associated with occupational therapy, physical therapy, and nursing. The next day, she was left on a commode with arm rails, with instructions not to reach for toilet paper, but to call when ready. The plaintiff, however, reached for the toilet paper on her own, and fell off the commode. She does not recall how the accident occurred.

The defendant argued that if the plaintiff had followed the instructions and called for assistance, the accident would not have occurred. The defendant further contended that the plaintiff had been alert and oriented on the date of the accident. The plaintiff sustained a fracture of the medial malleolus and was casted for approximately one month. The plaintiff claimed that as a result of the trauma of the fall, she damaged her peroneal nerve, resulting in drop foot. She currently has limitation of dorsiflexion on the foot, some degree of incapacity in the rest of the leg, and a slight incapacity to her upper body on the left side as a result of the stroke.

The plaintiff has subsequently returned to work. The defendant argued that the drop foot was the result of the stroke and noted that testing performed before the fall had indicated that while the plaintiff was paralyzed on the left side, the greatest disability was to the ankle and foot area.

The jury returned a plaintiff verdict of $325,000 for the plaintiff, reduced to $178,750 for 45 percent comparative negligence of the plaintiff.[9]

Nursing Implications

This case shows the necessity for complete and precise documentation of the patient's medical and mental status. In addition, it is impossible to err on the side of ensuring safety.

CASE

Axelrad v. Jackson (2004)

During a malpractice case against a physician, claiming a failure to diagnose diverticulitis and negligently prescribing an enema which ultimately caused an intestinal perforation, the plaintiff was accused of comparative negligence for failing to report important points in his medical history. The defense focused on the plaintiff's duty to divulge such information. But, if there is no duty, there is no negligence. Cited cases found that the patient has a responsibility to cooperate with the treating physician, but the patient may rely on the doctor to ask appropriate questions to guide him to disclosing information. The patient has the duty to respond accurately and truthfully. A duty to volunteer information only arises when a patient knows the significance of the unrevealed history and knows that the physician has failed to ascertain the history.

On appeal, the case was found for the physician, and the comparative negligence of the plaintiff supported. The court's opinion alleged that although a doctor has specialized knowledge to diagnose an illness, the diagnosis is often based on the exchange of information between the patient and his physician. The patient is in the best position to know exactly what his current symptoms are and his pertinent medical history. While a patient does not have a duty to diagnose his own illness, the patient does have a duty to cooperate with his treating physician. Patient conduct in communicating symptoms and history which does not display cooperation as an ordinary and prudent person would do under the same or similar circumstances, may result in a finding of comparative negligence.[10]

Nursing Implications

Although this case involved a physician, the points of law are just as relevant to the nurse. You must always do a careful nursing assessment, making sure that you ask the questions most appropriate to the clinical situation. Then be sure that this information is recorded, and accurately and completely communicated to the physician.

An important legal concept is *res ipsa loquitur* ("the thing speaks for itself"), a legal doctrine that gets around the need for expert testimony or the need for the plaintiff to prove the defendant's liability because the situation (harm) is self-evident even to a lay person. The defendant must prove, instead, that he or she is not responsible for the harm done. Before the rule of *res ipsa loquitur* can be applied, three conditions must be present: the injury would not ordinarily have occurred unless there was negligence; whatever caused the injury at the time was under the exclusive control of the defendant; and the injured person had not contributed to the negligence or voluntarily assumed the risk. Often such a situation occurs in the operating room. *Chin v. St. Barnabas* is a good example.

CASE

Chin v. St. Barnabas Medical Center (1999)

A patient's death was caused by the incorrect hook-up of a hysteroscope which introduced gas into her uterus and blood stream during a surgical procedure. Two nurses who had no experience, familiarity, or training on the Hystero-flow Pump were assigned to the procedure as scrub nurses. A third nurse, having some experience with the equipment, acted as circulating nurse. At the beginning of the surgical procedure, the circulating nurse removed the pack containing the sterile tubing from the operating room cabinet, opened it, and presented it to the scrub nurse. The circulating nurse was responsible for hooking up the gas line to the nitrogen gas regulator and hooking up the exhaust tube to the suction. One scrub nurse asked the other for a suction tube, and received the sterile end while the nonsterile end of the tube was to be connected to a suction canister. Through negligence, either the nonsterile end of the suction tube was improperly connected to the exhaust hose or the sterile end of the suction tube was improperly connected to the outflow part of the hysteroscope. Either of these connections could have caused the closed circuit resulting in the patient's death. The jury awarded the plaintiff $2 million in damages, assessed 20 percent against the physician, 20 percent against one of the inexperienced scrub nurses, 25 percent against the circulating nurse, and 35 percent against the hospital. The jury verdict was upheld on appeal.[11]

Nursing Implications

There is a simple moral here: realizing the seriousness of nursing, there is a need to be thoroughly oriented to procedures before you participate, and to refuse to participate unless you have been thoroughly trained to operate equipment and to minister to the specific clinical population. Further, the check and double-check process used in administering medications is also appropriate to procedures. We can additionally observe the chain of command in this situation, and the responsibility of the circulating nurse for whatever happens in the operating room.

In 1995, newspapers reported that a Superior Court jury in New Jersey ordered a doctor and two nurses to pay a woman $500,000 for leaving a pad inside her body during a cesarean section in 1990. She was forced to undergo several surgeries, first to remove the pad, and then, in 1993, to correct problems from that surgery. The nurses were blamed for miscounting the pads; they said the doctor was also responsible. Here, the nurses did not exercise the *due care* that they owed the plaintiff.

Another point to note is the length of time between the negligent action and the suit. The *statute of limitations* varies with states, but usually the length of time during which a person can sue begins when the injury is noted (*discovery*), which may be several years after the occurrence. In the case of infants, or children, it does not begin until age 18, the *long tail* concept.

Another case of *res ipsa loquitur*, reported in 1987, resulted in an award of over $2 million. A four-day-old infant suffered trauma to her head as a result of being dropped or mishandled by the nursing staff. The hospital and staff denied responsibility, although the baby had been under the exclusive control of the hospital staff throughout her stay. Even when the parents visited, staff were present. It appears that whoever caused the injury chose to cover up the incident. The hospital paid under the *respondeat superior* doctrine, since all the staff members were employees.

Assuming that you are at little risk because you don't work in the ICU, the emergency room, or some other high-pressure unit is a mistake. In reviewing cases in which nurses were found liable, the sad news is that most of the incidents were everyday situations in which nurses not only did not use nursing judgment but sometimes did not even use common sense. Quite often they neglected basic principles that they learned in their first year of nursing, such as how to give medications, or were careless about communication. Not only are RNs found liable, but also students. The following hypothetical situation (although based on fact) provides a useful illustration as well as applying several other legal principles.

A first-year student nurse was assigned by the instructor to care for a thin, very ill patient who required an intramuscular injection. The student had only practiced the procedure in the school laboratory. She injected the medication in the patient's sciatic nerve and caused severe damage. The patient sued the doctor, hospital, head nurse, student, faculty members, and school of nursing, an example of the *fishnet* principle. This was a case of *res ipsa loquitur*. The student was clearly negligent because she should have known the correct procedure and should have taken special precautions with an emaciated patient. The student is held to the standards of care (*standards of reasonableness*) of an RN if she is performing RN functions. If the student is not capable of functioning safely unsupervised, she should not be carrying out those functions. The doctor may or may not be held liable, depending on the court's notion about the *captain-of-the-ship doctrine*. However, this would have nothing to do with the drug and injection itself, assuming that it was an appropriate order. The hospital would probably be held liable under *respondeat superior*, because students, even if not employed, are usually treated legally as employees. Also applicable is the doctrine of *corporate liability*, which relates to the legal duty of a health care institution to provide appropriate facilities (staff and equipment) to carry out the purpose of the institution and to follow established standards of conduct. In addition, because the head nurse is responsible for all patients on the unit and presumably should have been involved in the student's assignment, or should have assigned an RN to such an ill patient, she too would be liable, because she did not make an appropriate assignment ("appropriate delegation of duties").

The instructor might be found liable, not on the basis of *respondeat superior*—just as the head nurse or supervisor would not be liable if the student had been an RN, because these nurses are not the employers in the legal sense—but on the basis of inadequate supervision. If a supervisor or other nurse assigns a task to someone not competent to perform that task and a patient is injured because of that individual's incompetent performance, the supervising nurse can be held personally liable because it is part of her or his responsibility to know the competence and scope of practice of those being supervised. (Although theoretically, in dealing with other than students, this nurse could rely on the subordinate's licensure, certification, or registration, if any, as an indication of competence, if there is reason to believe that the individual would nevertheless perform carelessly or incompetently and the nurse still assigns that person to the task, the nurse is held accountable, as is the employer under the doctrine of *respondeat superior*.) The school might be found liable in the case of the student, if the court believed the director had not used good judgment in employing or assigning the faculty member carrying out those teaching responsibilities. Nevertheless, the bottom line is that the student *is* responsible for her own actions, a basic principle of law.

Another case involving a student reinforces the principle of individual and teacher responsibility. In *Central Anesthesia Associates v. Worthy* (1985), Bonnie Castro, a senior student nurse anesthetist, was accused of administering anesthesia improperly, causing the patient to have a cardiac arrest and brain damage; the patient was still in a coma at the time of the case. Castro was under the supervision of a PA employed by the professional corporation that ran the nurse anesthetist program. The Supreme Court of Georgia held Castro, the PA, and the three anesthesiologist teachers liable. It rejected her argument that she should be held to the student standard; she was held to the standards of a certified nurse anesthetist (CNA). The teachers were not on the scene and had not delegated supervision properly. The PA either did not supervise adequately or was himself not capable. This case has implications for nursing students and their staff nurse preceptors when faculty are absent.

MAJOR CAUSES OF LITIGATION

Certain practices are more likely than others to result in nurses being sued or included in a malpractice case. Sometimes legal problems are caused by lack of knowledge, as when a nurse simply does not know the most current use or dangers of a drug or treatment or how to respond to a complication. For instance, $7.3 million was awarded to a husband in Illinois when his wife died because nurses did not recognize or handle an emergency correctly. A central venous pressure line, which had been inserted through the patient's internal jugular vein during surgery, perforated the wall of her heart, allowing fluid to accumulate in the pericardial sac. Even though in the first five postoperative hours the blood pressure became undetectable and her heart rate rose, the nurses failed to call the physician. The suit alleged inadequate postoperative care because of the nurses' failure to act.

Often problems result from poor nursing judgment, as when a nurse in the emergency room sends away a patient without consulting with or calling a physician, or does not question a doctor's order or behavior, despite having doubts that the action is correct. The amount of responsibility now put on nurses to judge the actions of the physician and (within their scope of practice or knowledge) to stop and/or report a questionable action is increasing. For instance, in one case, both nurse and physician knew that a baby was in footling breech position and the nurse observed symptoms of fetal distress, but the physician decided to perform a vaginal delivery anyhow. The nurse expressed her concerns to the physician (who ignored them), but she did not contact her supervisor or anyone else. The baby suffered brain damage. In the suit that followed, the courts ruled that the physician made an error, but that the nurse should have notified a supervisor immediately. The hospital was held responsible and the family was awarded damages. A large number of cases are the result of poor physician–nurse communication.

COMMUNICATION PROBLEMS

Do you have a responsibility to take action when a doctor writes an order that you think is incorrect or unclear? When he or she does not respond to a patient's worsening condition? When he or she does not come to see a patient even if you think it's urgent? When he or she does not follow accepted precautions in giving a treatment? What if the physician becomes angry and abusive? According to court decisions in the last few years, the answer to all these questions is that it *is* the nurse's responsibility to take action. The following case is illustrative.

CASE

Deerman v. Beverly California Corp. (1999)

A nurse hired as a Case Plan Coordinator in a California nursing home was sought out by family members of a patient who was losing weight, having hallucinations, and other symptoms of acute distress. She documented the patient's condition, and reported the situation to the responsible physician. She attempted to contact the physician by phone, but her calls were not returned. The patient was deteriorating and when the family asked for advice, the nurse advised that she would "reconsider the choice of physicians." Once the nursing home heard of the advice she had offered the family, she was fired. The nurse maintained that this was part of her responsibility both as a registered nurse and a Patient Case Coordinator. The nurse filed suit, and the County Superior Court found for the defendant. On appeal the judgment of the lower court was reversed, noting that the statement which led to her termination was offered in fulfillment of her "teaching and counseling" obligations as a licensed professional nurse. The court also recognized that, as Case Plan Coordinator, she was responsible for managing the medical care and treatment of all patients at the nursing home. Despite the fact that she documented and reported all of the patient's medical difficulties to the physician, the physician was unresponsive.[12]

Nursing Implications
The court thought it significant that the nurse was sought out by the patient's family, who solicited her opinion. She therefore had a responsibility to give accurate information and to direct them to appropriate resources. Her response to the inquiry of the family was regarded as "teaching and counseling" under the state's Nurse Practice Act, and not the unauthorized practice of medicine as alleged by the defendant. The nurse's case was based on a claim of wrongful discharge in violation of public policy, and did not contest the fact that the employer did have the right to terminate her as an employee for no reason, or for an arbitrary or irrational reason, but not for an unlawful reason.

There are also problems of communication when the nurse does not keep the supervisor and/or the physician informed. Although the nurse may have no liability, the situation could be disastrous for the patient and embarrassing for the institution, as in *Bellard v. Willis Knighton Medical Center.*

CASE

Bellard v. Willis Knighton Medical Center (2001)

Siblings of a psychotic patient, who was shot and killed in an armed confrontation with sheriff's deputies several hours after he left the emergency room of the hospital, allege that the ER nurse breached the standard of care by failing to notify the doctor and detain the patient for treatment, if necessary on a protective order. According to police who were in the ER, the patient was not acting in a violent or threatening manner, and the nurse did attempt to detain the patient. But the nurse did not have the authority to detain the patient involuntarily. The District Court entered a jury verdict for the hospital. Later the Appeals Court held that evidence supported the finding that the emergency room nurse did not breach the standard of care by failing to notify the doctor of the patient's condition and detain the patient.[13]

Nursing Implications

Just why didn't the nurse summon the physician on call? Busy doctor; busy nurse? Behavior that was not threatening or exceptional for a psychiatric patient? The fact that the patient had the right to leave? It is difficult to determine what the outcome would have been under different circumstances. Be cautious to communicate the details of such a clinical episode to your supervisor, to the physician, or ideally both. Regardless of the reception you get, you must report the incident, and record fully what happened. There is nothing worse to an administrator than being ignorant of a reportable event that occurred on your service.

You have a right to question the physician when in doubt about any aspect of an order, and the nursing service administration should support you. In fact, there should be a written policy on the nurse's rights and responsibility in such matters, so that there is no confusion on anyone's part and no danger of retribution for justifiable questioning when faced with an irate physician. What if the physician refuses to change the order? You should not simply refuse to carry out an order, for you may not have the most recent medical information and could injure the patient by *not* following the order. You should report your concern promptly to your administrative supervisor and record your action on the chart. Remember, a nurse who follows a physician's orders is just as liable as the physician if the patient is injured because, for instance, a medication was the wrong dose, given by the wrong route, or was actually the wrong drug. If the order is illegible or incomplete, it is necessary to clarify that order with the physician who wrote it. If you doubt its appropriateness, check with a reference source or the pharmacist, and always with the physician who wrote the order. A good collegial relationship and mutual courtesy can prevent or ease a doctor–nurse confrontation.

Verbal or telephone orders are another part of the problem. Although they are considered legal, the dangers are evident. In case of patient injury, either the doctor, or the nurse, or both will be held responsible. There frequently are or should be hospital, sometimes legal, policies to serve as guides. If telephone orders are forbidden and a patient is injured through confused orders, the situation could be considered negligence. If telephone orders are acceptable, precautions should be taken to ensure that they are clearly understood (and questioned if necessary), with the doctor required to confirm the orders in writing as soon as possible. Some hospital policies require a repetition of the order; it is not unheard of to have two nurses listen together to a telephone order, with the second nurse cosigning the order. In states where PAs' orders have been declared legal (as an extension of the physician), the same precautions must be taken, with the physician again confirming the order as quickly as possible.

An incident that repeatedly shows up in litigation is the failure of a physician to see a patient either on the unit or in the emergency room. Often the nurse is held liable for not following through. More and more often, it is suggested that a system (or a policy) be set up specifying who the nurse then contacts. If you neglect to call a doctor when the patient needs help or simply because you are not aware of the seriousness of the patient's condition, charting is not enough. This was clearly demonstrated in the *Darling* case; but charting is important. Even if a nurse swears in court that she did call a doctor and he denies it, the lack of charting has been noted by courts as raising questions about the nurse's credibility.

There are a number of actions you can take to resolve these problems of communication. Don't hesitate to call a physician; be persistent in tracking down the attending or substitute physician: stay on the phone until you get the information you need (use nursing judgment). Be especially careful about telephone orders. Make sure you're both talking about the same patient. Make certain you understand what the doctor is saying even if it requires repetition. Repeat the order. Document the order, noting physician's name, time, date, and name of the third party if there was a witness.

Still other judgments against the nurse have been given when a doctor has not followed through on appropriate technical procedures and the nurse knows it, such as the timely removal of an endotracheal tube. As noted earlier, if you know that a particular procedure is being done incorrectly or a wrong medication is ordered (because it is within the scope of your knowledge) and do nothing about it, you can be held liable as well as the physician. A nurse may also refuse to administer a drug or treatment because it is against hospital policy. However, it is important to have support from nursing management, if discussion with the physician ends with an impasse. It cannot be repeated too often: if the supervisor refuses to help, it will be necessary to go up the chain of command.

MEDICATION ERRORS

Medication errors are a particularly serious problem. A recent report from the Institute of Medicine (a private nonprofit entity providing health policy advice to the National Academy of Sciences under a Congressional mandate) revealed that between 44,000 and 98,000 people in this country die every year from medical errors. Even at the lower limit, this is more people than die from highway accidents, breast cancer, or AIDS.[14] The Institute for Safe Medication Practices (ISMP) claims that it is impossible to know the exact number of medication errors, projecting that only 5 to 7 percent of errors are even reported.[15] In January 2000, the Veterans Administration released a study documenting 3000 medical mistakes involving about 700 patients who died at VA facilities

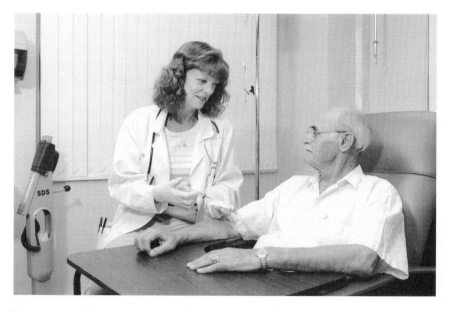

Because medication errors are a major cause of injury to patients, nurses must follow the appropriate procedure carefully. (*Courtesy of Palisades Medical Center, New York Presbyterian Healthcare System*)

during the first 19 months of a new mandatory reporting policy.[16] The whole issue of medication errors has created some intense debate. One dispute is between those who favor mandatory reporting systems which are inherently punitive, and others who support nonpunitive systems as an approach to identifying problems and focusing on prevention.

There are many legal cases based on medication errors, but actually it is generally agreed that those reported are the tip of the iceberg. Unless a patient has a serious adverse reaction, errors may not be reported or recorded. Common errors include: wrong drug, wrong dose, wrong route, and wrong time. In nursing school, correct administration of medications emphasized the five rights, instead of these wrongs, plus making sure that you have the right patient, verifying the name by checking his or her ID bracelet and asking the patient his or her name, if possible. There are many examples of how the wrongs led to trauma, and sometimes death, almost always resulting in legal suits involving nurses. These include a child receiving an adult dose of a potent drug; a nurse injecting a drug into the hip of an obese patient with too short a needle; a nurse delaying an antipsychotic drug for 2 hours, with the result that the patient jumped out a window; and a student nurse giving a patient Maalox intravenously, instead of orally.

An eight-figure settlement was recently secured in *Johnson v. Weiss Memorial Hospital* (March 2002). A woman was left in a persistent vegetative state after suffering a cardiac arrest and subsequent brain damage while hospitalized for treatment of an intestinal condition. The plaintiff alleged that nurses had negligently overdosed her on an intravenous version of the narcotic Dilaudid, while she was additionally medicated with two drugs that are contraindicated when giving Dilaudid, failed to ensure that the patient was carefully monitored after receiving this potent sedation, and failed to ensure that resuscitative equipment was readily available to her.[17]

Preventing medication errors is, in part, getting back to basics with the "five rights":

1. *Right drug.* Check the order, question any drug that seems inappropriate, and consult about any drug with which you are unfamiliar (drug references, drug inserts, or pharmacist). Listen to the patient who notes that the medication "looks different."
2. *Right patient.* Check the patient's identification band.
3. *Right dose.* Be sure that you understand all abbreviations and measurements used in your facility. Have a colleague recheck your calculations. Question any dose that you feel is incorrect.

4. *Right route.* Follow all procedures for each route of administration. If you question the route specified, clarify it *with the physician.*
5. *Right time.* Omit or delay a dose only when indicated by a specific time or condition. Record this.

If an order is illegible, guesswork is dangerous. Physicians are responsible for writing legible orders, with standard abbreviations. Computers are solving some of these problems, but it is still important to make sure the order is complete, including dose and route of administration. Preprinted standardized forms should be carefully reviewed, according to standard practices, so that the medication orders are not misunderstood.

What if you make an error? The patient should be observed for untoward results, the error should be reported, and documented on the chart, and an incident report filed. If necessary, the patient is treated. Then review what happened to prevent another error. The American Society of Hospital Pharmacists calls nurses "the final point of the checks and balances triad" that starts with the physician and pharmacist. Though to some degree repetitive of the classic "five rights," the Society offers the advice contained in Exhibit 12.1, which includes several additional dimensions for safety. *Green v. Long Island Medical College Hospital et al.* below depicts an especially obvious situation of malpractice.

Exhibit 12.1 Recommendations to Help Nurses Stop Medication Errors

- Review the medications of all patients, assessing drug interactions. If you have questions, get the information from pharmacists or other resources. If you're not satisfied, don't administer the medication until you've checked with the physician ordering it.
- Verify all new drug orders before you carry them out by checking the original order, the medication itself, and the patient's ID.
- Inspect the medication, checking expiration date and general appearance. If it doesn't look right, check with the pharmacist.
- Confirm calculations for drug dosage, flow rate, and anything else that requires a mathematical formula with another nurse or the pharmacist.
- Administer medications at the scheduled time. Don't remove identifying information until just before administration. Chart immediately.
- Follow up after administering a drug like an analgesic or antihypertensive to be sure it has had its intended effect.
- Check with pharmacy if the patient's medication hasn't arrived. Don't substitute or borrow from another patient's medication. Return all unfinished or discontinued drugs to the pharmacy.
- Question unusual orders, particularly for large dosages.
- Counsel patients and their caregivers about the prescribed medications, making sure they understand the purpose, how taken, and side effects to watch for.
- Listen to patients who question or object to the use of a particular drug. If concerns remain after you explain the medication's purpose, double-check the order and the dispensed medication with the doctor and pharmacy before giving it.

CASE

Green v. Long Island Medical College Hospital et al. (2005)

The plaintiff, a 35-year-old man, underwent hairline-revision surgery at the defendant hospital. During the procedure the defendant surgeon asked the assisting registered nurse to inject additional Xylocaine into plaintiff's scalp. The defendant nurse mistakenly injected epinephrine, a natural adrenaline hormone. Although epinephrine is sometimes balanced with larger does of Xylocaine, the plaintiff's Xylocaine dosage did not require epinephrine. The plaintiff sustained cardiac arrest following the injection. He was transferred to another hospital, where he remained for a week. The plaintiff suffered a second episode of cardiac arrest at home several months later. He claimed that the defendants' negligence created permanent serious damage to the substrates of his heart. According to the plaintiff, he is now at high risk for arrhythmia and Sudden Death Syndrome and has a reduced sex drive as a result of the medication which he takes. Published accounts claim the case settled before trial for $685,000.[18]

Nursing Implications

Giving medication by injection is a common procedure, but haste can cause serious damage. When you have basic knowledge like the need to maintain the sterility of equipment such as needles, dressings, or various catheters, but are careless about it, this can lead to court cases. But this is clearly not a matter of the need for esoteric knowledge or management of complex equipment, but simply carelessness.

OTHER COMMON ACTS OF NEGLIGENCE

Among the acts of negligence a nurse is most likely to commit in the practice of nursing are the following (not in order of importance):

- *Abandoning a patient.* Abandonment simply means leaving a patient when your duty is to be with him. One example would be leaving a child or incompetent adult without the protection you would have offered. This may include leaving a patient in the bathroom or on a chair or stretcher while attending to something else. Falls often bring on suits. The results of abandonment can be more serious than a broken bone.

- *Improper delegation and supervision.* Unless you work in a place that has all-RN staffing, you probably will be delegating certain patient assignments to an LPN or aide. Theoretically you can look to the LPN's licensure as evidence that this person is qualified to perform certain tasks. However, it is your responsibility to know an individual's competence before assigning an LPN or aide to patient care. The person, if not licensed, must be properly trained. In other words you cannot simply say "You take the patients on that side of the hall" if any one of those patients requires the care of an RN. Should a patient be injured, you can be held responsible.

○ *Failure to use adequate precautions to protect the patient against injury.* As a nurse, you are expected to know that drugs, or hot liquids, or potentially harmful implements, such as scissors, must be kept out of the reach of a young child or a delirious or confused patient. You know the danger of falls or slips when weak, elderly, or disabled patients are walking, left alone, or transferred from chair or stretcher to bed. Patients often fall when trying to get out of bed or using the bathroom. The case below explicates this point.

CASE

Heller v. Barnes-Jewish Hospital (2004)

The 74-year-old plaintiff alleged that while he was a patient at Barnes-Jewish Hospital, a nurse attempted to move him from his bed to a chair without assistance and during the transfer the plaintiff fell. The plaintiff claimed that the nurse failed to request assistance and that two attendants were required to move him because of his size and diminished mental capacity. The plaintiff also contended that there was a sign over his bed with specific instructions that he was only to be moved by two people. The plaintiff suffered soft tissue and internal injuries, resulting in retroperitoneal bleeding in the abdomen and femoral nerve palsy, resulting in decreased mobility.

The defendant argued that the nurse used proper techniques to move him from the bed to the chair near the bed. The defendant denied that there was any sign over the plaintiff's bed with instructions regarding transfers. The defendant also denied that the plaintiff's physical or mental condition made it unsafe for him to be moved from his bed to a chair by one nurse. A verdict for the defense was returned in this case.[19]

Nursing Implications

This is a relatively common situation. Nurses often find it easier to do something themselves rather than waiting for assistance. The primary concern should always be ensuring the safety of the patient, and additionally protecting yourself against ergonomic injuries.

○ Failure to respond, or to ask someone else to *respond, promptly to a patient's call light, signal, or request* if, because of such failure, a patient is injured (see *All Wrongful Death Beneficiaries et al. v. Diamond Care et al.* below).

CASE

Representative of All Wrongful Death Beneficiaries et al.
v. Diamond Care et al. (2001)

An 86-year-old nursing home resident began complaining of persistent nausea early one morning. This symptom was not unusual for this patient, who had a history of compression fractures, and who was being medicated for chronic pain relief with a drug that often upset her stomach. By 5:30 A.M. the patient was pale and complaining of pain in the chest and between her shoulders. Both feet were noted to have 3+ pitting edema and her blood pressure had dropped to 78/52. Furthermore, this patient, who was mentally alert and competent, made three direct requests between 5:20 A.M. and 6:00 A.M. to be transferred to the hospital. These requests were ignored until 6:10 A.M., when the charge nurse contacted the hospital emergency room, and began to initiate the paperwork for transfer. Although the patient's grandson was notified of the impending transfer at 6:10 A.M., EMS personnel were never called. The resident died within the nursing home ten minutes later at 6:20 A.M. This suit was brought by the decedent's two surviving sons. Their case was centered around three alleged acts of negligence: (1) failure of the charge nurse on duty to recognize classic signs and symptoms of a heart attack; (2) failure of the charge nurse on duty to perform a complete assessment of this patient-in-crisis when faced with classic signs of a heart attack; (3) failure of the charge nurse to call the attending physician and EMS in order to effectuate an immediate transfer of the patient to the hospital. The plaintiff maintained that the patient would probably have survived the heart attack had she been transferred to the hospital in a timely manner. The nurse admitted during her deposition that she had not called EMS personnel, or contacted the attending physician immediately.

The defendants contended that the decedent's history of compression fractures and chronic use of pain medication masked the symptoms which led up to her death. They argued that the nausea, paleness, shoulder pain, low blood pressure, and edema were all normal and expected recurring conditions, considering her medical history. According to the defense experts, the charge nurse named in this action was not negligent. They further argued that transfer of this patient to a hospital would not have changed the outcome owing to the fact that she was actually suffering from a pulmonary embolism, not a myocardial infarction. They argued that the decedent's pulmonary embolism was untreatable and imminently fatal.

The nursing home ultimately settled for $2,475,000.[20]

Nursing Implications
The basic problem here, of course, was poor nursing assessment. Ignoring the need to move quickly and expeditiously and the patient's pleas for transfer resulted in what was called *loss of chance,* that is, the patient might have

survived if someone summoned EMS personnel immediately and transferred her with haste. Ignoring call signals or waiting too long to respond is, unfortunately, not unusual in hospitals or nursing homes, especially with short-staffing. True, often the request is minor or trivial and could have waited, but you never know. A common mishap occurs when a patient gets tired of waiting, tries to get out of bed alone, and falls.

○   *Inadequate or dated nursing knowledge.* Since having current knowledge is a professional responsibility, there seems to be little excuse for this kind of negligence. However, on occasion, even the most competent nurse has a problem. If an entirely new type of treatment or piece of equipment is introduced on your unit, it is your responsibility, as well as that of the head nurse or supervisor, to get the appropriate information. The case below makes this point.

CASE

Guardian for Plaintiff v. Maurmanji Sangyo Co. et al. (2000)

The plaintiff was admitted to the hospital in July 1994 for induction of labor. Progress was slow and over the course of the first 24 hours, the child suffered variable decelerations noted on the fetal heart monitoring strips. The obstetrician was called to come in immediately. The mother had been receiving care from a midwife. An emergency cesarean section was performed by the obstetrician and the child was delivered with the cord wrapped tightly around his neck. Resuscitation was initiated immediately after birth with bag and mask ventilation and with brief intubation and suctioning. He was quite flaccid and pale. Apgar scores were 2, 3, and 7. The child was transferred to the newborn nursery and placed on supplemental oxygen with an umbilical artery catheter in place. A nurse placed a Medi-Heat crib warmer underneath the child's back about an hour later without orders to do so. The nurse had obtained the warmer at a seminar. The Medi-Heat warmer was removed an hour later and the child was noted to have a 102.3°F temperature and be warm to the touch. Three hours after the removal of the warmer the child was turned on his left side for a partial sponge bath and his entire back, from neck to sacrum, was deep red with two large fluid-filled blisters on the upper right side of his back. The blisters expanded in size over the next several hours. His blisters popped the next day and a yellowish fluid drained. He was then positioned on his side. He underwent debridement of his burns by a pediatrician and a few days later was taken to another hospital for emergency surgery on his back for the burns. The child suffered neurological injury, which the plaintiff claimed was due to perinatal asphyxia and the fluid and electrolyte loss due to the use of the Medi-Heat warmer. The child also suffers permanent scarring.

The defendant contended that there was no neurological impairment, and if there was, it was caused by the mother's poor prenatal care and poor care of her diabetes and her obesity. A $925,000 settlement was reached.[21]

Nursing Implications

It is never justified to institute a treatment without full understanding of its ramifications, and never without the physician's order unless standing orders or a clear clinical standard exist.

○ *Failure to teach a patient.* Nurses sometimes neglect to teach a patient in preparation for discharge, either because of the time it takes or because the physician objects. An increasing number of suits are being filed because such teaching was not done or not done thoroughly or understandably. Written instructions are often considered necessary to help the patient and family remember the information.

○ *Failure to make sure that faulty equipment is removed* from use, that crowded corridors or hallways adjacent to the nursing unit are cleared, that slippery or unclean floors are taken care of, and that fire hazards are eliminated. This is an area of negligence that, in most instances, would implicate others just as much as, or more than, the professional nurse. For example, the hospital administration would certainly share responsibility for fire hazards and dangerously crowded corridors, and the housekeeping and maintenance departments would not be blameless either. This does not lessen your responsibility for reporting unsafe conditions and following up on them or for checking equipment you use. Report persistent hazards in writing and keep a copy for personal protection.

LEGAL PROBLEMS IN RECORD-KEEPING

It is almost impossible to overemphasize the importance of records in legal action, especially nurses' notes. They are the only evidence that orders were carried out and what the results were; they are the only notes written with both the time and date in chronological order; they offer the most detailed information on the patient. Nurses' notes, like the rest of the chart, can be subpoenaed. No matter how skillfully you practice, if your actions and observations are not documented accurately and completely, the jury can judge only by what is recorded. If you are subpoenaed, comprehensive notes will not only give weight to your testimony, but will help you remember what happened. A case may not come up for years, and unless there was a severe problem at the time, it is difficult to

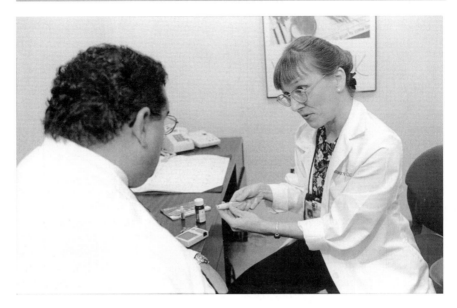

Teaching patients thoroughly can avoid malpractice claims. (*Courtesy of Robert Wood Johnson University Hospital, New Brunswick, New Jersey*)

remember exact details about one patient. General, broad phrases such as "resting comfortably," "good night," and "feeling better" are totally inadequate. How could a jury interpret them? How could another professional who did not know that patient interpret them?

Some of the most serious problems arising from poor charting concern lack of data, which have resulted in liability judgments against nurses and hospitals, although in each case it was contended that the right thing had been done. One judge noted that insufficient notes indicated substandard care. Moreover, there are instances when a patient might be legally harmed by inaccurate reporting, as in child or adult abuse or rape.

The correct way to chart, with legal aspects in mind, is probably to chart as you were taught and to follow good nursing practice.

Do:
- Be objective: write what you see, hear, smell, and feel.
- Be complete: for medications, record what, where, and how.
- Be accurate and write legibly: if a mistake is made, recopy or cross out, with the original copy attached; never use white-out (if paper charting).
- Be specific.
- Record the patient's progress and any change in condition.
- Record abnormal patient behavior.

- Document any patient teaching.
- Use only standard abbreviations.
- Be careful about how statements read. ("Bathed in wheelchair in lounge" can cause a legal problem.)
- Record the time and date of entries; chart the *correct time* when events occurred.
- Sign every entry.

Don't:
- Use a pencil.
- Make flip, derogatory, critical, or extraneous remarks about anyone or use labels to describe your patient's behavior, such as "noncompliant." (Describe what actually happened.)
- Omit data such as amounts and kind of fluids, oxygen, or the physician's visits.
- Guess at such things as output and vital signs.
- *Ever* lie or cover up for anyone. *Never* alter a record other than as described above; this has been shown to influence a jury negatively. Every good malpractice attorney calls on experts to examine charts for alterations, erasures, and additions. This can also lead to criminal charges.
- Let anyone chart for you or change what you have charted.
- Chart for anyone else. When you must chart what an aide or student says he or she did or what occurred when you have not personally seen it, add a statement that clarifies the fact to protect yourself.
- Fail to record verbal orders and have them signed.
- Chart your actions in advance to save time.
- Refer to staffing problems.
- Mention that an incident report has been filed. If you do, there could be an attempt to have it admitted as evidence. Do not include second-hand information, opinions, accusations, excuses, or suggestions for how to prevent future incidents in the incident report; they can be used against you if the report falls into evidence.[22]
- Use terms like "accidentally" or "somehow" to explain a mistake. Just record what happened.
- Air "dirty laundry"—disputes with colleagues or criticisms of nurses or doctors.
- Refer to another patient by name; use "roommate," initials, or bed number.
- Withhold important information, such as conversations with family or health professionals.

Computer records have changed correction procedures, since corrections can be made immediately. (Such "charting" does allow for more accurate, timely, and legible charting, but the issue of confidentiality discussed in Chapter 9 may present a problem.) Charting incorrect data in any form obviously does not give an accurate picture of your patient's condition, which could lead to life-threatening errors. It may also raise a question of fraud, so that your actions appear not just negligent, but criminal.

Some of the most serious problems arising from poor charting concern lack of data, such as omission of a temperature reading or other vital signs, lack of observations about a patient's condition, or no record of oxygen liter flow in a newborn infant; these and others have resulted in liability judgments against nurses and hospitals. Although it is often inaccurate, the statement "if it wasn't charted, it wasn't done" has evolved into a legal standard.

Court cases in which nursing documentation is inadequate are many and often result in a judgment for the plaintiff. While the current trend toward "charting by exception"—that is, charting only when something unusual or out of the ordinary happens—may save time, it frequently leaves gaps that raise questions about patient care.[23] A well-designed flowchart can be useful, but it should be consistent with the nurse's notes. You cannot simply check off what the nurses on the previous shift checked off. If you were sued, such discrepancies would damage your credibility. Moreover, you should not depend too heavily on flowcharts; it is still important to record the patient's *response* to care in your notes. Overall, any significant indicator of a change in the patient's condition, corresponding interventions, and the patient's response should be recorded. The chart must accurately reflect the patient's condition and progress. Cases such as the classic *Darling* one continue to occur. The case described below is a particularly good example of what can happen if charting by exception is taken too literally.

CASE

Holt v. Wesley Medical Center (2004)

The plaintiff was admitted to Wesley for an elective induction of labor. The baby was subsequently delivered by an emergency cesarean section. The baby was born limp and pale without spontaneous respirations and today suffers from permanent brain damage. Plaintiffs attribute this condition to negligence on the part of resident physicians, nurses, and other health care providers who participated in the labor and delivery. In addition, Mrs. Holt's uterus was ruptured and her bladder, cervix, and vagina were severely lacerated, resulting in her being unable to have other children. The plaintiffs also assert that they have sustained economic and noneconomic losses due to the continuing medical problems of mother and daughter.

Expert witnesses questioned the adequacy of professional monitoring during labor, given that the plaintiff was on a very high dose of pitocin. This case contained two interesting points of note to our discussion of record-keeping. First, when over 5 liters of fluid were given to the plaintiff during labor with almost no urine return, and subsequently only a small amount of grossly bloody fluid obtained, this information was not reported to the attending physician. This behavior was considered reckless by the court and far below the acceptable standard of care practices for any nurse. Subsequently, over three weeks after her hospitalization, the plaintiff's medical records were altered to include three specific reports of the low and bloody urine output to the attending physician. This was considered by the court as behavior in a most wanton manner.

An expert witness for the plaintiff testified that there was either nurse understaffing or bad nursing care at Wesley during the plaintiff's labor and delivery. This opinion was based on Mrs. Holt's medical chart, which showed that nurses failed to take and record vital signs as required by nursing policies. Further, staffing schedules proved that the nurses assigned to the plaintiff were also assigned to care for other patients during periods in the plaintiff's labor when one-to-one attention was necessary to assure safety.[24]

Nursing Implications

Although the hospital tried to discredit the sources of expert opinion, the evidence spoke for itself. The blatant violation of record-keeping, and the presence of records to document staffing assignments, were critical in this case. The failure of nurses to document and communicate early signs of impending complications put the patient at risk.

You should be very clear about what needs to be charted to document accurately the patient's condition, regardless of a hospital policy on charting. Saving time is not worthwhile if a patient suffers. As in so many other cases, taking short-cuts, even approved short-cuts, can be calamitous. First of all, however, your nursing assessment is the key to what to chart, and reporting as well as recording is essential. Should a situation arise when you do notify a physician about a problem and he denies it in court, your written documentation at the time of doing so generally carries weight over the doctor's testimony.

THE PROBLEM OF SHORT-STAFFING

Can an injury to a patient be excused on the basis of short-staffing? Not really. Even if there is a staff shortage, nurses have a responsibility to use good judgment.

In *Harrell v. Louis Smith Hospital* (1992), the plaintiff alleged negligence on the part of the hospital because of short-staffing, and the president of the hospital did make several statements that created some question as to whether certain units, such as the emergency room, were well staffed.

The court ruled that the hospital *must* provide staff "adequately trained to exercise a reasonable degree of care and skill when delivering healthcare." There is some feeling that with all the unlicensed assistive personnel being hired and a cutback of RNs today, this point will come up again. Short-staffing and cost containment are involved in the following case.

CASE

Adams v. Youville Health Care Center, Inc. (2000)

A nurse, employed on a subacute care unit, blows the whistle on unsafe health care practices. The nurse had become increasingly concerned about safety and quality as the hospital implemented staffing cuts and cost containment measures. He carefully documented the unsafe practice and correlated these instances with inadquate staffing, a substantial increase in assignments, and the lack of supervision. There were increased falls, serious medication errors, and instances where patients were left to lie in their own urine and feces. For three months this nurse and other colleagues followed the organization's procedures to communicate their concerns to administration. The administration offered no response, except to criticize him for collecting this information in the first place. In response, he decided to document what had not been done. He was eventually threatened with the loss of his job, in spite of previous excellent performance reviews, and was fired. The nurse sued and won his case. The hospital appealed and lost.[25]

Nursing Implications

The Adams case speaks to the situation faced by any nurse who acts to address unsafe practice conditions that conflict with his or her legal and ethical responsibilities as a registered nurse. The suit claims that in advocating for his patients and raising issues about their safety, Adams was doing what Massachusetts law says he is obligated to do as a licensed registered nurse.

If advocacy is the nurse's role, who protects the nurse? Legislative efforts are being set in place to offer protections to all health care workers who speak out on unsafe patient care.

Further problems can come from "floating." In these cases, you may be placed in a specialty area with which you are not familiar, with or without a more experienced nurse. There is no clear answer to this dilemma, since some courts have ruled that shifting staff is the employer's privilege and refusal can be considered insubordination. Express your reservations and explore alternatives, for instance, to delay such an assignment until you have received in-service training, or indicate a willingness to provide the care you are currently comfortable with. This is equally important if you are an inexperienced new graduate. The supervisor, of course, is also responsible for any damage done because he or she is supposed to delegate safely. The float nurse must be especially careful and report any change in a patient's condition. Perhaps the best defense if injury occurs is to be able to document that you recognized your knowledge gap, but did not know that specialty and had asked for help. Meanwhile, some union contracts and some individual agreements in hospitals specify that a nurse is not to be floated to an unfamiliar unit without some training in that specialty. (See also Chapter 15.) Regardless, as shown in the next case, you are responsible for your own actions.

CASE

Duplan v. Harper (1999)

This young woman, learning that she was pregnant, and given that she was employed in a setting where she was at risk of becoming infected with cytomegalovirus (CMV), which causes birth defects, was tested to determine whether she was immune to CMV. The patient and her husband had already agreed that if she were not immune they would abort the pregnancy, rather than risking having a child with CMV-induced birth defects. The test showed that the patient had an ongoing primary CMV infection, which created a significant risk of birth defects. The doctor directed a nurse to inform the patient of her test results. The nurse notified the patient that the CMV test was positive. The patient was unsure whether "positive" meant she was immune or that she was infected. The nurse incorrectly told the patient that it meant she was immune, and based on this information the patient decided not to abort the pregnancy. The patient gave birth to a son with serious CMV birth defects. The child will require custodial care throughout his life, and significant medical and rehabilitative services for any quality of life. The parents brought a wrongful birth suit, which was found for the parents. It was upheld on appeal. The district court awarded a settlement of over $3 million. In an interesting turn of events, that amount was reduced to $200,000 in the appeals court, citing that this was an adequate recovery to the parents for their emotional distress. Whereas the remainder of the settlement might have benefited the child, he was not the plaintiff in this case.[26]

Nursing Implications

One point this case demonstrates is that you are responsible for your own actions. The nurse should have been aware of the meaning of a "positive" test, and if not, should have referred the patient to the physician, and then made it her business to learn. This case also illustrates the need to communicate test results in writing, including a clear explanation of the meaning of those results. The importance of ensuring that patients not only have correct information but also actually understand its meaning cannot be overemphasized.

STANDARD OF CARE

The standard of care basically determines nurses' liability for negligent acts. (Note its importance in the cases cited previously.) This standard requires an individual to perform a task as any "reasonably prudent man [nurse] of ordinary prudence, with comparable education, skills, and training under similar circumstances" would perform that same function. Remember we are actually talking about malpractice here, which is more restricted, a specialized kind of negligence. It is the "violation of a professional duty or a failure to meet a standard of care or failure to use the skills and knowledge" that other professionals would use in similar circumstances. Who makes that judgment on what the "reasonably prudent" nurse would do?

In litigation, it is the judge or jury, based on testimony that could include the following:

- *Expert witnesses.* Did the nurse do what was necessary? A nurse with special or appropriate knowledge testifies on what would be expected of a nurse in the defendant's position in like circumstances. The expert witness would have the credentials to validate his or her expertise, but because the opposing side would produce an equally prestigious expert witness to say what was useful to them, the credibility of that witness on testifying is critical. A nurse would generally be judged by an expert in his or her particular specialization.
- *Professional literature.* Was the nurse's practice current? The *most current* nursing literature would be examined and perhaps quoted to validate (or invalidate) whether the nurse's practice in the situation was totally up to date.
- *Hospital or agency policies and protocols.* Were hospital policies, especially nursing policies (in-house law), followed? For example, if restraints were or were not used, was the nurse's action according to hospital policy? On the other hand, if a nurse followed an outdated policy or followed policy without using nursing judgment (according to the expert witness), it could be held against her or him.
- *Manuals or procedure books.* Did the nurse follow the usual procedure accurately? Example: if the nurse gave an injection that was alleged to have injured the patient, was it given correctly according to the procedure manual? If the procedure book is not up to date and the nurse followed it, she or he might still be liable on the basis of needing to be aware of current practice.
- *Drug enclosures or drug reference books.* Did the nurse check for the latest information? For example, if the patient suffered from a drug reaction that the nurse did not perceive, was the information

about the potential reaction in a drug reference book, such as the *Physicians' Desk Reference* (PDR) or a drug insert?

- *The profession's standards.* Did the nurse behave according to the published ANA standards, both general and in the specialty, if any?
- *Licensure.* Did the nurse fulfill her responsibilities according to the legal definition of nursing in the licensure law or the law's rules and regulations? For example, did she teach a diabetic patient about foot care?

If the judge or jury is satisfied that the standards were met satisfactorily, even if the patient has been injured, the injury that occurred would not be considered the result of the nurse's negligence. (If there is *no* injury, even if the health care provider was negligent, there is no tort.) Different judgments in different jurisdictions must be expected. The following cases are good examples.

CASE

Garley v. Columbia LaGrange Memorial Hospital et al. (2004)

The plaintiff's wife died from a pulmonary embolism three days after undergoing several abdominal surgeries. A wrongful death suit was filed against the hospital, based upon the conduct of its nursing staff and the attending surgeon in caring for Mrs. Garley both during and after surgery.

On the morning of surgery, the patient was admitted to the hospital, where she was to undergo several abdominal surgeries lasting approximately three hours. The patient was brought into the operating room and positioned in the lithotomy position (on her back with her legs elevated and separated) with the use of knee crutches. Though the length of the surgery, her weight, and her age placed Mrs. Garley at risk for developing a deep vein thrombus (DVT) or blood clot, no anticlotting device or medication was utilized or suggested during surgery. After surgery was completed, the surgeon ordered that Mrs. Garley be "ambulated with assistance" to decrease the risk that a DVT might develop. According to hospital records, the nurse unsuccessfully attempted to walk the patient in the late afternoon, about three hours after surgery. The patient was not ambulated on the operative day. On the first postoperative day, the patient was ambulated three times. On the second postoperative day, she ambulated twice, collapsing during the second ambulation and dying shortly thereafter.

The plaintiff based their case on negligence of the nursing staff. Three physician expert witnesses testified to the nurses not meeting the requisite standard of care by neglecting to ambulate her on schedule, not reporting her leg pain or the lack of ambulation to the attending physician, failing to comment on the position used for surgery, and the absence of anticlotting devices during surgery. Incidentally, all the nurses involved denied any complaints of leg pain from the patient.

The case was found for the plaintiff, but on appeal it was reversed and remanded granting a directed verdict for the hospital, based on the inappropriate expert opinion which was the backbone of the argument. The court described how physicians often have no first-hand knowledge of nursing practice except for observations made in patient care settings. In most situations, a physician would not be familiar with the standard of care or with nursing policies and procedures that govern the standard of care. Therefore, a physician's opinions would not be admissible in jurisdictions which hold that the expert must be familiar with the standard of care in order to testify as an expert.[27]

Nursing Implications

A nurse practicing in a specific specialty owes her patients the degree of knowledge and skill ordinarily possessed by other members of the profession who actively practice in that specialty, and further, to exercise those skills as would colleagues, using reasonable care and diligence. When there is reason to doubt that care and diligence, as in court, an expert opinion is necessary. A physician who is not licensed as a nurse is automatically incompetent to offer expert opinion about the nursing standard of care; his or her knowledge, experience, and level of expertise, no matter how extensive, are simply irrelevant.

CASE

Ferris v. County of Kennebec (1999)

On admission, an inmate at the county jail complained to the facility's nurse of abdominal pain and vaginal bleeding, and stated that she was pregnant and having a miscarriage. She made this statement with some previous experience, having had a miscarriage five years previously. The nurse took her pulse and told her she was menstruating, directing her to lie down. When her complaints continued, the nurse had her transferred to a cell where she had no contact with the nurse. Several hours later, the patient had a miscarriage. The patient subsequently filed suit. The U.S. District Court held that the nurse's behavior constituted deliberate indifference to serious medical needs. The case was found for the plaintiff.[28]

Nursing Implications

Providing an adequate standard of care is basic to the nurse's job. The nurse never even confirmed that the patient was pregnant. The nurse contended that a reasonably prudent nurse would have treated the patient in the same way. That is preposterous. It is important for nurses to treat patient complaints seriously, and take appropriate courses of action to provide reasonable care.

OTHER TORTS AND CRIMES

The average nurse probably will not get involved in criminal offenses, although in the last few years, a number of nurses have been accused of murder or other deliberate injury to patients. Nurses, like anyone else, may steal, murder, or break other laws, but they can also be falsely accused. Crimes most often committed are criminal assault and battery (striking or otherwise physically mistreating or threatening a patient); murder (sometimes in relation to right-to-die principles); and drug offenses. If found guilty of a felony, the nurse will probably also lose her or his license.

Whether the nurse is a perpetrator or victim, or simply has to deal with people who are, it is useful to know the definition and scope of the most common criminal offenses. These can be found in most nursing law texts. Several are discussed here. Not discussed but worth mentioning are some torts and crimes in which nurses occasionally are involved in their professional lives: *forgery*—fraudulently making or altering a written document or item, such as a will, chart, or check; *kidnapping*—stealing and carrying off a human being; *rape*—illegal or forcible sexual intercourse; and *bribery*—an offer of a reward for doing wrong or for influencing conduct. Other causes for action against nurses beyond negligence are false imprisonment (also discussed in Chapter 9), intentional infliction of emotional distress, and invasion of privacy.

ASSAULT AND BATTERY

Any attempt to use force and violence with an intent to injure, or put one in fear of injury, constitutes an *assault*, such as striking at a person with or without a weapon; holding up a fist in a threatening way near enough to be able to strike; or advancing with a hand uplifted in a threatening way with intent to strike or put someone in fear of being struck, even if the person is stopped before he or she gets near enough to carry out the intended action.

Battery, as distinguished from assault, is the actual striking or touching of a person's body in a violent, angry, rude, or insolent manner. Every laying on of hands is not a battery: the person's intention must be considered. To constitute a battery, intent to injure or put one in fear of injury must be accompanied by "unlawful violence." However, the slightest degree of force may constitute violence in the eyes of the law. Legal action can result from any of these acts unless they can be justified or excused.

This topic is covered from the perspective of the patient in Chapter 9.

DEFAMATION, SLANDER, AND LIBEL

As is true of so many legal terms, there is some overlapping of meaning and interpretation of the terms *defamation, slander,* and *libel.* In general, however, it is correct to consider *defamation* as the most inclusive term because it covers any communication that is seriously detrimental to another person's reputation. If the communication is oral, it is technically called *slander*; if written or shown in pictures, effigies, or signs (without just cause or excuse), it is called *libel.* All three are considered wrongful acts (torts) under the law, and a person convicted in court is ordered to make amends, usually by paying the defamed person damages in compensation.

In both slander and libel, a third person must be involved. For example, one person can make all kinds of derogatory statements directly to another without getting in trouble with the law *unless* overheard and understood by a third person. The remarks then become slanderous. Likewise a person can write anything she or he wishes to another, and the communication will not be considered libelous unless it is read and understood by a third person. A malicious and false statement made by one person to another about a third person also comprises slander.

Uncomplimentary statements are not necessarily slanderous or libelous. They must be false, damaging to the offended person's reputation, and tending to subject him or her to public contempt and ridicule. The best and often the only defense allowed under the law is proof that she or he told the truth in whatever type of communication used.

Given the many "ifs," "ands," and "buts" associated with defamation, slander, and libel, it is better to avoid becoming embroiled in such litigations. Be careful in what you say or write about anyone. Also, proceed with caution when you are the victim of slander or libel. Litigation is expensive and time-consuming and, in many instances, hardly worth the trouble. On the other hand, do not be overly meek in accepting unfair and untrue statements about yourself that are likely to adversely affect your reputation. There have been documented cases in which nurses were slandered by a physician, for instance, and collected damages.

HOMICIDE AND SUICIDE

Homicide means killing a person by any means whatsoever. It is not necessarily a crime. If it is unquestionably an accident, it is called *excusable homicide*. If it is done in self-defense or in discharging a legal duty, it is termed *justifiable homicide*. The accused must be able to prove justification, however. *Criminal homicide* is either murder or manslaughter; murder is usually with intent.

Suicide is considered criminal if the person is sane and of an age of discretion at the time of his or her action. A person who encourages another to commit suicide is guilty of murder if the suicide is successful. Statutes vary from state to state.

As a professional person, it is not unusual for a nurse to become involved in cases of murder and suicide, usually associated with patients. The following are a few suggestions for keeping as free of legal involvement as possible:

- Take seriously any indication on the part of any patient or employee that she or he has suicidal tendencies. Report this to the appropriate person.
- Generally, do not leave a patient with known suicidal inclinations alone unless completely protected from self-harm by restraints or confinement.
- Keep items that a depressed person might use for suicidal purposes out of reach.
- Make and report observations accurately on the patient's chart.
- Try to get help for individuals or their families immediately upon becoming aware of suicidal tendencies.
- Cooperate with the police and hospital authorities guarding a patient who is accused of homicide.
- Avoid unethical discussions of a homicide case involving a patient or employee.
- Keep complete and accurate records of all facts that might have a bearing on the legal aspects of a case.

DRUG CONTROL

In 1914, the United States adopted an antinarcotic law, the *Harrison Narcotic Act*, to be administered by a bureau of narcotics within the Department of the Treasury. It was amended frequently to meet the demands of changing times. The *Comprehensive Drug Abuse and Control Act of 1970 (Controlled Substances Act)* replaced virtually all earlier federal laws dealing with narcotics, stimulants, depressants, and hallucinogens. Sections of this law prohibit nurses (except APNs where allowed by state law) from prescribing controlled substances, but they may administer drugs at the direction of legalized practitioners (who are registered). All registrants must follow strict controls and procedures against theft and diversion of controlled substances. New state laws are based on the federal law, although there are variations. Controlled substances are identified as such in health care delivery sites. New drugs are also being given closer scrutiny because of misuse and consequent dangerous effects.

Knowledge of the laws controlling the use of drugs will help you to understand the reasons for the policies and procedures established by an institution or agency for the mutual welfare of the employer, employee, and patient. It will also help you to keep free of legal involvements and to direct and advise intelligently others whom you may supervise or who may look to you for guidance in such matters. Be alert to changes in drug laws at either the state or the national level.

GOOD SAMARITAN LAWS

The enactment of Good Samaritan laws in many states exempts doctors and nurses (and sometimes others) from civil liability when they give emergency care in "good faith" with "due care" or without "gross negligence." All states and the District of Columbia have Good Samaritan laws, but not all include nurses in their coverage. The law is intended to encourage assistance without fear of legal liability. As far as the law is concerned, there is no obligation or duty to render aid or assistance in an emergency. Only by statutory law can the rendering of such assistance be required. Emergency treatment in a health care setting, such as hospitals, clinics, and occupational health departments, is not covered under the Good Samaritan laws.

Because of the lack of clarity of terms and the many differences in the law from state to state, many health professionals are still reluctant to give emergency assistance. The following is good advice:[29]

- Don't give aid unless you know what you are doing.
- Stick to the basics of first aid.
- Offer to help, but make it clear that you won't interfere if the victim or family prefers to wait for other help.
- Don't draw any medical or diagnostic conclusions.
- Don't leave a victim you have begun to assist until you can turn his or her care over to an equally competent person.
- Whether you do or do not volunteer your services, be absolutely certain to call or have someone else call for a physician or emergency medical service immediately.

PROFESSIONAL LIABILITY (MALPRACTICE) INSURANCE

Almost all lawyers in the health field now agree that nurses should carry their own malpractice or, as it is increasingly called, *professional liability* insurance, whether or not their employer's insurance includes them. The employer's insurance is intended primarily to protect the employer; the nurse is protected only to the extent needed for that primary purpose. It is quite possible that the employer might settle out of court, without consulting the nurse, to the nurse's disadvantage. The nurse then has no control and no choice of lawyer.

There are a number of other limitations. The nurse is not covered for anything beyond the job in the place of employment during the hours of employment. If the nurse alone is sued and the hospital is not, the hospital has no obligation to provide legal protection (and may choose not to). Moreover, as noted earlier, if the nurse has been negligent, and carries no personal liability insurance, there is the possibility of subrogation. Should there be criminal charges, the employer or insurance carrier may choose to deny legal assistance, or the kind offered could be inadequate. However, some professional liability policies held by the nurse personally may also state that criminal action is not covered. Remember that no matter how trivial or how unfounded a charge might be, a legal defense is necessary and often costly, aside from the possibility of being found liable and having to pay damages.

Professional liability insurance should be bought with some care so that adequate coverage is provided. Certain features are optional. Decide which coverage meets your needs, but do not necessarily choose the least expensive. For instance, the most important distinction to be made in selecting insurance is whether it has an *occurrence-based* or a *claims-made coverage.* Occurrence-based policies cover injuries that occur during the period covered by the policy, even though the policy may no longer be active. Claims-made policies cover injuries only if they occur within the active policy period and the claim is reported to the insurer during the period that the policy is in force. If the insurance policy is allowed to lapse, an incident that occurred at the time of coverage will be covered in an occurrence-based policy but not in a claims-made policy. The latter may be less expensive but will require almost continuous coverage, which might be a problem for a nurse planning to interrupt practice for any reason or for one close to retirement.

Before deciding on a policy, check:

1. Is it occurrence-based or claims-made? What does it cover and for what amount? (A million dollars is reasonable coverage today—more if you are an APN.)
2. What, if any, is the deductible?

3. Is there a subrogation clause?
4. Are you covered for personal liability?
5. Will you be covered off the job?
6. What, if any, are the exclusions?
7. Under what circumstances will a lawyer be provided?
8. Can a settlement be made without your approval?
9. The term of the policy?
10. What affects renewability?
11. The cost?

Benefits usually include paying any sum awarded as damages, including medical costs, paying the cost of attorneys, and paying the bond required if appealing an adverse decision. Some policies also pay damages for injury arising out of acts of the insured as a member of an accreditation board or committee of a hospital or professional society, personal liability (such as slander, assault, or libel), and personal injury and medical payments (not related to the individual's professional practice).

Generally speaking, an ANA or CMA policy is the best buy. Premiums depend on the position of the nurse. Only nurse anesthetists and nurse–midwives are not covered, but NPs and nurses in private practice are, at a higher premium. In 1990, ANA also expanded its coverage to include students. Nurses who have retired are often advised to keep their professional liability insurance. Most nurses tend to help and advise neighbors, friends, and family about their health care. If the person advised feels that the advice was the cause of an emotional or physical problem later, he or she has been known to sue the nurse.

As noted earlier, most malpractice cases are settled out of court (although this still requires a lawyer) and multimillion-dollar awards are not as common as the newspapers may imply. However, for the careful nurse, professional liability insurance is a good investment, as well as being tax deductible.

IN COURT: THE DUE PROCESS OF LAW

Yes, you can be sued. What happens if you become involved in litigation? What steps should you take to try to make sure that the case will be handled to your best advantage throughout? The answers to these questions will depend on: whether you are accused of committing the tort or crime; whether you are an accessory, through actual participation or observance; whether you are the person against whom the act was committed; or whether you appear as an expert witness.

Assuming that this is a civil case, five distinct steps are taken:

- The filing of a document called a *complaint* by a person called the *plaintiff* who contends that his legal rights have been infringed by the conduct of one or more other persons called *defendants.*
- The written response of the defendants accused of having violated the legal rights of the plaintiff, termed an *answer.*
- Pretrial activities of both parties designed to elicit all the facts of the situation, termed *discovery.*
- The *trial* of the case, in which all the relevant facts are presented to the judge or jury for decision.
- *Appeal* from a decision by a party who contends that the decision was wrongly made. This step is optional.

The majority of persons who are asked to appear as witnesses during a hearing accept voluntarily. Others refuse and must be subpoenaed. A *subpoena* is a writ or order in the name of the court, referee, or another person authorized by law to issue the same, which requires the attendance of a witness at a trial or hearing under a penalty for failure to appear. Cases involving the care of patients often necessitate producing hospital records, x-rays, and photographs as evidence. A subpoena requiring a witness to bring this type of evidence to court contains a clause to that effect and is termed a *subpoena duces tecum.*

The plaintiff, defendant, and witnesses may be asked to make a *deposition,* an oral interrogation answering various questions about the issue concerned. It is given under oath and taken in writing before a judicial officer or attorney. Tips given by experts on how to handle yourself at a deposition are basically the same as for testifying. You may be cross-examined by the opposing lawyer; the only limitation on the scope of questioning is that the inquiry must be relevant to the subject under suit. Since the primary purpose is *discovery,* the procedure is sometimes referred to as a "fishing expedition."

The trial itself follows a certain format: choosing the jury; opening statements by both sides, with the plaintiff going first; testimony and cross-examination; possible request for dismissal; and closing arguments. An appeal to a higher court may be filed.

A witness has certain rights, including the right to refuse to testify as to privileged communication (extended to the nurse in only a few states) and the protection against self-incrimination afforded by the Fifth Amendment to the Constitution. The judge and jury usually do not expect a person on trial or serving as witness to remember all the details of a situation. Witnesses in malpractice suits are permitted to refer to the patient's record, which, of course, they should have reviewed with the attorney before the trial. Only under serious circumstances is someone accused (and convicted) of *perjury,* which means making a false statement under oath or one that the person neither knows nor believes to be true.

There are certain guidelines on testifying that are the same whether serving as an expert or other witness or if the nurse is the defendant:

- Be prepared; review the deposition, the chart, and technical and clinical knowledge of the disease or condition; discuss with the lawyer potential questions; educate the lawyer as to what points should be made. Trials are adversary procedures that are intended to probe, question, and explore all aspects of the issue.
- Dress appropriately; appearance is important.
- Behave appropriately: keep calm, be courteous, even if insulted: don't be sarcastic or angry; take your time (a cross-examiner attorney may try to put you in a poor light). Never argue with the attorney questioning you.
- Give adequate and appropriate information: if you can't remember, notes or the data source, such as the chart, can be checked. Answer fully, but don't volunteer additional information not asked for. Don't answer until you understand the question. Wait for the question to be completed before you respond. Think about your answer before responding.
- Don't use technical terminology, or, if use is necessary, translate it into lay terms. Enunciate clearly.
- Don't feel incompetent; don't get on the defensive; be decisive.
- Don't be obviously partisan (unless you're the defendant).
- Keep all materials; the decision may be appealed.

In the expert witness role, the same suggestions hold, but in addition the nurse should present her or his credentials, degrees, research, honors, and whatever else is pertinent, without modesty; the opposing expert witness will certainly do so. Expert witnesses are paid for preparation time, pretrial conferences, consultations, and testifying. Nurses are just beginning to act officially in this capacity, and several CMAs accept applications for those interested in placement on an expert witness panel, screen applicants in a given field for a specific case, submit a choice of names to attorneys requesting such information, and have developed guidelines and continuing education for nurse expert witnesses.

Should you be sued, here are some tips for defending yourself:[30]

- Cut off all communication with the claimant; simply tell whoever contacts you that your insurer will be in touch. (Then find out why they haven't already done so.)
- Educate the insurer; claims adjusters may know little about nursing.

- Keep tabs on the claim. Don't be afraid to ask questions.
- Be sure that your claim is supervised adequately. You have a right to ask that it be handled by an experienced and attentive professional.
- Seek input on settlement decisions. You may not have the right, but you can ask your insurer to check with you before making an offer.
- Remember that the defense attorney is *your* attorney. If you really think his or her qualifications are inadequate, ask for a change.
- Dictate all memories of the patient to the attorney. Do it as soon as possible but not until an attorney has been assigned to your case, or your information may not be considered "privileged."
- Retrieve medical records. You have access if you still work at the same place and can get access before the attorney does.
- Review the records.
- Compile a list of experts; the case may hinge on getting the best. [Although in some courts physicians have been allowed as expert witnesses on a nursing case, ordinarily it should be the nurse(s) who are most knowledgeable about the type of situation involved.]
- Have a reference list available.
- Speak up in court; you must project self-confidence.

Other attorneys also point out that you should not talk to anyone at your institution about the case except the risk manager, or with anyone involved in any way with the plaintiff, or to reporters. Certainly do not hide any information from your attorney, and *never* alter the patient's record.

RISK MANAGEMENT

No matter how strong the defense, everyone agrees that prevention is better than any suit. Therefore, hospitals have now adopted risk-management programs in which nurses are very much involved, as part of the team and also sometimes in one of the risk-management positions, including patient representative or advocate. Risk management must be a team effort involving everyone.

Risk management initiatives are now required by JCAHO and increasingly more often by state legislation. The purpose is not only to protect the interest of the hospital and its personnel but also to improve the quality of patient care. Risk management means taking steps to control the possibility that a patient will complain and minimizing any risks *before* complaints are filed. Nurses are often involved in risk management which includes focusing on the review and improvement of employee guidelines, personnel policies, incident reports, physician–nurse relationships, safety policies, patient records, research guidelines, and anything else that might be a factor in legal suits.

JCAHO urges facilities to voluntarily file reports of "sentinel events," defined as "an unexpected occurrence involving death or serious physical or psychological injury, or the risk thereof," and to conduct a "root-cause" analysis within 30 days. However, there is some fear that such a report is discoverable, and could lead to lawsuits.

Nevertheless, patient injuries do occur. In case of patient injury, most hospitals and health agencies require completion of an "incident report." The purpose is to document the incident accurately for remedial and correctional use by the hospital or agency, for insurance information, and sometimes for legal reasons. The wording should be chosen to avoid the implication of blame and should be totally objective and complete: what happened to the patient; what was done; what his condition is. The incident report may or may not be discoverable, depending on the state's law. It is considered a business record, not part of the patient's chart, but some courts rule that it is not privileged information. The incident *must* be just as accurately recorded in the patient's chart. This kind of omission casts doubt on the nurse's honesty if litigation occurs. However, *the fact that an incident report was filed should not be charted.*

Appropriate behavior by nurses and other personnel is often a key factor as to whether or not the patient or family sues after an incident, regardless of injury. Maintaining a good rapport and giving honest explanations as needed is very important.

AVOIDING LEGAL PROBLEMS

Malpractice continues to be an issue in health care from the point of view of both patient endangerment and cost. Physicians are said to practice "defensive medicine," that is, ordering every possible test to make sure that nothing was neglected that may eventually result in litigation. That and the rising cost of malpractice insurance add to the overall cost of health care. Nurses are also concerned about their liability as they care for patients who are sicker, with less help. While it may be possible to get some information from your employing agency's legal counsel or state licensing board in relation to specific aspects of your practice, observing some basic principles will also help to avert problems:

- Know your licensure law.
- Don't do what you don't know how to do. (Learn how, if necessary.)

- Keep your practice updated; continuing education is essential.
- Use self-assessment, peer evaluation, audits, and the supervisor's evaluations as guidelines for improving practice, and follow up on criticisms and knowledge/skill gaps.
- Don't be careless.
- Be considerate of patients and their significant others.
- Practice interdependently; communicate with others.
- Record accurately, objectively, and completely; don't erase.
- Delegate safely and legally; know the preparation and abilities of those you supervise.
- Help develop appropriate policies and procedures (in-house law).
- Carry professional liability insurance.

There are those nurses who defend their patients from harm and others whose substandard practices make them a target for litigation. Never forget that licensure is a privilege and a responsibility mandating accountability to the consumer it is intended to protect; therefore, you have a legal and moral obligation to practice safely.

KEY POINTS

1. Malpractice suits of any kind are often stimulated by how the patient and family were treated, as well as by the possible injury.
2. The standard of care by which a nurse is judged in a malpractice case is based on what the "reasonably prudent nurse" of the same background and in the same situation would do.
3. Negligence frequently occurs in giving medication and treatments because the nurse has inadequate knowledge or is careless.
4. *Darling v. Charleston Community Memorial Hospital* is a landmark case pinpointing the corporate liability of hospitals for the actions of their employees and physicians. For nurses, it underlines the legal responsibility to follow through and ensure that patients get competent care.
5. Poor communication between doctors and nurses, and among nurses themselves, can endanger patients and result in litigation.
6. To avoid problems in law, be accurate, complete, and objective in charting. Never falsify a record for any reason.
7. When selecting professional liability (malpractice) insurance, among the points to consider is whether it is occurrence-based or claims-made.
8. When testifying in a court of law, be prepared and calm; give appropriate information without jargon, and be accurate and honest.

9. To avoid malpractice, it is especially important to know your licensure law, stay up to date in your practice, communicate with others adequately, be careful, and practice humanistic nursing.

STUDY QUESTIONS

1. Develop a program to decrease the number of medication errors in your hospital.
2. You are uncomfortable with the drug dosage that the physician has ordered for your patient. The physician refuses to answer your questions and just orders you to give the medication. What should you do and why?
3. What is the rationale underlying "charting by exception" and what other systems must be in place to make it work properly?
4. What is the student's need for malpractice insurance?
5. Many nursing journals have columns on the law. Go to your college library, browse through these journals, and make a list of the types of problems that nurses are most typically confronted with.

REFERENCES

1. National Practitioner Data Bank. 2003 Annual Report: http://www.npdb-hipdb.com/pubs/stats/2003_npdb_Annual_Report.pdf. Retrieved April 24, 2005.
2. Showers JL. What you need to know about negligence lawsuits: http://www.westlaw.com. Accessed November 7, 2000.
3. *Darling v. Charleston Community Memorial Hospital*, Supreme Court of Illinois, 33 Ill.2d 326, 211 N.E.2d 253, 14 A.L.R.3d 860.
4. *Nurse's Legal Handbook*, 4th ed. Springhouse, PA: Springhouse, 2000, p 201.
5. *Nelson v. Trinity Medical Center*, Supreme Court of North Dakota, 419 N.W.2d 886.
6. *Danilczuk v. Hunterdon Medical Center*, Somerset County, Docket No. L-00124302.
7. *Lewis v. Lakeland Medical Center et al.*, Supreme Court of Wisconsin, No. 99-0001.
8. Ibid.
9. *Naya v. Mercy Medical Center, Nassau County*, Supreme Court of New York, Index No. 7676/98.
10. *Axelrad v. Jackson*, Court of Appeals of Texas, Houston (14th Dist.), No. 14-02-00518-CV.
11. *Chin v. St. Barnabas Medical Center*, New Jersey Superior Court, AD711, A2d, 352, 312.
12. Nurse advises "Reconsider choice of physicians." *Regan Rep* 40:7, December 1999.

13. *Bellard v. Willis Knighton Medical Center*, Court of Appeals of Louisiana (2d Circuit): http://web2.westlaw.com. Retrieved April 24, 2005.
14. Editor's Memo. Medical errors are making headlines. *Nurse Pract* 25:12–13, May 2000.
15. Farella C. Turning the tables on medication errors. *Nurs Spectrum*: http://www.nursingspectrum.com. Accessed March 30, 2000.
16. Health care errors report sparks major debate. *Am Nurse* 32:8, January–February 2000.
17. *Johnson v. Weiss Memorial Hospital*, Cook County Cir. Ct., No. 01 L 6581.
18. *William Green v. Long Island Medical College Hospital*, Kings County (NY) Supreme Court, Case No. 22941/00.
19. *Heller v. Barnes-Jewish Hospital*, St. Louis City (MO) Circuit Court, Case No. 012-9292.
20. *All Wrongful Death Beneficiaries et al. v. Diamond Care, Inc. et al.*, Ward County (TX) District Court, Case No. 00-05-19720-CVW.
21. *Gutierrez et al. v. Maurmanji Sangyo Co. et al.*, Lewis County (WA) Superior Court, Case No. 95-2-00497-9.
22. Satarawala R. Legal perils of IV therapy: http://westlaw.com. Accessed September 17, 2000.
23. Noone JM. Charting by exception. *J Nurs Admin* 30:342–343, July–August 2000.
24. *Holt v. Wesley Medical Center*, Supreme Court of the State of Kansas, No. 90,702.
25. Mass. nurses, docs spark healthcare revolution: http://nursingworld.org/tan. Accessed March 20, 2001.
26. Error in explanation of positive CMV: wrongful birth. *Regan Rep* 40:1, November 1999.
27. *Garley v. Columbia LaGrange Memorial Hospital*, Appellate Court of Illinois, 1st District, 4th Division, No. 1-02-2012.
28. Deliberate indifference constitutes deplorable care. *Regan Rep* 40:2, July 1999.
29. Brown SM. Good Samaritan laws: Protections and limits. *RN* 62:65–68, November 1999.
30. Quinley K. Twelve tips for defending yourself in a malpractice suit. *Am J Nurs* 90:37–38, 40, January 1990.

Updates can be found at

 http://www.JoelTheNursingExperience.com

HELPFUL WEBSITES FOR PART 4

The student should be aware that these sites serve as links to many other valuable sites.

Agency for Health Care Research and Quality: http://www.ahcpr.gov

American Association of Colleges of Nursing: http://www.aacn.nche.edu

American Association of Legal Nurse Consultants: http://www.aalnc.org

American Association of Retired Persons: www.aarp.org

American Bar Association Health Law Site: http://www.abanet.org/health
American Medical Association: http://www.ama-assn.org
American Nurses Association: http://www.nursingworld.org
American Society for Bioethics and Humanities: http://www.asbh.org
Center for Health Care Strategies: http://www.CHCS.org
Choice in Dying: http://www.choices.org
Electronic Policy Network (links to health policy information):
    http://epn.org/idea/hciclink.htmlro
Findlaw Legal Search Engine: http://www.findlaw.com
Health Care Financing Administration: http://www.hcfa.gov
Health Hippo (resources for health policy issues): http://hippo.findlaw.com
Last Acts (coalition to improve end-of-life care): http://www.lastacts.org
National Council of State Boards of Nursing: http://www.ncsbn.org
National Bioethics Advisory Commission: http://bioethics.gov
National Practitioner Data Bank: http://www.hrsa.dhhs.gov/bhpr/dqa
Nurses Service Organization: http://www.nso.com
The Nurse Practitioner: http://www.springnet.com/np/nursepract.htm
Nursing Spectrum: http://www.nursingspectrum.com
Patient Self-Determination Act: http://www.springnet.com/ce/m710a.htm
Revolution: The Journal of Nurse Empowerment: http://ideanurse.com/advon
Thomas (Library of Congress site for legislative information including links to
    congressional members' home pages): http://thomas.loc.gov

PART 5

TRANSITION INTO PRACTICE

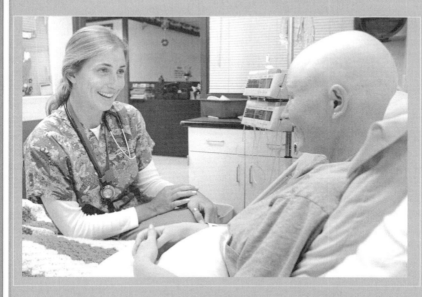

Your first job can set the tone of your nursing career. (*Courtesy of Robert Wood Johnson University Hospital, New Brunswick, New Jersey*)

Chapter 13

Nursing Organizations and Publications

OBJECTIVES

After studying this chapter, you will be able to:

1. *Compare and contrast the major organizations representing nurses.*
2. *Identify the value that NSNA holds for you.*
3. *Identify the mission of each of the major nursing organizations.*
4. *Detail key issues related to nursing organizations.*
5. *Discuss ways in which nursing organizations have sought unity in working together.*
6. *Identify aspects of the nursing literature with which nurses should be familiar.*

DIVERSITY AND DIFFERENCES

In 1952, when the six major nursing organizations decided to restructure, the ANA and NLN absorbed the activities of all but the American Association of Industrial Nurses (later renamed the American Association of Occupational Health Nurses), which maintained itself separately. Students became part of the newly formed National Student Nurses' Association, NSNA. In general, ANA was (and is) considered *the* professional organization, one that every RN can join and find some way in which to participate. RNs are also encouraged to join specialty associations, which are necessary to stay abreast of practice changes; and the NLN continues to offer membership to both RNs and the lay public who are interested in their mission.

There are several major differences between ANA and NLN. ANA membership is limited to RNs (through their local associations), but NLN includes anyone interested in the purposes of the organization, as well as agency members (health care facilities and educational programs in nursing). ANA is registered as a labor organization with the federal government, although it does not directly provide any workplace representation; rather, those services are provided by their local nurses associations. ANA, in its associated credentialing center, certifies clinical practitioners and nurse managers; it also has an accreditation program for continuing education (CE) programs and systems of nursing service. NLN is recognized for its services to academic faculty, and through its affiliate, accreditation of all kinds of nursing education programs. Both make policy statements about health and nursing; they also overlap in their public statements about nursing education. Over the past few years, they have come together often to speak "with one strong voice" on many issues, particularly public policy.

The first specialty organization, the American Association of Nurse Anesthetists, began in 1931. In the 1940s and 1950s several others were founded, but beginning in 1968, literally dozens were organized. They were usually splinter groups that broke off from ANA and formed their own association as the profession became more specialized. Later, still other organizations formed, as subspecialty groups or groups that felt they had certain needs that could be best met by uniting with the like-minded. These included ethnic nurses, male nurses, nurses with a certain philosophy of care or social concerns, and gay nurses. Some grew rapidly and acquired staff and headquarters. Others almost literally functioned out of a member's home or office. Special-interest groups seem to serve the same purposes: leadership development, certification, continuing education, peer support, and standard setting.

COOPERATIVE EFFORTS

The proliferation of nursing organizations, although meeting the special needs of some nurses, has also caused some confusion among nurses, other health workers, and the public. Do these organizations speak for nursing in addition to ANA? In place of ANA? Members of nursing organizations are also concerned. A perceived or real lack of unity in common health care interests can hamper the achievement of goals. Therefore, in November 1972, ANA hosted a meeting of ten specialty groups and NSNA to explore how the organizations could work toward more coordination in areas of common interest. It was found that concerns were similar and that such a meeting was generally considered long overdue.

In its second meeting, hosted by the American Association of Critical-Care Nurses (AACN), the participants accepted the importance of the specialty groups, at the same time recognizing the unique role of ANA. They agreed "in principle" to certain statements. In 1973, the group adopted a name: the Federation of Specialty Nursing Organizations and the American Nurses Association. There were 13 charter members.

Meetings were held on a semiannual basis in the following years, with the member organizations alternating as hosts, responsible for arranging and conducting the meeting and writing the minutes. The nursing press and auditors were permitted to attend meetings. The focus of the meetings was usually on current issues but was often related to CE accreditation procedures and certification, about which ANA and the other organizations seldom agreed. However, the Federation did support ANA on some issues.

In 1981, the title of the organization was changed to *National Federation for Specialty Nursing Organizations* (NFSNO), which more clearly defined the membership, not all of whom represented clinical specialties. By 1985, NFSNO had changed its requirements for membership, so that membership was exclusive to specialty nursing organizations. ANA, which had been a charter member, moved from member to auditor status. The purpose of NFSNO is now to foster excellence in specialty nursing practice by providing a forum for communication and collaboration and to assume a leadership position in activities that contribute to specialty nursing practice.

Another cooperative effort aimed at nurse specialists is the *National Alliance of Nurse Practitioners* (NANP), a coalition of nurse practitioner (NP) organizations formed in 1986. The purpose is to address the health care of the nation by promoting the visibility, viability, and unity of NPs. Among its major concerns is gaining reimbursement for NP services.

ANA also made a direct effort to bring together the various nursing organizations. A change in the 1982 by-laws provided for the formation of a *Nursing Organization Liaison Forum* (NOLF) to promote unified action of allied nursing organizations under the auspices of ANA. In December 1983, ANA invited 45 nursing organizations to come together to explore the possibilities. The meeting was cordial, but the results were somewhat noncommittal. There was a question of whether NOLF and NFSNO would be duplicative efforts, although ANA indicated that NOLF would focus on broad issues as opposed to specialty concerns. Over time, NOLF grew and flourished, uniting over 80 nursing organizations. It frequently spoke for both ANA and their specialty organization to the media, the Congress, and in a variety of instances. NOLF organizations have voluntarily shared their resources with ANA to help fund a variety of programs. In November of 2001, NOLF and NFSNO merged to form the new, independent *Nursing Organizations Alliance* (the Alliance).

The *Tri-Council for Nursing* represents another successful cooperative effort. The Tri-Council traces its roots to the ANA–NLN Coordinating Council, established with the ANA reorganization in the 1950s. In time, the American Association of Colleges of Nursing (AACN) and the American Organization of Nurse Executives (AONE) were added to this coalition. The Tri-Council agenda addresses broad-based issues such as public image, nursing shortages, recruitment to the field, and legislative and regulatory concerns. Despite the addition of AONE as a fourth member in 1986, the name of Tri-Council was retained. The presidents and executive directors of the Tri-Council organizations meet regularly and frequently engage in joint lobbying on the federal level.

Such collaborative activities among nursing organizations show a new maturity in nursing that recognizes the importance of joining together on major health issues. Cooperative action will enable nurses to be a stronger force for the nation's health.

The ANA and NSNA will be discussed in some depth, since they are the two associations of immediate interest to the student and new graduate. In addition, the International Council of Nurses (ICN) will be presented as our world-wide representative.

AMERICAN NURSES ASSOCIATION

The ANA was established in 1897 by a group of nurses who, even then, recognized the need for a membership association within which nurses could work together in concerted action. Its original name was the Nurses' Associated Alumnae of the United States and Canada, but in order to incorporate under the laws of the state of New York, it was necessary to drop the reference to another country in the organization's title. This was done in 1901; however, the name remained Nurses' Associated Alumnae of the United States until 1911, when it became the American Nurses Association. The Canadian nurses formed their own membership association.

History shows that ANA's primary concern has always been individual nurses and the public they serve. In its early years ANA worked hard for improved and uniform standards of nursing education, for registration and licensure of all nurses educated according to these standards, and for improvement of the welfare of nurses. Similar efforts continue today. ANA headquarters is 8515 Georgia Avenue, Silver Spring, MD 20910-3492, http://nursingworld.org.

MEMBERSHIP

ANA is made up of organizations and individuals who have member or affiliate status. Constituent member associations (CMAs) include state and territorial nurses associations, multi-state associations, an association for United States nurses overseas, and a federal nurses' association composed of members of the United States military on active duty. Most CMAs are made up of district nurses' associations (DNAs). Where the individual member belongs to a CMA, the CMA is the member of ANA, not the individual directly. Contingent on an agreement between ANA and the CMA, individuals may have the opportunity to join ANA directly. Individual membership is open only to registered professional nurses holding a currently valid license, new graduates as first-time writers of the licensing exam, and impaired nurses who have surrendered their license to practice. ANA also has organizational affiliates, which are national organizations that have applied for and been granted this status. They do not hold the same rights and responsibilities as the CMAs, and their members receive no privileges or services from ANA.

Only 8–10 percent of all RNs belong to ANA. Some belong to specialty or special-interest organizations, others to none. Why? Cost may be a factor; ANA/CMA dues are more than $200 a year in most states, considerably more than for other organizations. Some nurses are simply not interested in nursing issues and do not know why it is important to be represented in legislation or other policy making; and, of course, others disagree with ANA positions, such as entry into practice and collective bargaining.

GENERAL ORGANIZATION

The House of Delegates and Board of Directors carry on the business of the association. The House of Delegates, consisting of 630 individuals representing their CMAs and the individual member division (IMD), and including the ANA Board of Directors and representatives of the organizational affiliates, is the highest authority in the association. The number from each CMA and the IMD are based on the overall size of the membership of each. The House of Delegates, which meets yearly, with full conventions in even years, is the policymaking body of ANA. Between conventions, decisions based on House policies are made by the Board of Directors, which has been elected by the House. The board consists of 15 members, including the officers (president, first and second vice-president, secretary, and treasurer). Terms are staggered to prevent a complete turnover at any one time and to provide continuity of programs and action.

The ANA has a largely RN professional staff, with supporting clerical and secretarial staff. They carry out the day-to-day activities based on policies adopted by the House and ANA's general functions. The executive director, a nurse, is the chief administrative officer and works closely with the board and CMAs.

Like other large organizations, ANA has its *standing committees,* those that are written into the by-laws and that continue from year to year to assist with specific continuing programs and functions of the association. *Special committees* and *task forces* of the House or board are appointed on an ad hoc basis to accomplish special purposes.

Other structural units include the *Congress on Nursing Practice and Economics* and the *Constituent Assembly.* The Congress is a deliberative body that focuses on long-range policy development essential to the mission of the association. The Assembly is the representative body of the CMAs and the IMD that consults with and advises the Board of Directors on professional and organizational issues.

In 1999, the House of Delegates created a national labor entity, *United American Nurses* (UAN). The UAN is an associate organizational member of ANA that supports CMAs in their collective bargaining work. Members are those CMAs with active collective bargaining programs. The UAN is governed by a National Labor Assembly, and is advisory to the ANA Board of Directors on the labor implications of association policy. In a related action, the House of Delegates established the Center for American Nurses (CAN) as an associate organizational member concerned with workplace advocacy. Workplace advocacy is an array of services, products, and programs that support individual nurses to help them address their workplace challenges through policy research and advocacy, education, and communications.

MAJOR PROGRAMS AND SERVICES OF ANA

The programs and services of ANA represent the efforts of members, staff, and elected officers. These include meeting with members of other groups and disciplines; planning or convening institutes, workshops, conventions, or committee meetings; developing and writing brochures, manuals, position papers, standards, or testimony to be presented to

Congress; and implementing ongoing programs, planning new ones, or trying to solve the problem of how to serve the members best within the limitations of the budget. Every issue of the *American Journal of Nursing* and *The American Nurse* carries reports of these many and varied activities. Presented here are brief descriptions of some (but not all) of the major ANA programs and services.

Programs are implemented both through the internal administrative structure of ANA and in some cases by independent or affiliated organizational entities related to ANA. These allied structures are presented, following this discussion of ANA activities.

Nursing Education

The important ANA function of setting standards and policies for nursing education has been demonstrated in many ways. The 1965 Position Paper was the beginning of a series of specific actions toward implementing the position that education for entry into professional nursing practice should be at the baccalaureate level (see Chapters 2 and 5).

ANA endorses the concept of CE for all nurses as a vehicle to maintain competence, but believes that the responsibility for maintaining competence is personal and not an area for government intrusion. ANA puts emphasis on the role of the CMAs in providing and approving the quality of CE offerings. To facilitate this work, in 1975 the Association established an accreditation program which currently operates through the American Nurses Credentialing Center (ANCC).

Nursing Practice

Nursing is practice, and so many would say that ANA's work in this area drives all of the other association activities. ANA is responsible for developing and disseminating the *Standards of Clinical Nursing Practice* (see Chapter 4). ANA has collaborated with countless specialty associations to ensure that their standards are framed in the same model, and subsequently can be endorsed by ANA. Many excellent publications are part of the overall plan to assist CMAs and individuals in the utilization of the standards of practice. Workshops, seminars, and other programs are held to provide nurses with new knowledge to facilitate implementation and thereby improve nursing care. Major papers and/or proceedings of these conferences are made available. ANA's concern for quality nursing care is also manifested through its Center for Ethics and Human Rights and *Code for Nurses*. One of the center's purposes is to develop and disseminate information on ethical and human rights issues facing the profession of nursing. The center provides consultation and resources on

Exhibit 13.1 ANA Select Position Statements

Ethics and human rights
- Active Euthanasia
- Use of Placebos for Pain Management in Patients with Cancer
- Reduction of Patient Restraint and Seclusion in Health Care Settings
- Health Nutritional Screening for the Elderly
- Assisted Suicide
- Nurses' Participation in Capital Punishment
- Nursing Care and Do Not Resuscitate Decisions
- Forgoing Artificial Nutrition and Hydration
- Nursing and the Patient Self-Determination Act
- Promotion of Comfort and Relief of Pain in Dying Patients

Bloodborne and airborne diseases
- Guidelines for Disclosure to a Known Third Party About Possible HIV Infection
- Post-Exposure Programs in the Event of Occupational Exposure to HIV/HBV
- Education and Barrier Use for Sexually Transmitted Diseases (STDs) and HIV Infection
- Availability of Equipment and Safety Procedures to Prevent Transmission of Bloodborne Diseases
- Travel Restrictions for Persons with HIV/AIDS
- Support for Confidential Notification Services and a Limited Privilege to Disclose
- Personnel Policies and HIV in the Workplace
- HIV Testing
- HIV Infection and Nursing Students
- HIV Exposure from Rape and Sexual Assault
- Tuberculosis and HIV

Social causes and health care
- Physical Violence Against Women
- Lead Poisoning and Screening
- Childhood Immunizations
- Informal Caregiving
- Cessation of Smoking
- Environmental Tobacco Smoke
- Discrimination and Racism in Health Care

Drug and alcohol abuse
- Position Statement on Opposition to Criminal Prosecution of Women for Use of Drugs while Pregnant
- Drug Testing for Health Care Workers
- Support for Treatment Services for Alcohol and Drug Dependent Women of Childbearing Age
- Polypharmacy and the Older Adult
- Abuse of Prescription Drugs

Nursing practice
- Psychiatric Mental Health Nursing and Managed Care
- Adult Immunization

Exhibit 13.1 (*continued*)

- Protecting Patients' Safe Access to Therapeutic Marijuana/Cannabis
- Privatization and For-Profit Conversion

Nursing research
- Education for Participation in Nursing Research

Workplace advocacy
- Maintaining Professional and Legal Standards During a Shortage of Nursing Personnel
- Sexual Harassment
- Elimination of Manual Patient Handling to Prevent Work-Related Musculoskeletal Disorders
- Restructuring, Work Redesign, and the Job and Career Security of Registered Nurses
- The Right to Accept or Reject an Assignment
- Opposition to Mandatory Overtime
- Latex Allergy

Unlicensed assistive personnel
- Registered Nurse Utilization of Unlicensed Assistive Personnel
- Registered Nurse Education Relating to the Utilization of Unlicensed Assistive Personnel

Joint statements
- Maintaining Professional and Legal Standards During a Shortage of Nursing Personnel
- Computer-Based Patient Records

The above are a sample of current position statements, which are regularly reviewed and revised. The reader is referred to http://nursingworld.org/readroom/position for the full narrative of these statements and others not included here.

addressing practice dilemmas and controversies. For example, the center helps nurses and CMAs with application of the *Code for Nurses* and prepares documents such as the position statement on the nurse's role in end-of-life decisions. This is only one example of a variety of position papers which ANA has authored and approved to provide guidance for the practice of nursing. A list of current position statements is presented in Exhibit 13.1.

All of the programs of the ANA hold serious implications for practice. Some examples are the legislative and regulatory work to ensure advanced practice nurses staff privileges in health care facilities, prescriptive authority, and direct reimbursement for services rendered to the public. Much effort has also been expended in having the National Library of Medicine (NLM) recognize the classification systems which are unique to nursing practice: the North Atlantic Nursing Diagnosis Association (NANDA) classification of nursing diagnoses, the Nursing Intervention Classification (NIC), Nursing Outcome Classification (NOC), and the Omaha and Saba systems for classifying home care encounters (refer to Chapter 4). This is part of a broader goal to have the government incorporate data necessary to distinguish nursing in its mandatory reporting systems. All of these pieces come together in activities related to the minimum data set (MDS) for nursing. Not only does this work promise to have us recognized for our practice, but it also allows retrieval of information related to our practice both from government reporting systems and library databases.

Legislation and Legal Activities

ANA's legislative program is an important one that often affects, directly and indirectly, the welfare of both nurses and the public (see Chapter 10). ANA's legislative program has three main purposes: (1) to help CMAs promote effective nursing practice acts in their states in order to protect the public and the nursing profession from unqualified practitioners; (2) to offer consultation on other legislative and regulatory measures that affect nurses; and (3) to speak for nursing in relation to federal legislation for health, education, labor, and welfare, and for social programs such as civil rights.

The major responsibility for coordinating legislative information and action lies with the ANA's governmental affairs arm. The headquarters staff's responsibilities include lobbying (through its registered lobbyists); development of relationships with congressional members and their

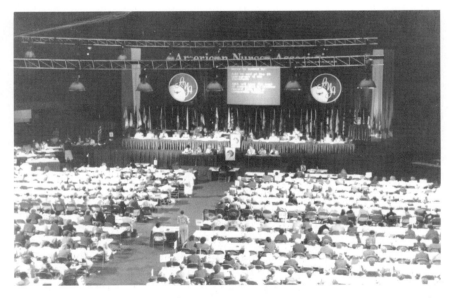

The ANA House of Delegates meets yearly to set policy for nursing in this country. (*Courtesy of the American Nurses Association*)

staffs and committee staffs; contacts with key figures in the executive branch of government; maintaining relations with other national organizations; preparing most of the statements and information presented to congressional committees; drafting letters to government officials; presenting testimony; acting as backup for members presenting testimony; and representing ANA in many capacities. Major newspapers and journals have commented on nursing's presence and influence.

Over the years, ANA has represented nursing with the federal government on numerous major issues: funds for nursing education, Social Security amendments, national health insurance, quality of care in nursing homes, collective bargaining rights, health hazards, civil rights, Federal Trade Commission authority and regulations, problems of nurses in the federal service, tax revision, workplace safety, pension reform, prescriptive authority and reimbursement for nurses, and general support for improvement of health care.

ANA has often cooperated and coordinated with other health disciplines, but has also faced areas of disagreement (such as opposition of AMA to reimbursement for advanced practice nurses). Such philosophical differences still occur, but there has been increasing cooperation with both health and other groups to achieve mutual legislative goals.

Communication about legislative matters is particularly important to help members keep abreast of key issues. The legislative staff of *The American Nurse* and *The American Journal of Nursing* prepare regular feature articles that highlight major legislative and related developments.

Legislative information and special communications are sent out from the ANA headquarters when membership support is needed for legislative programs. CMAs have a vital role in providing information and assistance to members on pertinent legislative issues, and in most CMAs there is a legislative staff, lobbyists, and perhaps a separate legislative newsletter for state activities.

In addition to specific legislative action, ANA becomes involved in various legal matters that affect the welfare of nurses. In some cases, ANA acts as a friend of the court, providing information about the issues involved. In other cases, ANA joins with a CMA if its issue has broader implications. One such situation was the class action litigation in the state of Illinois claiming salary inequity for women employed by the state, a large number of whom were nurses.

Economic and General Welfare

The ANA economic security program is often misunderstood by members, nonmembers, and others. Seeing that the economic security of its members is maintained is one of the classic roles of a professional association, and, especially in recent years, economic security has been seen as extending beyond purely monetary matters and conditions of employment to involvement of nurses in the decision-making aspects of nursing care. An example might be that, through an agreed-upon process, perhaps including a formal committee structure, nurses' objections to inadequate staffing and inappropriate job assignments would be instrumental in bringing about changes that would provide improved care.

Unions, which have been successful in organizing nonprofessional health workers and a number of professionals, have been giving priority to organizing nurses. There is serious concern that large unions with strong economic backing and single-purpose goals to increase monetary and working benefits may prove competitive, for nurses frequently do not see their professional organization as a strong or even appropriate bargaining agent. Because past experience has shown that unions have taken little action to negotiate contracts involving nurses in decisions that could improve patient care, and because many nurses are not even aware that such participation is possible, one of the most worthwhile purposes of collective bargaining could be lost. In 2001, CMAs represented over 100,000 RNs in 23 states, the District of Columbia and the U.S. Virgin Islands. Potential union members find the CMAs much more appealing as a workplace representative than traditional unions. This definitely places the CMAs at advantage as an amalgam of associations providing workplace representation. To add visibility and strength to the collective bargaining program, in 1999 a new labor entity, the United American Nurses (UAN), was established within ANA. In June 2001, registered nurse delegates to the UAN's National Labor Assembly (decision-making body) voted to affiliate with the AFL-CIO, forming an historic partnership with the federation's 64 unions. In 2000, the House of Delegates created the Commission on Workplace Advocacy to service those states without collective bargaining programs.[1] In 2003, both the UAN and the Center for American Nurses (CAN, formerly the Commission on Workplace Advocacy) became Associate Organizational Members of ANA, distancing their work from the parent association.

Human Rights Activities

ANA works toward integrating qualified members of all racial and ethnic groups into the nursing profession and tries to achieve sound human rights practices. From the time of its founding, ANA as a national organization has never had any discriminatory policies for membership in the association. Until 1964, however, a few of its constituent associations denied membership to black nurses. In these instances, ANA made provision for black nurses to bypass district and state associations and become members of ANA directly. At that point (1950), the National Association for Colored Graduate Nurses (NACGN) voluntarily went out of existence, on the basis that there was no longer a need for such a specialized membership association.

ANA's human rights activities are housed in the Center for Ethics and Human Rights. A major program with over 25 years of success is the Racial/Ethnic Minority Fellowship Program. The Program provides financial and personal support to minority candidates for doctoral study preparing for research or clinical practice in psychiatric and mental health nursing.

Communication and Information Services

ANA is a veritable goldmine of information. The association publishes *The American Nurse,* which reports recent activities and happenings important to the nursing community. Many of the staff units, as already described, have specific newsletters and websites that are updated on a regular basis. ANA is also a clearinghouse for information on the state-specific statutory requirements for nursing, and the prevailing demographics of practicing nurses, as some examples. The ANA Internet site is a comprehensive on-line source of current information about ANA and its affiliate structures, and also the home of the *On-line Journal of Issues in Nursing.*

American Nurses Publishing (an arm of ANA and ANF) publishes standards of practice, the *Code for Nurses,* major reports, monographs, papers presented at meetings, and certain publications of the AAN and ANCC. The association also publishes position statements, guidelines for practice, bulletins, manuals, and brochures for specialized groups within the organization and sends out news releases and announcements concerning activities of interest to the public. A periodically revised *Catalogue* is available on request, and a list of publications also exists on-line at http://www.nursingworld.org.

Other Activities and Services

Among other ANA benefits for nurses is insurance of various kinds, available at favorable group rates at national and state levels. Many educational programs, seminars, workshops, clinical conferences, scientific sessions, and so on are available at all levels of the association at reduced rates for members. They are geared to current issues and new developments in health and nursing.

Nurses are also increasingly interested in international nursing. ANA was one of the three charter members of the International Council of Nurses (ICN). Essentially, ICN is a federation of national associations of professional nurses (currently one from each country), and ANA is the member association for the United States.

ANA established an International Nursing Center in 1992 through the ANF. The center sponsors an international talent bank composed of nurses with expertise in international work and foreign language capability.

AMERICAN ACADEMY OF NURSING

A significant action taken by the 1966 House of Delegates was the creation of the American Academy of Nursing (AAN) to provide for recognition of professional achievement and excellence. It was established in 1973. The members, designated as Fellows of the American Academy of Nursing, are entitled to use the initials FAAN following their names. They are selected on the basis of their outstanding contributions to nursing and their potential for continued contributions. The Academy holds a yearly Scientific Session combined with business meetings.

The Academy was constituted as a self-governing affiliate of ANA to insulate its work from the inevitable politics of membership associations. The Academy has its own dues structure, by-laws, fund-raising capability, and elected officials. Using AAN as the vehicle, the leadership corps for the profession provides thinking on the critical issues confronting nursing. Their ability to create, speak, and disseminate intellectual products must be unencumbered by political pressure. The AAN has responded well to the challenge of shaping the future. The Magnet Hospital Study of 1983 (see Appendix 1) set the stage for the current Magnet Hospital Recognition Program instituted by ANCC to pay tribute to departments of nursing service that are exemplary. The Teaching Nursing Home Program contributed significantly to the nursing home reforms of 1987. The AAN Clinical Scholars Program accorded advanced practice nursing intellectual respect, and moved practice toward the level of distinction it currently enjoys. The faculty practice initiative of the 1980s gave credibility to service–education unification efforts that have since become the standard to bring the best of nursing to both students and patients. The AAN has accomplished its work through demonstration projects, annual meetings, smaller interest groups that are a mechanism for continuing problem solving and discussion around issues, dissemination of ideas through *Nursing Outlook* (the Academy's official journal), and the wide reach of its influential members.

For the Academy, knowledge is power, and this image has been augmented by the establishment of two scholar-in-residence programs, each cosponsored with a major governmental or quasi-governmental entity. The Agency for Healthcare Research and Quality (AHRQ)/AAN Scholar focuses on areas of investigation which integrate clinical nursing with cost, quality, and accessibility concerns. The Institute of Medicine (IOM)/ANF/AAN Scholar is concerned with health policy issues.[2]

THE AMERICAN NURSES FOUNDATION

The American Nurses Foundation (ANF) was created by ANA in 1955 to meet the need for an independent, permanent, nonprofit organization devoted to nursing research. This tax-exempt foundation was organized exclusively for charitable, scientific, literary, and educational purposes.

ANF has a Competitive Extramural Grants Program, funded through the contributions of both corporations and individuals, that provides small grants to nurse researchers. This annual competition provides funding for beginning and experienced nurse researchers in both clinical and academic settings. Since the first grants were awarded in 1955, more than 900 nurse researchers have benefited from more than $3 million in grants. Countless patients, hospital administrators, and consumers have benefited from the research of ANF Scholars who continue to impact health outcomes, improve the processes of the delivery of care, and enhance the quality of work life for nurses. In 2004, ANF's Board of Trustees again confirmed their support of this successful and evolving program by awarding 20 new grants to nurse researchers around the country.

ANF has been the overseer for several years of grants/contracts which have been funded externally. Some of the grants have been awarded to ANA and managed through ANF while others have been awarded directly to ANF. Funding has been received from private foundations such as W. K. Kellogg for a community coalition-building project and Robert Wood Johnson for smoking cessation. The Centers for Disease Control and Prevention, Division of Adolescent School Health, Maternal and Child Health Bureau, Substance Abuse and Mental Health Services Administration, Health Resources and Services Administration, and the Agency for Healthcare Research and Quality are examples of federal funding received by ANA/ANF. Projects focus on nurse staffing, workplace health and safety, continuing competency, and patient safety and health.

ANF is governed by its by-laws and directed by a nine-member board of trustees; all trustees are RNs. The executive director of ANA is also the executive director of ANF. There is a professional ANF headquarters staff involved in fund-raising and grant management.

THE AMERICAN NURSES CREDENTIALING CENTER

The ANA established a *certification* program in 1973 to recognize professional achievement in practice. More than 5000 applications were received for the first examination given in May 1973. This program provides a *credential* which is rewarded by salary increases, prestige, and promotion in many work settings, and recognized by many state governments as indicating competence in advanced practice. By 2005, 39 areas of certification were offered, with 17 of those being for advanced practice, and a total of over 145,000 individuals were certified by ANCC [3] (see Exhibit 13.2).

Three levels of certification are offered: competence in specialized areas of practice (generalist), and acknowledged achievement as a specialist. The latter calls for a master's degree. The former offers two separate certifications, one requiring the baccalaureate degree and the other for diploma and associate degree nursing practice. Each credential is based on the assessment of knowledge through examination, demonstration of current practice ability, and endorsement of colleagues. Once certified, the certification is valid for five years and may be renewed by fulfilling stipulated requirements for practice and continuing education or by retaking the examination. Specific information on eligibility criteria for each specialty area and the cost of the exam may be obtained by contacting ANCC or through the ANA website.

An *accreditation* program was established in 1974 by ANA as a voluntary system for accreditation of continuing education in nursing. The essential purpose of this system is to provide professional nursing judgment on the quality of CE offerings. An organization may be accredited as either an approver or a provider of CE in nursing.

The Magnet *Recognition Program* was introduced in 1994, and is built on the 1983 Magnet Hospital Study conducted by AAN. The goal of this program is to identify excellence in nursing services and to recognize health care facilities that act as a "magnet," creating a work environment that attracts and retains professional nurses. The first recipients of this status were the University of Washington Medical Center in Seattle and Hackensack University Medical Center in New Jersey (awarded in 1995). The program now recognizes over 100 "magnet" facilities. A listing of these organizations can be found at http://nursingworld.org/ancc/magnet/facilities.html.

Early certification and accreditation activities were conducted by ANA. In 1991, as a result of the action of the ANA House of Delegates, these credentialing programs were placed in a separately incorporated center (ANCC). The ANCC philosophy of credentialing is consistent with and based on the ANA ethical code, standards of practice, and

Exhibit 13.2 ANCC Current Certifications

Advanced Practice Certifications
  Acute Care Nurse Practitioner
  Adult Nurse Practitioner
  Family Nurse Practitioner
  Gerontological Nurse Practitioner
  Pediatric Nurse Practitioner
  Adult Psychiatric and Mental Health Nurse Practitioner
  Family Psychiatric and Mental Health Nurse Practitioner
  Clinical Specialist in Gerontological Nursing
  Clinical Specialist in Medical–Surgical Nursing
  Clinical Specialist in Pediatric Nursing
  Clinical Specialist in Adult Psychiatric and Mental Health Nursing
  Clinical Specialist in Child and Adolescent Psychiatric and Mental Health Nursing
  Clinical Specialist in Community Health Nursing
  Clinical Specialist in Home Health Nursing (last test administration May 14, 2005)
  Advanced Diabetes Management—Nurse Practitioner
  Advanced Diabetes Management—Clinical Nurse Specialist
  Nursing Administration, Advanced

Baccalaureate Level Certifications
  Cardiac/Vascular Nurse
  College Health Nurse (last test administration May 14, 2005)
  Community Health Nurse
  Gerontological Nurse
  Home Health Nurse (last test administration May 14, 2005)
  Informatics Nurse: Baccalaureate degree in nursing
  Informatics Nurse: Baccalaureate degree in other relevant field of study
  Medical–Surgical Nurse
  Nursing Professional Development
  Pediatric Nurse
  Perinatal Nurse
  Psychiatric and Mental Health Nurse
  Nursing Administration

Associate Degree / Diploma Level Certifications
  Cardiac/Vascular Nurse
  Gerontological Nurse
  Medical–Surgical Nurse
  Pediatric Nurse
  Perinatal Nurse
  Psychiatric and Mental Health Nurse

Other Specialty Certifications
  Ambulatory Care Nursing
  Nursing Case Management
  Pain Management (available October 2005)

positions on practice, education, and service. The separation of ANA and ANCC removes the threat of conflict of interest which can result when the entity establishing the standard intrudes in the work of evaluating the practitioner or program according to that standard.

AMERICAN NURSES ASSOCIATION POLITICAL ACTION COMMITTEE

Most professional organizations have a political action group that is independent of the organization but related to it. This is because a tax-exempt professional organization such as ANA is under definite legal constraints as far as partisan political action is concerned. In 1974, with a $50,000 ANA grant, a voluntary, unincorporated, nonpartisan political action group was formed. Initially called Nurses' Coalition for Action in Politics (N-CAP), the name was later changed to the American Nurses Association Political Action Committee (ANA–PAC). ANA provides some dollars for administrative support, but none for the campaigns of candidates for election. ANA–PAC has a single purpose: to promote the improvement of health care through political action. Its two major activities are education and endorsement of candidates for public office on the national level who support ANA's public policy positions. This requires major fund-raising efforts. Many CMAs have their own political action committees that support candidates for state office.

The ANA–PAC has enjoyed significant growth in recent years, and demonstrated significant success. Its candidate success rate has never been less than 70 percent and in some election cycles has been 98 percent. CMA members are more politically active than other citizen groups, giving many hours as well as dollars to political campaigns. About 58 percent donate to political campaigns and 91 percent are registered to vote.

The ANA–PAC is noted for its grassroots network, Nurses Strategic Action Team (N-STAT). N-STAT educates members of the Congress to nursing issues and provides an immediate response in areas where "time is of the essence." Members of the N-Stat *Leadership Team* are individually assigned to a Congressperson or Senator. Their forte is the relationship. It becomes their task to monitor the record of this legislator, educate them to nursing's issues, and seeing support for our positions, work to keep them in office. Other N-Stat volunteers constitute a rapid response network which provides the strength and volume to make legislators aware of nursing's opinion on specific issues as they arise.

ANA–PAC is governed by its own Board of Directors. ANA–PAC is headquartered at ANA's offices.

THE INDIVIDUAL NURSE AND ANA

A classic article by sociologist Robert Merton lists the functions of any professional organization as including social and moral support for individual practitioners to help them perform their role as professionals, to set rigorous standards for the profession and help enforce them, to advance and disseminate research and professional knowledge, to help furnish the social bonds through which society coheres, and to speak for the profession. In carrying out some of these functions, the association is seen as a "kind of organizational gadfly, stinging the profession into new and more demanding formulations of purpose."[4]

Not all members agree with their organization's goals. However, the key to the success of any organization is the participation of its actual and potential members. Even though ANA has only a small percentage of working nurses, it is still the largest organization representing American nurses. ANA speaks for nurses; nonmembers have no part in the organization and have no right to complain if it does not represent them. The strength in the organization and in nursing lies in thinking, communicating nurses committed to the goal of improving nursing care for the public and working together in an organized fashion to achieve this goal.

INTERNATIONAL COUNCIL OF NURSES

Nursing claims the distinction of having the oldest international association of medical professionals in the world, the International Council of Nurses (ICN). It antedates by many years the international hospital

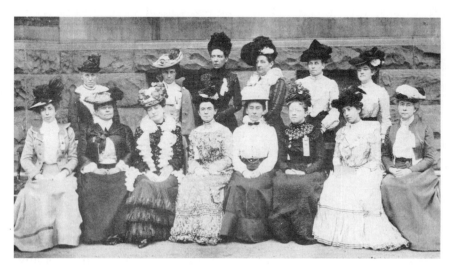

Foreign delegates and officers of the International Council of Nurses, Buffalo, New York, 1901. (*Courtesy of Lucie Kelly, private collection*)

and medical associations. The originator and prime mover of ICN was a distinguished and energetic English nurse, Ethel Gordon Fenwick, who first proposed the idea of an international nursing organization in July 1899.

ICN is a federation of national nurses' associations worldwide. The requirements for membership have been, essentially, that the national association be an autonomous, self-directing, and self-governing body, nonsectarian, with no form of racial discrimination, whose voting membership is composed exclusively of nurses and is broadly representative of the nurses in that country. Its objectives must be in harmony with ICN's stated objective: to provide a medium through which national nurses' associations may share their common interests, working together to develop the contribution of nursing to the promotion of the health of people and the care of the sick. A majority vote by the ICN's governing body determines the admission of national associations into membership.

ORGANIZATION

The governing body of ICN is the Council of National Representatives (CNR), consisting of the presidents of over 128 member associations.[5] This group, including ICN's board of directors, meets at least every two

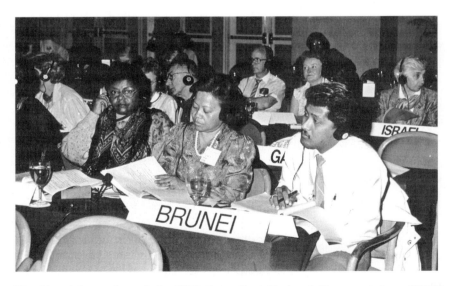

The biennial meeting of the ICN Council of National Representatives (CNR) brings together the representatives of over 128 countries. (*Courtesy of the International Council of Nurses, Geneva*)

years to establish ICN policies. Carrying out ICN's day-to-day activities is its headquarters staff—a group of professional nurses, including ICN's executive director, currently a Canadian nurse. These nurses represent ICN's executive staff, and in their relationships with and services to the member associations, they serve in an advisory and consultative capacity. Staff members are selected from various member countries.

ICN CONGRESSES

Once every four years, the ICN holds its Quadrennial Congress: a meeting of the members of the national nurses' associations in membership with ICN. Nursing students are eligible to attend ICN congresses. Students have been meeting as a Student Assembly during the congresses.

During the last several congresses, discussions and resolutions ranged from those focusing specifically on nursing issues to general social concerns. Included, for instance, were career ladders, socioeconomic welfare, educational and practice standards, research, autonomy, the nurse's role in safeguarding human rights, the nurse's role in the care of detainees and prisoners, and nurse participation in national health policy planning and decision making. Related to general health care were such topics as primary care, female genital mutilation, increased violence against patients and health personnel, the uncontrolled proliferation of ancillary nursing personnel, environment quality, care for the elderly, and workplace conditions. On an even broader scale were the concerns about refugees and displaced persons, nuclear war, poverty, and the status of women.

The activities at ICN congresses are reported in the *American Journal of Nursing (AJN)* and other nursing journals, including *International Nursing Review,* the ICN journal.

FUNCTIONS AND ACTIVITIES

From the very beginning, ICN has been concerned with three main areas: nursing education, nursing service, and nurses' social and economic welfare. Whenever possible, ICN has sought common denominators in education and practice throughout the world. One such common denominator, for instance, is the international Code of Ethics (see Chapter 8) adopted by ICN and equally applicable to nurses in every country. At the same time, ICN has always recognized the autonomy of its member associations and the principle that each country will develop the systems of education and practice best suited to its individual culture and needs.

Providing liaison for nurses with other international groups is one of ICN's most significant contributions to world nursing. Among the organizations, government and nongovernmental, with which ICN is associated in some way are the WHO, the World Federation of Mental Health, the International Labor Organization, the World Medical Association, the International Hospital Federation, the International Federation of Red Cross and Red Crescent Societies, the International Committee of the Red Cross, the United Nations Educational, Scientific and Cultural Organization (UNESCO), the Council of International Organizations of Medical Sciences (CIOMS), and the Union of International Associations.

ICN has sponsored a variety of projects to study issues critical for the development of nursing. Most recent ventures have been the International Classification of Nursing Project, the Regulation Project, costing nursing services, nursing and AIDS, nursing research, the use of assistive personnel, and mental health services, to name a few. Most of these initiatives produce publications that are available through headquarters, some free and others for a fee. More information is available through the ICN website, http://www.icn.ch.

PLANS FOR THE FUTURE

ICN has anchored its strategic plan for the future in two primary areas: creation of an *international knowledge network* and *advancing the global nursing and health agenda.*

The advent of instant communication and new technologies has made the pursuit and dissemination of raw knowledge among the most powerful tools in the world. With an electronic network that includes most of the national nurses' associations (NNAs) and translation into its three working languages (English, Spanish, and French), ICN is the only worldwide nursing exchange for the dissemination and interchange of information by nurses. Expansion plans for ICN's *international knowledge network* include:

- Innovations in accessing and exchanging information, new distance education programs, and networking structures whereby nurses with special interests can exchange information and offer expert advice on issues. Websites have already been established for nurse researchers, nurse regulators, and advanced practice nurses.
- Offering health information directly to the public via the Internet and new nursing publications.

- Establishing electronic links with all ICN member associations.
- Continuing the development of the ICNP—the International Classification for Nursing Practice. The ICNP is a landmark project that brings the profession closer to monitoring and comparing global trends and documenting the outcomes of nursing interventions. ICNP builds on a strong foundation of documented success and is one of ICN's greatest contributions of the century. The ICNP will make it easier to: (1) describe, measure, and compare what nurses do; (2) monitor global trends in nursing care; (3) compare nursing data across specialties, populations, settings, geographical areas, and time; and (4) document the outcomes of nursing interventions.
- The prominence of electronic technology does not eliminate the need for print materials for basic and continuing nursing education. ICN is also committed to creating a core library of nursing books and publications in every country.

ICN enjoys a privileged status in the international community. Nurses and nonnurses alike appreciate the trust that consumers place in nurses, and the influence that they hold with the public. Recent surveys indicate that 92 percent of patients trusted health care information given to them by registered nurses, a higher percentage than trusted any other single health care professional. This places nurses in an ideal position to shape health policy and nursing practice. However, the challenge will require research, information, and advocacy as well as the nurturing of leadership. ICN's plan for *shaping the world health agenda* includes:

- *Development of the family nurse.* For most of the world's people, health is dependent on community-based, primary care services. The concept of the "family nurse" includes these qualities and has been welcomed by the public. A key ICN initiative consists of studying a variety of "family nurse" practice models that have demonstrated good outcomes, defining the competencies of this role, and comparing the effectiveness between models. The family nurse as a community-based practitioner puts the emphasis on the nurse as the primary care provider and embraces the concepts of community development, health promotion, and collaborative practice. It establishes the nurse as the consumer's point of entry into the health care delivery system.
- *Implementation of the global study of the girl-child.* The Fourth UN World Conference on Women held in Beijing focused international attention on the girl-child, and ICN has identified an especially needy cohort within that population, the young urban girl. ICN is currently involved in a study to define the needs of young urban girls, and position the nursing profession to intervene on their

behalf. This unique and much-needed initiative combines research and policy development within a single project. It will discover and analyze information that will serve as a solid foundation for effective policies and programs to promote the healthy development of young girls.

- *Extension of the ICN leadership program.* This is an established program which teaches nurses how to exercise more effective leadership in shaping health policy as health care systems are reformed throughout the world. ICN plans to extend the program to new regions of the world and to expand offerings to currently and previously served areas.

ICN headquarters is located at 3 Place Jean Marteau, 1201 Geneva, Switzerland (mailing address: PO Box 42, CH-1201 Geneva 20, Switzerland).

NATIONAL STUDENT NURSES' ASSOCIATION

The National Student Nurses' Association, Inc. (NSNA), established in 1952, is the national organization for nursing students in the United States, its territories, and possessions.[6] The NSNA is autonomous, student financed, and student run. It is the voice of all nursing students speaking out on issues of concern to nursing students and nursing.

MEMBERSHIP

Students are eligible for active membership in NSNA if they are enrolled in state-approved programs leading to licensure as an RN or are RNs enrolled in programs leading to a baccalaureate degree in nursing. Students are eligible for associate membership if they are prenursing students enrolled in college or university programs designed to prepare them for programs leading to a degree in nursing. Associate members have all of the privileges of membership except the right to hold office as president and vice-president at state and national levels.

Application for membership is made directly to NSNA. Dues paid to NSNA are a combination of national and state association dues; the latter vary from state to state. The dues structure is decided by a vote of the membership.

NSNA also has two categories of membership not open to students. Sustaining membership is open at the national level to any individual or organization interested in furthering the development and growth of

NSNA. Sustaining members receive literature and other information from the NSNA office. Dues vary for sustaining members, which may include NSNA alumni, local organizations, and national organizations. Honorary membership is conferred by a two-thirds vote of the House of Delegates upon recommendation by the board of directors on persons who have rendered distinguished service or valuable assistance to NSNA. This is the highest honor NSNA can bestow upon an individual.

HISTORY

Just when or where the idea of a national association of nursing students originated will probably never be known. For many years, however, and in increasing numbers, students had been attending the national conventions of ANA and NLN, eager to learn of the activities of these two associations that would soon be affecting them as graduate nurses. Special sessions were arranged at these conventions so that students could meet together and discuss mutual problems. At the same time, some student nurses' organizations had been formed on the state level, giving students an awareness of both the strength and the values of group association and action. It was inevitable, of course, that sooner or later the idea of a national association would arise. Once it did, nursing students throughout the United States began to work enthusiastically in that direction.

In June 1952, approximately 1000 students attending the ANA nursing convention in Atlantic City, New Jersey, voted to form an organization under the sponsorship of the Coordinating Council of the ANA and NLN. A committee of nursing students and representatives of ANA and NLN worked on organization plans, and in June 1953 the NSNA was officially launched. By-laws were adopted and NSNA's officers were elected.

In its first few years, NSNA had little money, a small membership, no real headquarters of its own, and no headquarters staff. Its main assets at the time were the persistence, determination, and dedication of its members, plus financial and moral support from ANA and NLN. A year after NSNA's founding, these two organizations appointed (and paid) a coordinator to help NSNA function; many of the association's activities were transacted through correspondence. Each organization also provided a staff consultant to NSNA and helped finance the association's necessary expenses and publications. Among the latter were the by-laws and a newspaper. The next step was a headquarters office. Today, NSNA has offices at 45 Main Street, Brooklyn, New York 11201.

Even in its early years, NSNA was able to help finance itself; and year after year, NSNA's share of the costs increased. Membership grew, and annual dues, which had originally been 15 cents per year, were raised to 50 cents in 1957. Finally, in 1958, only five years after its inception, NSNA became financially independent. The original coordinator appointed in 1954, Frances Tompkins, became the executive director, and headed a staff of two. In 1959, NSNA became legally incorporated as the National Student Nurses' Association, Inc., a nonprofit association. Today, the association pays for headquarters offices, a staff, and all the other expenses incidental to running the business of a large association. It holds and finances its own annual convention. At the same time, it has also initiated and financed many important projects in the interests not only of its members but of the nursing profession as a whole.

GENERAL PLAN OF ORGANIZATION

The policies and programs of NSNA are determined by its House of Delegates, whose membership consists of elected representatives from the school and state associations. The delegates at each annual convention elect NSNA's three officers; six nonofficer directors, one of whom serves as editor of *Imprint*, the official journal of NSNA; and a four-member nominating committee. Officers serve for one year or until their respective successors are elected.

Two consultants are appointed, one each by the ANA and NLN, in consultation with the NSNA board of directors. They serve for a two-year period or until their respective successors are appointed. According to the by-laws, these consultants are charged with providing an interchange of information between their boards and NSNA. All consultants are expected to serve only as resource persons, consulting with officers, members, and staff and attending the meetings of the association.

The board of directors manages the affairs of the association between the annual meetings of the membership, and an executive committee, consisting of the president, vice-president, and secretary/treasurer, transacts emergency business between board meetings. There are two standing committees: the nominating and elections committee, and the resolutions committee. The board has the authority to establish other committees as needed. State and constituent organizations may or may not function in a similar manner; their by-laws must be in conformity with NSNA's by-laws.

PROJECTS, ACTIVITIES, SERVICES

NSNA has a wide variety of activities, services, and projects to carry out its purpose and functions. Even in its early years, the association sought participation in ANA and NLN committees and sent representatives to ICN.

Early projects were the Minority Group Recruitment Project (which has developed into Breakthrough to Nursing) and the Taiwan Project. The latter project, carried out in cooperation with the American Bureau for Medical Aid to China, grew out of NSNA members' interest in nursing students in other countries, coupled with a desire to assist whenever possible. After a firsthand report about the inadequate, overcrowded living conditions for nursing students at the National Defense Medical Center, Taiwan, delegates to the 1961 NSNA convention voted to raise $25,000 to build and equip a new dormitory for this group. By 1965, through vigorous fund-raising drives carried out at all levels of NSNA, the larger sum of $37,000 had been accumulated. The completed 50-student residence, named the NSNA Dormitory, was officially dedicated in March 1966, with American government officials cutting the traditional ribbon at the ceremony and representing both NSNA and the United States government.

Today, NSNA collaborates with many nursing and other health organizations. NSNA is a member of the Nursing Organization Alliance (the Alliance). The Alliance is composed of national nursing organizations and serves as a forum for networking and addressing nursing issues. NSNA is also a leading participant in the student assembly of the ICN. NSNA members are involved in community health activities such as hypertension screening, health fairs, child abuse, teenage pregnancy, and education on death and dying. Some of these activities are carried out in cooperation with other student health groups.

BREAKTHROUGH TO NURSING

NSNA has always been involved in recruiting qualified men and women into nursing. In 1965, however, NSNA launched a nationwide project directed toward the recruitment of ethnic and racial minorities, and members of other underrepresented groups, into the nursing profession. Known as the National Recruitment Project, this long-term effort grew out of an increasing awareness on the part of nursing students of their collective responsibility for supporting the civil rights movement, for recruiting to nursing, for alerting young men and women in minority groups to the opportunities in a nursing career, and in recognition of the value of such nurses in improving the care of their own ethnic groups.[7]

The national project was proposed at the 1965 NSNA convention by the 1964–1965 NSNA Nursing Recruitment Committee, whose recommendations were based on results of pilot projects conducted in

Colorado, Minnesota, and Washington, DC. The delegates voted to undertake the project on a national scale.

By early 1967 the project was well underway in many different areas of the country, with the state associations tackling the problem in various ways. In collaboration with other appropriate community groups—the Urban League, those associated with Head Start or other antipoverty programs, and civil rights groups—nursing students throughout the United States worked diligently not only to interest minority group members in nursing but also to help them financially, morally, and educationally to undertake such a career. In 1971, NSNA set the Breakthrough to Nursing Project, as it is now called, as a priority and secured funds to strengthen and expand the existing program. In order to sustain such a program, the involvement and support of nursing student volunteers, faculty, and heads of schools of nursing is essential. Student volunteers carry out such activities as career fairs, education of school counselors, working with schools and community groups to provide tutorial and counseling services, development and distribution of brochures, help with the application and registration procedures in colleges, and provision of information about financial resources.

Breakthrough to Nursing guidelines and materials are available for distribution nationally. Although there are still problems such as racial polarization and retention of students after recruitment, there is no doubt that the project has had an impact on nursing, on NSNA members, and on the community. Over the years, the Breakthrough to Nursing Project has evolved to reflect the needs of contemporary society. For example, in addition to those groups already cited, the Breakthrough to Nursing Project also focuses on nontraditional students (returning students) and encourages all qualified people to enter the profession.

LEGISLATION

One of the most impressive NSNA developments in recent years is the active and knowledgeable participation of NSNA members in legislation. Excellent resources on legislative activities and political education on a national level and assistance and support in legislation provided by NSNA to constituent associations resulted in legislative committees in most states. During the various crises of federal funding for health, students have testified before congressional committees and supported the passage of the Nurse Education Act by their active participation in the political process. They have also urged passage of social and health care reform legislation. Students are also encouraged to work with state nurses' associations (SNAs), state political action committees (PACs), and other groups on health legislation at the local and state levels, and to educate members in such areas as state nurse practice acts and political activism.

INTERDISCIPLINARY ACTIVITIES

NSNA has shown a forward-looking interest in the health and social problems of society, often combined with like interest in interdisciplinary cooperation. With the American Medical Student Association (AMSA), Student American Pharmaceutical Association (SAPhA), and American Student Dental Association (ASDA), individual nursing students have participated in Head Start, Appalachian and Indian health, migrant health, and Job Corps projects. Recently reinstated as the Coalition of Health and Professional Students, students from various health-related disciplines meet routinely to discuss mutual interests and concerns.

One major interdisciplinary activity in which NSNA participated was Concern for Dying's *Interdisciplinary Collaboration on Death and Dying.* This student program recruited representatives from the AMSA, the Law Student Division of the American Bar Association, and students from social work and theology schools. The Collaboration introduced students to a variety of professional perspectives on death and dying and created a dialogue among future professionals. Concern for Dying, now known as Choice in Dying, continues to provide NSNA members with information on nursing's role in death and dying issues.

SCHOLARSHIP FUNDS

The Foundation of the National Student Nurses' Association (FNSNA) administers its own scholarship program. The Foundation was established in 1969 to enable individuals and organizations to contribute funds to nursing education scholarships. The fund is incorporated and has obtained federal tax exemption. Scholarship monies are obtained from various organizations, and contributors have included both commercial enterprises and professional organizations. The FNSNA is establishing an endowed scholarship fund for undergraduate nursing education. This fund will ensure that money will always be available to support students seeking RN licensure as well as those in BSN completion programs.

PUBLICATIONS

Imprint, the official NSNA magazine, came into existence in 1968, and a subscription is given to members. Subscriptions are also available to other interested groups, schools, and individuals. *Imprint*, published five times during the academic year, is the only publication of its kind specifically for students. It is the only nursing magazine written by and for nursing students, and students are encouraged to contribute articles and letters.

Other publications include the *NSNA News*, a newsletter that keeps organization leaders at state and school levels informed of pertinent issues and activities; *The Dean's Notes*, a newsletter for deans and directors of schools of nursing; the *Business Book*, which serves as an annual report and is printed for the annual convention; *Getting the Pieces to Fit*, a yearly handbook for state and school chapters; and informational, supportive materials on students' rights. Most states and some schools also publish newsletters.

AN AGE OF ACTIVISIM

By the tenth anniversary of its founding, NSNA had accomplished a great deal. Before its thirtieth, it had become an involved group whose activities demonstrated committed professionalism. Gone were the talent shows and uniform nights of the early days. Students learned to conduct meetings and to use parliamentary procedure, they showed concern about their education and their future practice, and they showed concern for others. They were involved in many of the same issues as ANA and

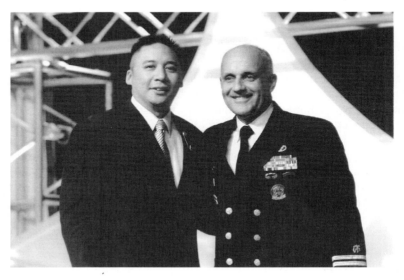

John Arce, 2004-05 NSNA President, with Vice Admiral Richard H. Carmona, United States Surgeon General. Admiral Carmona was a registered nurse early in his medical career. (*Courtesy of the National Student Nurses' Association*)

NLN and often seemed to show more foresight. With their fiftieth anniversary NSNA had reason to celebrate their history and their future.

Education has always been of prime interest, and among the issues discussed in meetings were curriculum planning, accreditation, entry into practice, and students' rights. In 1976, the NSNA House of Delegates recognized the need for baccalaureate education in nursing and encouraged greater availability of baccalaureate programs in nursing and increased enrollment of registered nurses in baccalaureate programs. NSNA urges the gradual movement of all programs preparing for practice as RNs to the baccalaureate level. NSNA also recognizes the contributions of associate, baccalaureate, diploma, generic master's, and doctoral programs that prepare students for RN licensure. As early as 1969, NSNA delegates also encouraged the development and demonstration of nursing education programs that would recognize an individual's previously acquired knowledge and skill. For the next decade, convention resolutions called for pathways for career mobility for AD and diploma nurses.

As in other fields, nursing students have also fought for their own rights, and NSNA has maintained a commitment to students' rights. In 1970, a guideline for a student bill of rights was distributed to all constituents, a mandate of the 1969 delegates. In 1975, a comprehensive *bill of rights*, responsibilities, and grievance procedures was accepted and published. The statement was adopted in schools throughout the country. The NSNA has also authored a *Code of Ethics* to address professional, academic, and clinical conduct. Both the Code of Professional Conduct and the Code of Academic and Clinical Conduct are available at www.nsna.org.

In the area of practice, students have taken positive stands on the concept of mandatory licensure, maldistribution of nurses, national standards for practice, substitution of unlicensed personnel for nurses, and use of student nurses as a substitute for nurses. They have supported economic security and the ANA position that in the event of a non-RN strike, students would not substitute for striking workers unless patients were endangered.

Finally, NSNA members have been involved in issues affecting the public's health—for instance, by participating in projects to educate children and young people about the dangers of drugs. NSNA has taken numerous positions on contemporary issues such as women's health and social issues, pregnancy, infant and child health, sexually transmitted diseases, AIDS–HIV prevention and education, smoking and health, drug and alcohol abuse, infection control, and promotion of a positive image of nursing. NSNA offers the opportunity for nursing students to be heard, becomes a forum for debates on health and social issues as well as nursing issues, provides opportunities for interdisciplinary contacts, and is a training ground for participatory leadership skills. Participation and involvement can be a meaningful and valuable part of the nursing student's education. Many involved NSNA members go on to leadership positions in nursing organizations and continue their lifelong commitment to advancing the profession of nursing.

HEALTH-RELATED ORGANIZATIONS

Many health-related organizations, both governmental and nongovernmental, frequently provide opportunities for participation by nurses through some form of membership, consultation, or inclusion on committees or programs. A number provide services specifically for nurses, such as workshops, conferences, publications, and audiovisual materials. Nurses may be invited to attend other program sessions, present papers, or serve on panels. Some examples include the American Cancer Society, the American Heart Association, the American Medical Association, and the Catholic Hospital Association.

There are also organizations in which there are large, active nursing components, such as the American Hospital Association and, particularly, the American Public Health Association (see Appendix 4). The American Red Cross, particularly, has many activities in which nurses are involved, including their disaster health services and educational programs. Nurses may give volunteer service and apply for enrollment as a Red Cross Nurse.

THE NURSING LITERATURE

Not long ago, text or reference books in nursing were generally limited to the major clinical fields. Now there is scarcely any area relating to nursing that does not have books on the subject. New titles show the extremely diverse nature of the subjects that nurses must read and write about today. Many of these books (this one, for instance) must be frequently revised and published in new, updated editions to keep up with new knowledge and expanding concepts.

Reading the book advertisements in the nursing magazines is almost an education in itself; by doing this, you are reminded of the "hot" topics of the day—or of tomorrow. Even more important is reading the reviews of these books, also published in the nursing journals or on the Internet. That way, you get a better knowledge of their content and the reviewer's estimate (and he or she is usually an expert in the field) of their value. It is then easier to decide whether to buy it, borrow it from the library, glance at it in the bookstore, or forget about it. It is impossible to read all the books published in the nursing field today, so you will want to select those that are most worthwhile for you.

It is the nursing journals, however, that will keep you up to date and well informed. Usually at least six months pass between the writing of a book and its appearance in print, and a few more months may pass before it is reviewed. However, the nursing journals, especially those that are published monthly, make available news, reviews, and information promptly. Within the past 15 years alone, there has been a remarkable increase in the numbers and kinds of nursing magazines, and many are available in electronic format. Some you will want to subscribe to and keep for reference, others to look at each month in the library or on the Internet. It is helpful to have at least an idea of the content, purpose, and approach of all of them, whether for reading purposes or sometime to publish in yourself. Writing for publication is becoming more important as changes in nursing and health care occur; therefore, learning how to write and publish is worth considering.

It is not feasible to review the content of all these periodicals; some are listed in Appendix 4, if they are associated with a professional organization. There are also other general and clinical journals, those owned by commercial publishers, others are nonprofit. There are journals of the CMAs, and national publications of other countries. It is worthwhile to review a cross-section of these works (they are not subscribed to by many libraries), as well as the other health-related journals, because they contain useful information. Direction to nursing and allied health periodicals can be obtained through an Internet search engine, or many are listed in the *Cumulative Index to Nursing and Allied Health Literature* (CINAHL), either in electronic or hard copy format. Other health-related journals are found in *Index Medicus* or through the *National Library of Medicine* at http://www.nlm.nih.gov.

OTHER REFERENCE SOURCES

Most schools of nursing today do not have a collection adequate to meet the needs of a serious scholar or even of someone who wants to go beyond the major nursing journals and books. Nevertheless, nurses who learn how to use the library, the interlibrary loan service, and the various computer information retrieval systems will find a new world of reference sources.

Other reference sources of interest to nurses, such as directories, handbooks, review texts, and manuals, are too numerous to list in these pages. A number of guides regularly provide libraries and nurses with lists of recommended journals, books, and other materials. For specific needs, it is advisable to consult a professional librarian.

You will not want to confine yourself to the limits of nursing's literature. The publications of medical and hospital groups, allied professions, education, administration, the social services, and other related fields frequently contain useful and interesting material. Social, economic, educational, and other issues are as important to understanding current and future changes in nursing as knowledge of medical and scientific progress.

Of course, all the reference sources in the world are of little value if you cannot use them properly. What follows are some of the ways students and professionals can maximize the benefit they receive from the library's services:

- Establish personal contact with a professional librarian in the institution's library. Information management is the librarian's expertise, and he or she can provide valuable support in meeting educational and clinical goals. Librarians want to meet information needs, but they can only do so if they know their patrons and their specific needs.
- Take advantage of library orientations and tours, and keep up with regular library newsletters. Internal library operations are fast becoming totally computerized, and knowing how to retrieve needed data quickly from on-line catalogs and other systems will prove advantageous. Some training is also needed to use the library's electronic systems for searching the databases mentioned previously. It is also valuable to know how to request copies of articles or books from other libraries.

KEY POINTS

1. The rapid increase in various specialty nursing organizations resulted in some initial lack of coordination in advancing nursing goals.
2. The Alliance, NANP, and the Tri-Council are examples of the way in which nursing organizations have established relationships that allow them to communicate and, at times, collaborate in areas of mutual interest.
3. ANA and its allied associations focus considerable attention on nurses' economic and general welfare, lobbying, standard setting, certification, accreditation of continuing education programs, and relationships with other groups.
4. ANA sees itself as speaking for America's nurses.

5. The NSNA grooms student nurses to enter the world of practice.
6. Specialty organizations include those that are clinical, have special interests in ethnic or other minority concerns, or maintain a scholarly, educational, or socially oriented focus.
7. Health-related organizations, such as AHA, the American Public Health Association (APHA), and the Red Cross, often have activities specially geared to nurses.
8. There are a number of aids for nurses that will help them find the kinds of references they need; nurses should seek them out and become familiar with the use of computers for this purpose.

STUDY QUESTIONS

1. Attend a local or state nurses' association meeting. What were the issues discussed? What were the strengths and weaknesses of the discussion?
2. Develop a strategic plan for increasing membership in the American Nurses Association and the National Student Nurses' Association.
3. Which association(s) is it most important for you to join on graduation? Build your case.
4. Is association membership more important to professionals in the United States than in other countries?
5. Explore the various databases available to nurses. Formulate an opinion as to which are most important to a student of your level.

REFERENCES

1. CAN: http://nursingworld.org/can. Retrieved April 20, 2005.
2. AAN: http://www.aannet.org/opportunities/scholarinresidence. Retrieved April 22, 2005.
3. American Nurses Credentialing Center: http://nursingworld.org/ancc/cert.html.
4. Merton R. The functions of the professional association. *Am J Nurs* 58:50–54, January 1958.
5. International Council of Nurses: http://www.icn.ch/abouticn.htm. Retrieved April 26, 2005.
6. NSNA: http://www.nsna.org/contact_us.asp. Retrieved April 26, 2005.
7. Johnson N: Recruitment of minority groups—A priority for NSNA. *Nurs Outlook* 14:29–30, April 1966.

Updates can be found at

 http://www.JoelTheNursingExperience.com

Chapter 14

Workplace Choices

OBJECTIVES

After studying this chapter, you will be able to:

1. *Assess your talents and interests in planning for your career.*
2. *Prepare for a job interview.*
3. *Put together a professional résumé.*
4. *Write an application letter.*
5. *Identify sources of information about jobs.*
6. *Terminate employment in an appropriate manner.*
7. *Deal with being fired or laid off.*

Graduation at last! And now what? For most nurses, "what" means it's now time to get a job. For some, the job is predetermined—commitment to the armed services, the Veterans Administration, or another agency that funded their education. Others may have decided early on exactly the kind of nursing they prefer and the place they want to do it. If all goes well and there are no problems, such as an oversupply of nurses for that specialty or geographical area, at least one major decision is made. For all graduates, however, choosing that crucial first job and preparing for it are big considerations.

A pandemic shortage of nurses has created many employment opportunities, although the place of employment preferred may not offer the exact hours, specialty, opportunities, or assistance wanted by a new graduate. The shortage is also characterized by maldistribution, with not enough nurses opting to work in isolated or inner city areas, although the need there is serious. In the midst of these circumstances, new and exciting nursing opportunities are constantly emerging (these are described in some detail in Chapter 6). How, then, can you decide what is the best job for you? How do you maximize the chances of getting it?

BASIC CONSIDERATIONS

PERSONAL AND OCCUPATIONAL ASSESSMENT

It's a good idea to start thinking about career choices while you are still in your educational program. Since most schools have rotations through the various clinical specialty areas, this gives you a chance to compare as you learn. Generally, there is also access to someone who can advise you about the pros and cons of certain types of nursing—or at least there's a more experienced nurse, often a faculty member, to talk to.

More important than anything else, though, is to take a considered look at yourself—your own qualities and what you want out of life. There are a variety of approaches to this sort of self-assessment that are interesting to explore in depth, and there are generally certain commonalities among choices. Some questions you might ask are:

- *What are my personality characteristics?* Do I like to do things with people or by myself? Am I patient? Do I like to do things quickly? Am I good at details, or do I like to take the broad view? Do I like a structured and quiet environment or one that is constantly changing? Am I relatively confident in what I undertake or do I look for support? Am I easily bored? Do I like to tackle problem situations or avoid them? Do I have a sense of humor? Am I emotional? Am I a risk taker? Do I care about the way I look? Do I care what others think of me?
- *What are my values?* Do I believe in the right to life or the right to die? Do I think everyone should have access to health care? Do I have a religious orientation? Do I think that too many people today are too rigid or too loose in their beliefs and behavior? Can I accept and work with those who have very different values? How do I feel about my responsibility to myself, my employer, my patient, the doctors, my profession, and society? Do I believe strongly that my way is the right way? Am I intolerant of others' beliefs?
- *What are my interests?* In the broad field of nursing? In certain specialties? In the health field? In my private and social life? In the community? Do I like to travel? Do I long for adventure?

○ *What are my needs?* Am I ambitious? Do I like to be the boss? Is money important to me? Status? Do I need intellectual stimulation? Is academic success important? What about academic credentials? Am I comfortable working where the majority of nurses have different educational credentials? Do I prefer working with a supervisor of the same or other sex? Am I willing to relocate? Does a city, suburb, or rural area fit my desired lifestyle? Is success in my field important? Am I willing to sacrifice personal and family time for success? Do I think that my first responsibility is to my family at this point? Do my spouse and I plan to have dual careers? Is part-time work an option? Do I want plenty of time for family, friends, and leisure activities? Do I see nursing as a career or a way to earn a living as long as that is necessary? Do I really like nursing? If not, why not, and what can I do about it?

○ *What kinds of abilities do I have?* In manual skills? In communication? In intellectual/cognitive skills? In analyzing? In coordinating? In organizing? In supervising? In dealing with people? Do I have a great deal of energy and stamina? Are there certain times, situations, or climate conditions in which I have less? Am I good at comforting

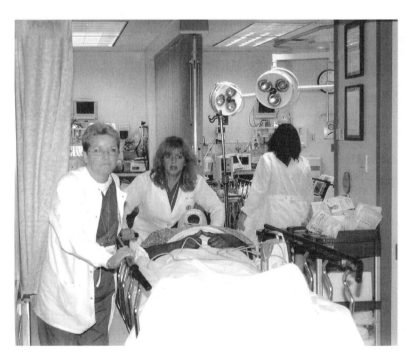

Hospital nursing assumes a fast pace and the constant presence of technology. (*Courtesy of Hackensack University Medical Center, Hackensack, New Jersey*)

people? Am I able to give some of myself to others? Am I more comfortable with or enjoy more caring for children, the elderly, the chronically ill, or some other group?

It's good to prioritize some of these lists, since life and a job are usually a compromise. What's most important? What would make you miserable? It might also be very helpful to share this list with others. Is this the way you are seen by them? Have you missed something? If some of your friends and peers are involved in their own decision making, get together with them and/or a trusted teacher or mentor to brainstorm about the possibilities in the field now or later in order to match your own profile most accurately with nursing opportunities. When compromises are necessary, you can decide ahead of time which ones are tenable or even perfectly acceptable at that point.

Since there will probably be economic constraints in the health care system for a long time, one way to look at the job market is in terms of future growth. For instance, you may choose a community hospital for a first job, but have you considered a university medical center or, later, a long-term care facility, home care, a one-day surgical center, a wound-care center, or an ambulatory-care outreach center? Each is part of the health care scene. You should examine those job prospects as carefully as any other. They may have aspects that do not fit in with your own self-assessment, but don't close doors because of preconceived notions.

It is also wise to be aware that there are both linear and nonlinear career routes. Historically, staff nurse led to charge nurse to assistant head nurse to head nurse to area coordinator or supervisor and up you go. Or, in a more contemporary fashion, staff nurse to senior staff nurse to clinical coordinator to case manager to advanced practice, assuming the requisite academic preparation. These are the traditional routes and they need sound planning. But are there other ways to conceptualize your career? Play to *your passions and individual talents* to create highly individualized career options. If you are articulate and persuasive with an insatiable interest in public policy, why should this be an avocation? How about work as a nurse lobbyist? You love to work with children, so have chosen pediatrics. In your leisure you spend every minute outdoors. Why keep the two apart? You could work in a child's camp or residential school. Be creative, and explore every option as crazy as it may seem... but know yourself first.[1]

LICENSURE

Regardless of the results of your self-study, a basic and essential step in your professional nursing career is becoming licensed, since you cannot practice in any state without an RN. Information about how to apply to take the state board examination leading to licensure is found in Chapter 11. The procedure for becoming licensed is very quick with the use of computerized adaptive testing and the ability to take the test any time of the year at any one of hundreds of testing centers. Some state boards of nursing permit nurses to practice temporarily while their application for licensure is being processed. Check with the board of nursing or your school. It may be possible to be employed as a *graduate nurse* until you pass the licensure exam. However, in reality, many hospitals will interview you but not employ you until you become licensed. The administration feels that the cost of orientation is too great to take a chance that the nurse will fail. If a nurse fails the test after employment, he or she may be dismissed or must work as some type of nursing assistant.

What if you decide not to work right away—for example, to stay home with your family or to take a long vacation? It's probably wise to study for and take the exam anyway. Unused knowledge has a way of disappearing from the mind, and it might be much more difficult to pass the exam later, without some ongoing learning and practice. Moreover, in most states, you are expected to take the exam within a certain time after graduation. Should you take a nursing board review course? It depends on the confidence you have in your nursing knowledge and test-taking ability. A good review course can be very helpful. However, be careful to select a reputable company. Remember that these are profit-making operations, expensive to you, and always attracting some borderline operators. Another way of preparing is to study with a group of peers, perhaps using board review workbooks or texts designed for that purpose.

PROFESSIONAL BIOGRAPHIES AND RÉSUMÉS

New nursing graduates today have a wider variety of personal and educational backgrounds than they did a few years ago. Many have held responsible positions in other fields, and even more have worked part or full time before or during their educational programs.

Therefore, the suggested procedures for application and resignation presented are just that. They review generally accepted ways to handle certain inevitable professional matters in a sophisticated and businesslike way, and may serve as a refresher for those already familiar with these or other equally acceptable ways of relating and communicating in business relationships. For the younger, less experienced nurse, this material provides a convenient reference and guide.

After self-assessment and thought about career alternatives, it's time to write a résumé. No matter how you obtain a position in nursing, you will probably be asked to submit a résumé or summary of your qualifications for the job before any interview is possible. In addition, a prospective employer may request a transcript of your educational record and names and addresses of references, but this may not occur until after the interview. Some universities and other educational programs maintain a file with updated information about your career provided by you, as well as references that you have solicited. This has the advantage of eliminating the need to ask for repeated references from teachers who may scarcely remember you or to write again and again to a variety of places for records. However, this service is gradually fading away and that may not be bad. As you and your career develop, a reference from your first teacher or your first staff position says little other than how you were evaluated at that time. Newer references may be far more useful. Your academic record or simply evidence of your graduation may still be requested, and your school always provides that information. Today, however, a well-prepared résumé is considered a must for a job applicant.

A résumé is a relatively short professional or business biography. In academia, a curriculum vitae (CV), which is somewhat lengthier and contains different and more detailed information, is the appropriate form of professional biography.

The résumé should be businesslike, prepared with a word processor (with no insertion of handwritten comments) on one side of good-quality paper—plain white, off-white, or light gray—measuring 8 by 11 inches, with adequate margins all around, and consistency of font (traditional, clear, and crisp) and format. The envelope should match. Proofread for any spelling and grammatical errors. Typographical errors are guaranteed to turn off any employer. Have someone read the document who has a critical eye.[2] No more than two pages are recommended, one is better. Some experts suggest that you have a professional printer duplicate your résumé on a photocopier that produces a sharp copy, absolutely free of dark areas or smudges. Quick-copy shops may specialize in making a résumé look good, doing layouts, typing, printing, and copying.

There are various ways to write a résumé; however, the content areas are generally the same. They start with name, mailing address, e-mail address, and telephone number, with the name written as you would sign it, but including appropriate degrees or credentials—for example, Mary Smith RN, BSN or RN, MSN, CCRN. Periods are not necessary in these abbreviations as long as you are consistent in their use. Some nurses prefer to put the degree before the RN. Be sure your address and telephone number are complete. Include your business address only if you can accept calls there, though this is commonly omitted when you are seeking another job. An answering machine may be useful so that important calls from potential employers are not missed.

Résumés are organized in a chronological or functional—sometimes called topical—format. In a chronological format, you list your experience in reverse chronological order. The functional format calls for separate categories, such as clinical experience, teaching, education, and so on. The most common format is probably a combination in which the various areas of work experience, education, honors, publications, and other activities are presented in separate sections, but items are listed in reverse chronological order in each section. Remember that a résumé is a marketing tool that should show you to advantage. Therefore, while you must never be dishonest, the way you present your talents and credentials, especially after you have accumulated some work experience, may make the difference between whether you are interviewed or ignored, especially in a competitive situation. Although format is a matter of taste and style, a sample résumé that might be used by a new graduate is shown in Exhibit 14.1.

The following points may also be helpful. Stating a professional objective is not a must, especially if you are not sure exactly what you want to do. If you choose to write one, it should match the job for which you are applying and thus may need to be changed accordingly. For instance, someone with a master's degree in perinatal nursing may be interested in either a teaching or a clinical specialist position. Both the objective and the emphasis in the résumé must focus on the position for which the person is applying. Needless to say, if you are applying for your first or second staff nurse position in a hospital, the decision on what to write is less complex.

All relevant work experiences should be included, with the most recent listed first. The usual format is to list the agency and date, followed by a brief description of duties performed, using "action" verbs—*developed, initiated, supervised*. Some experts suggest that if you have not had impressive positions, you should attempt to bury this fact in statements that focus on your personal qualities, such as: "Leadership—Demonstrated by ability to lead others—as night nurse on a pediatric unit at X hospital, such and such address." No one really knows whether this is more effective, but again, style is a matter of personal choice. Many new graduates describe their nursing school clinical experiences in their résumé. This nonessential information can contribute substance to an otherwise thin résumé. If the clinical experience section makes your résumé more than two pages in length, leave it out.[3]

The education section should also begin with the most recent academic credential, and should include the major and such additions as research projects, special awards, academic honors, extracurricular activities, and offices held. There is no need to go as far back as high school.

Exhibit 14.1 Sample Résumé

LESLIE B. SMITH
120 Pine Street   Home Phone (415) 456–7890
North Ridge, CA 01302   Message Phone (415) 482–6132

PROFESSIONAL
OBJECTIVE: Staff nursing in a community hospital.

EXPERIENCE:
September 2002   Central Hospital, Alton, California
to August 2003   Unit clerk on medical–surgical units, evening shift.
                                   Assisted charge nurse in (list activities); trained new clerks;
                                   developed end-of-shift report between clerks.

Summer 2002   Central Hospital, Alton, California
                                   Nurse's aide on medical–surgical units. Responsible for care
                                   of thirty patients under direction of RNs, including (list major
                                   activities).

EDUCATION:
2003–2005   Blank Community College
                                   Associate of Science in Nursing (to be awarded May 2005)

HONORS:
2003–2005   Dean's List

2004–2005   Member, Wings, college honor society
2003–2005   Honor Scholarship
2005   Outstanding Student Leader Award,
                                   Blank Community College

PROFESSIONAL ACTIVITIES:
2004–2005   Member, National Student Nurses' Association
2005   Chair, Program Committee, NSNA
May 2005   Presented paper "When Students Teach Patients,"
                                   Blank Hospital, Nurses' Day
June 2004   Attended ANA Convention
April 2004   Debate: "Be It Resolved: Everyone Has a Right to
                                   Health Care," Student Leadership Forum,
                                   Blank Community College

COMMUNITY ACTIVITIES:
1999–2005   Volunteer for public television telethon
1999–2005   Volunteer for March of Dimes
1998–2000   Candy-striper at Central Hospital, Alton, California

Information on other honors, professional memberships and activities, and community activities might also be given in separate sections. If you have certification in a specialty area, include this. (You may also put the appropriate initials after your name.) Don't put down a heading such as "honors" and then write "none." Just omit such categories.

Under federal law, you cannot be required to include personal data such as your age, marital status, place of birth, religion, sex, race, color, national origin, or handicap. In fact, there is some feeling that including irrelevant personal data such as this and including height, weight, hobbies, and interests, unless they contribute to your ability to do the job you've applied for, is a negative. If you choose to do so, decide whether this makes you a more desirable candidate. For instance, a second language or extensive travel might be a plus in certain situations. When you are licensed as an RN, or if you later become certified in a specialty, that can be listed as well.

It is not necessary to say "References on request"; you would hardly refuse to give them. If your school does maintain a file, you can state this later, giving the correct address. When you do give the references, include the full names, titles, and business addresses of three persons who are qualified to evaluate your professional ability, scholarship, character, and personal qualities. Most suitable are teachers and former employers. Ask permission to use their names as references in advance. Choose carefully. If the individual, no matter how prestigious, really doesn't know you, your talents, and your abilities, and the reference is noncommittal, it can do more harm than good. When you contact a reference, however, it is acceptable, even good sense, to offer to send a résumé to refresh that person's memory. For instance, almost everyone forgets the dates they knew you, as you are not likely to be the only student or employee they know. If the individual is reluctant, don't push; the result can be a reference that says nothing much, and the potential employer may read it as negative—and it may be. You should also keep in mind that prospective employers frequently telephone the reference, either because they want a quick answer or because they want to ask questions that are not on a reference form or to explore some aspect of the written reference (particularly if it was noncommittal). Therefore, if the individual you've chosen as a reference is inclined to be abrupt, unpleasant, or irritated on the phone, choose another. As a rule, don't ask for a "To whom it may concern" letter and have it recopied. Most sophisticated employers see that as an uninterested response. If you carry a reference with you to an interview, it may be regarded with some suspicion.

Suppose that you didn't get along with your last employer and, even though you left with appropriate notice, you fear a poor reference. Sometimes someone else who was your positional superior, or another person such as a clinical specialist who knows your work, can be substituted. (A peer's opinion may be discounted.) However, administrators often know each other, and your potential employer may know that you did not name the person who would be the usual reference and may check with him or her by phone. That could result in a really negative reference. Therefore, as lists of references are often not requested until after the interview, you could simply say then that you did not have a positive relationship. Be careful not to speak negatively of the former employer; try to be objective or neutral. Though references can be important, the impression you make in an interview can be much more important in the long run.

LOOKING OVER THE JOB MARKET

It's sensible to assess the potential for a particular job both before and after applying for and/or being offered a nursing position. Chapter 6 should be helpful as an overview of the opportunities available in terms of both specialties and professional development (career ladder, internships); but reading the literature, talking to practitioners in the field, and, if possible, getting exposure to the actual practice during your educational program will help answer some specific questions. Start thinking about that first job early, while you're a student. Start getting preliminary information and talking to people in your network.

Today, even if an employer is actively recruiting for nurses, an application, a formal letter of interest, and often a résumé are necessary before a position is actually offered. Although there are those who feel that going through the entire process is worthwhile for the experience alone, unless you have at least some interest, it is unfair to take an employer's time to review an application and go through an interview for nothing. Therefore, after self-assessment, do at least a potential job assessment in advance. The first logical consideration is a place with which you have already had experience.

Hospitals or other agencies affiliated with schools of nursing may offer new graduates staff positions. That has several advantages for the employer and usually for the student as well. Nurses who are familiar with the personnel, procedures, and physical facilities may require a shorter orientation period, which saves time and money, and, of course, to an extent, the former student is already known. There are also benefits for new graduates. During these first months after graduation, you can gain valuable experience in familiar surroundings. There are opportunities to develop leadership and teaching skills and to practice clinical skills under less pressure because the people, places, and routines will not be totally unknown. The potential trauma of relocating and readjusting your personal life is not combined with the tension of being both a new, untried graduate and a new employee. It may also be a wonderful place to work. Besides, if the job market is tight, making a good impression as a student (or even as a volunteer or employee in another capacity) may bring you a job offer or, at least, give you an advantage over another applicant.

However, if the experiences offered do not help you to develop, if the environment is one that eventually makes you resistant, resentful, indifferent, unhappy, or uninterested, you may be set for a lifetime of nursing jobs, not a professional career. Of course, that can also happen in other places, but if you're alert, you can often get a pretty good notion of how it would be to work at the agencies in which you have had student or work experience. Be observant; look at how care is being given, the interaction between staff and management, with physicians, with other departments, and generally, the work environment. This evaluation can be a little more difficult if you don't know a place at all, but the opinion of someone you respect, word-of-mouth information, the institution's newsletter and brochures, and even the way someone replies to your inquiry, provides indirect as well as direct information.

On a more concrete level, you can give some thought to what you are willing to accept in terms of salary, shifts, benefits, and travel time. (Don't underestimate the value of the fringe benefits, which may not be taxable.) Balancing these with other advantages and disadvantages as determined by your self-assessment is important, and realistically, if the job market is tight in the geographical area of your choice, your opportunities may be fewer.[4] Whether or not this is so, spend the time, effort, and sometimes money to research institutions in which you are interested. Call for their information pamphlet/brochure, and perhaps the annual report. All this is public information, available from the public/community relations office. The public library also has materials giving information about health care agencies. If you are considering relocation and are not familiar with the area, again check the library, write to that town's Chamber of Commerce, or get some copies of the local newspaper. However, some of your best information may come from your network, discussed later.

Remember that in any health care organization there are *critical indicators* that send a message about how highly nursing is valued. Collect some telling information:

- How is certification valued and rewarded? How many staff nurses are certified in their practice areas?
- Are staff nurses involved in policy development? How?
- What is the approximate salary of the highest paid staff nurse?
- What is the hospital's yearly attrition rate among nurses?
- Are there advanced practice nurses on staff? How many, and what is their availability to the staff nurse?
- What is the role of staff development; remedial and responding to deficiencies, regulations, new procedures, equipment, and processes; or is enrichment also included?
- Is there a career ladder? How is education rewarded?
- What is the quality of the nurse/physician relationship? Are there integrated patient records, joint care planning? Do any nurses hold

membership on the medical staff organization and what privileges do they have?

- Is there an active presence of nursing research?
- Where is the chief nurse executive in the organizational chart? (Nursing usually represents the single largest group of employees. If the nurse executive is buried somewhere down in the organizational hierarchy, this is a message about the respect given nursing.)

All of these factors must be considered seriously. You'll never have another first job in nursing, a job that could set the tone of your professional future. It's much better to act carefully and make sure that your choice is the best possible one for moving you toward your goal, whatever it may be.

SOURCES OF INFORMATION ABOUT POSITIONS

Two principal sources of information are available to nurses who are looking for a position: (1) personal contacts and inquiries, and (2) advertisements and recruiters, often found on the Internet. Commercial placement agencies can be of some help at a later stage of your search, although they may be more interested in nurses with advanced experience, education, or specialization.

PERSONAL CONTACTS AND INQUIRIES

The nursing service director or someone on the nursing staff of a student-affiliated agency, instructors, other nurses, friends, neighbors, and family members may suggest available positions in health agencies or make other job suggestions. Hospitals not affiliated with schools of nursing sometimes ask the heads of nursing schools to refer graduates to them for possible placement on their staff. Often, letters or announcements of such positions are posted on the school bulletin board or are available in a file. Your own inquiries are likely to be equally productive in turning up the right position.

Never underestimate the value of personal contacts—your network. People seldom suggest a position unless they know something about it. That gives you the opportunity to ask questions early on, and the information can help you decide as well as prepare you better for the interview. Moreover, if your contact knows the employer and is willing (better yet, pleased) to recommend you, your chances of getting the position are immediately improved.[5] (This kind of networking, discussed more fully in Chapter 7, will be useful throughout your career.) One business executive has said, "Eighty percent of all jobs are filled through a grapevine . . . a system of referrals that never sees the light of day." When equally qualified people compete for the same position, the network recommendation could make the crucial difference. Asking for job-seeking help is neither pushy nor presumptuous, but you should be prepared to discuss your interests intelligently. A résumé will help, too. Most people like to be asked for advice and want to be helpful, but they have to be asked. On the other hand, you need to use some common sense in deciding how much and how often you ask for help, and from whom.

Some aspects of networking are much less formal, but equally helpful. For instance, contacts you've made as a member of a national nursing organization, beginning with NSNA, can give you inside information on what it's like to work in a certain place and/or in a particular geographical region. They may help with anything from housing to introduction to professional, social, or community groups.

ADVERTISEMENTS AND RECRUITERS

Local newspapers and official organs of district and state nurses' associations often carry advertisements of positions for professional nurses. National and regional nursing magazines and papers list positions in all categories of employment, usually classified into the various areas of the country. National medical, public health, and hospital magazines also carry advertisements for nurses, but they usually are for head nurse positions or higher, or for special personnel such as nurse anesthetists or nurse consultants. The Internet has become a rich source of recruitment, but you are cautioned to be careful about the ethics of some recruiters.

All of these sources carry classified advertisements for information only, and, of course, as a source of revenue. Rarely, if ever, does the publisher assume responsibility for the information in the advertisement beyond its conformity to such legal requirements as may apply. If you accept an advertised position that does not turn out to be what was expected, you cannot hold the publication responsible. Read the advertisement very carefully. Is the hospital or health agency well known and of good reputation? Is the information clear and inclusive? Does it sound effusive and overstress the advantages and delights of joining the staff? What can be read between the lines? How much more information is needed before deciding whether the job is suitable? Some of these questions can be resolved through correspondence, a telephone contact, the Internet or your network. Naturally, advertisers are putting their "best foot forward." Unless you've been watching the advertisements for some time or know someone from that institution, you might not be aware, for example, that the turnover is high, generally a sign of some problems. Nevertheless, want-ads in both electronic and print media are one reasonable start to a job search.

At some time, you may want to place an advertisement in the "Positions Wanted" column of a professional publication or on the Internet. In that case, review the directions for submitting a classified advertisement. The editor will arrange the information to conform to the publication's style but will not change the material sent unless asked to. Therefore, all the information needed to attract a prospective employer within the limits of professional ethics should be included clearly and concisely.

Career directories published periodically by some nursing journals or other commercial sources are free to job seekers. They have relatively extensive advertisements with much more detailed information than appears in the usual ad. The other advantage is instant comparison and geographical separation. Directories are frequently available in the exhibit section of student and other nursing conventions. Some carry reprints of articles on careers, licensure, job seeking, and other pertinent information. Some journals also do periodic surveys on job salaries and fringe benefits that can be useful when considering various geographical areas and may have special sections describing job opportunities in certain regions of the country.

Recruiters for hospitals and other agencies are usually present at representative booths in the exhibit areas of conventions; some have hotel suites where they have an open house. Recruiters, who may or may not be nurses, also visit nursing schools and often arrange for space in a hotel for preliminary interviews. Notices are placed in newspapers or sent to schools. There are advantages to the personalized recruiter approach because your questions can be answered directly, and you can get "a feel" for the employer's attitude, especially if nurses accompany the recruiter. However, remember the recruiters are selected for their recruiting ability.

COMMERCIAL PLACEMENT AGENCIES

There are commercial placement agencies that maintain a list of nurses who are looking for part-time work or who are job hunting. As might be expected, some are reliable and some are not. They can be checked out with the Better Business Bureau and your network. Almost always a fee must be paid to the registry, sometimes based on a percentage of the nurse's earnings. At another level of job seeking—executive positions—well-known agencies of good reputation (headhunters) are used by both employers and potential employees to match the best possible person to a suitable position.

Temporary nurse service or a *supplemental staffing agency* is another option (see Chapter 6). These services commonly employ nurses and then, according to requests and a nurse's choices, send her or him to an institution or other agency for a specific period of time. Nurses are usually placed in short-term situations in hospitals, home care, or nursing homes. The single most important factor that seems to attract nurses to temporary nurse services is control over working conditions, including the time, place, type of assignment, and so on. New graduates may find this type of employment attractive as a temporary measure, since the absence of fringe benefits may not be important to them immediately (taxes are withheld but no other benefits are usually given). There is also an opportunity to try out different types of nursing, but for the new nurse, the lack of individual support and supervision is a disadvantage.

PROFESSIONAL CORRESPONDENCE

New nursing graduates today have a wider variety of personal and educational backgrounds than they did a few years ago. Many have held responsible positions in other fields, and even more have worked part- or full-time before or during their educational programs.

Therefore, the suggested procedures for application and resignation presented are just that. They review generally accepted ways to handle certain inevitable professional matters in a sophisticated and businesslike way and may serve as a refresher for those already familiar with these or other equally acceptable ways of relating and communication in professional business relationships. For the younger, less experienced nurse, this material provides a convenient reference and guide.

The first contact with a prospective employer is usually made by letter, followed by a personal interview, telephone conversation, and, occasionally, fax or e-mail. Every business letter makes an impression on its reader—an impression that may be favorable, unfavorable, or indifferent. To achieve the best effect, the stationery on which it is written should be in good taste; the message accurate and complete yet concise; the tone appropriate; and the form, grammar, and spelling correct.

STATIONERY AND FORMAT

If preparing a letter to post, it should be neatly and legibly presented in black ink on unlined white paper. Single sheets measuring 8½ by

11 inches are most suitable. Personal stationery is acceptable if it is of the right size and color (white or off-white) and used with unlined envelopes. Notebook paper should never be used for business correspondence; neither should someone else's personal stationery or the stationery of a hospital, hotel, or place of business. An e-mail attachment should be prepared with the same care, format, and attention to detail. The font used should be traditional, clear, and crisp.

Your letter should be typed or a word processor should be used. This is considered most desirable; in fact, some employers react very negatively to a handwritten letter, even if neatly printed. They feel that it is always possible to get a letter typed and not to do so shows lack of interest or professionalism. In addition, the letter, like the résumé, should be error-free. Always keep a copy for future reference.

Books on English composition and secretary's handbooks include correct forms for writing business letters. Two or more variations may be given; the choice is yours. One example is shown in Exhibit 14.2. If personal stationery on which the name and address are engraved or printed is used, this information should be omitted from the heading of the letter and only the date given. Another acceptable format is shown in Exhibit 14.3.

Exhibit 14.2 Sample Application Letter

Date of letter
Applicant's address
Applicant's phone number

Employer's name and title (Use complete title and address)
Employer's address

Salutation:

Opening paragraph: State why you are writing. Name the position or type of work for which you are applying. Mention how you learned of the opening.

Middle paragraph: Explain your interest in working for this employer and the specific reason for desiring this type of work. Describe relevant work experience, pointing out any other job skills or abilities that relate to the position for which you are applying. If appropriate, state your academic preparation and how it relates to the job description. Be brief but specific; your résumé contains details. Refer the reader to your enclosed résumé.

Closing paragraph: Have an appropriate closing to pave the way for an interview and indicate date and times of availability. A telephone number is useful. If you cannot be reached during the day, give a number for messages. Or you might also indicate a time and date in which *you* will call to check about making an appointment.

Sincerely,

Signature
Name typed

Enc. (probably your résumé)

Exhibit 14.3 Sample Letter of Resignation

240 North Street
San Diego, CA 00000
Date

Carol Winter, RN, MSN
Vice President of Nursing
West Central Hospital
20 California Avenue
San Diego, CA 00000

Dear Ms. Winter:

I will be relocating to Phoenix, Arizona, in May and have accepted a position there at General Hospital as head nurse of the pediatric unit. Therefore, I wish to resign effective April 19, 2005.

Being at West Central Hospital has been a very satisfying personal and professional experience. The atmosphere is one in which a nurse can grow, and I appreciate the support given by the staff of 4B and the head nurse, Melanie Jones. She has especially helped me to develop my managerial skills and encouraged me to take advantage of the hospital's tuition reimbursement. I expect to finish my degree in Phoenix. I am proud to have been a part of a group of clinicians and managers who are committed to compassionate, competent patient care.

If there is anything I can do to help in the transition, I will be happy to do so.

Sincerely,

(Signature)
Alan Collins, RN

cc: Melanie Jones
    Head Nurse 4B

In doing business correspondence, it is always advisable to address a person exactly as the name appears on her or his own letters. The full title and position should be used, no matter how long they may be. It is better to place the lengthy name of a position on the line below the addressee's name, and break up a long address, in the interest of a neat appearance, remembering to indent continuation lines.

It is always best to address your correspondent by name. If you are within reasonable telephoning distance, call and get the correct name, credentials, and title from the person's secretary, telephone operator, or other staff. However, if the name of the person to whom you are writing to inquire about a position is not known, the letter may be addressed to the recruiter, the director, or supervisor of the appropriate division, for example, "Director of the Department of Nursing." The salutation could then be "Dear Director," or "Dear Sir or Madam." Using "Dear Sir" or "Dear Madam" alone may be incorrect, since you don't know whether the recipient is male or female. The inside address and the envelope address should be identical. People are sensitive about their names and titles; be accurate. Again, a little extra effort is worthwhile and may pay off in the favorable impression you make: get the correct name and title. If you've done the necessary research about the institution in which you are interested, this kind of information is available. The Internet is another valuable source.

There is no agreement as to whether or not it is correct to give a title before the name in an address in the heading and on the envelope—or in the form of initials after the name—for example, "Dr. Constance E. Wright" rather than "Constance E. Wright, EdD." Both forms seem to be used. In a signature, however, it is preferable to place the degree initials after the name of the signer of the letter. Never use both the title and the initials in an address; "Dr. Constance E. Wright, EdD" or Ms. Mary Jones RN are incorrect.

It is quite suitable, and even desirable, for a (licensed) nurse to use "RN" after his or her name, particularly in professional correspondence. Many nurses with doctorates place after their names RN PhD or EdD RN to clarify that they are nurses as well as holders of a doctorate. They should be addressed as "Dear Dr. Whatever."

A professional or businesswoman (if married) usually does not use her husband's name at all in connection with her work. Probably most business or professional women without a doctorate prefer to be addressed as "Ms." in correspondence. However, she may use the title "Mrs." to identify herself as a person who is, or has been, married if she desires. "Mrs." goes in parentheses before her typed name under her signature. "Ms." or "Mr." are not used at this point in a letter as a rule.

CONTENT AND TONE

The information included in a business letter should be presented with great care, giving all pertinent data but avoiding unnecessary details. It is often helpful to outline, draft, and edit a business letter, just as you would a term paper. This requires you to think it through from beginning to end in order to ensure completeness and accuracy. It is also helpful to tailor it to fit a well-spaced single page, if possible, or two at the most.

Your writing style is your own, but how you word your message may be part of what you are judged on. The tone of a business letter has considerable influence on the impression it makes and the attention it receives. It is probably better to lean toward formality rather than informality. Friendliness without undue familiarity, cordiality without overenthusiasm, sincerity, frankness, and obvious respect for the person to whom the letter is addressed set the most appropriate tone for correspondence about a position in nursing. Although there are those who suggest very unusual dramatic, or "different" formats, the reality is that they may backfire.

If you feel that you need more information before seriously considering a position (for instance, whether tuition reimbursement is a benefit or a particular specialty area has an opening), you can indicate your interest in a letter beforehand, simply asking for the information, or ask directly within the same application letter. A courteous telephone call to the recruiter might take care of such questions more simply and avoid wasting time. The kind of response you get in terms of courtesy, promptness, and general tone will tell you a lot about the prospective employer.

If you decide not to apply for the position after all, or not to follow through with an interview, it is courteous to inform the person with whom you have corresponded. Specific reasons need be given (briefly) only if such a decision is made after first accepting the position. This is not only courteous but advisable, because you may wish to join that staff at another time or may have other contacts.

APPLICATIONS

Applications are not just routine red tape. Whether or not a résumé is requested or submitted, the formal application, which is developed to give the employing agency the information it wants, can be critical in determining who is finally hired. Even if the information repeats information offered in the résumé, it should be entered. It is usually acceptable to attach the résumé or a separate sheet if there is not adequate space to give complete information. It is a good idea to read the application first so that the information is put in the correct place. Neatness is essential. Erasures, misspellings, and wrinkled forms leave a poor impression. Abbreviations, except for state names and dates, or other standard abbreviations, should not be used as a rule.

If the form must be completed away from home, think ahead and bring anticipated data—Social Security and registration numbers, places, dates, and names. Although occupational counselors say that it is not necessary to give all the information requested (such as arrests, health, or race, some of which are illegal to request), it is probably not wise to leave big gaps in your work history without explanation. (See Chapters 9 and 15 regarding federal legislation on employment rights.)

PERSONAL INTERVIEW

An interview may be the deciding factor in getting a job. Anyone who has an appointment for a personal interview should be prepared for it physically, mentally, emotionally, and psychologically. The degree of preparation will depend on the purpose of the interview and what has preceded it. Assuming that you have written to a prospective employer about a position and an interview has been arranged, preparation might include the following:

○ *Physical preparation.* Be rested, alert, and in good health. Dress suitably for the job, but wear something in which you feel at ease. It is important to be well groomed. First appearances are important, and given a choice, no one selects a sloppy or overdressed person in preference to someone who is neat and appropriately dressed. Have enough money with you to meet all anticipated expenses. If you are to be reimbursed by the employing agency, keep an itemized record of expenses for submission later. Get accurate directions to the interview site. Arrive at your destination well ahead of time, but do not go to the human resource department or your prospective employer's office earlier than five minutes before the designated time.

○ *Mental preparation.* Read some articles about interviews and think about how you would answer potential questions. Review all information and previous communications about the position. Showing that you know about the hospital or agency is desirable and impressive. Make certain that you know the exact name or names of the persons you expect to meet and can pronounce them properly. (You can always ask the secretary.) Decide what additional information you want to obtain during the interview. Consider how you will phrase your leading questions, making notes if necessary. Think ahead about what you might need. Have your list of references with correct addresses typed on a separate sheet. You might also bring a copy of your transcript, although the interviewer may choose to send for it. Carry a small notebook or card on which you have listed data that you may need during the interview. If you bring an application form with you, place it in a fresh envelope, which you leave unsealed. Have it ready to hand to the interviewer when she or he asks for it; otherwise, offer it at an appropriate time. Some interviewers suggest that you bring another copy of your résumé, it *can* be lost.

○ *Emotional and psychological preparation.* If you have any worries or fears in connection with the interview, try to overcome them by thinking calmly and objectively about what is likely to take place. (Role playing an interview with a colleague who may have been through the experience can be helpful.) Be ready to adjust to whatever situation may develop during the interview. For example, you may expect to have an extended conversation with at least a nurse manager and find when you arrive that a personnel officer who is not a nurse will interview you. She or he may interview you in a very few minutes and in what seems to be an impersonal way. You may have visualized the job setting as quite different.

Accept things as you find them, reserving the privilege of making a decision after consideration of the total job situation. If a stimulating challenge is inherent in the position, you will sense it during the interview, or you may have reason to believe that it will develop. However, you cannot demand a challenge, and if one is "created" for you spontaneously by the interviewer, regard the promise with some reservations; an employment situation rarely adjusts to the new employee.

DURING THE INTERVIEW

Usually the interviewer will take the initiative in starting the conference and closing it. You should follow that lead courteously and attentively. Shake hands firmly. Be prepared to give a brief overview of your experiences and interests, if asked. At some point, you will be asked if you have any questions, and you should be prepared to request additional information if you would like to have it. Should the interviewer appear to be about to close the conference without giving you this opportunity, say, "May I ask a question, please?" It is perfectly acceptable to ask, before the interview is over, about salary, fringe benefits, and other conditions of employment if a contract or explanatory paper has not been given to you. In fact, it would be foolish to appear indifferent. A contract is desirable, but if that is not the accepted procedure, it is important to understand what is involved in the job. The job description should be accessible in writing, and it is best that you have a copy. You should know if the staff is unionized, which often affects the job description.

Most interviewers agree that an outgoing candidate who volunteers appropriate information is likeable. On the other hand, many use the technique of selective silence, which is anxiety-provoking to most people, to see what the interviewee will say or do. A good interviewer will try to make you comfortable, in part to relax you into self-revelation; most do not favor aggressive methods. Good eye-contact is fine, but don't stare. Be sensitive to the interviewer's being uninterested in a certain response; maybe it's too lengthy. Don't interrupt. Don't smoke. Don't mumble. Watch your body language (and the interviewer's). It can denote indifference, irritation, or even nervousness. Be enthusiastic but don't gush.[6]

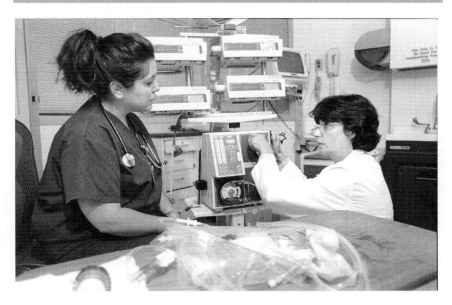

The extent and nature of the orientation period are important factors in considering a new job. (*Courtesy of Robert Wood Johnson University Hospital, New Brunswick, New Jersey*)

Some questions that are likely to be asked in an average interview are:[7]

- What position interests you most? (Be specific.)
- Why do you want to work here? (Know something positive.)
- What are your strengths and weaknesses? (Play up your strengths, and, although you should be honest, play down your weaknesses. Give examples, perhaps of what people say about you.)
- What sets you apart from all the other candidates who could do this job? (Show your decision-making and judgment skills.)
- What can you do for us? (Tell about your special qualities and experience.)
- Tell me about yourself. (Keep it short; don't give more information than necessary to reassure the interviewer that you are suitable for the job physically, mentally, and in terms of preparation. Stress your reliability.)
- What did you like most and least in school or on your last job? (Be honest, but don't list a series of gripes.)
- How would you describe your ideal job? (Take the opportunity to do so, but let the interviewer know that you know that nothing's perfect.)

○   Where do you think you'll be five years from now? (Emphasize goals that show your interest in growing professionally.)
○   Do you have any questions? (Be prepared.)

In a survey of directors of nursing service in various settings, the characteristics valued most highly in rating a nursing job applicant were punctuality, completion of the application prior to the interview, neatness and completeness of the application, well-groomed personal appearance, and questions asked. As other qualities that might be more important were bypassed, this list may show how important the external aspects of an interview can be.

When the interview is over, thank the interviewer, shake hands, and leave promptly. A tour of the facility may be offered before or after the interview. This gives you a chance to observe working conditions, ask questions, and, sometimes, note interpersonal relationships. You may or may not have been offered the position. If it was offered to you, it is usually well to delay your decision for at least a day or two until you have had time to think the matter over carefully from every practical point of view. Perhaps you will want more information, in which case you may write a letter, send a fax, a telegram, mailgram, or e-mail or make a phone call to your prospective employer. It is always courteous to send a thank-you letter.

FOLLOW-UP COMMUNICATIONS

Sometimes during the procedure of acquiring a position, you may have occasion to discuss some aspect of it over the telephone with the prospective employer. If you make the call, be brief, courteous, and to the point, with notes handy, if needed. It may be helpful to make notations on the conversation. It is sensible to listen carefully and not interrupt. If you receive a call and are unprepared for it, be courteous but cautious and, perhaps, ask for time to think over the proposal—or whatever may have been the purpose of the call.

Agreements about a position made over the phone should be confirmed promptly in writing. If it's your place to do so, you might say, while speaking with the person, "I'll send you a confirming letter tomorrow." If it's the responsibility of the other person to confirm an agreement but she or he doesn't mention it, ask, "May I have a letter of confirmation, please?"

After any interview or conversation, make notes about what happened for future use and reference. If any business arrangements are made by fax, e-mail, or letter, file this information with other related correspondence.

For positions sought through a registry or employment agency, the same courteous, thorough, and businesslike procedures used when dealing directly with a prospective employer are appropriate. A brief thank-you note or e-mail message for help received shows consideration of the agency's efforts on your behalf.

In her *Career Guide*, Eagles suggests that, at the conclusion of this process of fact finding, interviewing, and the back and forth that characterizes the job-seeking and searching process, there are some very basic questions that you must be able to answer for yourself:[8]

- What does this job require?
- Are my skills a "good match" for this job?
- Are these the kind of people that I would enjoy working with?
- What sets me apart from all the others who can do this job, and how can I convey this to those who matter, and who matters?
- How can I persuade you to hire me, and pay me the salary I want?

EVALUATION

What if you didn't get the job you wanted? There may simply have been someone better suited or better qualified. Still, it's helpful to review the experience in order to refine your interview skills. Were you prepared? Did you present yourself as someone sensitive to the employer's goals? Did you make known your personal strengths and objectives? Did you look your best? Sometimes discussing what happened with another person also gives you a different perspective, and there's no reason why you can't reapply another time.

CHANGING POSITIONS

It is generally expected that nurses should remain in any permanent position they accept for at least a year. Certainly, this is not too long—except in the most unusual circumstances—for you to adjust to the employment situation and find a place on the staff in which to use your ability and talents to their fullest. Furthermore, persons who change jobs too frequently may find that some employers are reluctant to hire them. However, should it be desirable or necessary to change positions, a number of points might be observed. Consider your employer and co-workers as well as yourself, and leave under friendly and constructive circumstances.

Depending on the reasons for leaving and how eager you are to make a change, some writers suggest that before you definitely accept a new position, the present employer should be informed about your desire to leave and why. It may be that, depending on the employer's concept of your value to the institution, a new, more desirable position might be offered. However, it is important to give reasonable notice of your intention to resign. If there is a contract, the length of the notice will probably be stipulated. Two weeks to a month is the usual period, depending principally on the position held and the anticipated difficulty in hiring a replacement. Do not tell anyone else before you tell your immediate superior, privately and courteously.

Try to finish any major projects you have started; arrange in good order the equipment and materials your successor will inherit; and prepare memos and helpful guides to assist the nurse who will assume your duties. Sometimes, you will be asked to help that person before you leave. Check out employment policies about benefits, including accrued vacation or sick leave.

A letter of resignation should state simply and briefly, but in a professional manner, your intention of leaving, the date on which the resignation will become effective, and the reasons for making the change. A sincere comment or two about the satisfactions experienced in the position and regrets at leaving will close the letter graciously. There should be no hint of animosity or resentment, because this will serve no constructive purpose and may boomerang. (See Exhibit 14.3.)

Don't burn your bridges. You may want to come back to that place at another time. At the least, you may need a reference, and if you appear vindictive or childish, the employer is unlikely to give you an enthusiastic reference, even if you did your job satisfactorily. In these days of litigation, nothing may be written specifically, but employers are adept at reading between the lines of a bland reference. The administrative network (via a personal phone call) may paint you as an undesirable employee, and you'll never know.

Terminal interviews are considered good administrative practice, and are sometimes used for a final performance evaluation and/or a means to determine the reasons for resignation. There is some question of how open employees are about discussing their resignation (unless the reason is illness, necessary relocation, and so on), perhaps because of fear of reprisal in references or even a simple desire to avoid unpleasantness. This is a decision you must make in each situation.

What if you're fired? The most common reasons for being fired are poor job performance, chronic tardiness, excessive absenteeism, or inappropriate behavior. Usually you are given a warning about any of these problems, and if you haven't done anything about correcting your problem (assuming that the charge is justified), you had better take a good look at yourself. Those kinds of uncorrected problems may make your future prospects look dim.

Whether or not you're caught by surprise when you're told, try to maintain your composure. If you can't pull your thoughts together, request another interview to ask questions and find out about the termination procedure. If you *are* at fault, make a clean, fast break. If you are *not* at fault, try to clarify the situation to avoid negative references. You may choose to contest the action and file a grievance, particularly if you are part of a union. However, weigh whether it's worth it. You may need to clear your name, but it might be unpleasant or impossible to stay in that setting and work productively.

In a period of downsizing in health care institutions, it will become more frequent to be laid off. Fewer patients and reduced budgets are major factors, especially as institutions are bought by for-profit chains or are consolidated or merged with others. Some close altogether.

If you're called into your manager's office and told that your position is being eliminated, don't take it personally, and even more important, don't get angry and lash out at the manager; the decision is often made at a higher level and quite impersonally. Again it's a matter of not burning bridges. Clear out your locker or office, turn in your key and name-tag, if that's appropriate, and take your personal belongings and files. Don't try to get even by deleting important computer documents or otherwise undermining projects. Don't discuss severance pay or other details at this point.

After you've had time to think, make notes about the original meeting. If possible, review your employment benefit manual and union contract. Then make an appointment with someone in the human resources department to go over your benefits. These might include retirement benefits, remaining vacation and sick-leave pay, and health insurance. Federal legislation concerning health benefits gives you the right to pay to remain insured for up to 36 months after you've been laid off, but you need the correct forms and information. If you are eligible for outplacement, human resources personnel can help with techniques of job hunting and contacts. Negotiate for severance pay, asking for twice as much as you expect to get (usually one week per year of service). If this is not forthcoming, try for additional vacation or sick-leave payout, outplacement services, or job counseling. At the same time, check on who will provide reference information and what will be said.

Immediately, start planning your job hunt, but also apply for unemployment benefits—that process takes a while. Many of the same suggestions presented earlier about initiating a job search apply here. It's good if you have a "nest egg," so that you are not immediately pressed financially and don't feel desperate enough to take the first offer. Don't let the lay-off period become a time to simply "sleep-in" or avoid social gatherings, professional meetings, and colleagues. All these can be useful in your job search. Use your support system of family and friends to help you psychologically and practically. Keep a positive attitude about yourself. Opportunities will come!

When leaving a job is not your choice, it sometimes helps to talk with a supportive person, to ventilate and analyze what happened. Choose someone you can trust but who can help you see things as objectively as possible. Then it's time to get back to career planning. Perhaps you should look at the possibility of further education or training in a different kind of nursing. If not, be sensible about conserving your economic resources until you find another job. Try to select the next job, keeping in mind what made you unhappy in the last one and, of course, correcting those problems that got you fired, if that occurred. You need not volunteer to your prospective employer that you were fired, but if asked, don't lie. Just say that you were asked to leave and why. Don't criticize your previous employer and try to be as positive as possible about your last job. Your honesty and determination to do well could be a plus.

It's doubtful that you will stay in the same institution throughout your career. This is a very mobile society, and there are many job opportunities for nurses throughout the country (and world). Without closing the doors to unexpected opportunities, beginning early to think in terms of a career will make nursing more satisfying and interesting in the long run.

KEY POINTS

1. Assessing yourself in terms of abilities, interests, characteristics, and values is a good idea before starting a job hunt.
2. A professional résumé and appropriate letters of application are factors in being selected for a job.
3. Some of the best sources of information about the job market are advertisements in both electronic and print media, personal contacts, job fairs, and recruiters.
4. In interviewing for a job, it is important to be prepared physically and psychologically and to know, or get, as much information as possible about the position and environment.
5. Consideration of its effect on future employment is an important factor in how a job should be terminated.

STUDY QUESTIONS

1. Develop a hypothetical search for your preferred first job: review sources of advertising, write an introductory letter, develop a résumé, and prepare questions for your interview.

2. The varied roles and specialties available in nursing offer something to suit every personality. Characterize the qualities which one job demands as opposed to another.

3. Interview nurses in various practice settings. Find out what prepared them for their positions, and what are the satisfactions and dissatisfactions of their work on a day-to-day basis.

4. Use the Internet to find out about a job you like, and the environment within which it exists.

REFERENCES

1. Anderson C, Bednash G. Nursing as a launching pad for other options—A variety of nurses' paths to other roles. In Andersen C (Ed.): *Nursing Student to Nursing Leader.* Albany, NY: Delmar, 1999, pp 228–238.
2. Feery B, Tierney C. Résumés: The recruiter's perspective. *Nursing Spectrum 2003* Career Fitness Guide, pp 18–21.
3. Ibid.
4. Mason D. No shortage of opportunities. Career Guide: *Am J Nurs*, January 2002, p 13.
5. Barba S. Help from your friends. *Nursing Spectrum 2003* Career Fitness Guide, p 88.
6. Restifo V. Interviewing for career advancement. *Nursing Spectrum 2003* Career Fitness Guide, pp 32–35.
7. Eagles Z. *The Nurses' Career Guide.* San Luis Obispo, CA: Sovereignty, 1997, pp 144–147.
8. Ibid.

Updates can be found at

    http://www.JoelTheNursingExperience.com

Chapter 15

Career Management

OBJECTIVES

After you have studied this chapter you will be able to:

1. Anticipate the socialization process through which you may go in moving from the role of student to graduate nurse.
2. Define biculturalism.
3. List five symptoms of burnout.
4. Identify four things you can do to combat burnout.
5. Explain what strategies you can use to adjust successfully to the work world.
6. Discuss two workplace rights that are guaranteed to employees by the law.
7. Describe the major activities available to maintain your practice competence.
8. List funding sources for continuing your formal education.
9. Identify ways in which you can enhance your professional and personal lives as a nurse.
10. Develop your own career map even if there are major areas of uncertainty.

RESOCIALIZATION

Eventually, graduation *does* come, and for most nurses, the next step, with hardly a break, is that first nursing job. What can you expect?

The student has spent two to four years being socialized into nursing in the education setting; now resocialization into the work world is necessary. Socialization into a new role is not usually a conscious process, although both the individual being socialized and those doing the socializing consciously make certain efforts.

In reality, the educational experience for any field of work will differ from the expectations when you are being compensated for your services. For the most part, students are not integral to the systems of care, look to faculty for their cues and rewards, and are allowed to falter somewhat in their practice. Further, the socialization–resocialization phenomenon (student to full-fledged professional) is often presented as a one-time occurrence. In fact, given today's rapidly changing health care system with the movement from hospitals into community practice, and new markets for health services, nurses will be confronted with resocialization many times during their career life.

All of these circumstances caution that the only way to accomplish a comfortable transition time after time after time is to know yourself and the dynamics of a situation. There is nothing so unexpected or mystical about role transition and socialization. All of us have been through the process at least once (but really many times) as we took on the role of a participating member of society.

Role is an abstract idea that can be assumed only through the presence of certain cues allowing you to infer its presence. A role is a constellation of rights and responsibilities that characterize a social position. Since the individual role occupant is embedded in a social structure, the role behaviors are derived from the expectations of both the individual and the social systems with which that individual interfaces. Socialization is the process by which an individual acquires the behaviors necessary for acceptance by these interfacing groups or systems. This is accomplished through a reciprocal process of role shaping and role taking, with the eventual incorporation of the behaviors within one's self as follows:[1]

- *Step 1.* Interaction with primary groups who mirror the expected behaviors (exposure).
- *Step 2.* Development of an interpersonal attachment with significant others from that group (identification).
- *Step 3.* Clarity on expectations; covert messages are made overt (empathy).
- *Step 4.* Negotiations to resolve differences between the ideal and the real, and determine how much freedom there is to modify the role to personal preference (role shaping).
- *Step 5.* Continuing support to allow the new behaviors to become established (role taking).

Successful role transition is greatly enhanced where there is a good feeling (chemistry) between you and your group of peers (staff nurses). This alerts you to the need to meet the people you will be working with on a day-to-day basis when applying for a position. The best of organizations go further, providing a preceptorship or "buddy" arrangement with someone who is senior in the staff nurse role. Make sure you ask questions until you fully understand what is expected of you, and be cautious in bending the rules until you have established yourself. However, make inquiries that help predict how much personal role shaping will be possible. Some cues of an organization that allows little flexibility in role development are:

- Highly precise and detailed job descriptions.
- Management by memo in situations where personal communication would have sufficed.
- Guarded interdisciplinary boundaries that hamper smooth operation.
- A hierarchy that is an obstacle as opposed to facilitating your work.
- Policies, procedures, and documentation systems that are cumbersome and even inconsistent with current practice.
- Absence of staff nurse autonomy in caring for patients.
- Verbalized discontent from staff, but no evidence of any attempt to change things.
- High turnover rate.

Successful role transition includes identifying with the right group, interpreting their expectations accurately, negotiating to the extent that is possible while maintaining your unique identity, and merging with the group on terms that are mutually acceptable. This is the best of worlds. In less perfect situations, you have parties that refuse to tolerate any variance; individuals who are unable to "read" the expectations accurately or refuse to become fully involved.

DEALING WITH REALITY SHOCK

For all but a few graduates, the first job is as an employee in some bureaucratic setting, the antithesis of professionalism. For instance, a bureaucracy has specialized roles and tasks; professionals have specialized competence with an intellectual component. The bureaucracy is organized into a hierarchical authority structure; professionals expect extensive autonomy in exercising their special competence. The bureaucracy's orientation is toward rational, efficient implementation of specific goals and tends toward impersonality; professionals have influence and responsibility in the use of their specialized competence and make decisions governed by internalized standards. On these differences alone, and there are others, professionals in a bureaucracy find themselves in conflict.

Some years ago, Kramer identified the problems of new graduates in resolving their role in a bureaucratic–professional conflict and called it *reality shock*, "the specific shock-like reactions of new workers when they find themselves in a work situation for which they have spent several years preparing and for which they thought they were going to be prepared, and then suddenly find that they are not."[2] Reality shock is different from, but related to, both culture shock and future shock.

Thus, when the new nurse, who has been *in* the work setting but not of it, embarks on the first professional work experience, there is not an easy adaptation of school-learned attitudes and behaviors, but the necessity for an entirely new socialization. Kramer has described this process, which is still relevant:[3]

- *Skills and routine mastery.* The expectations are those of the employment setting. A major value is competent, efficient delivery of procedures and techniques to clients, not necessarily including psychological support. New graduates immediately concentrate on skill and routine mastery.
- *Social integration.* This involves getting along with the group and being taught by them how to work and behave: the "backstage" reality behaviors. New graduates who continue to focus on routine mastery may not be seen as competent peers. Those who try to incorporate some of the professional concepts of the educational setting and adhere to those values may alienate the group.
- *Moral outrage.* Given the differences between what was taught and what is identified and labeled, new graduates feel angry and betrayed by both their teachers and their employers. They were not told how it would be, and they are not allowed to practice as they were taught.
- *Conflict resolution.* The graduates may and do change their behavior but maintain their values; change both values and behaviors to match the work setting; change neither values nor behavior; or work out a relationship that allows them to keep their values but begin to integrate them into this new setting.

The individuals who make the first choice in conflict resolution have selected what is called behavioral capitulation. They may be the group with potential for making change, but they simply slide into the bureaucratic mold, or more likely they withdraw from nursing practice altogether. Those who choose bureaucracy (value capitulation) may either become "rutters" (staying in a rut), with an "it's a job" attitude, or they may eventually reject the values of both. Others become organization men and women, who move rapidly into the administrative ranks and totally absorb the bureaucratic values. They are those who will change neither values nor behavior, what might be called "going it alone." They either seek to practice where their professional values are accepted or try the "academic lateral arabesque" (also used by the first group), going on to advanced education with the hope of new horizons or escape. The most desirable choice, says Kramer, is the last, which she calls *biculturalism*.

It has been documented that new graduates do indeed go through variations of the socialization process described. That there has been little change in the adjustment process for decades can be seen by reviewing journals in the interim and by the nomadic patterns of nursing that must reflect deep-seated job dissatisfaction. Turnover and absenteeism are signs of boredom, lack of involvement, and apathy.

Why is this still happening? Some say that the gap in communication between educators and nursing service administrators is part of the problem; no matter how fine the students' education is, not enough schools have prepared students for evolving needs such as specialization. Educators answer that in no other professional field is the new practitioner expected to be a finished product; all have periods of training and support. In fact, the attitude of the administration is too often echoed by the staff, who may be critical, not helpful, and do not provide the kinds of role models new graduates need. Not all behave in this way, of course, and seasoned nurses talk about how their first job was horrible or great, often depending on the kind of support they got.

Workplace enrichment programs can greatly enhance the retention of nurses. This has been proven with each shortage cycle. Enrichments most commonly take the form of strategies to professionalize the workplace, and presumably decrease the bureaucratic–professional conflict:

- Clinical ladders to recognize competence in direct care positions
- Peer review
- Shared governance and participatory management
- Increased practice autonomy
- Decentralization of operations
- Integrated documentation systems

The realities of the workplace, albeit generally a bureaucracy, could certainly be softened if faculty were to bring more of these insights to their students, or if students had more chances for "rehearsal."

The following deserve consideration:

- A synthesis semester at the end of the educational experience that incorporates, as far as legally possible, all the ingredients of full-time employment.
- Work-study programs that alternate semesters with work placements in your anticipated field.
- A curriculum that progresses toward more independence and personal accountability with students and faculty moving to a collegial relationship, as opposed to superiors and subordinates.
- Service–education partnerships with faculty teaching students on their own panels of patients.
- Summer externships, and new graduate internships or residencies.
- Patient areas exclusively dedicated to the clinical learning needs of students.
- Assignment of each student to a staff nurse.
- Preceptor or "buddy" systems involving agency staff.
- An experience with interdisciplinary or at least multidisciplinary education.

STRESS AND STRAIN: THE PERSISTING OCCUPATIONAL HAZARD

Stress and strain are synonymous with nursing, stress being the factors external to you and strain being those internal feelings of frustration and tension. Sometimes stress creates strain. Some individuals have the capacity to tolerate stressful conditions, putting them in perspective. In other instances strain is internally triggered and the search for external blame is fruitless. There are endless experts who can tell you how to deal with these frustrations and tensions. From Selye,[4] the father of the concept of stress, to Peplau,[5] the pioneer of psychiatric nursing, to Kobasa,[6] who introduced the descriptor of "hardiness" to explain why some people rise above it all, interpretations vary. There is little predictability about who will respond negatively to stressful situations, but group cohesiveness or interpersonal support seem to have a positive effect. Your best protection against stress and strain is to be alert to those situations which usually hold jeopardy:

- A lack of clarity of your responsibilities and reporting relationships.
- A poor fit between your ability, attitudes, or values and the expectations of your employer or co-workers.

- Contradictory expectations of what your job responsibilities are.
- Being caught in a situation where you are underloaded or overloaded.
- Feelings of being under- or overqualified for a position.

The stress and strain that come with most of the service occupations can lead to codependency or burnout. In codependency, a person controls through the assurance that he or she is needed, and works to keep things that way. "Unable to determine who owns a problem, they become angry and intolerant. The natural impulse to feel for their patients and occasionally bring home their frustrations is played out with exaggeration, and eventually rejected. Where once they felt too much, they now feel too little in defense of their ego. The result is poor judgment, insensitivity and burnout."[7] The codependent personality is particularly at high risk for burnout and the severe loss of self-esteem as one's clinical competence is questioned.

There is no one prescription for coming to terms with an unmanageable personal or professional life. The problems are relative to the personality of the afflicted, and solutions must be individualized. "The ultimate goal is to establish control and identity that is driven by internal strength" rather than be captive to the volatility of the environment. Given that your best investment is in self-care, consider:[8]

- Learning to use distance therapeutically. Allow people to fail and learn from their own mistakes. Find a comfortable and private place to retreat when you are stressed. If you cannot physically distance yourself, try meditation techniques.
- Decide who owns a problem. If you don't own it, you have no obligation to fix it, especially if it requires self-sacrifice.
- Examine the quality of the peer support you give and get, and correct the situation if needed. Sometimes support systems become habits as opposed to helps.
- Invest in upgrading yourself. Expose yourself to new experiences; learn new skills. Plan your self-care as seriously as you plan your patient care.
- Consciously schedule routine tasks, and those requiring physical exertion, as a break from complex and stressful activities.
- Learn to trust your instincts. Every problem does not have a rational and logical solution. Sometimes think in terms of what could be the worst consequence.
- Identify one person who would be willing to serve as your objective sounding board. This may be one way to find out how you come across to people.

- Make contact with your feelings about situations. Feelings are neither good nor bad; they just are.
- Create options for yourself. Identify those circumstances that you need to personally control, those that are just as well controlled for you, and those that you choose to wait out.

THE WORKPLACE: RIGHTS AND HAZARDS

The prevailing theme of this chapter is successful career management through personal control. Aspects of that control are to understand how you successfully establish yourself in your role, and how you deal with stress and strain while protecting a personality that may be vulnerable. An additional dimension of control is to know your rights and responsibilities as an employee—and to confront the hazardous conditions that will affect your work life from start to finish as a nurse. You have protections under the law.

A comprehensive overview of workplace rights would include issues of minimum wage, unemployment and disability, workmen's compensation, family leave, continuing health benefits after termination of employment, discrimination, job safety, pensions, unfair labor practices, and collective bargaining. The growing number of workplace concerns addressed through legislation and the courts has contributed to the general decline in unionization. Unions appeared on the American scene when there were few legal workplace protections.

Given the broad range of issues, the focus here will be on the most common questions:

- Can I be fired without reason?
- Is it possible to refuse an assignment?
- Are there any protections for whistle-blowing?
- What protections do I have against discrimination?
- Do I have a right to withhold information about myself from an employer?
- Are there laws that guarantee fringe benefits including health insurance, pension, and family leave?
- How dangerous is the work of nursing?

CAN I BE FIRED WITHOUT REASON?

Most employment relationships are not protected by any formal contract and are for an indefinite period of time. Such an arrangement is termed *employment-at-will*, and the relationship may be terminated by either the employee or employer at any time, with cause or for no cause at all. A growing number of court decisions in such situations have recognized employee handbooks and a variety of other internal employer-generated documents as having a quasilegal status. Thus, where an at-will dismissal violates one of these policies, the employer could be held liable. Even though you may have nothing at all in writing, an expressed contract takes shape as you discuss the terms and conditions of employment. Above and beyond this presumed contractual protection, a number of states are moving forward to protect at-will employees through legislation.

No employer is justified in an *arbitrary dismissal of an employee*. It is important to note what circumstances will cause an episode of dismissal to be found in favor of the employee if the situation goes to grievance, arbitration, or court. The most common conditions for a successful appeal on the employee's behalf are:

- The charges for the termination are not proved.
- The severity of the consequence is inappropriate to the charge.
- The reason for dismissal is unrelated to job performance.
- Proper or customary disciplinary procedures were not used.

Most dismissals come as a result of growing dissatisfaction between employee and employer, not a single episode. The situation should have produced documentation, and a series of warnings, written notices, attempts to counsel, and so on.

IS IT POSSIBLE TO REFUSE AN ASSIGNMENT?

That is not an idle question today, as we deal with clinical situations that may be contrary to our personal conscience, hazardous, or require our participation in circumstances that are potentially unsafe for patients. This last situation is particularly common with reduced staffing, the substitution of less prepared personnel in order to cut costs, and the perils of floating to services where you do not feel completely at ease or competent.

Nursing administration has the right to assign you where needed (providing you don't have a written contract that says otherwise), but they also have the responsibility of assigning duties appropriately. Courts have considered nurses' rights in such situations. In a 1992 case, *Winkelman v. Beloit Memorial Hospital*, a nurse with experience in pediatrics was ordered to float to a geriatric unit. She refused and was terminated. The court found that the hospital wrongfully discharged the nurse and offered several pertinent comments:[9]

> A nurse is not necessarily qualified or competent to practice in any area of nursing simply because the nurse has graduated from a school of nursing and has passed a licensure exam.... If a particular area is not a nurse's major area of employment, the nurse has a right to refuse assignment to the questionable area. If an employer wants a nurse to rotate to an area that is not the nurse's usual area of assignment, then the employer should provide for the nurse's further education and training to prepare the nurse to work in the area.

In a 1986 case, *Francis v. Memorial General Hospital*, a New Mexico nurse was instructed to float from the intensive care unit to the orthopedics unit. He refused and was suspended for two days. On his return, he informed his supervisor that he would not float if he felt incompetent. He was offered the opportunity of being oriented to all those units he might be required to cover. He declined the offer and was indefinitely suspended. The court found that the hospital was authorized to discharge the nurse, and made the following observations:[10]

> Prior to his discharge, [the nurse] was presented with the opportunity for orientation to floors where he might "float" in the future to overcome his feeling of incompetence. This was done in deference to his ethical scruples, yet [the nurse] refused to find out whether he could ever become comfortable with "floating." Because he declined this deference to his scruples, he cannot complain now that he was fired for following them.

These cases show that you have the right to refuse to *float* if you think you are unqualified and you can request orientation and training if the administration insists that you do. In fact, the Joint Commission on Accreditation of Healthcare Organizations requires facilities to have a systematic plan for *cross-training* to ensure competency. However, if orientation or training is offered and you continue to refuse, you run the risk of termination.

You also run the risk of a lawsuit and of disciplinary action by the state board of nursing. Further, agreeing to float and then presumably practicing at a level lower than your license, let's say as a nurse's aide, is unacceptable. You were hired and expected to adhere to the standard of your job description.

Mandatory overtime is often commingled with this issue, and is becoming an increasingly difficult problem for RNs and health care facilities. Because of inadequate RN staffing, employers have used mandatory overtime to staff facilities often as a cost-saving factor. Nurses are concerned about the health effects of long-term overtime and the quality of care being provided. Organized nursing has been working tirelessly for several years for the enactment of mandatory overtime legislation on both the federal and state levels. This is not a situation that involves the RN alone. By the end of 2003, 11 states had enacted legislation/regulations, and 21 additional states had introduced legislation/regulations to limit the amount of overtime a nurse would be required to work, and prevent employers from penalizing or dismissing those who refuse excess overtime.[11] Clearly, the battle is being waged on a state-by-state basis.

In some workplaces there are labor contracts to prevent inappropriate assignment or compulsory overtime. Others have developed a form that says, in essence, that in the nurse's professional judgment, the current assignment is unsafe and places the patients at risk, but that it will be carried out under protest. The form documents the assignment, number, and condition of patients and number and type of staff. The legality of this process has not yet been tested, and there are some other concerns. If a nurse has stated that an assignment is unsafe and then takes it, she or he is vulnerable in case of a later negligence suit. And, of course, the use of the form can be abused. Conversely, if you refuse an assignment, one of the dangers is being accused of abandoning your patients. Just what that means in any specific case is not clear, but it could result in the loss of your license. You should discuss any assignment that you see as inappropriate with your supervisor to put her or him on notice about your limitations; identify your options (sharing or trading the assignment); and document the situation. In the end, it is your decision, and not an easy one; but it is almost inevitable in many institutions. It's best to think it through ahead of time.

One situation that has been gaining attention is fair treatment for nurses who cannot work on certain days for *religious reasons*. As might be expected, rulings have differed, but in 1985, the U.S. Supreme Court ruled that there was no constitutional right involved; that, in fact, it was unconstitutional for a state to legislate an unqualified right not to work on the Sabbath. From a practical point of view, the nurse may be willing to accept alternatives, such as working on other holidays or on weekend days.

ARE THERE ANY PROTECTIONS FOR WHISTLE-BLOWING?

Whistle-blowing is a moral action of last resort, and "indicative of an ethical failure at the organizational level."[12] Whistle-blowers are employees who disclose information about an organization's violation of a law, rule, or regulation; mismanagement; gross waste of funds; abuse of authority; or a substantial and specific danger to the public health or safety. The range of situations for whistle-blowing is obviously broad, and in many situations the protections are few. It is critical to have your facts straight. Since whistle-blowers must often proceed on good faith, every effort should be made to verify the correctness of the information. By the end of 2003, 19 states had enacted legislation to protect whistle-blowers, and additionally 29 states had introduced such legislation. New Jersey enacted a whistle-blower statute that specifically protects health care workers who speak out about quality of care and patient safety problems. Other states have measures that protect anyone who blows the whistle on health-related issues, regardless of whether that person is a health care worker or not. In Virginia, for example, it is illegal for a nursing facility to retaliate against any person who complains about or provides information on its patient care practices. Laws have been passed by the U.S. Congress to preempt state laws and provide mandatory protection where no state laws apply. Whistle-blower protections are included in the Homeland Security Bill of 2002.[13]

A noteworthy case occurred in 1996. Barry Adams, a registered nurse (RN) working on a subacute care unit in a New England hospital, blew the whistle on unsafe health care practices that he observed in his work setting. Adams became increasingly concerned about the quality, safety, and dignity of patient care as the hospital implemented staffing cuts and cost containment measures. He carefully documented unsafe practices and correlated these with inadequate staffing and a lack of adequate supervision of inexperienced nurses. There was an increased incidence of patient falls, instances where patients were left to lie in their own urine and feces, treatments not being completed, and serious medication errors. These incidents resulted from a substantial increase in the nurses' patient assignments.

For three months, Adams and other nurses followed precisely the process outlined by the organization to communicate concerns to hospital administrators. He soon realized that the administrators were not interested in using the information he provided to correct the situation; in fact, he was harshly criticized for collecting this information. He then decided to proceed with a variation of the traditional saying: "If it's not documented, it's not done" and, instead, adopted the approach: "If it's not done, document it!"

Adams was threatened with the loss of his job and, in spite of previous performance reviews that were excellent, he was eventually fired. He sued and won his case. The hospital appealed and lost again.[14]

The following are some necessary conditions that should be established before one undertakes whistle-blowing, and it seems that Adams met them all:[15]

1. The reason the whistle-blower is blowing the whistle is because he or she sees a grave injustice or wrongdoing occurring in his or her organization that has not been resolved despite using all appropriate channels within the organization.

2. The whistle-blower morally justifies his or her course of action by appeals to ethical theories, principles, or other components of ethics, as well as relevant facts.
3. The whistle-blower thoroughly investigates the situation and is confident that the facts are as she or he understands them.
4. The whistle-blower understands that her or his primary loyalty is to client(s) unless other compelling moral reasons override this loyalty.
5. The whistle-blower ascertains that blowing the whistle most likely will cause more good than harm to client(s); that is, clients will not be retaliated against because of the whistle-blowing.
6. The whistle-blower understands the seriousness of his or her actions and is ready to assume responsibility for them.

WHAT PROTECTIONS DO I HAVE AGAINST DISCRIMINATION?

A host of discriminatory areas could be involved in your workplace relations. Besides the protections for race and ethnicity, gender and age are of particular interest in nursing. The discrimination against male nurses continues, especially in obstetric practice. The U.S. District Court in Arkansas gave the opinion that "The fact that the plaintiff is a health care professional does not eliminate the fact that he is an unelected individual who is intruding on the obstetrical patient's right to privacy. The male nurse's situation is not analogous to that of the male doctor who has been selected by the patient."[16]

There has been significant progress through federal and state laws that protect against *age discrimination* in the workplace. Some laws have no upper limits; others specify protection until a certain age, perhaps 65, 70, or 75. The burden of proof in age discrimination is often difficult, and nurses should be vigilant wherever there is a trend to cut back on the numbers of nurses on staff. A typical case is reported from California where the courts awarded damages to two nurses who sued on the basis of age discrimination. These nurses, 59 and 60, respectively, were 30-year employees of the same hospital. Each had been publicly recognized for the quality of her practice. When a clinical ladder was put in place, they consciously decided to remain at a lower level of the clinical nurse category. After being told that it was mandatory for them to participate in a career advancement program and qualify for a higher status, they were both dismissed on grounds of the inability to demonstrate the competencies for the new level. Both of these nurses are now successfully employed elsewhere.[17] There is fear that these will no longer be isolated cases in nursing. This becomes an especially significant issue with the current "aging" of nurses.

The Americans with Disabilities Act of 1990 extends protection in employment to individuals with HIV/AIDS, and also to people who are regarded to be infected, or in close association with persons with HIV/AIDS. The ANA has assumed the leadership role for over a decade in providing policy direction to nurses and other health care professionals in dealing with HIV/AIDS. Nursing's continuous presence on the health care scene and commitment to comprehensive care created the need for ANA to speak out early and loudly in the course of this pandemic. Issues of testing and disclosure of HIV status are closely linked with discrimination.[18]

> ANA opposes perpetuation of the myth that mandatory testing and mandatory disclosure of the HIV status of patients and/or nurses is a method of preventing the transmission of HIV disease, and therefore does not advocate mandatory testing or mandatory disclosure of HIV status. ANA supports the availability of voluntary anonymous or confidential HIV testing that is conducted with informed consent, and pre and posttest counseling.

In every situation, the nurse's first concern is the protection of the patient. Therefore, the following policy provides direction for the HIV-infected nurse:[19]

> Nurses who know they have a transmissible blood-borne infection should voluntarily avoid exposure-prone invasive procedures that have been epidemiologically linked to HIV or other blood-borne infection transmission. The nurse has a duty to report exposure of a patient to blood-borne infection. Support and protection of the nurse with a seropositive status has been a long-standing position of ANA. The association supports the confidentiality of all information about the HIV-infected nurse.

An additional dimension of the HIV-infected health care provider issue involves *offers of employment.* An employer may require a physical examination, including serology with HIV testing, once a conditional promise of employment has been made, but not before the promise of employment. If the anticipated employee tests HIV positive, the offer may not be withdrawn based on the positive status unless the results indicate that the employee is not qualified to perform the essential job functions. The results must be kept strictly confidential.[20] There can often be a narrow line of interpretation here, and the possibility of frequent abuse. Some states are expanding their civil rights acts to prohibit employers from requiring HIV testing. Again, state-specific inquiries are in order.

Sexual harassment is a form of sex discrimination and a violation under Title VII of the Civil Rights Act of 1964, as affirmed by the U.S. Supreme Court in 1986. The standard for sexual harassment has been made clearer by the Equal Employment Opportunity Commission (EEOC), defining it as unwelcomed sexual advances, requests for sexual favors, and verbal or physical conduct of a sexual nature. These behaviors become harassment when they are a term or condition of employment; a criterion for employment decisions; interfere with the victim's job performance; or create a hostile, intimidating, or offensive work environment. Based on these definitions and circumstances, there are two categories of sexual harassment, "quid pro quo" and "hostile environment." In the former, employment or employment conditions are contingent on submission. In the latter, the harassment creates a situation which is offensive and intimidating or seriously interferes with job performance.

Neither the high profile of this issue in recent years nor laws prohibiting sexual harassment seem to have reduced its prevalence among nurses. The following studies, although some involve small samples, should cause us to stop and consider the true extent of this form of discrimination and the responses that are most effective in confronting this type of abuse. In a survey of critical care nurses, 46 percent of the respondents had been harassed, most frequently by offensive sexual remarks and unwanted physical contact. In 82 percent of the incidents, the harassers were physicians, and 80 percent of the nurses claimed that they had neither been trained to deal with the situation nor did policies exist to facilitate documentation or reporting. A more recent nationwide survey of hospital human resources managers reveals that, despite the actions of the courts and legislation in intervening years, allegations of sexual harassment in hospitals are increasing. Reported statistics for a 4½-year period show that nurses continue to bring the largest number of charges. Most are "hostile environment" allegations, and most formal charges are levied against coworkers. When compared to data gathered in earlier surveys, these statistics show an alarming trend. A significant increase in allegations occurred in 1999 and 2000, corresponding to two U.S. Supreme Court rulings that clarify an employer's responsibility to eliminate this form of sexual discrimination from the workplace.[21]

Besides some disagreement about whether a harassing incident actually occurred, nurses were generally reluctant to report these situations because of a disparity in status and power between the offender and the victim. Where incidents were reported, they were often dismissed or ignored. More assertive action was effective in most cases but not all. The suggested response is to:

1. Confront the harasser and label the behavior.
2. Report the incident and document the incident.
3. Seek support from others.

Most victims who confronted the offender put a stop to the behavior, others found themselves isolated, and still others gained nothing but additional hardship for their courage. Action offers the most hope of change, silence perpetuates the victimization. Sexual harassment policies, procedures, and training to handle these situations effectively are necessary for a safe workplace environment. Much clarity was given to this whole area by the U.S. Supreme Court decision of June 1998. The Court held that an employee who resists a supervisor's advances need not have suffered a tangible job loss or detriment to be able to pursue a lawsuit against an employer. But such a suit cannot succeed if the company has an anti-harassment policy with an effective complaint procedure in place and the employee has unreasonably failed to use it. In other words, the employer is responsible for the development, maintenance, and dissemination of strong and fair policy, and the employee is bound to use due process.[22]

DO I HAVE THE RIGHT TO WITHHOLD INFORMATION ABOUT MYSELF FROM AN EMPLOYER?

The *degree of privacy* guaranteed to an employee is directly related to the information in question and its relation to the employer's interest. The need for information is considered reasonable when it relates to the employee's competence, reliability, and honesty as a worker, or when required by the government. There are both limitations on the right to privacy and on the intrusions into that right. Some examples will help:

- An employer can contact a former employer and check references provided by the employee about work history.
- Employers must notify an employee and provide a report of any investigative report about an employee's credit or financial position.
- An employer can search an employee for theft of company property, but the circumstances of the detection must be reasonable (if not, the employer may be liable for false imprisonment).
- Employees can be expected to take a lie detector test, except in states where employee permission is required.
- Many employers are subject to a law that requires mandatory drug testing of their employees under certain circumstances. (Your state nurses' association will be able to advise you on the laws which apply in your situation.)
- An employer may only require a physical (including HIV testing) after a conditional promise of employment has been made, and the offer of employment may not be withdrawn unless the results interfere with the ability to perform essential job functions.

Each situation is judged on the standard of reasonableness and relevance, and interpretations vary; however, more and more case law and legislation surfaces daily. Many privacy situations are commingled with protection under civil rights and the *Americans with Disabilities Act*. State laws are also at issue here.

ARE THERE LAWS THAT GUARANTEE FRINGE BENEFITS?

Fringe benefits and pension are of growing importance to nurses. Although most employers provide fringe benefit packages, there is no federal or state requirement, with the exception of employer contributions to Social Security, workers compensation, and unemployment insurance. However, there are a number of legislative protections that the employee should be aware of. The *Family Leave Bill* of 1993 requires that employees be allowed a limited period for a new baby, adoption, or to care for a disabled family member. You are assured the right to return to a position comparable with the one you left, and your health benefits must be continued for the period of the leave. In a similar fashion, you are given the right to pay personally for the continuation of your health insurance for up to 36 months after you leave a job. Over the years, pensions have also increased in their protections for the worker. Benefit plans, including pensions, must satisfy nondiscriminatory requirements, treating men and women equitably. Pension benefits have mandatory vesting schedules, guaranteeing 100 percent nonforfeiture of accrued benefits after five years of service, or the option to phase in 100 percent vesting over three to seven years. In short, no benefits or pensions are guaranteed with the exception of Social Security, but where these fringes are provided there are increasing protections.

Ideally there should be a written employment contract that details conditions of employment such as salary, vacation, sick leave, holidays, pension, and duration of the contract. More usually, these things are shared verbally, and may be found written in personnel policies.

HOW DANGEROUS IS THE WORK OF NURSING?

Health care personnel, including nurses, are exposed to the environmental dangers of toxic chemicals, radiation, and infectious agents. Nurses are also at high risk for muscle strain, back injuries, cuts, bruises, and needle punctures. Psychological stress is a constant, due both to the nature of the work and to the demands of the workplace (shift rotation, overtime, and so on). Violence has also become a more frequently occurring workplace situation.

The converse of patient exposure to the *HIV*-infected provider is the risk of infection to the provider from the patient. This risk has been compounded by the significant incidence of *tuberculosis* in HIV-infected

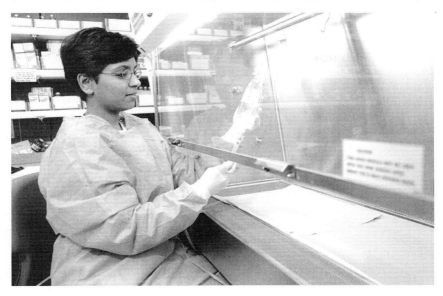

Modern diagnostics and treatment can represent workplace hazards for the nurse. (*Courtesy of Robert Wood Johnson University Hospital, New Brunswick, New Jersey*)

individuals. The cutback in public health funds to allow proper follow-up of TB patients, and the presence of HIV-infected individuals with compromised immune systems and frequent drug therapy, has resulted in the development of *multidrug-resistant strains of TB* (MDR-TB).

MDR-TB and HIV/AIDS have increased our awareness of workplace hazards. Nurses have for the most part accepted the inherent risk that comes with their practice. However, recent years have prompted a new philosophy on the part of health workers that places a high value on their own physical and psychological well-being. This has already been acted out in the U.S. Supreme Court. In an 1998 decision (*Bragdon v. Abbott*, 66 U.S.L.W. 4601), the court held that under the ADA, patients with HIV/AIDS deserved treatment comparable to that given other patients. Here, a dentist refused to treat an HIV/AIDS patient without extraordinary protections, and the court found the precautions discriminatory.

The obligation of the employer is to provide environmental safety, work practice controls, and personal protective equipment to minimize or prevent exposure, and postexposure programs including counseling. The Center for Disease Control and Prevention (CDC) has developed guidelines for the management of health care workers following occupational exposure to HIV. A program would include information, immediate evaluation, prophylactic intervention, counseling, and supportive care. The nurse who seroconverts should be guaranteed workers' compensation and continued health insurance coverage. Workmen's compensation still presents difficulty due to probable under-reporting and the burden of proving occupational transmission. Some occupational groups such as firefighters and coal miners have been successful in legislation that assumes occupational transmission for certain conditions and places the burden of proof on the employer to prove that the condition is not work-related. The important observations for the new employee are what policies exist for postexposure manage-ment and whether adequate precautions are in place to reduce the risk of exposure. MDR-TB prevention requires "a high index of suspicion for TB and early recognition of symptoms which may trigger the need for respiratory precautions. . . . All efforts boil down to containing the infectious agent from becoming airborne."[23] When this is impossible, most facilities are using disposable particulate respirators that fit snugly around the face.

For the protection of both patients and workers against transmission from one another, *universal precautions* should be used when dealing with blood and other body fluids including semen, vaginal secretions, cerebrospinal fluid, and synovial fluid, among others. The precautions include guidelines for handling sharps and laboratory specimens, use of gloves and gowns, hand washing, protective eyewear, disposal of linen, resuscitation procedures, and care of reusable equipment.

Over one million injuries due to *sharp instruments*, including *needle sticks*, occur in the United States annually, exposing health care workers to potentially lethal blood-borne pathogens such as HIV and hepatitis viruses. In October 2000, the U.S. Congress passed legislation providing needle stick protection under the Occupational Safety and Health Administration (OSHA). The Needle Stick Safety and Prevention Act requires the use of safety devices to prevent sharps injuries, input from nonmanagerial workers responsible for direct patient care in selecting work practice controls, and maintenance of a sharps injury log to document details of any sharps injury incident. This issue continues to be addressed on the state level with legislation to strengthen needle stick protections for nurses and other health care providers. Some states have introduced legislation to cover state and municipal employees who are not covered by the Needle Stick Safety and Prevention Act. Other states are pushing for protections that go beyond the federal needle stick law. By the end of 2003, 25 states had enacted legislation to offer needle stick injury prevention, and 15 additional states had introduced such legislation. New Jersey legislation would require workers compen-sation benefits for public safety workers (including nurses) who are exposed to blood and bodily fluids during employment and contract a disease.[24]

Ergonomic hazards, though less dramatic, are job and process design problems that are common and harmful. Examples are improper work methods and inadequate work and rest patterns or repetitive tasks that result in musculoskeletal damage such as back injuries, and carpal tunnel syndrome. Such situations affect up to one-third of all nurses. There is no way to safely lift an average adult patient without assistive devices. Effective measures exist to perform these tasks, but few health care employers have voluntarily implemented them. Although the Occupational Safety and Health Administration (OSHA) has made little progress on this issue, the Veterans Health Administration has begun intensive applied research in the area of ergonomic injury prevention which may promote voluntary implementation of safe patient handling and movement programs.[25] Legislation was introduced in eight states during 2002 to address ergonomic standards designed to reduce repetitive injuries in the workplace; however, the only state enacting policy was Rhode Island. In 2003, four states introduced legislation to impose standards or establish commissions to study the ergonomic problems. In the state of Washington, ergonomic rules that existed were repealed. In 2003, OSHA released guidelines to avoid ergonomic injuries in nursing homes, but these are not regulations, nor are they mandatory. This is addressed in Chapter 10. In 2003, ANA initiated the *Handle with Care* campaign to mount a profession-wide effort to prevent back and other musculoskeletal injuries through greater education and training, and increased use of assistive equipment and patient-handling devices. The campaign also seeks to reshape nursing education, and federal and state ergonomics policy, by highlighting the ways in which technology-oriented safe patient handling benefits patients and the nursing workforce. The slow progress and controversy over policy is obvious.[26]

Violence has been a constant threat to nursing in the workplace. Incidents have rarely been reported because of the poor public image it would create for the health care facility. Currently caught in violent times, the incidence of workplace violence is increasing. Weapons that are easy to obtain, deinstitutionalized chronically mentally ill, substance abuse, and a generally angry underclass all contribute to the increasing danger of violence and assault. In Los Angeles, 25 percent of trauma patients were found to be carrying lethal weapons. Assaults on inpatient units account for 13 percent of incidents in hospitals. In 2000, there were 1.7 million episodes of violence in the workplace and 48 percent involved health care workers.[27] According to ANA, as violence in health care escalates, nurses are the workers at greatest risk because: a high percentage of nurses are women; the nature of the work involves close physical contact, and people under stress; work is in shifts; and the worksite is highly accessible and may not be secure. A comprehensive review of the literature identified the following factors to be associated with assault in the health care workplace:[28]

○ Inexperienced health care workers are at increased risk of assault.
○ The largest number of injuries occur while attempting to contain patient violence.
○ Short staffing and temporary staffing have been associated with increased assaults.
○ Assaults seem to occur during times of high activity and high emotion on patient units.

The presence of policies that show sensitivity to these factors is necessary, as is the establishment of peer assistance and post-assault assistance programs in environments where the incidence of violence is high.[29]

The most rapidly escalating workplace hazard is *latex allergy*. Latex represents a threat not only to health care workers, but also to our patients. There are over 40,000 latex products on the market; the majority are medical devices, and the most common is the latex glove. In 1987, the CDC introduced universal precautions and the use of latex gloves increased dramatically. The allergic response is due to latex protein, which may differ as much as 400 percent product to product. Allergic reactions to latex range from contact dermatitis to fatal anaphylaxis. The National Institute for Occupational Safety and Health (NIOSH) recommends that if latex gloves are worn, they should be powder-free and low allergen. It is possible to decrease the allergen in manufacturing and powder releases dangerous levels of protein-laden dust into the air. A latex-free environment is impossible, but precautions are possible. Nonlatex, low-allergen, and powder-free gloves should be available. Employee policies should provide for latex allergy screening, and education on the subject.[30] The goal is to heighten awareness, understand your personal risk, if any, and provide options for safe practice.

COLLECTIVE BARGAINING: THE PROCESS AND THE ISSUES

Some employment issues are resolved by collective bargaining. The process of collective bargaining, because it is set by law, is similar regardless of who the bargaining agent is, and details can be found in any book on labor relations. In the context of constituent member associations (CMA) of ANA as collective bargaining agents, the following is presented as a brief overview. The same process applies in the outreach to any collective bargaining agent.

○ The nurses (or group of nurses) in an institution, discontented with a situation or conditions, and having exhausted the usual channels for correction or improvement, ask the CMA for assistance.

○ A meeting is held outside the premises of the institution and always on off-duty time. CMA staff and the nurses explore the problems, and the nurses are given advice about reasonable, negotiable issues and how to form a unit; for instance, they are told who can be included in a unit. Administrative nurses are excluded, but the question of supervisors is still being debated in some places.

○ Authorization cards, which designate the CMA to act as the nurses' bargaining representative, must be signed by at least 30 percent (and some unions require more) of the group to be represented. Membership forms are also suggested because the CMA cannot provide service without funds. All collective bargaining activity must be carried out in nonwork areas where the employee is protected from employer interference. (There are a series of National Labor Relations Board [NLRB] rules governing authorization card distribution and solicitation.)

○ If sufficient cards are signed, the CMA notifies the employer that an organizing campaign is in process, calling attention to the fact that the activity is protected. Copies of the notice are distributed to the nurses so that they know they are protected.

○ An informational meeting is held for all nurses and CMA staff.

○ If it is agreed that the CMA will represent the nurses, a bargaining unit is formed and officers are elected.

○ To seek voluntary recognition of the unit by the employer, a majority of the nurses must sign designation cards; this will probably be checked by a mutually accepted third party.

○ If the employer chooses not to recognize the unit, or if the designation is challenged by another union, a series of actions takes place, including an NLRB-conducted election. To petition for election, any union must have authorization cards signed by 30 percent of the nurses in the proposed unit. The election is won or lost by the majority of nurses *voting*. They may vote for a particular union or specify none at all. The NLRB then certifies the winner as the exclusive bargaining agent. If the majority of nurses vote against *any* bargaining agent, the NLRB certifies this as well.

○ Assuming that the CMA wins the election, the CMA representative, at the direction of the unit, attempts to settle the problems and complaints of the nurses by negotiating with administration. There are specific rules about what is negotiable. *Mandatory* subjects include salaries, fringe benefits, and conditions of employment, and both sides must bargain in good faith about these issues. *Voluntary* subjects can be almost anything else that both sides want to discuss, except for *prohibited* or illegal subjects such as requirements for mandatory membership in the union by all employees. It should be remembered that the nurse executive, both through position and under law, is an administrator. Even though the person might be in complete support of the nurses' demands, he or she cannot join them. Quite often the director has previously tried unsuccessfully to help them achieve their goals.

An agreement may or may not be reached, probably with some compromise on both sides. If there is agreement, a contract is voted on and signed outlining agreed-upon conditions and the responsibilities of each group. Contracts are renegotiated after set periods, usually of several years. If no agreement can be reached, the dispute may be referred to binding or nonbinding arbitration by an outside person, or some job action such as picketing or a strike may occur. Picketing may be merely informational, to communicate the issues to the community, or it may be intended to prevent other employees or services from entering the institution. The latter, combined with a strike, is the very last resort, to be used when all other efforts fail. If such action is decided upon, sufficient notice is given to allow planning for maintenance of essential patient services. Even if strikes are successful, there is often a lingering, unpleasant feeling between participants and nonparticipants. However, as ANA members agreed, as they gradually removed no-strike clauses from ANA and CMA policies, the strike is the ultimate weapon that may be necessary when the employer refuses any attempt to resolve issues.

Once a labor contract is in place, there are times when individual nurses are in dispute with the employer. A grievance procedure is generally used to resolve the problem. A grievance may be caused by "an alleged violation of a contract provision, a change in a past practice, or an employer decision that is considered arbitrary, capricious, unreasonable, unfair, or discriminatory." Simple complaints are not considered grievances. If informed discussion does not resolve the issue, a grievance procedure is followed. The steps include (1) written notice of the grievance, with a written response within a set time; (2) if the response is not satisfactory, an appeal to the director of nursing follows; (3) the employee, CMA representative, grievance chairperson, and/or delegate, director of nursing, and director of personnel meet; (4) if no resolution occurs, the final step is arbitration by a neutral third party selected by both parties involved. The technique for carrying out the process involves interpersonal, adversarial, and negotiating skills.

For nurses, the collective bargaining environment has always been covered with landmines. Nurses are predominately professional employees. Employee–employer issues were historically settled internal to the workplace, and health care workers were of little interest to traditional trade unions in the heyday of the labor movement. With increasing government control of unions, the declining industry and manufacturing market, and the 1974 repeal of the Tyding Amendments that since 1947 exempted the nonprofit health care industry from the requirements of the National Labor Relations Act (the right to organize for collective bargaining), health care workers were targeted for organizing. While unionization has declined from a one-time high of over 30 percent of American labor to a current low of less than 15 percent, over 20 percent of health care workers are represented, with a significant increase in the last decade. The largest single constituency in health care is RNs. They have traditionally avoided unionization, but when forced to seek more leverage through collective bargaining, their preferred choice for representation has been the state affiliate of the ANA.

The uniqueness of nurses, the frequent choice of the CMA as their bargaining agent, and their practice patterns create some special problems in labor representation. You are referred to Chapter 30 in *Dimensions of Professional Nursing* (8th edition) for a more extensive discussion. A summary of these areas of concern is included here, but these brief statements should not minimize the seriousness or complexity of these issues:

- Nurses, both employees and managers, have always come together in their professional associations. When those associations offer labor representation, opponents are quick to claim supervisory domination when nurse-managers hold office.
- The RN-only bargaining unit has proved the most appropriate for the registered nurse. The Supreme Court agreed.
- Since nurses carry out many of their functions through other people, for example nursing assistants, there is the risk that they could be considered supervisors (managers) and lose their protected status as employees. A relevant Supreme Court decision of May 1994, involving licensed practical nurses, found them to be managers.
- Human resource techniques that build cooperation between labor and management are critical for our failing industries and health care facilities. In nursing, this observation has given rise to decentralization approaches and shared governance as discussed in Chapter 6. This necessary movement from the traditional

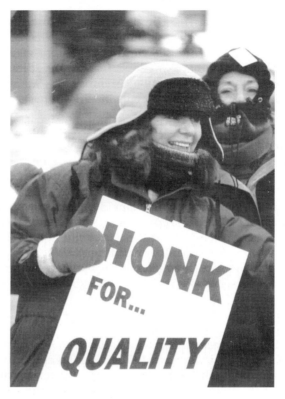

Nurses have been militant and brought their message to the public where quality of care or patient safety is in jeopardy. (*Courtesy of the American Nurses Association*)

adversarial relation in collective bargaining again challenges the employee status of nurses, and their right to unionize.

CAREER MAPPING

You have sought the best educational preparation to enter the field of nursing. You have hopefully done so with the intent of building a career. No field offers such variability or such opportunity to advance. Each decision you make can strategically build toward your long-term goal. Additionally, for the professional there is the obligation to remain current, which is no simple task given the rate at which the science of nursing is expanding.

THE VALUE OF EXPERIENCE

You have already reviewed the process of searching and courting employment in Chapter 14. You have also been counseled to take time for a personal assessment. Identify the route in nursing you would like to take. Given today's complex clinical environment, your competence as a generalist will be short-lived.

The half-life of today's knowledge in the basic sciences is no longer than 18 months in many cases. As an applied science, can nursing hope for too much more? With your first position, you begin to develop competencies in a specialized area of practice. Given even a short time, you are unable to shift comfortably to new populations. For this reason it is important that you have some idea of the area of nursing which offers you the most satisfaction. Seek out a position with that population and resolve to provide the best possible care to those patients, growing through experience and keeping current with a well-planned program of continuing education. It is just as acceptable to have a vision of a lateral move into education, and formal schooling that stretches on for many years, and perhaps many degrees. It is also acceptable to fail, to reconsider, and change courses many times. The only thing that is unacceptable is to have no goals at all.

While you are considering your lateral moves and vertical climbs, pay proper respect to the fact that nursing is a practice discipline. You definitely grow in your ability to care as you minister to patients and as you invest hours and years in your art. Experience is not a myth, but one essential ingredient in clinical sophistication.

CONTINUED COMPETENCE

Process is content in this new millennium. Your educational experience is adequate only if it taught you how to think and where to go to find the information you need. Most of the content you currently hold will be outdated in five years. The most established professions have learned that lesson. Case material in law only provides the substance through which to cultivate analytic skills. The activities that constitute your role will be no more stable than your knowledge. During your career lifetime, the activities that are part of your practice will shift. Some will disappear, and others will be delegated by you to lesser prepared individuals. New role functions currently foreign to you will become part of your day-to-day repertoire. Beyond your own personal security and flexibility to move with the times, you need reliable sources of continuing education, and access to information. Besides what your employer provides on their own behalf to ensure your safety and currency, it is your personal obligation to maintain a curiosity and thirst for better ways to nurse.

The term "continuing education" has been interpreted many ways. Most agree that it includes any learning activity after the basic educational program. Courses of study or programs leading to an academic degree are separated out. The basic and overriding purpose of continuing education in nursing is the maintenance of continued competence so that the care of the patient is safe and effective. Continuing education is provided through your employing agency, or you may choose (or the employer may encourage you) to seek outside programs. The variety of programs is limitless. The secret is to be a discerning consumer and select those which are most immediately valuable to your practice. Continuing education need not be only clinically oriented. You must also remain conversant with current issues in the discipline, and with the thinking of nursing leaders. Employer funding and time off for education is often a workplace benefit. The types of educational experiences that staff are approved to attend are often an indication of how administration views nursing, as a technical or professional field. From another perspective, it provides insights on the staff who will be your peers. The professions have always recognized the fact that learning for practice was lifelong. Florence Nightingale was eloquent on the subject:

> Nursing is a progressive art, in which to stand still is to go back. A woman who thinks to herself, "Now I am a full nurse, a skilled nurse, I have learnt all there is to be learnt"—take my word for it, she does not know what a nurse is, and never will know; she is gone back already. Progress can never end but with a nurse's life.

With continuing education programs proliferating (and getting more expensive), better give some thought to what is worth spending time and money on. One suggested plan for diagnosing your needs is to develop a model of required competencies, assessing your practice in relation to the model, and identifying the gaps between your knowledge and skills and those required. Some of this preliminary testing can be done by taking some of the tests in journals, and by carefully evaluating your own practice and getting feedback from peers and supervisors as well.

Other methods of continued learning, besides formal classes or conferences, are well worth investigating, although, of course, there is often the added value of interaction with other nurses in group activities. Many nursing journals offer monthly self-study programs, and Internet courses are becoming common. These are usually offered by local universities.

Another aspect of maintaining competence is the ability to locate the information you need for your practice, and access those information sources. Your educational program should have prepared you to find the information you need, and impressed on you that you are responsible for the changing standard of practice. In some situations, physicians are being held liable for not conducting literature searches when appropriate; nurses are similarly at risk.

You will find your most updated indexes of the nursing and allied health literature in computerized databases. With the technical aspects of reviewing the literature computerized, searching becomes a highly exciting learning experience, and librarians, health care professionals, and students increasingly conduct computerized literature searches. The databases most commonly used in nursing are the Cumulative Index to Nursing and Allied Health Literature (CINAHL) and MEDLINE. MEDLINE and CINAHL are computerized, and available both on-line or in CD-ROM format.

MEDLINE is provided free by the National Library of Medicine (NLM). MEDLINE is a massive, world-renowned biomedical database. MEDLINE is updated twice a month. Some 360,000 citations from 3500 journals are added to MEDLINE each year. It contains citations as far back as 1966. Its print counterpart is *Index Medicus*. CINAHL is available for a fee. Its on-line version is updated monthly, the CD-ROM every two months. The CINAHL collection started in 1956 and is also available in print form. Both databases contain abstracts of many articles.

The NLM provides access to 40 additional databases which would be of interest to nurses, some are: AIDSLINE (AIDS and related topics), AIDSDRUGS (AIDS drugs in clinical trials), BIOETHICSLINE (ethics and related public policy issues in health care), CANCERLIT (cancer topics), DIRLINE (directory of resources providing information services), HealthSTAR (clinical and nonclinical issues in health care), HISTLINE (history of medicine and related sciences), HSRPROJ (health service research including clinical practice guidelines), POPLINE (family planning, maternal/child health in developing countries, primary health care), SPACELINE (space life sciences), TOXLINE (toxicology), and more. All of these databases are free. The Internet address is http://www.nlm.nih.gov.

FORMAL HIGHER EDUCATION

Besides participating in continuing education programs, you may want to give serious consideration to formal education leading to another degree (or a first one, if you have none). Educational standards for all positions in nursing are growing steadily higher. If you really want to advance professionally to positions of greater scope and challenge, you will need an advanced degree, at least a baccalaureate. The process of obtaining this and higher degrees will not only serve you well professionally, but will also add considerably to the enrichment of your personal life and interests. In fact, these are the reasons given by many nurses who pursue further formal education.

Because baccalaureate programs with a nursing major have not always been available (or affordable) to nurses in a particular geographical area, a number of programs have sprung up offering a degree in nursing or another field, giving credit for the lower-division nursing courses, but offering no upper-division nursing. Evaluate them in relation to your career goals. These programs are *not* usually acceptable for future graduate studies in nursing. You may not be able to enroll in a graduate program without having taken upper-division nursing courses. Some nurses have found it necessary to complete a second baccalaureate program, this time with a nursing major, in order to qualify for graduate study. The master's in nursing has become consistently necessary for advancement in nursing; the exceptions are few. In selecting a baccalaureate program, be sure to select one that is NLN or CCNE accredited.

RNs will find that they receive varying amounts of recognition or credit for their basic nursing courses, but ever more nursing programs are offering some form of educational articulation or challenge opportunities to give full credit for previous knowledge, skill, and ability. The external degree is such a program. There are also a large number of baccalaureate programs that only admit RN students.

Many of the same points apply to graduate education. Consider carefully what you want from a program and prepare yourself for this more competitive admission procedure. Some nurses complete graduate programs in the various sciences or education, with or without any nursing courses. Again, you must consider your specific career goals. Someone with a nursing major may be given preference in a position requiring a graduate degree. Many state boards of nursing require faculty in basic nursing education programs to have a graduate degree with a major in nursing. Or if you are hired now, there is no guarantee that later, when there are more nurses with graduate nursing degrees, you may not be bypassed for promotion or may be required to take a second graduate degree in nursing in order to hold the current position. These are practical considerations presented here for information. You must still make the educational decisions you wish, but with as complete a knowledge of the pros and cons as possible.

Suppose you simply don't want any degree? Or suppose you enroll in an accredited nursing program but then, in time, drop out? That's your decision. There is no reason why you cannot function at an acceptable level of competence, maintaining and improving your knowledge and skill through continuing education, thereby making a valuable contribution to the profession and society. If, however, you withdraw because of disappointment or lack of interest in a particular program, it may well be that the program is not congruent with your philosophy. Consider a second try, taking time to determine whether a program's philosophy, objectives, approaches to teaching, and attitudes are what you want. Some of this information can be obtained from the catalog, the faculty, or adviser interviews, or by informal contact with students or *recent* graduates (programs do change). Sometimes, if some courses may be taken without need for full matriculation, a sampling of courses will prove especially informative.

Sources of Financial Aid

The problem of finances is one of the most common blocks to advanced education for able nurses. Review your financial resources realistically. If you are going to request financial aid, you will need to estimate as accurately as possible your expected income and expenses. Major educational expenses will include tuition, books, educational fees, and perhaps travel. Related personal expenses depend on where and how you live. Economizing may mean enrolling in a community college for the liberal arts and later transferring to a local or state college. Economy should not include enrolling in a poor program. Graduating from a nonaccredited nursing program may create difficulties in advancing to the next higher degree. Not all nonaccredited programs are poor, but this risk does exist.

The major sources of income for a self-supporting RN in a formal educational program are savings or other personal resources, part-time work, scholarships, and loans. If you plan to do part-time work while attending college, make reasonably sure that a position is available at a satisfactory salary and that it seems to be professionally suitable, including offering enough flexibility to make it possible to take courses. Consider also your mental and physical health under this double load. Can you manage? One answer is cooperative education, which is part work and part school; some higher education programs function in this mode.

There are a number of scholarships, fellowships, and loans earmarked for educational purposes for which nurses are eligible. Some sources of financial assistance are well known and are used regularly; others are not used simply because people do not know about them. The financial aid officer at the institution where you plan to enroll is an excellent source of information. The Federal Student Financial Aid Information Center at (800)-433-3243 provides explanations on government loans and grants and requirements to qualify. You can also make contact through the Internet at www.studentaide.ed.gov.

Exhibit 15.1 Sources of Financial Aid for Education

Local	National/international
School alumni associations	Federal government—DHHS; Dept. of Education
District and CNAs of ANA	Nurses Educational Funds
District and regional Leagues	American Nurses' Foundation
Other local or state nursing organizations	Sigma Theta Tau
State government	Other national nursing organizations
Chapters of national fraternities/sororities	National Student Nurses' Association Foundation
Fraternal organizations (Elks, Amvets)	Veterans Administration
Local foundations	Private foundations
Hospital associations	Military
Your place of employment	World Health Organization
College or university loans or scholarships	Large corporations
Bank loans	
Local companies	
Women's groups	

The professional nursing journals frequently carry news items and articles about such funds, which can be found through the annual and cumulative indexes. Most college catalogs also list sources of student financial support. Exhibit 15.1 lists some of the possible sources of funds. Some give relatively small amounts of money, but these sums do add up. Check also for special funding for ethnic and minority students.

How you apply for financial assistance may have considerable bearing on whether or not you obtain it. Correspondence, personal interviews, application forms, and references should all show the same meticulous attention that is given to an application for a new position.

PROFESSIONAL AND COMMUNITY ACTIVITIES

Active participation in community activities is very rewarding. Some activities are directly related to nursing, such as attending alumni and nurses' association meetings and accepting appointments to committees and offices. Others include volunteer work on a regular or special basis, such as participating in student nurse recruitment programs or career days, soliciting donations for various health organizations, helping with the Red Cross blood program, assisting with inoculation sessions for children, acting as adviser to a Future Nurse Club, or volunteering time at a free clinic.

The importance of nursing input into the various community, state, and national joint provider–consumer groups that study means of improving the health care delivery system is discussed in Chapter 7. Although participation at the state or national level may not be immediately feasible for a nurse who has not yet achieved professional recognition, just showing interest and volunteering your services will often open doors at a local level. That's an important foot in the door!

Consumer activism has resulted in the formation of many groups concerned with health delivery, and nurses offering their expertise and understanding of health care service problems can make valuable contributions. Sometimes you need to convince these groups that you have a sincere interest in improved health care services and are willing to work cooperatively. In some areas, ethnic and minority groups are especially suspicious of professional health workers outside of their own group, because unfortunate experiences have shown some of them to be more concerned with defending their own interests than the consumer's well-being, as the consumer sees it. In these groups, it is even more important to listen than to talk. Participation can lead to development of free clinics, health fairs, health teaching classes, recruitment of minority students for nursing programs, tutoring sessions for students, liaison activities with health care institutions, programs for the aged, and legislative activities directed toward better health care. The opportunities, challenges, and satisfactions are unlimited.

Consumer health education is being stressed more and more today, and in what better area can nurses offer their expertise? Classes can be held under the auspices of health care institutions, public health organizations, and public and private community groups, and include teaching for wellness as well as teaching those with chronic or long-term illnesses. Nurses who like to teach and are skilled and enthusiastic can participate in programs already set up and, equally important, can work to develop other programs and involve others on the health team.

Keeping the public informed about nursing and the changes that have occurred in recent years in both education and practice is a contribution to the community. Offers to present programs about nursing are often welcome in the many community, social, business, professional, and service groups that meet frequently and are interested in community service. And yes, you *can* become a good speaker.

Activities such as these involve you in the community and are stimulating and satisfying. They also require time, effort, and often patience. But besides having the satisfaction of being useful, you'll gain in personal development as a nurse and as an individual.

AS YOU ANTICIPATE THE FUTURE

Nursing is noble work, and you have chosen it wisely. You enter the profession in times of upheaval and paradox, but also at a point of its renaissance. This book has tried faithfully to portray the picture of a profession that is moving with the times. It is a profession that has often been the conscience of health care, speaking out on social issues with a fervor that has sometimes been self-destructive. Our past has been greatly influenced by the women's movement and the growth of modern medicine and the health care industry. Through all of the change that has characterized human affairs, nursing has stayed positioned at the bedside, in the home, in the community ... often the only human link between our patients and an intimidating experience in the health care delivery system.

Nursing will give you many benefits and allow you many options if you are only alert to them. In selecting nursing, you receive a distinctive role, social status, and the choice of a job or a career. For some, fuller involvement in nursing may be limited by other life circumstances such as family, school, or personal interests. For others, nursing is the work of their lives. This does not eliminate the possibility of a full family, community, and social life. Nurses have always balanced multiple and competing demands, and many have done so with the nagging feeling that they never do anything quite as well as they would like. Especially for women, there have been some significant changes. More attention is being given to working women and to the need for family support. Careerism is a real choice today for the nurse who wants it all.

The relatively brief accounts of civic and political opportunities have been included with a purpose. Selecting nursing as a career means more than "being a good nurse." It means bringing the sensitivities of nursing to the community in a variety of volunteer capacities and presenting yourself as a nurse.

Given the time and effort you have invested in your education, you should want to manage your future actively, yet some of you will move haphazardly through your life in nursing, neglecting to orchestrate opportunities, taking things as they come. However unwise that may be, it can offer excitement of its own. Take nursing seriously, but not so seriously that you deny yourself time to appreciate the honorable work you do.

KEY POINTS

1. There has historically been an incongruity between what you expect of the nursing workplace before graduation, and what you find when you get there.
2. Accepting that you hold different values from those in a bureaucracy and working out a relationship that accommodates both your values

and the reality of the workplace is a healthy way to adjust to "reality shock."

3. Nurses are considered a very costly resource and are being held to rigorous standards for actively managing the clinical care of their patients.

4. Burnout occurs when the various pressures of a job and dissatisfaction with the work situation seem to be impossible to cope with.

5. Being good to yourself, allowing for personal activities, as well as working with a support group, can relieve some aspects of stress and burnout.

6. Nursing is physically and psychologically dangerous work; many of these hazards are being addressed by state and federal legislation.

7. Continuing education for nurses may include in-service programs, self-learning, and programs offered by educational institutions and professional organizations.

8. The primary purpose of continuing education is to ensure your competence in practice.

9. You should proceed with care in selecting the right educational program, whether for continuing education or for a degree, so that you do not waste your time or money.

10. Funding for formal nursing education is available from a variety of sources, but it saves time to consult first with the financial officer of the school in which you are interested.

11. Participating in nursing and community organizations is a way to enrich your life as a nurse and as a person.

STUDY QUESTIONS

1. Describe how your socialization experiences in school have modified your image of nursing.

2. Interview several new graduates. How are they handling the transition from student to graduate? What have you learned from them that will help in your own transition?

3. What questions would you ask in an interview to determine the degree of flexibility you would have in a workplace?

4. How do you deal with stress and strain and what new approaches have you learned from this text?

5. What precautions do you routinely take to guarantee your own safety in nursing?

6. Trace the history of collective bargaining and nurses.

REFERENCES

1. Hardy ME, Conway ME. *Role Theory*. Norwalk, CT: Appleton & Lange, 1988, pp 73–110.
2. Kramer M. *Reality Shock*. St. Louis: Mosby, 1974, pp vii–viii.
3. Ibid, pp 155–162.
4. Selye H. *Stress Without Distress*. Philadelphia: J.B. Lippincott, 1974.
5. Peplau HE. Peplau's theory of interpersonal relations. *Nurs Sci Q* 10:162–167, Winter 1997.
6. Kobasa S, et al. Effectiveness of hardiness, exercise and social support as resources against illness. *J Psychosom Res* 29:525–533, May 1985.
7. Joel LA. Maybe a pot watcher but never an ostrich. *Am J Nurs* 94:7, April 1994.
8. Ibid.
9. Gobis L. Workplace Rights: The Perils of Floating. http://nursingworld.org/ajn/2001/sept/ajn_wr09.htm. Retrieved August 15, 2002.
10. Ibid.
11. ANA. State Government Relations: Mandatory Overtime. http://nursing world.org/gova/ state.htm. Accessed April 17, 2005.
12. Fletcher J et al. Whistleblowing as a failure of organizational ethics. *Online Journal of Issues in Nursing*, December 31, 1998: http://nursingworld.org/ojin/topic8/topic8_3.htm. Retrieved August 5, 2002.
13. Government Accountability: http://www.whistleblower.org. Retrieved August 17, 2002.
14. Barry Adams' struggle for justice for all nurses. *Am Nurs*, May/June 2000, 32(3): http://www.medi-smart.com/advo_barry.htm. Retrieved April 16, 2005.
15. Fletcher et al., op cit.
16. Ketter J. Sex discrimination targets men in some hospitals. *Am Nurs* 26:3,24, April 1994.
17. Workplace rights: If you're replaced by a younger nurse. *Am J Nurs* 100(3), March 2000: http://nursingworld.org/ajn/2000/mar/wrights.htm. Retrieved July 10, 2002.
18. ANA. Position Statements: HIV Testing. http://nursingworld.org/readroom/position/blood/bltest.htm. Retrieved April 4, 2005.
19. ANA. Position Statements: HIV Infected Nurse, Ethical Obligations and Disclosure. http://nursingworld.org/readroom/position/blood/bltest.htm. Retrieved April 4, 2005.
20. ANA. Position Statements: Personnel Policies and HIV in the Workplace. http://nursingworld.org/readroom/position/blood/blpers.htm. Retrieved April 2, 2005.
21. Kinard J, Little B. Sexual harassment in the health care industry: a follow-up inquiry. *Health Care Mgmt* 20(4):46–52, June 2002.
22. Court spells out rules for finding sex harassment. *New York Times* 147:A1, 10–12, June 27, 1998.
23. ANA. Positions Statements: Tuberculosis and HIV. http://nursingworld.org/readroom/position/blood/blhvtb.htm. Retrieved April 4, 2005.

24. ANA. State Government Relations: Needlestick Injury Prevention. http://nursingworld.org/gova/ state.htm. Accessed April 17, 2005.
25. ANA. *Making Patient Handling and Movement Safer.* Washington, DC: The Association, 2002.
26. ANA. State Government Relations: Ergonomics. http://nursingworld.org/gova/state/2002/ergo.htm. Retrieved April 10, 2005.
27. United States Department of Justice: http://www.ojp.usdoj.gov/bjs. Retrieved April 17, 2005.
28. McPhaul K, Lipscomb J. Work place violence in health care: Recognized but not regulated. *On-Line Journal of Issues in Nursing* 9(3):7, September 2004: http://nursingworld.org/ojin/topic25/tpc25_6.htm. Retrieved April 2, 2005.
29. Ranson D. Workplace violence in health care. *J Law Med* 12(1):14–16, August 2004.
30. Gritter M. The latex threat. *Am J Nurs* 98:26–32, September 1998.

Updates can be found at

 http://www.JoelTheNursingExperience.com

HELPFUL WEBSITES FOR PART 5

American Association of Colleges of Nursing: http://www.aacn.nche.edu
American Nurses Association: http://www.nursingworld.org
The above may also serve as a gateway to other nursing organizations.
Center for Disease Control and Prevention: http://www.cdc.gov
Global RN Website: http://nurseweb.ucsf.edu/www/globalrn.htm
International Council of Nurses: http://www.icn.ch
Lippincott Publishers: http://www.nursingcenter.com
Links to endless nursing websites:
National League for Nursing: http://www.nln.org
National Student Nurses' Association: http://www.nsna.org
Sigma Theta Tau International: http://www.nursingsociety.org

Bibliography

This bibliography is organized in a way that should make it easy to find appropriate resources.

1. With rare exceptions, citations already appearing in each chapter reference list are not reprinted in the bibliography.
2. As a rule, works published prior to 2002 are not included, the exceptions being those that the author considers "classic" or of historical significance. Other useful works are cited in the bibliography for Kelly's *Dimensions of Professional Nursing*, 9th edition, which can be accessed through the Internet at http://www.books.mcgraw-hill.com/medical/kelly. Works from earlier periods are also included in previous editions of *The Nursing Experience*.
3. The selection of books and journals is broad in order to include fields other than nursing, so that readers who are interested may explore some other perspectives.
4. Many of the sources cited have extensive bibliographies.

CHAPTER 1   Care of the Sick: How Nursing Began

Buchanan T. Nightingalism: haunting nursing history. *Collegian* 6(2):28–33, April 1999.
Denehy J. A tribute to nurses and Florence Nightingale. *J Sch Nurs* 18(3):125–127, June 2002.
Harris MD. Remembering Florence Nightingale. *Home Healthc Nurse* 20(5):291–293, May 2002.
Helmstadter C. "A real tone": professionalizing nursing in nineteenth-century London. *Nurs Hist Rev* 11:3–30, 2003.
Meehan T. In the shadows of nursing history. *Leadership* 31(2):32–33, Second Quarter 2005.
Melchior F. Feminist approaches to nursing history. *West J Nurs Res* 26(3):340–355, April 2004.
Russell D. Roundway, Wiltshire County Asylum attendants and nurses, 1881–1905: a window onto Victorian sobriety. *Int Hist Nurs J* 5(3):14–21, Summer 2000.

Selanders LC. Florence Nightingale and the transvisionary leadership paradigm. *Nurs Leadersh Forum* 6(1):12–16, Fall 2001.

CHAPTER 2   Nursing in the United States: American Revolution to
            Nursing Revolution

Brush BL. Caring for life: nursing during the Holocaust. *Nurs Hist Rev* 10:69–81, 2002.

Buhler-Wilkerson K. No place like home: a history of nursing and home care in the U.S. *Home Healthc Nurse* 20(10):641–647, October 2002.

Dawley K. Perspectives on the past, view of the present: relationship between nurse-midwifery and nursing in the United States. *Nurs Clin North Am* 37(4):747–755, December 2002.

Evans GD. Clara Barton: teacher, nurse, Civil War heroine, founder of the American Red Cross. *Int Hist Nurs J* 7(3):75–82, Spring 2003.

Frantz A. Nursing pride: Clara Barton in the Spanish–American War. *Am J Nurs* 98:39–41, October 1998.

Grando VT. The influence of economic forces on American nursing. Post World War II—1945 to 1950. *Reflections* 3(3):24–25, 3d–4th Quarter 1997.

Grando VT. Making do with fewer nurses in the United States, 1945–1965. *Image J Nurs Sch* 30(2):147–149, 1998.

Helmstadter C. "A real tone": professionalizing nursing in nineteenth-century London. *Nurs Hist Rev* 11:3–30, 2003.

Holder VL. From handmaiden to right hand—the Civil War. *AORN J* 78(3):448–450, 453–458, 461–464, September 2003.

Holder VL. From handmaiden to right hand—the infancy of nursing. *AORN J* 79(2):374–382, 385–390, February 2004.

Houwling I. Image, function, and style: a history of the nursing uniform. *Am J Nurs* 104(4):40–48, April 2004.

Kaiman C. PTSD in the World War II combat veteran. *Am J Nurs* 103(11):32–41, November 2003.

Kalisch PA, Kalisch BJ. Nurses under fire: the World War II experiences of nurses on Bataan and Corregidor. *Nurs Res* 44(5):260–271, September–October 1995.

Levasseur JJ. The proving grounds: combat nursing in Vietnam. *Nurs Outlook* 51(1):31–36, January–February 2003.

Lewenson SB, Keith KA, Kelleher C, Polansky E. Carrying on the legacy of Lillian Wald: partnership with the Henry Street Settlement and the Lienhard School of Nursing at Pace University. *Nurs Leadersh Forum* 5(4):116–121, Summer 2001.

Macduff C. Meeting the mother man: rediscovering Walt Whitman, writer and nurse. *Int Hist Nurs J* 3(2):32–44, Winter 1997.

McBride AB. Nursing and the women's movement: the legacy of the 1960s. *Reflections* 23(3):38–41, 3d–4th Quarter 1997.

Monahan EM, Neidel-Greenlee R. And if I perish: nurse leadership in World War II. *Nurse Educ* 29(6):229–236, November–December 2004.

Nelson S. Invisible radicals. Although rarely given credit for it, Catholic women religious were instrument in creating U.S. health care. *Health Prog* 84(2):27–37, 65, March–April 2003.

Patai F. Heroines of the good fight: testimonies of U.S. volunteer nurses in the Spanish Civil War, 1936–1939. *Nurs Hist Rev* 3:79–104, 1995.

Poslusny SM. Feminist friendship: Isabel Hampton Robb, Lavinia Lloyd Dock and Mary Adelaide Nutting. *Image J Nurs Sch* 21(2):63–68, Summer 1989.

Ruby J. History of higher education: educational reform and the emergence of the nursing professorate. *J Nurs Educ* 38:23–27, January 1999.

Sarnecky MT. Julia Catherine Stimson: nurse and feminist. *Image J Nurs Sch* 25(2):113–119, Summer 1993.

Scannell-Desch EA. Lessons learned and advice from Vietnam war nurses: a qualitative study. *J Adv Nurs* 49(6):600–607, March 2005.

Schmidt CK. One vision followed by thousands: Clara Barton turned caring into global call to action. *Am J Nurs* 104(8):36–37, August 2004.

Shampo MA, Kyle RA. Jane Delano—organizer and recruiter of nurses. *Mayo Clin Proc* 77(10):1026, October 2002.

CHAPTER 3   The Health Care Delivery System

Biedrzycki BA. Telenursing: nursing care without geographic boundaries? *ONS News* 20(3):9–10, March 2005.

Billings DM, Skiba DJ, Connors HR. Best practices in web-based courses: generational differences across undergraduate and graduate nursing students. *J Prof Nurs* 21(2):126–133, March–April 2005.

Chamberlain-Webber J. Start the public health revolution. *Prof Nurse* 20(6):12–17, February 2005.

Chang MY, Wang SY, Chen CH. Effects of massage on pain and anxiety during labour: a randomized controlled trial in Taiwan. *J Adv Nurs* 38(1):68–73, April 2002.

Clausing SL, Kurtz DL, Prendeville J, Walt JL. Generational diversity—the Nexters. *AORN J* 78(3):373–379, September 2003.

Connolly C, Wilson D, Missett R, Dooley WC, Avent PA, Wright R. Associate degree nursing in a community-based health center network: lessons in collaboration. *J Nurs Educ* 43(2):78–80, February 2004.

Deaton C. Outcomes measurement and evidence-based nursing practice. *J Cardiovasc Nurs* 15(2):83–86, January 2001.

Ekerdt DJ. Assisted living: a place to manage uncertainty. *J Gerontol Nurs* 31(1):38–39, January 2005.

Fried TR, et al. Who dies at home? Determinants of site of death for community-based long-term care patients. *J Am Geriatr Soc* 47:25–29, January 1999.

Gilliland AL. Beyond holding hands: the modern role of the professional doula. *J Obstet Gynecol Neonatal Nurs* 31(6):762–769, November–December 2002.

Harrison JP, Ford D, Wilson K. The impact of hospice programs on U.S. hospitals. *Nurs Econ* 23(2):78–84, 90, March–April 2005.

Hartford K. Telenursing and patients' recovery from bypass surgery. *J Adv Nurs* 50(5):459–468, June 2005.

Heinschel JA. A descriptive study of the interactive guided imagery experience. *J Holist Nurs* 20(4):325–346, December 2002.

Hu J, Herrick C, Hodgin KA. Managing the multigenerational nursing team. *Health Care Mgmt* 23(4):334–340, October–December 2004.

Kim S, Hohrmann JL, Clark S, Munoz KN, Braun JE, Doshi A, Radeos MS, Camargo CA Jr. A multicenter study of complementary and alternative medicine usage among ED patients. *Acad Emerg Med* 12(4):377–380, April 2005.

Kupperschmidt BR. Understanding Net Generation employees. *J Nurs Admin* 31(12):570–574, December 2001.

Lechich AJ. Home care in jeopardy. The impact of severe fiscal pressures on patients, management, and staff: the perspective of management and staff. *Care Mgmt* 2(2):128–131, Summer 2000.

Mantle F. The use of complementary therapies. *J Holist Nurs* 20(4):323–324, December 2002.

Monarch K. The quality of care provided in nursing homes: nurses can help facilities do the right things. *Am J Nurs* 105(5):70–72, May 2005.

Morgan P, Strand J. What about physician assistants? *Health Aff (Millwood)* 24(3):886–887, May–June 2005.

Moylan LB. Alternative treatment modalities: the need for a rational response by the nursing profession. *Nurs Outlook* 48(6):259–261, November 2000.

Nield-Anderson L, Ameling A. The empowering nature of Reiki as a complementary therapy. *Holist Nurs Pract* 14(3):21–29, April 2000.

O'Brien BL, Anslow RM, Begay W, Sister Benvinda A Pereira, Sullivan MP. 21st century rural nursing: Navajo traditional and Western medicine. *Nurs Admin Q* 26(5):47–57, Fall 2002.

Oliver NR. Complementary and alternative therapies and SCI (spinal cord injury) nursing. *SCI Nurs* 18(3):127–133, Fall 2001.

O'Mathuna DP. Evidence-based practice and reviews of therapeutic touch. *J Nurs Scholarsh* 32(3):279–285, 2000.

Parsons LC. Converging values: matures, boomers, Xers, and nexters in the health care workforce. *SCI Nurs* 19(1):25–27, Spring 2002.

Pearson L. *Healthy People 2010* and protecting children. *Nurse Pract* 25(7):12, 14, 17, July 2000.

Roe B, Daly S, Shenton G, Lochhead Y. Development and evaluation of intermediate care. *J Clin Nurs* 12(3):341–350, May 2003.

Russell C. *The Master Trend: How the Baby Boom Generation is Remaking America*. New York: Plenum Press, 1993.

Santos SR, Cox KS. Workplace adjustment and intergenerational differences between matures, boomers, and Xers. *Nurs Econ* 18(1):1–13, January 2000.

Sloman R. Relaxation and imagery for anxiety and depression control in community patients with advanced cancer. *Cancer Nurs* 25(6):432–435, December 2002.

Smith DB. Racial and ethnic health disparities and the unfinished civil rights agenda. *Health Aff (Millwood)* 24(2):317–324, March–April 2005.

Stefanacci RG, Podrazik PM. Assisted living facilities: optimizing outcomes. *J Am Geriatr Soc* 53(3):538–540, March 2005.

Tedesco P, Cicchetti J. Like cures like: homeopathy. *Am J Nurs* 101(9):43–50, September 2001.

Thomas DV. Aromatherapy: mythical, magical, or medicinal? *Holist Nurs Pract* 16(5):8–16, October 2002.

Treloar LL. Integration of spirituality into health care practice by nurse practitioners. *J Am Acad Nurse Pract* 12(7):280–285, July 2000.

Turkeltaub M. Nurse-managed centers: increasing access to health care. *J Nurs Educ* 43(2):53–54, February 2004.

Turris SA. Unpacking the concept of patient satisfaction: a feminist analysis. *J Adv Nurs* 50(3):293–298, May 2005.

Velsor-Friedrich B. *Healthy People 2000/2010*: Health appraisal of the nation and future objectives. *J Pediatr Nurs* 15(1):47–48, February 2000.

Ward D, Berkowitz B. Arching the flood: how to bridge the gap between nursing schools and hospitals. *Health Aff (Millwood)* 21(5):42–52, September–October 2002.

Yeh SC, Wan TT, Neff-Smith M. Subacute care in nursing homes. *J Nurs Admin* 32(7–8):369–370, July–August 2002.

Zahourek RP. Trance and suggestion: timeless interventions and implication for nurses in the new millennium. *Holist Nurs Pract* 15(3):73–82, April 2001.

The Alan Guttmacher Institute at http://www.agi-usa.org/ publishes useful information on population and family planning, including *Perspectives on Sexual and Reproductive Health, International Family Planning Perspectives,* and *The Guttmacher Report on Public Policy.* Also useful is *Population Reports.* This quarterly journal is published by the Information and Knowledge for Optimal Health (INFO) Project of the Johns Hopkins Bloomberg School of Public Health's Center for Communication Programs (CCP). *Population Reports* is supported by the United States Agency for International Development (USAID).

The Chronicle of Higher Education is a weekly newspaper that presents reports and discussions of the trends and issues in the field of education.

Both the *American Journal of Public Health,* http://www.ajph.org, and *The Nation's Health,* http://www.apha.org/journal/nation/tnhhome.htm, publications of the American Public Health Association, publish numerous articles and reports on population, environmental hazards, and other aspects of public health.

Good reference sources for current issues, problems, and trends in organized settings for care are *Hospital and Health Network,* the AHA journal, *Health Progress,* the Catholic Hospital Association journal, and the publications of the Group Health Association of America (GHAA), which represents managed care.

There are additionally journals from every segment of the industry, including home health, occupational health, hospice, and rehabilitation, to name a few. All include nontechnical articles. The *Journal of Family and Community Health* is a practical quarterly which presents creative, multidisciplinary perspectives and approaches for effective public health programs. Almost every issue has several pertinent articles.

The best and most up-to-date source of current, comprehensive data on health resources is the U.S. Department of Health and Human Services through its website, http://www.dhhs.gov.

For more information about trends in the health professions, the journals of each occupation and profession are the best sources. They are usually available in health professions' libraries. Most allied health professions also have websites.

CHAPTER 4   The Discipline of Nursing

Aquilino ML, Keenan G. Having our say: nursing's standardized nomenclatures. *Am J Nurs* 100(7):33–38, July 2000.

Astedt-Kurki P, Isola A. Humour between nurse and patient, and among staff: analysis of nurses' diaries. *J Adv Nurs* 35(3):452–458, August 2001.

August-Brady M. Prevention as intervention. *J Adv Nurs* 31(6):1304–1308, June 2000.

Barrett EA, Malinski VM, Ann M, Phillips JR. The nurse theorists: 21st century updates—Martha E. Rogers. *Nurs Sci Q* 16(1):44–51, January 2003.

Benner PE. *From Novice to Expert*. Menlo Park, CA: Addison-Wesley, 1984.

Benner P. Designing formal classification systems to better articulate knowledge, skills, and meanings in nursing practice. *Am J Crit Care* 13(5):426–430, September 2004.

Benner P. Extending the dialogue about classification systems and the work of professional nurses. *Am J Crit Care* 14(3):242–272, May 2005.

Benner PE, Wrubel J. *The Primacy of Caring*. Menlo Park, CA: Addison-Wesley, 1989.

Boling A. The professionalization of psychiatric nursing: from doctors' hand-maidens to empowered professionals. *J Psychosoc Nurs Ment Health Serv* 41(10):26–40, October 2003.

Brush, BL. Has foreign nurse recruitment impeded African American access to nursing education and practice? *Nurs Outlook* 47(4):175–180, July–August 1999.

Buerhaus PI, Auerbach D. Slow growth in the United States of the number of minorities in the RN workforce. *Image J Nurs Sch* 31(2):179–183, 1999.

Buerhaus PI, Donelan K, Norman L, Dittus R. Nursing students' perceptions of a career in nursing and impact of a national campaign designed to attract people into the nursing profession. *J Prof Nurs* 21(2):75–83, March–April 2005.

Burtt K. Male nurses still face bias. *Am J Nurs* 98(9):64–65, September 1998.

Faust C. Orlando's deliberative nursing process theory: a practice application in an extended care facility. *J Gerontol Nurs* 28(7):14–18, July 2002.

Fawcett J. The nurse theorists: 21st-century updates—Dorothea E. Orem. *Nurs Sci Q* 14(1):34–38, January 2001.

Fawcett J. The nurse theorists: 21st-century updates—Rosemarie Rizzo Parse. *Nurs Sci Q* 14(2):126–131, April 2001.

Fawcett J. The nurse theorists: 21st-century updates—Madeleine M. Leininger. *Nurs Sci Q* 15(2):131–136, April 2002.

Fawcett J. Conceptual models of nursing: international in scope and substance? The case of the Roy adaptation model. *Nurs Sci Q* 16(4):315–318, October 2003.

Fawcett J. Criteria for evaluation of theory. *Nurs Sci Q* 18(2):131–135, April 2005.

Fitzpatrick JJ. "I stood taller than the rest"—Hildegard Peplau. *Nurs Educ Perspect* 23(5):213, September–October 2002.

Herdtner S. Using therapeutic touch in nursing practice. *Orthop Nurs* 19(5):77–82, September–October 2000.

Hyun S, Park HA. Cross-mapping ICNP with NANDA, HHCC, Omaha System and NIC for unified nursing language system development. *Int Nurs Rev* 49(2):99–110, June 2002.

Ingersoll GL. Evidence-based nursing: what it is and what it isn't. *Nurs Outlook* 48(4):151–152, July–August 2000.

Jones SA, Brown LN. Alternative views on defining critical thinking through the nursing process. *Holist Nurs Pract* 7(3):71–76, April 1993.

King IM. The nurse theorists: 21st-century updates—Imogene M. King. *Nurs Sci Q* 14(4):311–315, October 2001.

Kreau SD. Using nurse-sensitive outcomes to improve clinical practice. *Crit Care Nurs Clin North Am* 13(4):487, December 2001

Lee T, Mills ME. The relationship among medical diagnosis, nursing diagnosis, and nursing intervention and the implications for home health care. *J Prof Nurs* 16(2):84–91, March–April 2000.

Leininger MM. Transcultural nursing: an imperative for nursing practice. *Imprint* 46(5):50–52, 61, November–December 1999.

Letvak S. Retaining the older nurse. *J Nurs Admin* 32(7–8):387–392, July–August 2002.

Letvak S. The experience of being an older staff nurse. *West J Nurs Res* 25(1):45–56, February 2003.

Lunney M, Delaney C, Duffy M, Moorhead S, Welton J. Advocating for standardized nursing languages in electronic health records. *J Nurs Admin* 35(1):1–3, January 2005.

Martinez LA. Self-care for stoma surgery: mastering independent stoma self-care skills in an elderly woman. *Nurs Sci Q* 18(1):66–69, January 2005.

Neuman B. The nurse theorists: 21st-century updates—Betty Neuman. *Nurs Sci Q* 14(3):211–214, July 2001.

Roy C. The nurse theorists: 21st-century updates—Callista Roy. *Nurs Sci Q* 15(4):308–310, October 2002.

Tanner CA. Critical thinking: beyond nursing process. *J Nurs Educ* 39(8):338–339, November 2000.

Watson J. The nurse theorists: 21st-century updates—Jean Watson. *Nurs Sci Q* 15(3):214–219, July 2002.

CHAPTER 5   Education and Research for Practice

Arslanian C. How to read a nursing research article. *Orthop Nurs* 19(3):43–44, May–June 2000.

Beck CT. Trends in nursing education since 1976. *MCN Am J Matern Child Nurs* 25(6):290–294, November–December 2000.

Beyea SC. Getting started in nursing research and tips for success. *AORN J* 72(6):1061–1062, December 2000.

Beyea SC et al. Is it research or quality improvement? *AORN J* 68:117–119, July 1998.

Buerhaus PI, et al. Implications of an aging registered nurse workforce. *JAMA* 283:2948–2987, November 22, 2000.

Care WD, Scanlan JM. Meeting the challenge of developing courses for distance delivery: two different models for course development. *J Contin Educ Nurs* 31(3):121–128, May 2000.

Casey K, Fink R, Krugman M, Propst J. The graduate nurse experience. *J Nurs Admin* 34(6):303–311, June 2004.

Cummings GG, Mallidou AA, Scott-Findlay S. Does the workplace influence nurses' use of research? *J Wound Ostomy Continence Nurs* 31(3):106–107, May–June 2004.

Dawley K. Perspectives on the past, view of the present: relationship between nurse-midwifery and nursing in the United States. *Nurs Clin North Am* 37(4):747–755, December 2002.

Fink R, Thompson CJ, Bonnes D. Overcoming barriers and promoting the use of research in practice. *J Nurs Admin* 35(3):121–129, March 2005.

Hegge M, Powers P, Hendrickx L, Vinson J. Competence, continuing education, and computers. *J Contin Educ Nurs* 33(1):24–32, January–February 2002.

Heller BR, Oros MT, Durney-Crowley J. The future of nursing education: ten trends to watch. *Nurs Health Care Perspect* 21(1):9–13, January–February 2000.

Im EO, Chee W. Issues in Internet research. *Nurs Outlook* 51(1):6–12, January–February 2003.

Lee MB, Tinevez L, Saeed I. Linking research and practice: participation of nurses in research to influence policy. *Int Nurs Rev* 49(1):20–26, March 2002.

Leeman J, Goeppinger J, Funk S, Roland EJ. An enriched research experience for minority undergraduates—a step toward increasing the number of minority nurse researchers. *Nurs Outlook* 51(1):20–24, January–February 2003.

Mahaffey EH. The relevance of associate degree nursing education: past, present, future. *Online J Issues Nurs* 7(2):3, 2002.

Malinski VM. Art in nursing research. *Nurs Sci Q* 18(2):105, April 2005.

McBride AB. Breakthroughs in nursing education: looking back, looking forward. *Nurs Outlook* 47(3):114–119, May–June 1999.

McCaughan D, Thompson C, Cullum N, Sheldon TA, Thompson DR. Acute care nurses' perceptions of barriers to using research information in clinical decision-making. *J Adv Nurs* 39(1):46–60, July 2002.

Merrill EB. Culturally diverse students enrolled in nursing: barriers influencing success. *J Cult Divers* 5:58–67, Summer 1998.

Mion LC. Evidence-based health care practice: addressing geriatric nursing practice. *J Gerontol Nurs* 25:5–6, December 1998.

Nelson S. The fork in the road: nursing history versus the history of nursing? *Nurs Hist Rev* 10:175–188, 2002.

Reisinger PB. Trends in qualitative nursing research. *SCI Nurs* 21(4):217–218, Winter 2004.

Rosenfeld P, et al. Engaging staff nurses in evidence-based research to identify nursing practice problems and solutions. *Appl Nurs Res* 13(4):197–203, November 2000.

Rudy E, Grady P. Biological researchers: building nursing science. *Nurs Outlook* 53(2):88–94, March-April 2005.

Sitzia, J. Barriers to research utilization: the clinical setting and nurses themselves. *Intensive Crit Care Nurs* 18(4):230–243, August 2002.

Sweeney JF. Historical research: examining documentary sources. *Nurse Res* 12(3):61–73, 2005.

Thurgood G. Legal, ethical and human-rights issues related to the storage of oral history interviews in archives. *Int Hist Nurs J* 7(2):38–49, Summer 2002.

Vanhanen L, Janhonen S. Changes in students' orientations to nursing during nursing education. *Nurse Educ Today* 20(8):654–661, November 2000.

Wallen GR, Rivera-Goba MV, Hastings C, Peragallo N, de Leon Siantz ML. Developing the research pipeline: increasing minority nursing research opportunities. *Nurs Educ Perspect* 26(1):29–33, January–February 2005.

Weeks SK, Satusky MJ. Demystify nursing research. *Nurs Mgmt* 36(2):42–43, 45–47, February 2005.

Whall AL, Hicks FD. The unrecognized paradigm shift in nursing: implications, problems, and possibilities. *Nurs Outlook* 50(2):72–76, March–April 2002.

Yoder-Wise PS. State and certifying boards/associations: CE and competency requirements. *J Contin Educ Nurs* 36(1):3–11, January–February 2005.

Zytkowski ME. Nursing informatics: the key to unlocking contemporary nursing practice. *AACN Clin Issues* 14(3):271–281, August 2003.

CHAPTER 6   Career Opportunities

Aiken LH, Havens DS, Sloane DM. The magnet nursing services recognition program. *Am J Nurs* 100(3):26–36, March 2000.

Aiken LH, et al. Hospital nurse staffing and patient mortality, nurse burnout, and job dissatisfaction. *JAMA* 288(16): 1987–1993. Retrieved from the World Wide Web, November 30, 2002: http://jama.ama-assn.org/issues/v288n16/abs/joc20547.html.

Benefield LE. Critical competencies for nurses in the new millennium. *Home Healthcare Nurse* 18(1):17–21, January 2000.

Berliner HS, Ginzberg E. Why this hospital nursing shortage is different. *JAMA* 288(21):2742–2744, December 4, 2002.

Boland CD. Parish nursing: addressing the significance of social support and spirituality for sustained health-promoting behaviors in the elderly. *J Holist Nurs* 16:355–368, September 1998.

Brennan PF, et al. Nursing practice models. *J Nurs Admin* 28:26–32, October 1999.

Buerhaus PI. Aging nurses in an aging society: long-term implications. *Reflect Nurs Leadersh* 27(1):35–36, 46, 2001.

Buerhaus PI. Shortages of hospital registered nurses: causes and perspectives on public and private sector actions. *Nurs Outlook* 50(1):4–6, January–February 2002.

Buerhaus PI, Needleman J, Mattke S, Stewart M. Strengthening hospital nursing. *Health Aff (Millwood)* 21(5):123–132, September–October 2002.

Capps L. Congresswoman Lois Capps speaks out on the nursing shortage. *Clin Nurse Spec* 15(3):136, May 2001.

Clarke SP, Aiken LH. Failure to rescue. *Am J Nurs* 103(1):42–47, January 2003.

Dayhoff NE, Moore PS. Think like an entrepreneur. *Clin Nurse Spec* 19(2):65–66, March–April 2005.

Deyoung S, Bliss J, Tracy JP. The nursing faculty shortage: is there hope? *J Prof Nurs* 18(6):313–319, November–December 2002.

Evans AM, Wells D. Scope of practice issues in forensic nursing. *J Psychosoc Nurs Ment Health Serv* 39(1):38–45, January 2001.

Ferrell BR, Coyle N. An overview of palliative nursing care. *Am J Nurs* 102(5):26–32, May 2002.

Furillo J, Kercher L. Should nurse-to-patient staffing ratios be mandated by legislation? *MCN Am J Matern Child Nurs* 26(4):176–177, July–August 2001.

Greene J. What nurses want. Different generations. Different expectations. *Hosp Health Netw* 79(3):34–38, 40–42, March 2005.

Havens DM. Nurse on Capitol Hill. *Semin Nurs Mgmt* 6:15–17, March 1998.

Kramer M, Schmalenberg CE. Magnet hospital staff nurses describe clinical autonomy. *Nurs Outlook* 51(1):13–19, January–February 2003.

Meadows G. The nursing shortage: can information technology help? *Nurs Econ* 20(1):46–48, January–February 2002.

Meadows G. Nursing informatics: an evolving specialty. *Nurs Econ* 20(6):300–301, November–December 2002.

McAuliffe MS, et al. Survey of nurse anesthesia practice, education, and regulation in 96 countries. *AANA J* 66:273–286, June 1998.

Minnick AF. Retirement, the nursing workforce, and the year 2005. *Nurs Outlook* 48(5):211–217, September–October 2000.

Needleman J, Buerhaus P, Mattke S, Stewart M, Zelevinsky K. Nurse-staffing levels and the quality of care in hospitals. *N Engl J Med* 346(22):1715–1722, May 30, 2002.

Parsons RJ, et al. Attributes of successful nurse executives: survey of nurses and their mentors. *J Nurs Admin* 28:10–13, July–August 1998.

Porter-O'Grady T. The making of a nurse entrepreneur. *Semin Nurse Mgmt* 6:34–40, March 1998.

Rogers B. Occupational health nursing expertise. *AAOHN J* 46:477–483, October 1998.

Sarnecky MT. Army nurses in "the forgotten war." *Am J Nurs* 101(11):45–49, November 2001.

Seago JA, Ash M, Spetz J, Coffman J, Grumbach K. Hospital registered nurse shortages: environmental, patient, and institutional predictors. *Health Serv Res* 36(5):831–852, October 2001.

Smith AP. Responses to the nursing shortage: policy, press, pipeline, and perks. *Nurs Econ* 20(6):287–290, November–December 2002.

Sochalski J. Nursing shortage redux: turning the corner on an enduring problem. *Health Aff (Millwood)* 21(5):157–164, September–October 2002.

Stechmiller JK. Nursing shortage in acute and critical care settings. *AACN Clin Issues* 13(4):577–584, November 2002.

Tanner CA. Education's response to the nursing shortage: leadership, innovation, and publication. *J Nurs Educ* 41(11):467–468, November 2002.

Unruh L. Licensed nurse staffing and adverse events in hospitals. *Med Care* 41(1):142–152, January 2003.

Possibly hundreds of articles on APNs (NPs, CNSs, CRNAs, CNMs) have appeared in nursing, medical, hospital, and public health journals, including information on education and practice, and evaluation research. In addition, specialty journals carry articles on the role of their constituency, and many of their websites are included throughout this book and in Appendix 4. Readers are also referred to the Career Guides published annually by the *American Journal of Nursing, Nursing Spectrum*, and the National Student Nurse Association.

CHAPTER 7   Leadership for an Era of Change

Anderson CA. Our obligation to the next generation. *Nurs Outlook* 48(4):149–150, July–August 2000.

Bennis WG. The seven ages of the leader. *Harv Bus Rev* 82(1):46–53, 112, January 2004.

Bowles A, Bowles NB. A comparative study of transformational leadership in nursing development units and conventional clinical settings. *J Nurs Mgmt* 8(2):69–76, March 2000.

Charters A. Role modelling as a teaching method. *Emerg Nurs* 7(10):25–29, March 2000.

Conger CO, Johnson P. Integrating political involvement and nursing education. *Nurse Educ* 25(2):99–103, March–April 2000.

Corser WD. The contemporary nurse–physician relationship: insights from scholars outside the two professions. *Nurs Outlook* 48(6):263–267, November–December 2000.

Coyle SK, Mills ME. Nurse executives champion change in integrated health systems. *Nurse Mgmt* 31(2):32–34, February 2000.

David BA. Nursing's gender politics: reformulating the footnotes. *ANS Adv Nurs Sci* 23(1):83–93, September 2000.

Doherty C, Hope W. Shared governance—nurses making a difference. *J Nurs Mgmt* 8(2):77–81, March 2000.

Dombeck MT. The mentor relationship. *Res Nurs Health* 22:1–2, February 1999.

Dziabis SP, et al. Building partnerships with physicians: moving outside the walls of the hospital. *Nurs Admin Q* 22:1–5, Spring 1998.

Fonville AM, et al. Developing new nurse leaders. *Nurs Econ* 16:83–87, March–April 1998.

Glass N, Walter R. An experience of peer mentoring with student nurses: enhancement of personal and professional growth. *J Nurs Educ* 39(4):155–160, April 2000.

Holt FM. Nurse–physician partnerships. *Clin Nurse Spec* 12:121, May 1998.

Iwi E, et al. The self-reported well-being of employees facing organizational change: effects of an intervention. *Occup Med* 48:361–368, September 1998.

Laurent CL. A nursing theory for nursing leadership. *J Nurs Mgmt* 8(2):83, March 2000.

Lowry LW, Burns CM, Smith AA, Jacobson H. Compete or complement? An interdisciplinary approach to training health professionals. *Nurs Health Care Perspect* 21(2):76–80, March–April 2000.

Milstead JA. *Health Policy and Politics*. Gaithersburg, MD: Aspen, 1999.

Neary M. Supporting students' learning and professional development through the process of continuous assessment and mentorship. *Nurse Educ Today* 20(6):463–474, August 2000.

Nielsen J. Take a colleague under your wing. *Nursing* 30(8):68–69, August 2000.

Perry MA. Reflections on intuition and expertise. *J Clin Nurs* 9(1):137–145, January 2000.

Rocchiccioli JT, Tilbury MS. *Clinical Leadership in Nursing*. Philadelphia: W.B. Saunders, 1998.

Rosenstein AH. Original research: nurse–physician relationships: impact on nurse satisfaction and retention. *Am J Nurs* 102(6):26–34, June 2002.

Schaffer B, Tallarica B, Walsh J. Win–win mentoring. *Nurs Mgmt* 31(1):32–34, January 2000.

Simpson RL. Bridging the nursing–physician gap: technology's role in interdisciplinary practice. *Nurs Admin Q* 22:87–90, Spring 1998.

Tourigny L, Pulich M. A critical examination of formal and informal mentoring among nurses. *Health Care Mgmt* 24(1):68–76, January–March 2005.

Vance C, Olson RK. Mentoring in the academic setting. *Imprint* 46(4):43–45, 78, September–October 1999.

VanNiekerk LM, Martin F. The impact of the nurse–physician professional relationship on nurses' experience of ethical dilemmas in effective pain management. *J Prof Nurs* 18(5):276–288, September–October 2002.

Wills CE, Kaiser L. Navigating the course of scholarly productivity: the protégé's role in mentoring. *Nurs Outlook* 50(2):61–66, March–April 2002.

CHAPTER 8   Ethical Issues in Nursing and Health Care

Abbadessa K. Creating a forum for ethical decision-making. *Caring* 19(8):34–36, August 2000.

Ahern K, McDonald S. The beliefs of nurses who were involved in a whistleblowing event. *J Adv Nurs* 38(3):303–309, May 2002.

Aveyard H. The requirement for informed consent prior to nursing care procedures. *J Adv Nurs* 37(3):243–249, February 2002.

Bassetti S. Culturally relevant genetic counseling: nurses play a critical role in helping women and families. *AWHONN Lifelines* 6(3):254–257, June–July 2002.

Bilsen JJ, Vander Stichele RH, Mortier F, Deliens L. Involvement of nurses in physician-assisted dying. *J Adv Nurs* 47(6):583–591, September 2004.

Charles J. Mandatory overtime: conflicts of conscience? *JONAS Healthcare Law Ethics Regul* 4(1):10–12, March 2002.

Cignacco E. Between professional duty and ethical confusion: midwives and selective termination of pregnancy. *Nurs Ethics* 9(2):179–191, March 2002.

Clover A, Browne J, McErlain P, Vandenberg B. Patient approaches to clinical conversations in the palliative care setting. *J Adv Nurs* 48(4):333–341 (review), November 2004.

Cooper RW, Frank GL, Gouty CA, Hansen MC. Key ethical issues encountered in healthcare organizations: perceptions of nurse executives. *J Nurs Admin* 32(6):331–337, June 2002.

Corley MC. Nurse moral distress: a proposed theory and research agenda. *Nurs Ethics* 9(6):636–650, November 2002.

Curtin LL. The case against mandatory overtime. *Semin Nurse Mgmt* 10(4):274–278, December 2002.

Dethloff SB. A family decision to discontinue dialysis treatment for a parent: an advanced practice nurse (APN) guided process. *Nephrol Nurs J* 31(4):443–444, July–August 2004.

Drought T. The privilege of bearing witness. *Nurs Ethics* 9(3):238–239, May 2002.

Erlen JA. When there are limits on health care resources. *Orthop Nurs* 21(4):69–73, July–August 2002.

Ersek M. Assisted suicide: unraveling a complex issue. *Nursing* 35(4):48–52, April 2005.

Gamble D, Thompson JB. Is recruitment of foreign nurses a viable or ethical component of strategies to solve the current nursing shortage in U.S.? *MCN Am J Matern Child Nurs* 28(1):8–9, January–February 2003.

Garzon N. Questions concerning changes in the nursing ethics scene. Interview by Anne J Davis. *Nurs Ethics* 9(6):579–582, November 2002.

Georges JJ, Grypdonck M. Moral problems experienced by nurses when caring for terminally ill people: a literature review. *Nurs Ethics* 9(2):155–178, March 2002.

Glaski S. Nurse tracking systems: do the benefits to nurse managers outweigh risks to nurses' privacy? *MCN Am J Matern Child Nurs* 27(2):72–73, March–April 2002.

Goldberg S. Do-not-resuscitate orders in the OR—suspend or enforce? *AORN J* 76(2):296–299, August 2002.

Haddad A. Ethics in action: honoring a daughter's wish to donate her organs. *RN* 65(5):33–36, May 2002.

Haddad A. Ethics in action: fairness, respect, and foreign nurses. *RN* 65(7):25–28, July 2002.

Hamric AB. What is happening to advocacy? *Nurs Outlook* 48(3):103–104, May–June 2000.

Higgins PA, Daly BJ. Knowledge and beliefs of nurse researchers about informed consent principles and regulations. *Nurs Ethics* 9(6):663–671, November 2002.

Husted G, Husted J. Ethical balance versus an ethical anomaly. *Adv Pract Nurs Q* 4:51–53, Summer 1998.

Jacobson PD. The Supreme Court's view of the managed care industry's liability for adverse patient outcomes. *JAMA* 284(12):1516, September 27, 2000.

Jezewski MA, Brown J, Wu YW, Meeker MA, Feng JY, Bu X. Oncology nurses' knowledge, attitudes, and experiences regarding advance directives. *Oncol Nurs Forum* 32(2):319–327, March 5, 2005.

Jezuit DL. Suffering of critical care nurses with end-of-life decisions. *Medsurg Nurs* 9(3):145–152, June 2000.

Killen AR. Stories from the operating room: moral dilemmas for nurses. *Nurs Ethics* 9(4):405–415, July 2002.

LaDuke S. Ethical issues in pain management. *Crit Care Nurs Clin North Am* 14(2): viii, 165–170, June 2002.

Locsin RC, Purnell MJ. Intimate partner violence, culture-centrism, and nursing. *Holist Nurs Pract* 16(3):1–4, April 2002.

Maas ML, Kelley LS, Park M, Specht JP. Issues in conducting research in nursing homes. *West J Nurs Res* 24(4):373–389, June 2002.

McClain K, Perkins P. Terminally ill patients in the emergency department: a practical overview of end-of-life issues. *J Emerg Nurs* 28(6):515–522, December 2002.

Mechanic D. Managed care and the imperative for a new professional ethic. *Health Aff (Millwood)* 19(5):100–111, September–October 2000.

Murray MA, Miller T, Fiset V, O'Connor A, Jacobsen MJ. Decision support: helping patients and families to find a balance at the end of life. *Int J Palliat Nurs* 10(6):270–277, June 2004.

O'Keefe ME, Crawford K. End-of-life care: legal and ethical considerations. *Semin Oncol Nurs* 18(2):143–148, May 2002.

Okie S. Physician-assisted suicide—Oregon and beyond. *N Engl J Med* 352(16):1627–1630, April 21, 2005.

Panke JT. Difficulties in managing pain at the end of life. *Am J Nurs* 102(7):26–33 (quiz 34), July 2002.

Phillips J. Whistleblowing as a failure of organizational ethics. *Online J Issues Nurs* 7, 2002.

Porter T, Johnson P, Warren NA. Bioethical issues concerning death: death, dying, and end-of-life rights. *Crit Care Nurs Q* 28(1):85–92, January–March 2005.

Roberts M. Do-not-resuscitate orders in the OR—do they work for the patient? *AORN J* 76(2):242–244, August 2002.

Roosevelt M. Choosing their time. The next contentious end-of-life issue: assisted suicide: how Oregon offers a way out. *Time* 165(14):31–33, April 4, 2005.

Runeson I, Hallstrom I, Elander G, Hermeren G. Children's participation in the decision-making process during hospitalization: an observational study. *Nurs Ethics* 9(6):583–598, November 2002.

Scanlon C. A professional code of ethics provides guidance for genetic nursing practice. *Nurs Ethics* 7(3):262–268, May 2000.

Scanlon C. Ethical concerns in end-of-life care. *Am J Nurs* 103(1):48–55, January 2003.

Shelstad K. Landmark United States biomedical ethics cases: a selected bibliography. *Med Ref Serv Q* 18(2):27–53, Summer 1999.

Silva M, Ludwick R. Domestic violence, nurses, and ethics: what are the links. *Online J Issues Nurs* 7(2):6, 2002.

Silva MC, Ludwick R. Ethical issues in complementary/alternative therapies. *Online J Issues Nurs* 7(1):7, 2002.

Smith KV. Ethical issues related to health care: the older adult's perspective. *J Gerontol Nurs* 31(2):32–39, February 2005.

Stanley KJ. Silence is not golden: conversations with the dying. *Clin J Oncol Nurs* 4(1):34–40, January–February 2000.

Swenson CJ. Ethical issues in pain management. *Semin Oncol Nurs* 18(2):135–142, May 2002.

Tiblets C. National policy on confidential student information. *Nurse Educ* 27(3):102, May–June 2002.

Tolle S. A study in what not to do: Schiavo case reveals dangers of letting strangers make end-of-life decisions. *Mod Healthc* 35(14):22, April 4, 2005.

Tolson J. Wrestling with the final call. When it comes to end-of-life decisions, taking an ethical path isn't always easy. *US News World Rep* 138(12):22–23, April 4, 2005.

Tumolo J. To the rescue: considering the risks and rewards of being a good Samaritan. *Adv Nurse Pract* 10(2):68–70, February 2002.

Turkoski BB. Ethical dilemma: HIV and the elderly lovers. *Home Healthc Nurse* 20(11):707–709, November 2002.

Ulrich CM, Wallen GR, Grady C. Research vulnerability and patient advocacy: balance-seeking perspectives for the clinical nurse scientist? *Nurs Res* 51(2):71, March–April 2002.

Valente SM. End-of-life challenges: honoring autonomy. *Cancer Nurs* 27(4): 314–319, July–August 2004.

White C. An exploration of decision-making factors regarding advance directives in a long-term care facility. *J Am Acad Nurse Pract* 17(1):14–20, January 2005.

Wilmot S, Legg L, Barratt J. Ethical issues in the feeding of patients suffering from dementia: a focus group study of hospital staff responses to conflicting principles. *Nurs Ethics* 9(6):599–611, November 2002.

Wood BA. Caring for a limited-English proficient patient. *AORN J* 75(2):305–308, February 2002.

CHAPTER 9 Patients' Rights; Students' Rights

Annas GJ. "Culture of life" politics at the bedside—the case of Terri Schiavo. *N Engl J Med* 352(16):1710–1715, April 21, 2005.

Aveyard H. The requirement for informed consent prior to nursing care procedures. *J Adv Nurs* 37(3):243–249, February 2002.

Bernat J. A defense of the whole-brain concept of death. *Hastings Center Rep* 28:14–23, March–April 1998.

Bogan LM, Rosson MW, Petersen FF. Organ procurement and the donor family. *Crit Care Nurs Clin North Am* 12(1):23–33, March 2000.

Bragadottir H. Children's rights in clinical research. *J Nurs Scholarship* 32(2):179–184, 2nd Quarter, 2000.

Calloway SD, Venegas LM. The new HIPAA law on privacy and confidentiality. *Nurs Admin Q* 26(4):40–54, Summer 2002.

Dobbins EH. Helping your patient to a "good death." *Nursing* 35(2):43–45, February 2005.

Emanuel EJ. Living wills: are durable powers of attorney better? *Hastings Center Rep* 34(6):5–6, November–December 2004.

Enders SR, Paterniti DA, Meyers FJ. An approach to develop effective health care decision making for women in prison. *J Palliat Med* 8(2):432–439, April 2005.

Hobson JE. How the system functions: the roles of the United Network of Organ Sharing, the organ procurement and transplantation network, and the organ procurement organization in heart transplantation. *Crit Care Nurs Clin North Am* 12(1):11–21, March 2000.

Jezewski MA, Meeker MA, Robillard I. What is needed to assist patients with advance directives from the perspective of emergency nurses. *J Emerg Nurs* 31(2):150–155, April 2005.

Konur O. Access to nursing education by disabled students: rights and duties of nursing programs. *Nurse Educ Today* 22(5):364–374, July 2002.

Lo B, Dornbrand L, Dubler NN. HIPAA and patient care: the role for professional judgment. *JAMA* 293(14):1766–1771, April 13, 2005.

Mayer DM, Torma L, Byock I, Norris K. Speaking the language of pain. *Am J Nurs* 101(2):44–50, February 2001.

Mazanec P, Tyler MK. Cultural considerations in end-of-life care. *Am J Nurs* 103(3):50–59, March 2003.

Osinski K. Due process rights of nursing students in cases of misconduct. *J Nurs Educ* 42(2):55–58, February 2003.

Panke JT. Difficulties in managing pain at the end of life. *Am J Nurs* 102(7):26–34, July 2002.

Pinch WJ. Confidentiality through a feminist lens. Reaction piece. *AAOHN J* 47(12):569–573, December 1999.

Rivera-Andino J, Lopez L. When culture complicates care. *RN* 63(7):47–49, July 2000.

Selekman J. Nursing students with learning disabilities. *J Nurs Educ* 41(8):334–339, August 2002.

Simmonds KE, Likis FE. Providing options counseling for women with unintended pregnancies. *J Obstet Gynecol Neonatal Nurs* 34(3):373–379, May–June 2005.

Sullivan EE. Issues of informed consent in the geriatric population. *J Perianesth Nurs* 19(6):430–432, December 2004.

Veatch RM. The topic of potential conflict between advance directives and surrogate decisions. *J Clin Ethics* 11(3):284, Fall 2000.

CHAPTER 10   Politics and Public Policy

Coffman JM, Seago JA, Spetz J. Minimum nurse-to-patient ratios in acute care hospitals in California. *Health Aff (Millwood)* 21(5):53–64, September–October 2002.

Fradd L. Political leadership in action. *J Nurs Mgmt* 12(4):242–245, July 2004.

Glaessel-Brown EE. Use of immigration policy to manage nursing shortages. *Image* 30:323–327, 4th Quarter, 1998.

Hodges LC, Williams BG, Carman DD. Taking political responsibility for nursing's future. *Medsurg Nurs* 11(1):15–24, February 2002.

Inglehart JK. The American health care system—Medicare. *New Engl J Med* 340:327–332, January 28, 1999.

Long RE. From revelation to revolution: critical care nurses' emerging roles in public policy. *Crit Care Nurs Clin North Am* 17(2):191–199, June 2005.

Rosenbaum S. The impact of United States law on medicine as a profession. *JAMA* 289(12):1546–1556, March 26, 2003.

Williamson GR, Prosser S. Action research: politics, ethics and participation. *J Adv Nurs* 40(5):587–593, December 2002.

Many publications of nursing and health care organizations cover legislation and politics on a regular basis. The *Congressional Record* (verbatim transcript of the proceedings of the Senate and House) is a useful government publication. Access to this and other federal documents can be found through: http://www.gpoaccess.gov/crecord/index.html. Major newspapers and news magazines always carry political–legislative news, with or without editorials.

CHAPTER 11   Health Care Credentialing and Nursing Licensure

Beckstead JW. Reporting peer wrongdoing in the healthcare profession: the role of incompetence and substance abuse information. *Int J Nurs Stud* 42(3):325–331, March 2005.

Benner J. How to navigate specialty certification. *Nursing* 30(8):52–53, August 2000.

Blumenreich GA. The importance of being certified. *AANA J* 68(1):9–12, February 2000.

Cary AH. Original research: certified registered nurses. *Am J Nurs* 101(1):44–52, January 2001.

Giddens J, Gloeckner GW. The relationship of critical thinking to performance on the NCLEX-RN. *J Nurs Educ* 44(2):85–89, February 2005.

Hales A. Perspectives on prescribing: pioneers' narratives and advice. *Perspect Psychiatr Care* 38(3):79–88, July–September 2002.

Havens DS, Johnston MA. Achieving magnet hospital recognition: chief nurse executives and magnet coordinators tell their stories. *J Nurs Admin* 34(12):579–588, December 2004.

Mikos CA. Beware the consequences of license relinquishment. *Nurs Mgmt* 35(10):16, 18, 52, October 2004.

Miller JC. Tips on taking the NCLEX-RN. *Imprint* 52(1):28–30, 32, January 2005.

Murphy EK. The multistate licensure compact. *AORN J* 71(4):878–881, April 2000.

Phillips SJ. A comprehensive look at the legislative issues affecting advanced nursing practice. *Nurse Pract* 30(1):14–47, January 2005.

Spector N, Hellquist K. Questions and answers about your nursing license and mobility. *Imprint* 52(1):38–39, 41, January 2005.

Thomas SA, Barter M, McLaughlin FE. State and territorial boards of nursing approaches to the use of unlicensed assistive personnel. *JONAS Healthcare Law Ethics Regul* 2(1):13–21, March 2000.

Tumolo J. The obstacle course of NP prescribing: 40 years later, fair practice landscape remains elusive. *Adv Nurse Pract* 13(1):41–42, 44, January 2005.

The most up-to-date information on credentialing is found on the websites of the National Council of State Boards of Nursing, http://www.ncsbn.org, the American Nurses Credentialing Center, http://www.nursingworld.org/ancc, and the Commission on Graduates of Foreign Nursing Schools, http://www.cgfns.org. The Commission deals with immigration issues.

CHAPTER 12   Legal Aspects of Nursing Practice

Allen J, et al. Legal documentation: a case study in basic concepts. *Adv Nurse Pract* 8(1):67–68, January 2000.

Baker SK. Minimizing litigation risk: documentation strategies in the occupational health setting. *AAOHN J* 48(2):100–105, February 2000.

Cavell GF. Drugs: the nurse's responsibility. *Prof Nurse* 15(5):296, February 2000.

Chappel HW, et al. Nursing law violations: a threat to competent and safe nursing practice. *JONAS Healthcare Law Ethics Regul* 1(3):25–32, September 1999.

Cornock M. *Nursing Law and Ethics*, 2nd edition. *J Adv Nurs* 49(6):688, March 2005.

Crane M. NPs and PAs: what's the malpractice risk? *Med Econ* 77(6):205–208, 215, March 20, 2000.

Fetter MS. Medical errors: medical–surgical nurses speak. *Medsurg Nurs* 9(2):58, 68, April 2000.

Fiesta J. Liability for falls. *Nurs Mgmt* 29:24–26, March 1998.

Frank-Stromborg M, Christiansen A. The undertreatment of pain: a liability risk for nurses. *Clin J Oncol Nurs* 4(1):41–44, January–February 2000.

Hampton S. The role of the expert witness. *J Wound Care* 13(10):435–436, November 2004.

Health care errors report sparks major debate. *Am Nurse* 32(1):8, January–February 2000.

Ignatavicius DD. Asking the right questions about medication safety. *Nursing* 30(9):51–54, September 2000.

Murray RB. The subpoena and a day in court: guidelines for nurses. *J Psychosoc Nurs Ment Health Serv* 43(3):38–44, March 2005.

Noone JM. Charting by exception. *J Nurs Admin* 30(7–8):342–343, July–August 2000.

Oddi LF, Oddi AS. Student–faculty joint authorship: ethical and legal concerns. *J Prof Nurs* 16(4):219–277, July–August 2000.

Thobaben M. Policy implications of medication errors. *Home Care Provid* 5(5):160–161, October 2000.

The areas of law, regulation, and ethics are constantly changing, and some of the best instruments to remain current are electronic. Lexis-Nexis, and Westlaw are databases and research services available to users for a significant fee. Students may have access through their school library. Though including information on a variety of subjects, Lexis-Nexis and Westlaw are particularly noted for their information and commentaries on law, ethics, and related materials.

CHAPTER 13 Nursing Organizations and Publications

All of the organizations in this chapter and in Appendix 4 have journals, newsletters, and other published material that are identified here. Many have websites and they are also noted.

CHAPTER 14 Workplace Choices

Andrica DC. Answering tough questions on interview. *Nurs Econ* 18(1):45, January–February 2000.

Bowles C, Candela L. First job experiences of recent RN graduates: improving the work environment. *J Nurs Admin* 35(3):130–137, March 2005.

Hawke M. Building a secure financial future. *Nursing Spectrum Career Fitness Guide* 87–98, 2001.

Impollonia M. How to impress nursing recruiters to get the job you want. *Imprint* 51(1):11–13, 15, January 2004.

Lindell C. Four steps to better search results on the Internet. *Nursing Spectrum Career Fitness Guide* 182–184, 2001.

Morgan J. Demystifying the application and interview process. *Emerg Nurse* 11(8):17–20, December 2003–January 2004.

Powers L. Anatomy of an interview. *AORN J* 72(4):671–674, October 2000.

Spivak M. A world of opportunities—the challenges and benefits of working overseas. *Emerg Med Serv* 29(3):47–52, March 2000.

Stepanski LM. Becoming a nurse-writer: advice on writing for professional publication. *J Infus Nurs* 25(2):134–140, March–April 2002.

Zurlinden J. Resuscitate your interviewing skills. *Nursing Spectrum Career Fitness Guide* 48–50, 2001.

CHAPTER 15 Career Management

Abu al Rub R. Legal aspects of work related stress in nursing: exploring the issues. *AAOHN J* 48(3):131–135, March 2000.

Almost J, Laschinger HK. Workplace empowerment, collaborative work relationships, and job strain in nurse practitioners. *J Am Acad Nurse Pract* 14(9):408–420, September 2002.

Blazys D. Asthma and latex allergy. *J Emerg Nurs* 26(6):583–585, December 2000.

Blumenreich GA. More help for whistleblowers. *AANA J* 71(2):89–91, April 2003.

Bruder P. Verbal abuse of female nurses: an American medical form of gender apartheid? *Hosp Top* 79(4):30–34, Fall 2001.

Budd KW, Warino LS, Patton ME. Traditional and non-traditional collective bargaining: strategies to improve the patient care environment. *Online J Issues Nurs* 9(1):9, January 31, 2004.

Clark DA, Clark PF, Day D, Shea D. The relationship between health care reform and nurses' interest in union representation: the role of workplace climate. *J Prof Nurs* 16(2):92–96, March–April 2000.

Cook MJ. The renaissance of clinical leadership. *Int Nurs Rev* 48(1):38–46, March 2001.

de Castro AB. Handle with care: the American Nurses Association's campaign to address work-related musculoskeletal disorders. *Online J Issues Nurs* 9(3):3, September 30, 2004.

DeMarco R. Two theories/a sharper lens: the staff nurse voice in the workplace. *J Adv Nurs* 38(6):549–556, June 2002.

Demerouti E, Bakker AB, Nachreiner F, Schaufeli WB. A model of burnout and life satisfaction amongst nurses. *J Adv Nurs* 32(2):454–464, August 2000.

Evans M. On the job: nurses reveal most, least enjoyable aspects of work. *Mod Healthcare* 35(14):14–15, April 4, 2005.

Foley BJ, Kee CC, Minick P, Jennings BM. Characteristics of nurses and hospital work environments that foster satisfaction and clinical expertise. *J Nurs Admin* 32(5):273–282, May 2002.

Forman H, Davis GA. The anatomy of a union campaign. *J Nurs Admin* 32(9):444–447, September 2002.

Forman H, Grimes TC. The "new age" of union organizing. *J Nurs Admin* 34(3):120–124, March 2004.

Garrett DK, McDaniel AM. A new look at nurse burnout: the effects of environmental uncertainty and social climate. *J Nurs Admin* 31(2):91–96, February 2001.

Gates DM. Stress and coping: a model for the workplace. *AAOHN J* 49(8):390–397, August 2001.

Jeffries E. Creating a great place to work: strategies for retaining top talent. *J Nurs Admin* 32(6):303–305, June 2002.

Johnson CL. Come together: nurses representing nurses. *Am J Nurs* 100(9):81–82, September 2000.

Kalliath T, Morris R. Job satisfaction among nurses: a predictor of burnout levels. *J Nurs Admin* 32(12):648–654, December 2002.

Keely BR. Recognition and prevention of hospital violence. *Dimens Crit Care Nurs* 21(6):236–241, November–December 2002.

Kinard J, Little B. Sexual harassment in the health care industry: a follow-up inquiry. *Health Care Mgmt* 20(4):46–52, June 2002.

Kinderman K. Unionization of health care professionals. *J Med Pract Mgmt* 18(3):162–164, November–December 2002.

Kramper MA. Latex allergy: a nursing update. *ORL Head Neck Nurs* 18(3):7–11, Summer 2000.

Lambert VA, Lambert CE. Literature review of role stress/strain on nurses: an international perspective. *Nurs Health Sci* 3(3):161–172, September 2001.

Lang TA, Hodge M, Olson V, Romano PS, Kravitz RL. Nurse–patient ratios: a systematic review on the effects of nurse staffing on patient, nurse employee, and hospital outcomes. *J Nurs Admin* 34(7–8):326–337, July–August 2004.

Laposa JM, Alden LE, Fullerton LM. Work stress and posttraumatic stress disorder in ED nurses/personnel. *J Emerg Nurs* 29(1):23–28, February 2003.

Lin SM, Yin TJ, Li IC. An exploration of work stressors and correlators for nurse's aides in long-term care facilities. *J Nurs Res* 10(3):177–186, September 2002.

Manojlovich M, Spence Laschinger HK. The relationship of empowerment and selected personality characteristics to nursing job satisfaction. *J Nurs Admin* 32(11):586–595, November 2002.

McBride EL. Employee satisfaction: code red in the workplace? *Semin Nurse Mgmt* 10(3):157–163, September 2002.

McCullough C, et al. Collective bargaining and workplace advocacy: three states present their views. *Imprint* 47(1):29–33, January 2000.

McDonald S, Ahern K. Physical and emotional effects of whistleblowing. *J Psychosoc Nurs Ment Health Serv* 40(1):14–27, January 2002.

McPhaul KM, Lipscomb JA. Workplace violence in health care: recognized but not regulated. *Online J Issues Nurs* 9(3):7, September 30, 2004.

Meier E. Is unionization the answer for nurses and nursing? *Nurs Econ* 18(1):36–37, January–February 2000.

Michael JE. Don't strike out in union negotiations. *Nurs Mgmt* 34(11):15–16, November 2003.

Peter EH, Macfarlane AV, O'Brien-Pallas LL. Analysis of the moral habitability of the nursing work environment. *J Adv Nurs* 47(4):356–364, August 2004.

Polovich M. Safe handling of hazardous drugs. *Online J Issues Nurs* 9(3):6, September 30, 2004.

Ruggiero JS. Health, work variables, and job satisfaction among nurses. *J Nurs Admin* 35(5):254–263, May 2005.

Santucci J. Facilitating the transition into nursing practice: concepts and strategies for mentoring new graduates. *J Nurses Staff Dev* 20(6): 274–284, November–December 2004.

Schraeder M, Friedman LH. Collective bargaining in the nursing profession: salient issues and recent developments in healthcare reform. *Hosp Top* 80(3):21–24, Summer 2002.

Shirey MR. Social support in the workplace: nurse leader implications. *Nurs Econ* 22(6):313–319, November–December 2004.

Trofino J. Power sharing: a transformational strategy for nurse retention, effectiveness, and extra effort. *Nurs Leadership Forum* 8(2):64–71, Winter 2003.

Tumolo, J. All in a day's work? NPs combat workplace violence. *Adv Nurse Pract* 10(9):57–60, 74, September 2002.

Ward D, Berkowitz B. Arching the flood: how to bridge the gap between nursing schools and hospitals. *Health Aff (Millwood)* 21(5):42–52, September–October 2002.

Watson CA. Understanding the factors that influence nurses' job satisfaction. *J Nurs Admin* 32(5):229–231, May 2002.

Wilmot S. Nurses and whistleblowing: the ethical issues. *J Adv Nurs* 32(5):1051–1057, November 2000.

As practice becomes your work, and competence your responsibility, the following website is particularly useful: http://www.guidelines.gov [National Guideline Clearinghouse (NGC), a public resource for evidence-based clinical practice guidelines].

Appendixes

1. Major Studies of the Nursing Profession
2. Major Health Care Personnel
3. State Boards of Nursing (2005)
4. Major Nursing and Related Organizations
5. Specialty Certifications
6. Basics of Parliamentary Procedure
7. Distinguished Nurses of the Past:
   Fifty Nurses Who Made a Difference

Appendix 1 Major Studies of the Nursing Profession*

Study	Year	Sponsor; Project director	Key points; Recommendations; Impact
The Educational Status of Nursing	1912	American Society of Superintendents of Training Schools for Nurses; M. Adelaide Nutting, RN	Revealed many appalling working and living conditions of students, limited and poor teaching. No real action taken, but set precedent for later studies. Highlighted need for nursing schools to be independent of hospitals.
Nursing and Nursing Education in the United States	1923	Rockefeller Foundation; Josephine Goldmark (nonnurse researcher)	Found poor education practices and often poor quality of teachers and students. Education for public health nursing should include postgraduate courses in public health nursing. High educational standards should be maintained. The average hospital school does not adequately prepare high-grade nurses; university schools should be developed and strengthened. Resulted in founding of Yale School of Nursing.
Nurses, Patients, and Pocketbooks (first study)	1928	Committee on Grading of Nursing Schools, with members from major nursing and health care organizations; partly funded by nurses; Dr. May Ayres Burgess (statistician)	Showed oversupply of nurses; serious unemployment and maldistribution; low salaries and poor working conditions; some serious incompetence, but both the public and physicians generally satisfied with nurses' services (primarily private duty). Should secure public support for nursing education; replace student nurses with graduates in hospitals.
An Activity Analysis of Nursing (second study)	1934	Committee on Grading of Nursing Schools; Ethel Johns and Blanche Pfefferkorn (lay persons)	First large-scale attempt to find out what nurses were actually doing on the job. Included an explanation of what constitutes good nursing care and a description of basic conditions calling for the services of a nurse.
Nursing Schools Today and Tomorrow (third study)	1934	Committee on Grading of Nursing Schools; Ethel Johns	Proposed characteristics of what a "professional" nurse should know and be able to do. Set forth conditions essential for growth and functioning of professional school, including types of control, funding, and qualifications of faculty.

Study	Year	Sponsor; Project director	Key points; Recommendations; Impact
Study of Incomes, Salaries and Employment Conditions Affecting Nurses (exclusive of those engaged in public health nursing)	1938	American Nurses Association (ANA)	Data from 11,000 questionnaires returned by private-duty, institutional, and office nurses. Had considerable bearing on the development of the ANA economic security program.
Administrative Cost Analysis for Nursing Service and Nursing Education	1940	National League of Nursing Education (NLNE); American Hospital Association (AHA); ANA	Provided data on the cost of a school of nursing to the hospital and the economic value of services rendered by students. No real action taken.
The General Staff Nurse	1941	ANA, NLNE, AHA, Catholic Hospital Association (CHA) (joint committee)	Indicated that staff nurses had little status, as reflected by their hours of duty (often split shifts), salaries, and personnel policies. Gave impetus to the movement to upgrade staff nurses' status.
Nursing for the Future	1948	Carnegie Foundation; Russell Sage Foundation; National Nursing Council (representatives of various health organizations); Esther Lucile Brown, PhD (social anthropologist)	Pointed out continued inadequacies of schools of nursing; emphasized need for official examination of all, with publication of names of accredited schools and pressure to eliminate those not accredited. Found nursing education "not professional." Nursing education should be part of the mainstream of education. Nurses could be divided into "professional" and "practical" categories. Mixed reviews. Similar recommendations given in other reports 20 years later.
Nursing Schools at the Mid-Century	1950	National Committee for the Improvement of Nursing Services (committee of members of all six national nursing organizations); Russell Sage Foundation; Margaret Bridgman, RN EdD (former Academic Dean)	Reported on practices of over 1000 schools of nursing (organization, cost, curriculum content, clinical resources, student health). Gave schools the opportunity to evaluate their performance; stimulated improvement in baccalaureate schools.
Twenty Thousand Nurses Tell Their Story	1958	ANA and American Nurses Foundation (ANF); Dr. Everett C. Hughes (professor of sociology)	Part of a five-year sequence of 34 studies of nursing functions. Funded in part by individual nurses. Intended to produce better patient care; revealed what nurses actually did, their attitudes about the job, and job satisfaction. Formed basis for development of ANA nursing functions, standards, and qualifications.

Appendix 1 (*continued*)

Study	Year	Sponsor; Project director	Key points; Recommendations; Impact
Community College Education for Nursing	1959	Institute of Research and Service in Nursing Education Teachers College, Columbia University; Mildred Montag, RN EdD (nursing professor)	Report of five-year Cooperative Research Project in Junior and Community College Education for Nursing, based on Montag's doctoral study. Included evaluation of seven two-year nursing programs leading to an associate degree (AD) in nursing. A second part presented data from 811 graduates. Influenced establishment of more AD programs.
Toward Quality in Nursing: Needs and Goals	1963	Consultant Group on Nursing—panel of nurses, others in the health field and the public; Apollinia Adams, RN (special assistant to Division of Nursing Chief)	Report to U.S. Surgeon General to advise him on nursing needs and to identify the role of the federal government in ensuring adequate nursing service for the nation. Noted qualitative and quantitative shortages of nursing personnel, problems in recruiting and retaining nurses, need for more nursing research, and improvement of nursing education and administration. Recommended study of nursing education and federal funding for nursing.
An Abstract for Action (Report of the National Commission on Nursing and Nursing Education)	1970	ANA, ANF, National League for Nursing (NLN), Avalon (Mellon) and Kellogg Foundations; Jerome Lysaught EdD (nonnurse educator)	Analyzed current practices and patterns of nursing and assessed future needs. Included observations and analysis of findings from other studies. Feedback from various groups reiterated many of Brown's findings and recommendations from 1948. Recommended joint practice committees of physicians and nurses, state master planning committees for nursing education, federal funding for nursing research and education, different approaches to nursing curriculum, degree programs in diploma schools. Got mixed reviews. Followed by new federal funding (for a short time), short-term joint practice committees. Later follow-up showed little lasting impact.

Study	Year	Sponsor; Project director	Key points; Recommendations; Impact
Extending the Scope of Nursing Practice: A Report of the Secretary's Committee to Study Extended Roles	1971	U.S. Department of Health Education and Welfare (DHEW); Faye Abdellah, RN, EdD (Assistant Surgeon General)	Appointed by Secretary Elliott Richardson. Reviewed current responsibilities of nurses; noted nurses' role on the health team. Recommended: curricular innovations demonstrating physician–nurse team concept in health care delivery; financial support for educating nurses in extended role; economic studies to assess impact of extended nursing practice on health care system. Resulted in federal funding and growth of nurse practitioner programs.
The Study of Credentialing in Nursing: A New Approach	1979	ANA; Inez Hinsvark, RN, EdD (nursing professor)	Consisted of a comprehensive review of credentialing, especially health care and nursing. (Contains excellent information.) Followed by appointment of a Task Force to implement recommendations. Reaffirmed earlier recommendation to establish free-standing credentialing center for nursing. Not accepted by nursing organizations.
Magnet Hospitals: Attraction and Retention of Nurses	1983	American Academy of Nursing (AAN), AAN Task Force on Nursing Practice; Margaret McClure, RN, EdD, chair (nurse executive)	Identified U.S. hospitals able to attract and retain RNs. Studied 41 (questionnaires, interviews). Findings included the importance of well-prepared nurse managers and chief nurse executives; good nurse executives (seen as strong, supportive, visible); clearly enunciated high standards; participatory management; good personnel policies and competitive salaries; career development opportunities.

Appendix 1 (continued)

Study	Year	Sponsor; Project director	Key points; Recommendations; Impact
Nursing and Nursing Education; Public Policies and Private Actions	1983	DHHS contracted to the Institute of Medicine (IOM) Study Committee; included some nurses; Dr. Katharine Bauer (nonnurse)	Mandated by PL 96-76, the Nurse Training Act Amendments of 1979, to determine whether further substantial outlays of federal monies for nursing education were needed to ensure an adequate supply of nurses. Recommended in part that various combinations of public and private support be applied to financial aid for nursing students in basic programs, graduate programs and students in NP programs, to upgrade skills of RNs, LPNs, and aides in LTC facilities; improvement of supply and job tenure by addressing employment conditions; continued support for collection and analysis of nursing data; establishment of a federal organizational entity for nursing research. Seen as influential in establishment of National Center for Nursing Research (NCNR).
National Commission on Nursing Study	1983	American Hospital Association (AHA); Hospital Research and Educational Trust; American Hospital Supply Corporation. Independent Commission; members from various fields, including nursing; Marjorie Beyers, RN, PhD	Primarily initiated in response to the nursing shortage. Final report much weaker than initial report, probably due to need for compromise to further implementation. Stated need for all types of nursing programs, with baccalaureate education as an "achievable goal"; promoted educational mobility. Omitted statement urging utilization of nurses according to educational background. Other recommendations: high priority for nursing research; strong affiliations between academic institutions and practice settings; involvement of nursing in hospital policymaking; recognition of nursing as a clinical practice; salaries and benefits commensurate with nurses' education, experience, and performance.

Study	Year	Sponsor; Project director	Key points; Recommendations; Impact
Secretary's Commission on Nursing	1988	DHHS; Lillian Gibbons, RN, PhD	Established in response to widespread nursing shortage, to advise the DHHS Secretary, Dr. Otis Bowen. Documented pervasive and serious nursing shortage and reinforced themes of previous nursing shortage studies concerning need for improvement of status and working conditions of nurses. Demand for nurses seen as increasing. To increase supply, saw need for increased financial support for education, improved program accessibility, promoting nursing as a career.
Nursings' Vital Signs: Shaping the Profession for the 1990s Report of the National Commission on Nursing Implementation Project (NCNIP)	1989 1991	Tri-Council, made up of ANA, NLN, American Association of Colleges of Nursing (AACN), American Organization of Nurse Executives (AONE); Vivien De Back, RN, PhD	NCNIP was launched (1984–1991) with Kellogg Foundation funding to implement selected recommendations of the IOM and the National Commission on Nursing Reports. Described innovative approaches and strategies developed by the work groups on education, management and practice, research, and development. Distributed a number of brochures and documents offering recommendations for the future of nursing. Also noted that NPs and CNMs not used to fullest, in part due to lack of reimbursement. Held number of conferences on differentiated practice (nursing assignments according to competence, experience, and educational background); nursing information systems; and nurses' contribution to health care. Developed proposal for Advertising Council to clarify image of nursing. Successful National Nursing Image Campaign seen as partially responsible for increasing nursing school enrollments. Project concluded in 1991; seen as fostering coalitions between nursing and other groups.

Appendix 1 (*continued*)

Study	Year	Sponsor; Project director	Key points; Recommendations; Impact
Secretary's Commission on the National Nursing Shortage (CONNS)	1990	DHHS; 15-member committee representing nursing, other providers, third-party payers, data policy field representatives, the public, and ex-officio government representatives; Caroline Burnett, RN ScD.	Appointed for one year by DHHS Secretary, Dr. Louis Sullivan, to advise federal officials on projects to implement the recommendations of the 1988 report. Analyzed ongoing public and private sector initiatives related to 3 focal areas; developed 4 projects and 10 recommendations. First project focused on recruitment, educational pathways, retention, and career development in long-term care facilities. Two projects in second focal area (restructuring nursing service, use of nursing personnel, information systems and related technology): one, a study of nurse-midwives in primary care settings; the other on case management. Recommendations were made related to the third focal area, data collection and analysis requirements as well as first two areas. Follow-through on recommendations not evident, perhaps because nursing shortage eased.
Health Professions Education for the Future: Schools in Service to the Nation	1993	Pew Health Professions Commission (funded by Pew Charitable Trusts); E.H. O'Neill	Follow-up on 1991 report that declared education and training of health professions not adequate to meet health needs of American people. This report reinforced that belief, with sections on various health professions, including nursing. Listed competencies needed for 2005. Pointed out difficulties in making these changes, particularly reluctance of academics. Cited value of nurse-midwives and nurse practitioners, importance of nurses in care of aging, in health promotion and disease prevention, in providing cost-effective care, and in management of care. Proposed 6 strategies for nursing education. Also made strong policy recommendations for federal and state governments, the health professions, and higher education.

Study	Year	Sponsor; Project director	Key points; Recommendations; Impact
Reforming Health Care Workforce Regulation: Policy Considerations for the 21st Century	1995	Pew Health Professions Commission, Task Force on Health Care Workforce Regulation; E.H. O'Neill	This second phase of the Pew Commission work focused on the need to re-regulate professional practice to make it more responsive to a rapidly changing health care environment. This requires a flexible, rational, and cost-effective system which promotes effective working relationships among health care workers, and facilitates professional and geographical mobility of competent providers. The Task Force proposed that the following regulatory adjustments are necessary to achieve these ends:

- Uniformity of standards and disciplinary procedures across states.
- Mutual recognition/endorsement.
- Licensure based on initial and continued competence.
- An active program of competence reassessment which uses random review and "triggers" to indicate who needs reassessment.
- Challenges to the exclusive scope of practice of any professional group.
- Recognition of alternative educational pathways for role preparation.
- Respect for the public's right to choose from a range of safe options.
- Inform the public about the outcome of investigations and disciplinary procedures.
- Partnerships between state, federal, and private regulatory systems.
- Redesign of regulatory boards to improve public membership and provide interdisciplinary oversight.

Pew has funded projects in regulatory reform, and by the end of 2000, 12 states had legislated the right to enter into interstate nurse licensure compacts. Public disclosure laws had also become more common, and governmental recognition of private sector credentials more frequent. State requirements for certification of advanced practice nurses is one example of the latter. |

Appendix 1 (continued)

Study	Year	Sponsor; Project director	Key points; Recommendations; Impact
Critical Challenges: Revitalizing the Health Professions for the 21st Century	1995	Pew Health Professions Commission: E.H. O'Neill	Third Pew Report offering specific recommendations on the way health professionals are educated and trained:

- Enlarge the scientific base of all programs to include psychosocial behavioral sciences and population and health management sciences in an evidence-based approach to clinical work.
- Integrate key areas of preclinical and clinical training across professional communities.
- Prepare students to use sophisticated information and communication technology to promote health and prevent disease.
- Educate for practice in more intensely integrated and managed systems.
- Ensure that students represent the rich ethnic diversity of our society, and that cultural sensitivity is part of the educational experience that touches every student.
- Develop education–service partnerships.

For nursing specifically:

- Recognize the value of multiple entry points to practice.
- Consolidate the professional nomenclature so that there is a single title for each level of nursing preparation and service.
- Distinguish between the practice responsibilities of different levels of preparation for nursing.
- Strengthen existing career ladder programs.
- Decrease the number and size of nursing education programs by 10–20%, reducing the associate degree and diploma programs and favoring geographical areas of shortage.
- Increase the number of nurse practitioner programs by increasing the level of federal funding.

The most highly controversial statement is the need to decrease the numbers of practicing nurses. This is open to many interpretations.

Study	Year	Sponsor; Project director	Key points; Recommendations; Impact
Nursing Staff in Hospitals and Nursing Homes: Is It Adequate?	1996	Institute of Medicine, responding to a legislative mandate: Carolyne Davis, co-chair	Although the Committee members expressed "shock" at the lack of current data relating to the quality of care, they presented a number of key conclusions (selected):

- The aggregate number of nurses is adequate, but their distribution and mix is inadequate.
- The roles of RNs in hospitals are changing, requiring increased professional judgment in the management of complex systems of care.
- Nursing assistants, under the direction of the RN, are assuming increased responsibility for care, but are often not satisfactorily trained.
- There is need to monitor the impact of the changing delivery system on the quality of care and well-being of staff.
- Although RN-rich staffing is sometimes associated with improved outcomes, they are essentially proxy measures for organizational attributes that grant nurses greater status, autonomy, and control over their practice.
- Although it has improved somewhat in recent years, nursing home care still leaves much to be desired.
- The presence of nurses on all shifts, and an RN-rich nursing ratio, are related to improved quality of nursing home care and potential long-term cost savings.

Recommendations (selected):
- Hospitals should expand the use of advanced practice nurses.
- Involve nursing personnel (RNs, LPNs, NAs) who are directly affected by organizational redesign and staffing reconfigurations in the process of planning and implementation.
- The NINR and other agencies should develop a research agenda on quality of care, and the relationship between quality of care and nurse staffing.
- Congress should require a 24-hour presence of RN coverage in nursing facilities.

Appendix 1 (*continued*)

Study	Year	Sponsor; Project director	Key points; Recommendations; Impact
			• Nursing facilities should use advanced practice nurses in gerontology. • Screen applicants for nursing assistant positions for a past history of abuse and criminal records.
Strengthening Hospital Nursing: A Program to Improve Patient Care	1996	Robert Wood Johnson Foundation and Pew Charitable Trusts: Barbara Donaho, MA, RN, FAAN	This project required an interdisciplinary approach to create innovative systems to strengthen patient care. Grantees pursued their goals by varying projects, and their efforts were reported in over 100 publications in nursing and other health care journals. A clear challenge was the ever-present demand to "do it better with less." Summaries give an excellent overview of what can be accomplished, problems notwithstanding.
Colleagues in Caring	Since 1997	Robert Wood Johnson Foundation: Mary F. Rapson, PhD, RN, CS	An attempt to control the market-driven changes of health care which create the periodic shortages–surpluses in the nurse workforce. The key was seen as regional collaboration among all levels of nursing practice and education. Regional recipients of grant awards were expected to: • Assess current and projected nursing care needs in the area. • Develop a system for estimating future needs. • Analyze capacity of region to meet these needs, and of educational infrastructure to produce the numbers and types of nurses required. • Develop a regional nursing workforce consortium to address supply–demand issues. • Establish a mechanism to keep the consortium in place over time. Grantees were joined by a number of independently funded program sites who are moving their own collaboratives toward implementing permanent systems of nursing workforce planning. Although RWJ funding was terminated, many of these projects continued with other governmental and private dollars.

Study	Year	Sponsor; Project director	Key points; Recommendations; Impact
			In many ways, this project tries to solve a political problem technically. There is an assumption that the nursing community will come together and control many personal needs in favor of a common cause. The jury is still out on this ongoing project.
Crossing the Quality Chasm: The IOM Health Care Quality Initiative	1996	Institute of Medicine	In 1996, the Institute of Medicine (IOM) launched a concerted, ongoing effort focused on assessing and improving the nation's quality of care, which is now in its third phase. The first phase of this "Quality Initiative" documented the serious and pervasive nature of the nation's overall quality problem, concluding that the burden of harm conveyed by the collective impact of all of our health care quality problems is staggering. Two of the studies stemming from this initiative are of particular importance to nursing and summarized below.
To Err Is Human: Building a Safer Health System	2000	Institute of Medicine	Innumerable health care groups have concerned themselves with the alarming number of errors and mishaps in health care practice. This recent Institute of Medicine (IOM) Report catalyzed the attention of virtually every health care stakeholder group in the country. Nurses and physicians as well as many patients and their families appreciate best the impetus behind the IOM Report. A whole "cascade" of victimized patients can be linked to catastrophic medical mistakes. And, for each heartbreaking incident, for the most part, there are not one but several "interlocking factors." Errors of any nature seldom occur in isolation, but rather, one flaw begets another. Documentation of these "medical errors" or "mishaps" describes a chain of events involving an array of health care providers practicing in a faulty, fragmented health care system.

Appendix 1 (*continued*)

Study	Year	Sponsor; Project director	Key points; Recommendations; Impact
			With the advent of managed care and the downsizing and restructuring of the health care environment with a focus on bottom line profits as opposed to quality and patient safety, it is little wonder that as many as 44,000 to 98,000 people die in hospitals each year from medical errors and/or medical mishaps, placing error as the 8th leading cause of death. Some challenge these statistics (which reflect only hospital-based data), stating that the numbers are greatly exaggerated. Nonetheless, in over 30 research studies collectively analyzed in the IOM Report, the results reveal that errors are a significant cause of injury and death. And any "significant" number is unacceptable. The IOM Report is a comprehensive, detailed account of the cost of health care errors and mishaps, not only in human lives and dollars (estimated at $37.6 billion annually, $17 billion of which is preventable), but also at the expense of trust between patients and providers, and between providers and professional colleagues; the loss of morale among providers; and the increased frustrations, to say nothing of the myriad ethical principles that are violated. All of these demand a "break of the cycle of inaction" and that is the goal of the IOM's Report—"to break the cycle of inaction."

Study	Year	Sponsor; Project director	Key points; Recommendations; Impact
Keeping Patients Safe: Transforming the Work Environment of Nurses	2004	Institute of Medicine: Donald M. Steinwachs, PhD, Chair; Ada Sue Hinshaw, PhD, RN, Vice-chair	According to a new report from the Institute of Medicine (IOM), nurses and nursing assistants in all health-care settings—including long-term care—must be empowered to practice principles that protect residents from medical errors, such as incorrect medications or wrong doses. The need for nurse empowerment is especially critical in long-term care, where residents are older, frailer, and sicker than in past decades, and where nearly half have some type of dementia. The IOM report indicates that not only are many long-term care residents unable to participate in their own safety, but many have behavioral problems that endanger their safety and challenge medical management. A critical issue that emerges from this report is that nurses and nursing assistants, such as certified nurse aides, should not work shifts longer than 12 hours per day because it can lead—not surprisingly—to fatigue and ultimately cause unintended errors.

*Considerable detail on these studies is found in Joel and Kelly's *Dimensions of Professional Nursing*, 9th ed. New York: McGraw-Hill, 2003, Chapter 5.

Appendix 2 Major Health Care Personnel

Occupation/ Profession	Estimated number of jobs[a]	Basic education[b]				Median salaries[d] ($ per yr/2005)	State regulation:[e] licensure; certification; registration	Major issues and trends
		One year or less	Associate degree, or 2-3-year program	Baccalaureate	Professional/ graduate[c]			
Primary care								
Chiropractor (DC)	49,000			2–4 years	4 years	77,320	×	Not accepted as legitimate by some health care providers, especially MDs. After battle, recognized in all states as primary care providers, with reimbursement, including Medicare and Medicaid.
Clinical psychologist	57,000			×	4 years +	71,067	×	Competing with psychiatrists and others in mental health for patients. Seeking prescriptive authority.
Dentist (DDS)	160,000			3 years min.	3–4 years +	113,319	×	Oversupply. Some dental schools closing or admitting fewer. Emphasis on specialization, notably preventive dentistry.
Doctor of medicine (MD/DO):	577,000			3 years min.	5 years +	135,000	×	Oversupply predicted, especially specialists. Others encroaching on their practice. Less control. More becoming employees. More are marketing services.

Profession	(number)			(number)		Comments
Family Practice (no OB)				175,000		
Pediatrics OB/GYN				261,000		
Doctor of optometry (OD)	38,000	3 years min.	4 years	90,609	×	Education expanding to prepare better for diagnosis and treatment; MDs object. Growth in pediatric, rehabilitative, and geriatric optometry.
Doctor of podiatric medicine (DPM) (Podiatrist)	14,000	3 years min.	4 years	168,000	×	Struggling with MDs to expand practice. Residency programs (advanced training) expanding, although not required. Want more liberal hospital privileges. Concern about wages, autonomy, federal funding.
Nurse-midwife (CNM)	6,000	(×)	(×)	78,565	×	More middle-class women want their services; more MDs trying to limit their practice. Major insurance crisis with soaring rates resulted in first nurse self-insurance. Most practice in hospitals. Lay midwives have secured legal recognition.

(continued)

Appendix 2 (continued)

Occupation/Profession	Estimated number of jobs[a]	Basic education[b]				Median salaries[d] ($ per yr/2005)	State regulation:[e] licensure; certification; registration	Major issues and trends
		One year or less	Associate degree, or 2-3-year program	Baccalaureate	Professional/graduate[c]			
Nurse practitioner (NP)	49,000			×	×	71,241 (institutional practice) 94,313 (private practice)	×	All states allow prescriptive authority, reimbursement, and clinical privileges. Still difficult to have an independent practice. MD opposition continues. New employment market in hospitals.
Nursing (except primary care)								
Registered nurse (RN)	Approximately 2.7 million		(×)	(×)		56,451	×	Greater movement to higher education. New opportunities outside of hospitals. Cyclical shortage continues, mostly attributed to an aging workforce, dissatisfying working conditions, and a scarcity of nurse educators.
Licensed practical nurse (LPN)	692,000	×				35,568	×	Fewer being employed in hospitals. Nursing homes major employer. Longer educational program being suggested. More continuing to RN.

Occupation							Comments
Clinical nurse specialist (CNS)	58,185		X	X	71,544	X	Expanded practice, reimbursement, prescriptive authority, and clinical privileges. Both CNSs and NPs have been included under the title of advanced practice registered nurse. Mostly salaried in health care facilities, and often seen as a threat to MD practice.
Nurse anesthetist (CRNA)	25,000		X	X	121,698	X	Proven history of safety and effectiveness, but constant struggle to remain free of anesthesiologist oversight.
Nursing assistant (NA), home health aid (not including mental health)	1.4 million	X			24,731		Many in nursing homes. Low salaries continue. Some increase in hospital employment to reduce numbers of higher paid workers. Being encouraged to continue education to LPN, then RN level. Requirements for training and certification to work in nursing homes and as home health aides in some states.

Others providing direct services or therapy

Occupation							Comments
Dental hygienist	143,000	(x)	(x)	(x)	64,500	X	More seeking independent practice, not controlled by dentist, and role expansion; dentists objecting. Some giving anesthesia.

(continued)

Appendix 2 (continued)

Occupation/Profession	Estimated number of jobs[a]	Basic education[b]				Median salaries[d] ($ per yr/2005)	State regulation:[e] licensure; certification; registration	Major issues and trends
		One year or less	Associate degree, or 2-3-year program	Baccalaureate	Professional/graduate[c]			
Dieticians and nutritionists	54,000			(×)	×	45,552		Some see need for licensure; achieved in few states. Concern about image, third-party reimbursement.
Emergency medical technician (EMT) and paramedics	150,000	(×)	(×)			31,326	×	Some struggle with nursing because of their use as nurse substitutes, especially in emergency rooms.
Pharmacist: Clinical Pharmacist	185,000			×	(PharmD)	87,110 92,144	×	Looking for ways to expand role. PharmD wanted as entry-level degree. External degree programs for pharmacists who want PharmD. Lobbying for prescriptive authority. The complexity of drug interaction has created a significant role for the clinical pharmacist to serve in a consulting capacity.
Pharmacy assistant/technician	170,000	(×)	(×)			27,000 (02)		

Occupation						Remarks
Physician's assistant (PA)	66,000	(x)	(x)	76,252	x	Programs expected to grow. Being used in hospitals instead of residents. Must work under direction of MD. Many states permit prescribing. Some competition with NPs. Some going on to nursing or public health. Now equal number of women and men.
Psychiatric mental health technician	95,000	(x)	(x)	24,617		Much used in state, local government hospitals. RN concern about overuse, competence. Low salary
Respiratory therapist	86,000	(x)	(x)	46,201	x	Disagreement as to whether nurses should reassume some of these responsibilities. Increased demand in hospitals.
Surgical technologist/technician	54,000	(x)	(x)	34,031		Disagreement as to whether OR nursing should include this role; report to nurse or MD. Improving salary.

Diagnostic services

Occupation						Remarks
Clinical laboratory/medical technician	313,000			37,295	x	Clinical Laboratory Scientists, also known as medical technologists, play a major role in the detection, diagnosis, and treatment of diseases. Acting as health detectives, they use sophisticated laboratory equipment to analyze body fluids, tissues, and cells.

(continued)

Appendix 2 (continued)

Occupation/ Profession	Estimated number of jobs[a]	Basic education[b]				Median salaries[d] ($ per yr/2005)	State regulation:[e] licensure; certification; registration	Major issues and trends
		One year or less	Associate degree, or 2-3-year program	Baccalaureate	Professional/ graduate[c]			
Cardiovascular technologists/ technicians	33,000	(×)	(×)			35,400		Meet the ever-growing need for cardiac services. Low salaries.
Nuclear medicine technologist	14,000		×			47,680		More complex technology.
Radiologic technologist (x-ray technician)	162,000	(×)	(×)	(×)		47,840 (01)	×	Becoming more complex with subspecialization in field. Major shortage, due to increase in nonintrusive testing.
Administration, business, record-keeping								
Health information technicians/ medical records administrator	92,000			(×)	(×)	35,464	×	Great need predicted, especially because of importance of records for reimbursement, and computer-based patient records.
Medical secretary—unit clerk	NA	(×)	(×)			30,162		Computer affecting how a job is done.

Rehabilitation, counseling, and social support

Occupational therapist (OT)	73,000	(x)	(x)	52,432	x	More needed in home care. Major shortage now.
Optician (dispensing)	71,000	(x)	(x) or apprenticeship	37,435		
Physical therapist (PT)	120,000		x	61,048	x	Great demand; many have private practices; more needed in home care where they often assume the role of primary provider. Major shortage, yet admissions to educational programs are very competitive; study has moved to the doctoral level. Cardiac rehab and sports medicine are growth areas.
Recreational therapist	39,000	(x)	(x)	38,804		Some competition with other rehabilitation groups. Has moved to graduate preparation.
Rehabilitation/Vocational counselor	NA	(x)	(x)	25,840 (02)		Some competition with social workers; governmental positions may decrease with budget cuts; low salaries.
Speech pathologist/audiologist	105,000	(x)	(x)	54,902	x	Growing fields; more with graduate education.

(continued)

Occupation/ Profession	Estimated number of jobs[a]	Basic education[b]				Median salaries[d] ($ per yr/2005)	State regulation:[e] licensure; certification; registration	Major issues and trends
		One year or less	Associate degree, or 2–3-year program	Baccalaureate	Professional/ graduate[c]			
Medical social worker	NA			(×)	(×)	40,235	×	Looking for ways to expand role. Competing with nurses in case management. Move toward doctorate.

[a] Figures cited are from the *Occupational Outlook Handbook*, 2000–01 Edition. Washington, DC: DOL, BLS, January 2000.

[b] (×) indicates optional routes to occupational preparation. An absence of brackets denotes the prevailing or required education for entry into practice.

[c] Usually assumes liberal arts or other baccalaureate that does not include clinical work; thus, number of years of preprofessional study or a cross, indicating the completion of an undergraduate degree, will also appear.

[d] Salaries derived from multiple sources including: Allied Physicians, Los Angeles Times & Rand McNally: http://www.allied-physicians.com/salary_surveys; Salary Wizard: http://swz.salary.com/salarywizard; Wage Access: Compensation Survey: http://www.wageaccess.com; and the occupational/professional associations representing these groups. The variation in salaries based on geography, specialization, and employer (public/private sector/self-employed) was significant, but there was an attempt to average across areas. Where official information gave hourly earnings, they were converted to an annual salary to allow comparison between groups. The assumption in that case was a 40-hour week and a 52-week year.

[e] Either voluntary or mandatory credentialing in at least one state. States can vary dramatically.

Appendix 3 State Boards of Nursing (2005)

Alabama
Alabama Board of Nursing
RSA Plaza, Suite 250
770 Washington Avenue
Montgomery, AL 36130-3900
Phone: (334) 242-4060
FAX: (334) 242-4360
Web Site: http://www.abn.state.al.us/

Alaska
Alaska Board of Nursing
Dept. of Commerce and Economic Development
Div. of Occupational Licensing
550 W. 7th Avenue, Suite 1500
Anchorage, AK 99501-3567
Phone: (907) 269-8161
FAX: (907) 269-8196
Web Site: http://www.dced.state.ak.us/occ/
pnur.htm

American Samoa
American Samoa Health Services
Regulatory Board
LBJ Tropical Medical Center
Pago Pago, AS 96799
Phone: (684) 633-1222
FAX: (684) 633-1869

Arizona
Arizona State Board of Nursing
1651 E. Morten Avenue, Suite 210
Phoenix, AZ 85020
Phone: (602) 331-8111
FAX: (602) 906-9365
Web Site: http://www.azboardofnursing.org/

Arkansas
Arkansas State Board of Nursing
University Tower Building
1123 S. University, Suite 800
Little Rock, AR 72204
Phone: (501) 686-2700
FAX: (501) 686-2714
Web Site: http://www.arsbn.org/

California
California Board of Registered Nursing
400 R Street, Suite 4030
Sacramento, CA 95814-6239
Phone: (916) 322-3350
FAX: (916) 327-4402
Web Site: http://www.rn.ca.gov/

California
California Board of Vocational Nurse
    and Psychiatric Technician Examiners
2535 Capitol Oaks Drive, Suite 205
Sacramento, CA 95833
Phone: (916) 263-7800
FAX: (916) 263-7859
Web Site: http://www.bvnpt.ca.gov/

Colorado
Colorado Board of Nursing
1560 Broadway, Suite 880
Denver, CO 80202
Phone: (303) 894-2430
FAX: (303) 894-2821
Web Site: http://www.dora.state.co.us/
nursing/

Connecticut
Connecticut Board of Examiners for Nursing
Division of Health Systems Regulation
410 Capitol Avenue, MS# 12HSR
PO Box 340308
Hartford, CT 06134-0328
Phone: (860) 509-7624
FAX: (860) 509-7553
Web Site: http://www.state.ct.us/dph/

Delaware
Delaware Board of Nursing
861 Silver Lake Blvd
Cannon Building, Suite 203
Dover, DE 19904
Phone: (302) 739-4522
FAX: (302) 739-2711
Web Site: http://
www.professionallicensing.state.de.us/
boards/nursing/index.shtml

District of Columbia
District of Columbia Board of Nursing
Department of Health
717 14th Street, NW
Suite 600
Washington, DC 20005
Phone: (202) 724-4900
FAX: (202) 727-8241
Web Site: http://www.dchealth.dc.gov/

Florida
Florida Board of Nursing
Mailing address:
4052 Bald Cypress Way, BIN C02

Appendix 3 (continued)

Tallahassee, FL 32399-3252
Physical address:
4042 Bald Cypress Way
Room 120
Tallahassee, FL 32399
Phone: (850) 245-4125
FAX: (850) 245-4172
Web Site: http://www.doh.state.fl.us/mqa

Georgia
Georgia State Board of Licensed
   Practical Nurses
237 Coliseum Drive
Macon, GA 31217-3858
Phone: (478) 207-1300
FAX: (478) 207-1633
Web Site: http://www.sos.state.ga.us/ebd-lpn/

Georgia
Georgia Board of Nursing
237 Coliseum Drive
Macon, GA 31217-3858
Phone: (478) 207-1640
FAX: (478) 207-1660
Web Site: http://www.sos.state.ga.us/ebd-rn/

Guam
Guam Board of Nurse Examiners
Regular mailing address:
PO Box 2816
Hagatna, GU 96932
Street address (for FedEx & UPS):
651 Legacy Square Commercial Complex,
South Route 10, Suite 9
Mangilao, GU 96913
Phone: (671) 735-7406
 (671) 725-7411
FAX: (671) 735-7413

Hawaii
Physical address:
Hawaii Board of Nursing
King Kalakaua Building
335 Merchant Street, 3rd Floor
Honolulu, HI 96813
Mailing address:
PO Box 3469
Honolulu, HI 96801
Phone: (808) 586-3000
FAX: (808) 586-2689
Web Site: http://www.state.hi.us/dcca/pvl/
areas_nurse.html

Idaho
Idaho Board of Nursing

280 N 8th Street, Suite 210
PO Box 83720
Boise, ID 83720
Phone: (208) 334-3110
FAX: (208) 334-3262
Web Site: http://www2.state.id.us/ibn

Illinois
Illinois Department of Professional Regulation
James R. Thompson Center
100 West Randolph, Suite 9-300
Chicago, IL 60601
Phone: (312) 814-2715
FAX: (312) 814-3145
Web Site: http://www.dpr.state.il.us/

Indiana
Indiana State Board of Nursing
Health Professions Bureau
402 W Washington Street, Room W041
Indianapolis, IN 46204
Phone: (317) 234-2043
FAX: (317) 233-4236
Web Site: http://www.state.in.us/hpb/boards/
isbn/

Iowa
Iowa Board of Nursing
RiverPoint Business Park
400 SW 8th Street, Suite B
Des Moines, IA 50309-4685
Phone: (515) 281-3255
FAX: (515) 281-4825
Web Site: http://www.state.ia.us/government/
nursing/

Kansas
Kansas State Board of Nursing
Landon State Office Building
900 SW Jackson, Suite 551-S
Topeka, KS 66612
Phone: (785) 296-4929
FAX: (785) 296-3929
Web Site: http://www.ksbn.org

Kentucky
Kentucky Board of Nursing
312 Whittington Parkway, Suite 300
Louisville, KY 40222
Phone: (502) 429-3300
FAX: (502) 429-3311
Web Site: http://www.kbn.state.ky.us/

Louisiana
Louisiana State Board of Practical Nurse
  Examiners
3421 N Causeway Boulevard, Suite 203
Metairie, LA 70002
Phone: (504) 838-5791
FAX: (504) 838-5279
Web Site: http://www.lsbpne.com/

Louisiana
Louisiana State Board of Nursing
3510 N Causeway Boulevard, Suite 501
Metairie, LA 70003
Phone: (504) 838-5332
FAX: (504) 838-5349
Web Site: http://www.lsbn.state.la.us/

Maine
Maine State Board of Nursing
158 State House Station
Augusta, ME 04333
Phone: (207) 287-1133
FAX: (207) 287-1149
Web Site: http://www.maine.gov/boardofnursing/

Maryland
Maryland Board of Nursing
4140 Patterson Avenue
Baltimore, MD 21215
Phone: (410) 585-1900
FAX: (410) 358-3530
Web Site: http://www.mbon.org/

Massachusetts
Massachusetts Board of Registration in Nursing
Commonwealth of Massachusetts
239 Causeway Street
Boston, MA 02114
Phone: (617) 973-0800, (800) 414-0168
FAX: (617) 973-0984
Web Site: http://www.state.ma.us/reg/boards/rn/

Michigan
Michigan CIS/Office of Health Services
Ottawa Towers North
611 W Ottawa, 4th Floor
Lansing, MI 48933
Phone: (517) 335-0918
FAX: (517) 373-2179
Web Site: http://
www.michigan.gov/healthlicense

Minnesota
Minnesota Board of Nursing
2829 University Avenue SE, Suite 500
Minneapolis, MN 55414
Phone: (612) 617-2270
FAX: (612) 617-2190
Web Site: http://
www.nursingboard.state.mn.us/

Mississippi
Mississippi Board of Nursing
1935 Lakeland Drive, Suite B
Jackson, MS 39216
Phone: (601) 987-4188
FAX: (601) 364-2352
Web Site: http://www.msbn.state.ms.us/

Missouri
Missouri State Board of Nursing
3605 Missouri Blvd.
PO Box 656
Jefferson City, MO 65102-0656
Phone: (573) 751-0681
FAX: (573) 751-0075
Web Site: http://pr.mo.gov/nursing.asp

Montana
Montana State Board of Nursing
301 South Park
PO Box 200513
Helena, MT 59620-0513
Phone: (406) 841-2340
FAX: (406) 841-2305
Web Site: http://
www.discoveringmontana.com/dli/bsd/
license/bsd_boards/nur_board/
board_page.htm

Nebraska
Nebraska Health and Human Services System
Dept. of Regulation and Licensure, Nursing
  Section
301 Centennial Mall South
PO Box 94986
Lincoln, NE 68509-4986
Phone: (402) 471-4376
FAX: (402) 471-1066
Web Site:http://www.hhs.state.ne.us/crl/
nursing/nursingindex.htm

Nevada
Nevada State Board of Nursing
5011 Meadowood Mall #201
Reno, NV 89502-6547
Phone: (775) 688-2620
FAX: (775) 688-2628
Web Site: http://
www.nursingboard.state.nv.us

Appendix 3 (continued)

New Hampshire
New Hampshire Board of Nursing
21 South Fruit Street, Suite 16
Concord, NH 03301-2341
Phone: (603) 271-2323
FAX: (603) 271-6605
Web Site: http://www.state.nh.us/nursing/

New Jersey
New Jersey Board of Nursing
124 Halsey Street, 6th Floor
PO Box 45010
Newark, NJ 07101
Phone: (973) 504-6586
FAX: (973) 648-3481
Web Site: http://www.state.nj.us/lps/ca/
medical.htm

New Mexico
New Mexico Board of Nursing
6301 Indian School Road, NE
Suite 710
Albuquerque, NM 87110
Phone: (505) 841-8340
FAX: (505) 841-8347
Web Site: http://www.state.nm.us/clients/nursing

New York
New York State Board of Nursing
State Education Department
Education Bldg.
89 Washington Avenue
2nd Floor West Wing
Albany, NY 12234
Phone: (518) 474-3817, Ext. 280
FAX: (518) 474-3706
Web Site: http://www.nysed.gov/prof/nurse.htm

North Carolina
North Carolina Board of Nursing
3724 National Drive, Suite 201
Raleigh, NC 27602
Phone: (919) 782-3211
FAX: (919) 781-9461
Web Site: http://www.ncbon.com/

North Dakota
North Dakota Board of Nursing
919 S 7th Street, Suite 504
Bismarck, ND 58504
Phone: (701) 328-9777
FAX: (701) 328-9785
Web Site: http://www.ndbon.org/

Northern Mariana Islands
Commonwealth Board of Nurse Examiners
PO Box 501458
Saipan, MP 96950
Phone: (670) 664-4812
FAX: (670) 664-4813

Ohio
Ohio Board of Nursing
17 South High Street, Suite 400
Columbus, OH 43215-3413
Phone: (614) 466-3947
FAX: (614) 466-0388
Web Site: http://www.nursing.ohio.gov/

Oklahoma
Oklahoma Board of Nursing
2915 N. Classen Boulevard, Suite 524
Oklahoma City, OK 73106
Phone: (405) 962-1800
FAX: (405) 962-1821
Web Site: http://www.youroklahoma.com/
nursing

Oregon
Oregon State Board of Nursing
800 NE Oregon Street, Box 25
Suite 465
Portland, OR 97232
Phone: (503) 731-4745
FAX: (503) 731-4755
Web Site: http://www.osbn.state.or.us/

Pennsylvania
Pennsylvania State Board of Nursing
124 Pine Street
PO Box 2649
Harrisburg, PA 17101
Phone: (717) 783-7142
FAX: (717) 783-0822
Web Site: http://www.dos.state.pa.us/bpoa/
cwp/view.asp?a=1104&q=432869

Puerto Rico
Commonwealth of Puerto Rico
    Board of Nurse Examiners
800 Roberto H. Todd Avenue
Room 202, Stop 18
Santurce, PR 00908
Phone: (787) 725-7506
FAX: (787) 725-7903

Rhode Island
Rhode Island Board of Nurse
   Registration and Nursing Education
105 Cannon Building
Three Capitol Hill
Providence, RI 02908
Phone: (401) 222-5700
FAX: (401) 222-3352
Web Site: http://www.health.ri.gov/

South Carolina
South Carolina State Board of Nursing
110 Centerview Drive, Suite 202
Columbia, SC 29210
Phone: (803) 896-4550
FAX: (803) 896-4525
Web Site: http://www.llr.state.sc.us/bon.htm

South Dakota
South Dakota Board of Nursing
4300 South Louise Ave., Suite C-1
Sioux Falls, SD 57106-3124
Phone: (605) 362-2760
FAX: (605) 362-2768
Web Site: http://www.state.sd.us/dcr/nursing/

Tennessee
Tennessee State Board of Nursing
426 Fifth Avenue North
1st Floor—Cordell Hull Building
Nashville, TN 37247
Phone: (615) 532-5166
FAX: (615) 741-7899
Web Site: http://www.tennessee.gov/health

Texas
Texas Board of Nurse Examiners
333 Guadalupe Street, Suite 3-460
Austin, TX 78701
Phone: (512) 305-7400
FAX: (512) 305-7401
Web Site: http://www.bne.state.tx.us/

Texas
Texas Board of Vocational Nurse Examiners
333 Guadalupe Street, Suite 3-400
Austin, TX 78701
Phone: (512) 305-8100
FAX: (512) 305-8101
Web Site: http://www.bvne.state.tx.us/

Utah
Utah State Board of Nursing
Heber M. Wells Bldg., 4th Floor
160 East 300 South
Salt Lake City, UT 84111
Phone: (801) 530-6628
FAX: (801) 530-6511
Web Site: http://www.commerce.state.ut.us/

Vermont
Vermont State Board of Nursing
81 River Street
Heritage Building
Montpelier, VT 05609-1106
Phone: (802) 828-2396
FAX: (802) 828-2484
Web Site: http://vtprofessionals.org/nurses/

Virgin Islands
Virgin Islands Board of Nurse Licensure
Veterans Drive Station
St. Thomas, VI 00803
Phone: (340) 776-7397
FAX: (340) 777-4003

Virginia
Virginia Board of Nursing
6603 W Broad Street, 4th Floor
Richmond, VA 23230
Phone: (804) 662-9909
FAX: (804) 662-9512
Web Site: http://www.dhp.state.va.us/

Washington
Washington State Nursing Care Quality
   Assurance Commission
Department of Health
HPQA #6
310 Israel Road SE
Tumwater, WA 98501-7864
Phone: (360) 236-4700
FAX: (360) 236-4738
Web Site: http://www.doh.wa.gov/nursing/

West Virginia
West Virginia State Board of Examiners for
   Licensed Practical Nurses
101 Dee Drive
Charleston, WV 25311
Phone: (304) 558-3572
FAX: (304) 558-4367
Web Site: http://www.lpnboard.state.wv.us/

Appendix 3 (continued)

West Virginia
West Virginia Board of Examiners for Registered
　Professional Nurses
101 Dee Drive
Charleston, WV 25311
Phone: (304) 558-3596
FAX: (304) 558-3666
Web Site: http://www.wvrnboard.com/

Wisconsin
Wisconsin Department of Regulation and
　Licensing
1400 E. Washington Avenue
PO Box 8935
Madison, WI 53708
Phone: (608) 266-0145
FAX: (608) 261-7083
Web Site: http://www.drl.state.wi.us/

Wyoming
Wyoming State Board of Nursing
2020 Carey Avenue, Suite 110
Cheyenne, WY 82002
Phone: (307) 777-7601
FAX: (307) 777-3519
Web Site: http://nursing.state.wy.us/

Appendix 4 Major Nursing and Related Organizations

Organization and year established[a]	Membership eligibility[b]	Primary purpose	Membership size (approximate)	Certification/ Accreditation[d]	Standards set and published	Legislative activities[e]	Research activities[f]	Publications[h] (journals, newsletters)
					Activities[c]			
General Nursing Organizations								
American Nurses Association (ANA) 8515 Georgia Ave., Silver Spring, MD 20910 [1897] http://www.nursingworld.org/	Members may be either associations or individuals. Constituent member associations (CMAs) include state and territorial nurses' associations, multi-state associations, an association for U.S. nurses overseas, and a federal nurses association composed of members of the U.S. military on active duty. Where the individual member belongs to a CMA, the CMA is the member of ANA, not the individual directly. Contingent on an agreement with the CMA, individuals have the opportunity to join ANA directly.	Work for improvement of health standards and availability of care for all; foster high standards for nursing; stimulate and promote professional development of nurses and advance their economic and general welfare.	155,000 and 53 constituent associations	×	×	×	×	American Nurse; American Journal of Nursing; Capital Update; Center for Ethics and Human Rights Communiqué; Legal Developments; E&GW Update

(continued)

Appendix 4 (continued)

Organization and year established[a]	Membership eligibility[b]	Primary purpose	Membership size (approximate)	Activities[c]				
				Certification/ Accreditation[d]	Standards set and published	Legislative activities[e]	Research activities[f]	Publications[h] (journals, newsletters)
International Council of Nurses (ICN) 3 Place Jean-Marteau, 1201 Geneva, Switzerland [1900] http://icn.ch/	National nurses' associations (NNAs).	Ensure quality nursing care for all, sound health policies globally, the advancement of nursing knowledge, and the presence worldwide of a respected nursing profession and a competent and satisfied nursing workforce.	124 national nurses associations		×		×	International Nursing Review
National League for Nursing (NLN) 61 Broadway, 33rd Floor, New York, NY 10006 [1893] http://nln.org/	Agency members include education institutions, health care agencies, and allied/public agencies. In addition, individuals and graduate students may join.	Assert leadership in faculty development, respond to the systemic changes ahead, and lead the way to excellence in nursing education.	1,143 nursing schools and health care organizations; 17,000 individual nurse educators, graduate students, and consumers; 20 state-affiliated leagues for nursing	×	×	×	×	Nursing Education Perspectives; Shaping the Future; Update

Organization	Eligibility	Purpose	Membership				Publications
National Student Nurses' Association (NSNA) 45 Main Street, Suite 606, Brooklyn, NY 11201 [1953] http://nsna.org/	Students are eligible for active membership in NSNA if they are enrolled in state-approved programs leading to licensure as an RN or are RNs enrolled in programs leading to a baccalaureate degree in nursing. Students are eligible for associate membership if they are prenursing students enrolled in college or university programs. Sustaining and honorary memberships are available to nonstudent members.	Organize, represent, and mentor students preparing for initial licensure as registered nurses, as well as those nurses enrolled in baccalaureate completion programs.	45,000	X	X	X	Imprint; Dean's Notes

Specialty Nursing Organizations

Organization	Eligibility	Purpose	Membership				Publications
Academy of Medical–Surgical Nurses (AMSN) East Holly Ave., Box 56, Pitman, NJ 08071 [1992] http://amsn.inurse.com/	RNs, LPNs, LVNs, clinical nurse specialists, nurse practitioners, educators, researchers, administrators, and students.	Advance the practice of medical–surgical nursing through continuing education, establishing standards, providing peer support and a forum for the management of issues.	5,000 and 20 local chapters	X		X	Med–Surg Nursing; AMSN News

(continued)

Appendix 4 (continued)

Organization and year established[a]	Membership eligibility[b]	Primary purpose	Membership size (approximate)	Activities[c]				Publications[h] (journals, newsletters)
				Certification/ Accreditation[d]	Standards set and published	Legislative activities[e]	Research activities[f]	
Air & Surface Transport Nurses Association [1998] (formerly the National Flight Nurses Association in 1981) http://www.astna.org	RNs, and affiliate members such as respiratory therapists, paramedics; pilots, aircraft vendors/operators, etc., also belong to the association.	The voice of clinical care, with regard to patient and provider advocacy in the transport medical field.	1,750 from 12 countries	×	×	×	×	The Air Medical Journal; Wings, Wheels & Rotors
American Association of Critical-Care Nurses (AACN) 101 Columbia, Aliso Viejo, CA 92656 [1969] http://aacn.org/	RNs, LPNs, students and all those interested in care of the acutely and critically ill and their families.	Improve practice; provide CE for critical-care nurses; promote environments that facilitate comprehensive nursing practice for people with critical illness or injury.	78,000 in over 240 chapters in 50 states and 2 foreign countries	×	×	×	×	Critical Care Nurse; American Journal of Critical Care; AACN Clinical Issues: Advanced Practice; Monthly Newsletter; eNewsletter

Organization	Membership	Purpose	Membership count				Publications
American Association of Diabetes Educators (AADE) 100 West Monroe Street, Suite 400, Chicago, IL 60603-1901 [1973] http://www.aadenet.org/	Multidisciplinary professional membership organization.	Dedicated to advancing the practice of diabetes self-management training and care as integral components of health care for persons with diabetes, and lifestyle management for the prevention of diabetes.	10,032 in over 100 local chapters	✕	✕	✕	✕	e-FYI Newsletter; The Diabetes Educator
American Association of Neuroscience Nurses (AANN) 224 N Des Plaines Street, Suite 601, Chicago, IL 60661-1134 (related to World Federation of Neurosurgical Nursing) [1968] http://aann.org/	RNs interested in the specialty.	Foster and promote interest, education, research, and high standards in neurosurgical nursing and promote growth of nursing.	3,400 in 60 regional chapters	✕	✕	✕	✕	Journal of Neuroscience Nursing; Synapse
American Association of Nurse Anesthetists (AANA) 222 South Prospect Ave., Park Ridge, IL 60068 [1931] http://www.aana.com/	Certified Registered Nurse Anesthetists (CRNAs) and student NAs.	Advance science and art of anesthesia; promote cooperation with other disciplines; CE; develop standards.	28,625 (over 95% of CRNAs are members)	✕[9]	✕	✕	✕	AANA Journal; AANA Newsletter

(continued)

Appendix 4 (continued)

Organization and year established[a]	Membership eligibility[b]	Primary purpose	Membership size (approximate)	Certification/ Accreditation[d]	Standards set and published	Legislative activities[e]	Research activities[f]	Publications[h] (journals, newsletters)
						Activities[c]		
American Association of Occupational Health Nurses (AAOHN) 2920 Brandywine Road, Suite 100, Atlanta, GA 30341 [1942] http://aaohn.org/	RNs employed in occupational health.	Maintain professional excellence in OHN through education and research programs; promote OHN; stimulate interest and provide forum for issues in field.	13,000 with 184 local, state, and regional constituent associations	×	×	×	×	AAOHN Journal; AAOHN News
American Association of Spinal Cord Injury Nurses (AASCIN) 75–20 Astoria Blvd., Jackson Heights, NY 11370-1178 [1983] http://www.aascin.org/	RNs engaged in care of patients with spinal cord injury.	Promote excellence in meeting needs of those with spinal cord injury; disseminate information; promote education and research.	1,500		×	×	×	SCI Nursing

Organization	Membership	Purpose	Members					Publications
American College of Nurse Midwives (ACNM) 818 Connecticut Ave., Washington, DC 20006 [1955: 1929 AANM 1955 merger] http:// www.acnm.org/	ACNM certified nurse-midwives or RN students in accredited nurse-midwifery programs.	Set standards for education and practice and evaluate these. Facilitate efforts of CNMs who provide quality service to individuals and child-bearing families. Promote research.	4,800	x[9]	x	x	x	Journal of Nurse Midwifery; Quickening
American Holistic Nurses Association (AHNA) PO Box 2130, Flagstaff, AZ 86003-2130 [1980] http:// www.ahna.org/	Nurses and others interested in holistically oriented health care.	Promote education of nurses in concepts and practice of the health of the whole person; serve as an advocate of wellness.	2,100	x	x	x	x	Journal of Holistic Nursing; Beginnings Newsletter
American Nephrology Nurses Association (ANNA) East Holly Ave., Box 56, Pitman, NJ 08071 [1969] http://www. annanurse.org/	RNs interested in care of patients with renal disease; Associate: dieticians, social workers, LPN/LVNs, technicians.	Develop and update standards of practice in this field; promote individual growth, promote research and development in field; CE.	11,900 in 112 local chapters	x	x	x	x	Nephrology Nursing Journal

(continued)

Appendix 4 *(continued)*

Organization and year established[a]	Membership eligibility[b]	Primary purpose	Membership size (approximate)	Activities[c]				
				Certification/ Accreditation[d]	Standards set and published	Legislative activities[e]	Research activities[f]	Publications[h] (journals, newsletters)
American Psychiatric Nurses Association (APNA) 1555 Wilson Blvd., Suite 515, Arlington, VA 22209 http://www.apna.org/	RNs in the field.	Advance the practice of psychiatric nursing through continuing education, setting standards, peer support, and providing a forum for management of issues.	4500 members; 35% basic level psychiatric nurses, 59% advanced practice nurses, and about 5–6% doctorally prepared	×	×	×	×	*Journal of the American Psychiatric Nurses Association*
American Public Health Association (APHA) Public Health Nursing Section, 800 I Street, Washington, DC 20001-3710 http://www.csuchico.edu/~horst/	RNs practicing or interested in PH nursing.	Improve nursing service and education in broad perspective of public health.	1,700		×	×	×	*American Journal of Public Health; Nation's Health*
American Radiological Nurses Association (ARNA) 7794 Grow Drive, Pensacola, FL [1981] http://arna.net/	RNs.	Define the functions, qualifications, and educational criteria for radiology nurses; recommend standards; evaluate practice; disseminate research.	1,393	×	×		×	*Journal of Radiology Nursing*

Organization	Purpose	Members				Publication
American Society for Parenteral and Enteral Nutrition (ASPEN) 8630 Fenton St., Suite 412, Silver Spring, MD 20910-3805 [1975] http://www.nutritioncare.org/	Multidisciplinary; MDs, RNs, dieticians, pharmacists; Associate: students and individuals who do not belong to core disciplines.	Promote quality patient care, education, and research in field of nutrition and metabolic support.	6,000	×	×	× Journal of Parenteral and Enteral Nutrition; Nutrition in Clinical Practice
American Society of Ophthalmic Registered Nurses (ASORN) PO Box 193030, San Francisco, CA 94119 [1976] http://www.asorn.org/	RNs engaged in ophthalmic nursing.	Unite RNs in field to promote excellence in ophthalmic nursing; CE.	1,800	×	×	Insight
American Society of Plastic Surgical Nurses (ASPSN) East Holly Ave., Box 56, Pitman, NJ 08071 [1975] http://www.aspsn.com/	LPNs, RNs engaged in field of plastic and reconstructive surgery.	Promote highest professional standards for better and safer care; CE.	1,700	×	×	× Plastic Surgical Nursing

(continued)

Appendix 4 (continued)

Organization and year established[a]	Membership eligibility[b]	Primary purpose	Membership size (approximate)	Activities[c]					
				Certification/ Accreditation[d]	Standards set and published	Legislative activities[e]	Research activities[f]	Publications[h] (journals, newsletters)
American Society of PeriAnesthesia Nurses (ASPAN) 10 Melrose Ave., Cherry Hill, NJ 08003 [1980] http://www.aspan.org/	RNs with primary practice in post-anesthesia care.	CE. Upgrade standards of care; promote professional growth; facilitate cooperation with others in field; encourage specialization and research.	11,087 in 40 state, regional, and international constituencies	×	×	×	×	Breathline; Journal of Post Anesthesia Nursing
Association for Professionals in Infection Control (APIC) 1275 K Street, NW, Suite 1000, Washington, DC 20005-4006 [1972] http://www.apic.org/	All individuals involved in infection control activities.	Improve patient care, support development of effective and rational infection control programs, promote quality research in field.	10,000	×	×	×	×	American Journal of Infection Control; newsletter

Organization	Membership	Purpose	Size					Publication
Association of Women's Health, Obstetric and Neonatal Nurses (AWHONN) 2000 L Street, NW, Suite 740, Washington, DC 20036 [1969] http://www.awhonn.org/	RNs interested in the field.	Promote excellence in nursing practice with women and newborn.	28,000 in 11 geographical districts	X	X	X	X	AWHONN Voice; Journal of Obstetric, Gynecological and Neonatal Nursing
Association of Nurses in AIDS Care (ANAC) 11250 Roger Bacon Drive, Suite 8, Reston, VA 20190-5202 [1987] http://www.anacnet.org/	RNs; Associates: LPNs and students.	Develop this area of specialty practice and promote quality care for patients.	2,600 in 33 chapters and 3 international affiliates	X	X	X	X	HIV Nurse
Association of PeriOperative Registered Nurses (AORN) 2170 S. Parker Rd., Suite 300, Denver, CO 80231 [1954] http://aorn.org/	Nurses employed in perioperative practice, education, research.	Enhance professionalism of perioperative nurses; improve their performance; provide a forum for interaction and idea exchange.	41,000 in 340 chapters and 12 specialty assemblies	X	X	X	X	AORN Journal

(continued)

Appendix 4 (continued)

Organization and year established[a]	Membership eligibility[b]	Primary purpose	Membership size (approximate)	Activities[c]					Publications[h] (journals, newsletters)
				Certification/ Accreditation[d]	Standards set and published	Legislative activities[e]	Research activities[f]		
Association of Pediatric Oncology Nurses (APON) 4700 W. Lake Ave., Glenview, IL 60025-1485 [1976] http://www.apon.org/	RNs in the U.S., Canada, and foreign countries interested in or engaged in pediatrics, oncology, pediatric oncology.	Promote optimal care of children with cancer and their families.	2,000	×	×	×	×		Journal of Pediatric Oncology Nursing
Association of Rehabilitation Nurses (ARN) 4700 W. Lake Ave., Glenview, IL 60025-1485 [1974] http://www.rehabnurse.org	RNs in rehabilitation nursing.	Advance quality of rehabilitation nursing; CE.	6,000 in 63 national chapters and 10 special interest groups	×	×	×	×		Rehabilitation Nursing Journal; ARN Network

Organization	Membership	Objective	Members					Focus/Publications
Dermatology Nurses' Association (DNA) East Holly Ave., Box 56, Pitman, NJ 08071 [1982] http://dna.inurse.com/	RNs, LPNs, and technicians in dermatology nursing.	Develop and foster highest standards of dermatologic nursing care; enhance professional growth through education and research; promote interdisciplinary collaboration; enhance communication.	3,000 in 25 chapters	X		X	X	Focus; Dermatology Nursing
Developmental Disabilities Nurses' Association (DDNA) 1733 H Street, Suite 330, PMB 1214, Blaine, WA 98230 [1992] http://ddna.bluestep.net/	RNs practicing in or having interest in the field.	Support practice with the developmentally disabled as a specialty.	880	X		X	X	International Journal of Nursing in Intellectual and Developmental Disabilities; newsletter; DDNA News Network
Emergency Nurses' Association (ENA) 915 Lee Street, Des Plaines, IL 60016-6569 [1970] http://www.ena.org	RNs in emergency care with special skills or knowledge in emergency nursing. Associate: any other health professional.	Provide optimum care to patients in emergency departments.	23,350 in 20 countries		X	X	X	Journal of Emergency Nursing; Journal of Trauma Nursing; ENA Connection Newsletter; Disaster Management and Response; ENA NewsBytes Online
Infusion Nurses Society (INS) 220 Norwood Park South, Norwood, MA 02062 [1973] http://www.insl.org/	RNs in specialty practice of IV therapy.	Enhance the practice of an IV nurse through research, education, and standards.	9,100 in 50 chapters	X		X	X	Infusion Nursing; INS Newsline

(continued)

Appendix 4 (continued)

Organization and year established[a]	Membership eligibility[b]	Primary purpose	Membership size (approximate)	Certification/ Accreditation[d]	Standards set and published	Legislative activities[e]	Research activities[f]	Publications[h] (journals, newsletters)
						Activities[c]		
International Society of Psychiatric-Mental Health Nurses (ISPN) 2810 Crossroads Drive, Madison, WI 53718 http://www.ispn-psych.org	RNs in specialty.	Unite and strengthen the presence and voice of specialty psychiatric-mental health nurses; promote equitable quality care for individuals and families with mental health problems.	4 Divisions (Child & Adolescent, International Consultation-Liaison, Education & Research, and Geropsychiatry), 4 Councils (Practice, Research, Education, and Legislation)		×	×	×	Archives of Psychiatric Nursing, Journal of Child and Adolescent Psychiatric Nursing, Perspectives in Psychiatric Care; Connections Newsletter
National Association of Neonatal Nurses (NANN) 4700 W. Lake Ave., Glenview, IL 60025-1485 [1984] http://www.nann.org/	RNs; Associates: other health care workers.	Advance the practice of neonatal nursing and safeguard the quality of care to the consumer.	13,000	×	×	×	×	Advances in Neonatal Care; Central Lines

Organization	Membership	Mission	Members					Journals
National Association of Nurse Practitioners in Women's Health (NANPWH) 505 C Street, NE, Washington, DC 20002 [1980] http://www.npwh.org/	NPs in obstetrics, gynecology, family planning, reproductive health, endocrinology, and infertility practice.	Ensure quality reproductive health services that guarantee reproductive freedom, and protect and promote service delivery by NPs.	2,000	x[9]	x	x	x	*The Monthly Cycle; Contemporary Nurse Practitioner; Nurse Practitioner World News; American Journal of Nurse Practitioners*
National Association of Orthopaedic Nurses (NAON) East Holly Ave., Box 56, Pitman, NJ 08071 [1980] http://orthonurse.org/	RNs/LPNs involved in orthopedic nursing.	Enhance personal and professional growth of members through continuing education.	7,000	x	x	x	x	*Orthopaedic Nursing*
National Association of Pediatric Nurse Associates and Practitioners (NAP-NAP) 1101 Kings Hwy Rd., Suite 206, Cherry Hill, NJ 08034 [1973] http://www.napnap.org	RNs who are primary care specialists in pediatrics.	Support legislation to improve the quality of health care to children and adolescents.	6,700 in 50 chapters	x	x	x	x	*Journal of Pediatric Health Care; The Pediatric Nurse Practitioner*

(continued)

Appendix 4 (continued)

Organization and year established[a]	Membership eligibility[b]	Primary purpose	Membership size (approximate)	Activities[c] Certification/ Accreditation[d]	Standards set and published	Legislative activities[e]	Research activities[f]	Publications[h] (journals, newsletters)
National Association of School Nurses (NASN) Eastern Office: Box 1300, 163 Route One, Scarborough, ME 04070–7300. Western Office: 1416 Park Street, Suite A, Castle Rock, CO 80109 [1969] http:// www.nasn.org	School nurses employed by boards of education, institutions of higher learning, and state departments of education.	Strengthen education of children by providing leadership in promotion and delivery of adequate health services by qualified school nurses.	10,000 in 51 affiliate school nurse organizations	×	×	×		Journal of School Nursing; NASN Newsletter
National Gerontological Nursing Association (NGNA) 7794 Grow Drive, Pensacola, FL 32514 [1984] http:// www.ngna.org	RNs, students, nursing assistants; Associate: nonnurses.	Provide a forum in which gerontological nursing issues are identified and explored; public education.	1,700	×	×	×	×	Geriatric Nursing; SIGN Newsletter (Supporting Innovations in Gerontological Nursing)

Organization	Membership	Mission/Purpose	Number					Publications
Oncology Nursing Society (ONS) 125 Enterprise Drive, RIDC Park West, Pittsburgh, PA 15275-1214 [1975] http://www.ons.Org/	RNs and other health care providers engaged in or interested in oncology.	Promote excellence in oncology nursing and quality cancer care.	32,000 in 206 local chapters, 29 national special interest groups, and 100 chapter special interest groups	X	X	X	X	Oncology Nursing Forum; Clinical Journal of Oncology Nursing; ONS News
Respiratory Nursing Society (RNS) 11 Cornell Rd., Latham, NY 12110 [1990] http://www.respiratorynursingsociety.org/	RNs and associate members who are interested in the specialty of respiratory care.	Promote coordinated, comprehensive, high-level nursing care for respiratory patients through fostering nurses' development.	NA	X	X		X	Perspectives in Respiratory Nursing; RNS Bulletin
Society for Vascular Nursing (SVN) 7794 Grow Drive, Pensacola, FL 32514 [1982] http://www.svnnet.org/	Licensed nurses; Associate: nonnurse health professionals; corporate members.	Promote excellence in the compassionate and comprehensive management of persons with vascular disease.	900	X	X		X	Journal of Vascular Nursing; SVN . . . prn
Society of Gastroenterology Nurses and Associates (SGNA) 401 N. Michigan Ave., Chicago, IL 60611 [1974] http://www.sgna.org/	RNs, LP/LVNs, medical technologists, x-ray technicians, PAs.	Advance the science and practice of the specialty through education, research, advocacy, and collaboration.	6,500	X	X		X	Gastroenterological Nursing

(continued)

Organization and year established[a]	Membership eligibility[b]	Primary purpose	Membership size (approximate)	Activities[c]					
				Certification/ Accreditation[d]	Standards set and published	Legislative activities[e]	Research activities[f]	Publications[h] (journals, newsletters)
Society of Otorhinolaryngology and Head-Neck Nurses (SOHN) 116 Canal Street, Suite A, New Smyrna Beach, FL 32168-7004 [1976] http://www. sohnnurse.com/	RNs working in the field.	Support the development of the specialty in the public interest.	1,100	×	×		×	ORL-Head and Neck Nursing; Update
Society of Pediatric Nurses (SPN) 7794 Grow Drive, Pensacola, FL 32514 [1990] http://www. pedsnurses.org/	RNs, LPNs, and graduate and undergraduate students interested in pediatrics.	Promote excellence in nursing care of children and their families through support of its members' clinical practice, education, research, and advocacy.	2,000		×		×	SPN Newsletter; SPN Journal

Organization / Address	Eligibility	Purpose	Number of Members				Publication
Society of Urologic Nurses and Associates (SUNA) East Holly Ave., Box 56 Pitman, NJ 08071 http://www.suna.org/	RNs working in the field.	Support the development of the specialty in the public interest.	4,000 and 36 local chapters		×	×	Urologic Nursing Journal; Uro-Gram
Wound, Ostomy and Continence Nurses Society (WOCN) 4700 W. Lake Ave., Glenview, IL 60025 [1968] http://www.wocn.org/	RNs working in the field.	Promote educational, clinical, and research opportunities to advance the practice and guide the delivery of expert health care to individuals with wounds, ostomies, and incontinence.	4,000	×	×	×	Journal of WOCN; WOCNews
Organizations Related to Leadership							
Alpha Tau Delta, National Fraternity for Professional Nurses 5207 Mesada St., Alta Loma, CA 91701 [1921] http://www.atdnursing.org/	Students in accredited baccalaureate or higher degree programs; based on scholarship, personality, and character. Also alumnae chapters.	Further professional and education standards, develop leadership, encourage excellence.	6,000				Captions of Alpha Tau Delta

(continued)

Appendix 4 (continued)

Organization and year established[a]	Membership eligibility[b]	Primary purpose	Membership size (approximate)	Certification/ Accreditation[d]	Standards set and published	Activities[c]			Publications[h] (journals, newsletters)
						Legislative activities[e]	Research activities[f]		
American Academy of Nursing (AAN) 555 E. Wells St, Suite 1100, Milwaukee, WI 53202-3823 [1973] http:// www.aannet.org/	Elected by current members. Based on contributions to nursing; members are called fellows (FAAN).	Advance role of nursing in health care delivery; identify and explore issues in health care, the professions, and society, and propose resolutions; disseminate scholarly concepts; formulate strategies to improve health care.	1,700			×	×		*Nursing Outlook;* newsletter
Sigma Theta Tau International Honor Society of Nursing 550 W. North St., Indianapolis, IN 46202 [1922] http:// www.stti.iupui.edu/	High academic achievement and leadership qualities as student in baccalaureate and higher degree programs. Also community leaders.	Recognize superior achievement, leadership qualities, foster high professional standards, encourage creative work; support scholarliness in nursing.	260,000 members in 72 countries				×		*Image: The Journal of Nursing Scholarship; Reflections*
Chi Eta Phi Society 3029 13th St. NW, Washington, DC 20029 [1932] http://www. chietaphi.com/	Interested RNs and students in U.S. and Africa; focus is on black nurses.	Recruit into nursing, identify corps of nursing leaders who will be agents of social change.	8,000 in 78 graduate and 38 undergraduate chapters in the U.S., U.S. Virgin Islands, and Africa						Newsletter

Organization	Membership	Purpose				Publication
American Assembly for Men in Nursing (AAMN) 11 Cornell Road, Latham, NY 12110 [1971] http://aamn.org/	Men nurses.	Provide support to men nurses; encourage men into nursing.	NA			*Interaction*
National Association of Hispanic Nurses (NAHN) 1501 Sixteenth St., NW, Washington, DC 20036 [1975] http://www.the-hispanicnurses.org/	Hispanic nurses, any RN interested.	Improve care of Hispanic patients; educate about health care needs; recruitment and retention of Hispanic students; ensure equal opportunities for Hispanic nurses.	NA	X	X	*Hispanic Health Care International*
National Black Nurses' Association (NBNA) 8630 Fenton Street, Suite 330, Silver Spring, MD 20910-3803 [1971] http://www.nbna.org	RNs, LPNs, students.	Improve care for black consumers; influence legislation about Blacks; recruit Blacks into nursing; unify black nurses.	Represents approximately 150,000 African-American nurses from the U.S.A., Eastern Caribbean, and Africa, with 76 chartered chapters nationwide.	X		*NBNA Journal; NBNA Newsletter*

(continued)

697

Appendix 4 (continued)

Organization and year established[a]	Membership eligibility[b]	Primary purpose	Membership size (approximate)	Activities[c]				Publications[h] (journals, newsletters)
				Certification/ Accreditation[d]	Standards set and published	Legislative activities[e]	Research activities[f]	
Philippine Nurses Association of America (PNAA) 20127 Avenida Pomplona, Cerritos, CA 90703 [1980] http:// www.pnaa03.org/	RNs and others interested in the issues of Filipino nurses.	Uphold the image and foster the welfare of Filipino nurses as a professional group.	26 chapters			×		Philippine-American Nurse
Job-Related Special Interest Groups								
American Academy of Ambulatory Care Nursing (AAACN) East Holly Ave., Box 56, Pitman, NJ 08071 [1978] http://www. aaacn.inurse.com/	Any RN interested in ambulatory nursing care.	Promote high standards of ambulatory care nursing administration and practice through education, exchange of information, and scientific investigation.	2,700		×		×	Viewpoint
American Association of Colleges of Nursing (AACN) One Dupont Circle, Suite 530, Washington, DC 20036 [1969] http://www. aacn.nche.edu/	Institutions with baccalaureate or higher degree nursing programs represented by dean or comparable chief administrator.	Promote academic leadership in nursing; disseminate information about higher education in nursing; advance the quality of baccalaureate and higher nursing education; promote research.	550 schools of nursing	×	×	×	×	Journal of Professional Nursing; AACN Newsletter; Syllabus

Organization	Objectives	Members				Publication
The American Association of Nurse Attorneys (TAANA) Box 515, Columbus, Ohio 43216-0515 [1982] http://www.taana.org/	Facilitate information sharing; develop the profession; educate nurses about law; influence health policy.	600		×	×	Inside TAANA
American Association of Office Nurses (AAON) 109 Kinderkamack Rd., Montvale, NJ 07645 [1988] http://www.aaon.org/	Development of the specialized field of the office nurse.	4,000	×			Office Nurse; Nurses Exchange Office News
American Organization of Nurse Executives (AONE) 840 North Lake Shore Dr., 10E, Chicago, IL 60611 [1967] http://www.aone.org/	Provide leadership for advancement of nursing practice and patient care in organized health care systems, through achievement in excellence in nurse executive practice; shape policy in health care.	4,800		×	×	The Nurse Executive

(continued)

Organization and year established[a]	Membership eligibility[b]	Primary purpose	Membership size (approximate)	Activities[c]				
				Certification/ Accreditation[d]	Standards set and published	Legislative activities[e]	Research activities[f]	Publications[h] (journals, newsletters)
Home Health Nurses Association (HHNA) Box 91486, Washington, DC 20090 [1993] http:// www.hhna.org/	RNs in any aspect of home health care.	Develop the specialty of home care nursing in pursuit of quality services for the public.	3,000	×	×		×	Home Healthcare Nurse Journal; Caring
Hospice and Palliative Nurses Association (HPNA) Penn Center West One, Suite 229, Pittsburgh, PA 15276 [1986] http:// www.hpna.org/	RNs in hospice practice; Associate and student membership.	Exchange information, experiences, and ideas; to promote understanding of the specialties of hospice and palliative nursing; and to study and promote hospice and palliative nursing research.	7,000	×	×		×	Journal of Hospice and Palliative Nursing; HPNA Nursing Assistant Newsletter; HPNA e-newsletter
International Association of Forensic Nurses (IAFN) East Holly Ave., Box 56, Pitman, NJ 08071 http:// forensicnurse.org/	RNs in forensic work; Associatee, student, and retired statuses.	Access information about the science of forensic nursing.	2,500	×	×			Journal of Forensic Nursing; On the Edge

Organization	Membership	Purpose	Number			Recruitment Directions / Issues
National Association for Health Care Recruitment (NAHCR) PO Box 531107, 307 Park Lake Circle, Orlando, FL 32853-1107 [1975] http://www.nahcr.com/	Those working in hospitals or health care agencies actively involved in health care recruiting.	Promote and exchange principles of professional health care recruitment.	850		X	Recruitment Directions
National Association of Directors of Nursing Administration in Long Term Care (NADONA/LTC) 10999 Reed Hartman Hwy., Suite 229, Cincinnati, OH 45242 http://www.nadona.org/	Nurses in long-term care administration or management.	Support development of the practice area.	2,800	X		NA
National Council of State Boards of Nursing 676 N St. Clair, Suite 550, Chicago, IL 60611 [1978] http://www.nesbn.org/	Boards of nursing in states and territories.	Develop licensing exams; assist boards in administering them; develop model licensure laws and regulations; disseminate information.	61 boards of nursing		X	X Issues

Appendix 4 (*continued*)

Organization and year established[a]	Membership eligibility[b]	Primary purpose	Membership size (approximate)	Activities[c]					Publications[h] (journals, newsletters)
				Certification/ Accreditation[d]	Standards set and published	Legislative activities[e]	Research activities[f]		
National Nurses in Business Association (NNBA) 56 McArthur Ave., Staten Island, NY 10312 [1985] http://www.nnba.net/	RN-entrepreneurs.	Support for nurse-owned businesses.	1,000						*NNBA ezine*
National Nursing Staff Development Organization (NNSDO) 7794 Gros Drive, Pensacola, FL 32534-1350 [1989] http://www.nnsdo.org/	Nurses in staff development practice.	Foster the art and science of staff development through research, standard setting, and issues management.	NA	X	X		X		*Trendlines; Journal for Nurses in Staff Development*

Organization	Membership	Purpose	Members				Publication
American Association for the History of Nursing (AAHN) PO Box 90803, Washington, DC 20090 [1982] http://www.aahn.org/aahn.html/	Anyone interested in purpose of the association.	Educate public about history and heritage of nursing; support historical research; promote development of centers for preservation of historical materials; disseminate information on nursing history.	NA			X	*Bulletin*
North American Nursing Diagnosis Association (NANDA) 1211 Locust St., Philadelphia, PA 19107 [1981] http://www.nanda.org/	Any RN interested in nursing diagnosis.	Develop a taxonomy of nursing diagnosis.	900		X	X	*Nursing Diagnosis*

Related Organizations

National Association for Practical Nurse Education and Service (NAPNES) 1400 Spring St., Suite 310, Silver Spring, MD 20910 [1941] http://www.napnes.org/	LPNs/LVNs, RNs, nurse educators, physicians, administrators, and consumers interested in practical nursing; agency members.	Improve and extend PN education to meet public needs.	NA	X	X	X	*Journal of Practical Nursing*

(continued)

Appendix 4 (continued)

Organization and year established[a]	Membership eligibility[b]	Primary purpose	Membership size (approximate)	Certification/ Accreditation[d]	Standards set and published	Legislative activities[e]	Research activities[f]	Publications[h] (journals, newsletters)
					Activities[c]			
National Federation of Licensed Practical Nurses (NFLPN) 1418 Aversboro Rd., Garner, NC 27529 [1949] http://www.nflpn.com/	State organizations made up of LPNs/LVNs and individual LPNs.	Secure recognition and effective utilization of LPNs; promote LPN welfare; improve standards of practice and education.	NA		×	×	×	Licensed Practical Nurse

[a] The organization may have been established under another name.

[b] Many organizations have associate membership for students and interested LPN/LVNs or others, and corporate membership. Some of these special categories have been noted; for more detailed information on others, make direct contact.

[c] All organizations have meetings or conventions, provide continuing education, and carry out public relations activities of some sort to educate or influence the public about themselves. Many offer other benefits such as insurance, credit cards, travel discounts, and so on.

[d] Certification/accreditation is often done by a separately incorporated organization.

[e] Legislative activities usually include staying on top of legislative and governmental issues and actions, informing members on these affairs, and providing information to legislators. Not all organizations actively lobby (often inappropriate to their mission or tax status). Others have lobbyists on staff or subcontract for these services.

[f] Research activities may include data collection and/or dissemination, research projects, funding for research, and educating on research.

[g] Accreditation also done (this may be through a separate corporation).

[h] Write to the organization for more details on the frequency of periodicals, and a complete list of other publications.

Note: This list is not all-inclusive. An extensive list of nursing organizations is available electronically at: http:www.nursingcenter.com/ or http://www.nursingworld.org/. Other information on organizations can also be found in Joel LA, Kelly's *Dimensions of Professional Nursing,* 9th ed. New York: McGraw-Hill, 2003 (Chapters 26 and 27).

Appendix 5 Specialty Certifications[a]

Specialty	Credential	Eligibility[b]	Certifying organization	Recertification	Numbers certified (2004)	Fee[c]
Addictions Nursing	CARN	Practicing as RN for 3 years, 4000 hours in addiction practice in last 5 years	Addictions Nursing Certification Board, 11 Glenwood Avenue, Suite A, Raleigh, NC 27603 www.IntNSA.org	Every 4 years	963 (both credentials)	$175–260
	CARN-AP	Current CARN cert., or CARN eligible; master's degree, and 500 hours supervised clinical experience				$275–375
Case Manager (multidisciplinary)	CCM	For nurses: RN, 12/24 months of specific experiential requirements; a post-secondary degree program in a field that promotes the psychosocial or vocational well-being of consumers	Commission for Case Management Certification (CCMC), 1835 Rohlwing Road, Suite D, Rolling Meadows, IL 60008 http://www.ccmcertification.org/	Every 5 years	26,000 (majority RNs)	$275
Childbirth Education (multidisciplinary)	LCCE (formerly ACCE)	Experienced childbirth educator, or midwife or midwifery student, or have successfully completed the Lamaze Childbirth Educator Program	Lamaze International, 2025 M Street, NW, Suite 800, Washington, DC 20036-3309 http://www.lamaze.org/	N/A	3,600	$160–325

(continued)

Specialty	Credential	Eligibility[b]	Certifying organization	Recertification	Numbers certified (2004)	Fee[c]
Critical Care Nursing	CCNS		American Assoc. of Critical Care Nurses Cert. Corp., 101 Columbia, Aliso Viejo, CA 92656 http://www.certcorp.org/	Every 4 years	415	$325–425
• Acute/Critical-Care Clinical Nurse Specialist		Master's degree; 500 hours in direct clinical practice in master's degree program or augmented with faculty supervision.				
• Acute/Critical Care to Adult, Neonatal, or Pediatric Patients (each awarded separately)	CCRN	1750 hours in specialty in last 2 years, with half of hours during most recent year		Every 4 years	42,337 (adult) 530 (neonatal) 1,324 (peds)	$220–300
Dermatology Nursing	DNC	Have a minimum of 2 years of dermatology nursing experience as an RN; minimum of 2000 hours of work experience in dermatology nursing within the past 2 years in a general staff, administrative, teaching, or research capacity	Dermatology Nursing Certification Board, East Holly Ave., Box 56, Pitman, NJ 08071-0056 http://www.dnanurse.org/	Every 3 years	200	$175–250
Developmental Disabilities Nursing	CDDN	4000 hours of practice in the last 5 years	Developmental Disabilities Nurses Association, 1733 H St., Suite 330, PMB 1214, Blaine, WA 98230 http://ddna.bluestep.net/	N/A	N/A	N/A

Specialty	Credential	Requirements	Certifying Body	Renewal	Number	Cost
Diabetes Educator (multidisciplinary)	CDE	2 years professional practice in diabetes self-management training with a minimum of 1000 hours of diabetes self-management training, and current employment as a diabetes educator of at least 4 hours weekly	National Certification Board for Diabetes Educators, 330 East Algonquin Road, Suite 4, Arlington Heights, IL 60005 http://www.ncbde.org/	Every 5 years	13,987	$250
Dialysis Nursing • Hemodialysis • Peritoneal	CHN CPDN	One year of specialty or ESRD facility experience	Board of Nephrology Examiners, Nursing and Technology, PO Box 15945-282 Lenexa, KS 66285 http://www.goamp.com/bonent/	Every 4 years	4,000 (both credentials)	$195
Emergency Nursing	CEN	2 years experience in specialty recommended	Board of Certification for Emergency Nursing, 915 Lee Street, Des Plaines, IL 60016-6569 http://www.ena.org/bcen/	Every 4 years	26,000	$220–340
Flight Nursing	CFRN	2 years experience in specialty recommended	Board of Certification for Emergency Nursing, 915 Lee Street, Des Plaines, IL 60016-6569 http://www.ena.org/bcen/	Every 4 years.	1,200	$230–370
Gastroenterology Nursing	CGRN	4000 hours or 2 years of full-time practice in a GI specialty in the last 5 years	Certifying Board of Gastroenterology Nurses and Associates, 401 N. Michigan Ave., Chicago, IL 60611-4267 http://www.cbgna.org/	Every 5 years	3,000	$300–385

(continued)

Specialty	Credential	Eligibility[b]	Certifying organization	Recertification	Numbers certified (2004)	Fee[c]
Health Care Quality (multidisciplinary)	CPHQ	For RN, medical records technologist, physicians. Minimum of associate degree; practiced 2 years in health care quality: case-, utilization-, and/or risk management activities in last 5 years by date of exam	Healthcare Quality Certification Board, Box 19604, Lenexa, KS 66285-9604 http://www.cphq.org/	Every 2 years	7,600	$370–440
HIV/AIDS Nursing	ACRN	At least 2 years of experience in clinical practice, education, management, or research related to HIV/AIDS nursing are recommended	HIV/AIDS Nursing Certification Board, Professional Testing Corporation (PTC), 1350 Broadway, 17th Floor, New York, NY 10018 http://www.ptcny.com/	Every 4 years	N/A	$260–400
	AACRN	Master's degree or higher in nursing; a minimum of 3 years experience as a registered nurse; and a minimum of 2000 hours of advanced HIV/AIDS nursing practice in the past 5 years			N/A	$350–450
Holistic Nursing	HNC	Minimum of BSN; 1000 hours or 1 year practice as a holistic nurse; minimum of 48 contact hours of CE in holistic nursing in last 2 years	American Holistic Nurses' Certification Corporation, 811 Linden Loop, Cedar Park, TX 78613 http://ahna.org/edu/certification.html/	Every 5 years	112	$150–210

Specialty	Credential	Requirements	Certifying Organization	Recertification	Number Certified	Cost
Hospice and Palliative Care Nursing	CHPN APRN, BC-PCM	2 years hospice and palliative care experience. Advanced practice, minimum of a master's degree and experiential requirements	National Board for Certification of Hospice Nurses, Medical Center East, Suite 375, 211 N. Whitfield Street, Pittsburgh, PA 15206-3021 http://www.nbchpn.org/	Every 4 years Every 4 years	8,200 (both credentials)	$245–345
Infection Control (multidisciplinary)	CIC	Practice in area for 2 years with a minimum of 800 hours in practice as defined as infection control; RN, or baccalaureate in health care field, or waiver	Certification Board of Infection Control and Epidemiology, 8310 Nieman Road, Lenexa, KS 66285-9554 http://www.cbic.org/	Every 5 years	5,000	$295
Infusion Nursing	CRNI	1600 hours IV experience in last 2 years	IV Nurses Certification Corp., 220 Norwood Park, South Norwood, MA 02062 http://www.ins1.org/	Every 3 years	3,600	$225–400
Lactation Consultant	IBCLC	BSN needs 2500 hours experience; others with less education require 4000 hours experience	International Board of Lactation Consultant Examiners, 7309 Arlington Blvd., Suite 300, Falls Church, VA 22042-3215 http://www.iblce.org/	Every 5 years	8,000	$395
Legal Nurse Consultant	LNCC	Practiced 5 years as an RN; have evidence of 2000 hours of legal nurse consulting experience within the 3 years prior to the application.	American Legal Nurse Consultant Board, 401 N. Michigan Ave., Suite 2200, Chicago, IL 60611-4267 http://www.aalnc.org/	Every 5 years	4,000	$275–375

(continued)

Appendix 5 (continued)[a]

Specialty	Credential	Eligibility[b]	Certifying organization	Recertification	Numbers certified (2004)	Fee[c]
Managed Care Nursing	CMCN	Must have 1 year full-time employment as RN/LPN in areas of managed care; or 2 years as RN/LPN providing direct or indirect care in an acute care, outpatient, skilled nursing, or mental health facility or other health care organization, or as an educator or consultant; or 1 year acceptable case management employment experience.	American Board of Managed Care Nursing, 4435 Waterfront Drive, Suite 101, Glen Allen, VA 23060 http://www.abncm.org/	Every 3 years	2,000	$225–395
Nephrology Nursing	CNN	2 years nephrology experience in last 3 years; 30 CE credits in nephrology nursing	Nephrology Nursing Certification Board, East Holly Ave,, PO Box 56, Pitman, NJ 08071-0056 http://nncc-exam.org/	Every 3 years	N/A	$175–225
Neuroscience Nursing	CNRN	2 years in specialty and active clinical practice	American Board of Neuroscience Nursing, 4700 W. Lake Ave,, Glenview, IL 60025 http://www.aann.org/credential/	Every 5 years	1,500	$215–300
Nurse Administrator— Long-Term Care	CDONA/ LTC	Director of nursing (DON) or assistant DON administrator in a long-term care setting for at least 12 months in the past 5 years. Former DONs and assistant DONs are eligible to take the exam.	NADONA/LTC Certification Registrar, 10101 Alliance Drive #140, Cincinnati, OH 45242 http://www.nadona.org/	Every 5 years	4,000	$150–225

Specialty	Certification	Requirements	Certifying Body	Renewal	Number	Fee
Nurse Anesthetist	CRNA	Graduate of accredited educational program (post-baccalaureate)	Council on Certification of Nurse Anesthetists, 222 S. Prospect Ave., Park Ridge, IL 60068 http://www.aana.com/	Every 2 years	28,000	$600
Nurse Midwifery and Midwifery (multidisciplinary for midwifery)	CNM CM	Graduate of accredited or preaccredited educational program	American College of Nurse-Midwives Certification Council, 8201 Corporate Drive, Suite 550, Landover, MD 20785 http://www.accmidwife.org/	Every 8 years	8,400	$567
Nutrition Support Nursing	CNSN	2 years experience in specialty	National Board for Nutrition Support Certification, 8630 Fenton St., Suite 412, Silver Spring, MD 20910 http://www.nutritioncertify.org/	Every 5 years	161	$200–275
Women's Health/Primary Care Nursing	Check website for other certifications in this area	Specific clinical practice and in some instances educational requirements; for all categories, practice/experience/employment is defined as direct patient care, education, administration, and/or research	National Certification Corporation for OB, GYN, Neonatal Nursing Specialities, Box 11082, Chicago, IL 60611-0082 http://www.nccnet.org/	Every 3 years		$135–185
• Breastfeeding	BF				121	
• Electronic Fetal Monitoring	EFM				1,074	
• Inpatient OB	RNC, INPT				28,763	
• Lo-Risk Neonatal	RNS, LRN				3,779	
• Material Newborn	RNC, NM				1,919	
• Neonatal Intensive Care	RNC, NIC				10,158	

(continued)

Appendix 5 (*continued*)[a]

Specialty	Credential	Eligibility[b]	Certifying organization	Recertification	Numbers certified (2004)	Fee[c]
• Neonatal Nurse Practitioner	RN, C	Advanced practice			3,143	$300
• Women's Health Care Nurse Practitioner	RNC	Advanced practice			10,707	$300
Occupational Health						
• Occupational Health Nursing	COHN	Specific courses related to occupational health nursing in past 5 years, 2 years (4000 hours) in occupational health nursing practice Additionally, requires BSN	American Board for Occupational Health Nurses, Inc., 201 East Ogden, Suite 114, Hinsdale, IL 60521-3652 http://www.abohn.org/	Every 5 years	6,700 (both credentials)	$300
• Occupational Health Nursing Specialist	COHN-S					
• Occupational Health Nurse Case Manager	COHN/CM COHN-S/CM	COHN or COHN-S and 10 CE hours in case management in last 5 years		Every 5 years	N/A	$150
Oncology Nursing						
• Generalist	OCN	12 months of RN practice in last 3 years; 1000 hours of oncology in last 30 months	Oncology Nursing Certification Corporation, 125 Enterprise Drive, Pittsburgh, PA 15275-1214 http://www.oncc.org/	Every 4 years	19,045	$220–320

Specialty	Abbreviation	Requirements	Certifying Body	Renewal	Number	Cost
• Advanced	AOCN	30 months of RN practice in last 5 years; 2000 hours of oncology in last 5 years; master's degree or higher		Every 4 years	1,276	$250–350
Ophthalmic Nursing	CBNO	4000 hours experience in specialty	National Certifying Board for Ophthalmic Registered Nurses, 655 Beach St., Box 193030, San Francisco, CA 94119 http://www.asorn.org/	Every 5 years	250	$275–350
Orthopaedic Nursing	ONC	2 years experience as RN, 1000 hours in specialty in last 3 years	Orthopaedic Nurses Certification Board, East Holly Ave., Box 56, Pitman, NJ 08071 http://www.orthonurse.org/	Every 5 years	3,300	$205–285
Otorhinolaryngology and Head-Neck Nursing	CORLN	Recommended at least 3 years practice in the specialty area	The National Certifying Board of Otorhinolaryngology and Head–Neck Nurses, 116 Canal Street, Suite A, New Smyrna Beach, FL 32168 http://www.sohnnurse.com/	Every 5 years	300	$275–375
Pain Management (multidisciplinary)	FAAPM	Diplomate, fellow, or clinical associate status, requiring doctorate, master's, or bachelor's degree respectively and experience	American Academy of Pain Management, 13947 Mono Way #4, Sonora, CA 95370 http://www.aapainmanage.org/	Every 4 years	N/A	$275
Pediatric Nursing • General	CPN	2 years or 3600 hours in pediatric nursing practice	National Certification Board of Pediatric Nurse Practitioners and Nurses, 800 South Frederick Ave., Suite 104, Gaithersburg, MD 20877-41150 http://www.pnpcert.org/	Annually	5,000	$280
• Nurse practitioner	CPNP	Master's or post-master's PNP program		Annually	9,000	$375

(continued)

Appendix 5 (continued)[a]

Specialty	Credential	Eligibility[b]	Certifying organization	Recertification	Numbers certified (2004)	Fee[c]
Pediatric Oncology Nursing	CPON	12 months experience as RN in last 3 years; 1000 hours in pediatric oncology within last 30 months	Oncology Nursing Certification Corporation, 125 Enterprise Drive Pittsburgh, PA 15275-1214 http://www.oncc.org/	Every 4 years	802	$250–350
Perianesthesia Nursing		1800 hours direct perianesthesia practice in last 2 years	American Board of Post-Anesthesia Nursing Certification, 475 Riverside Dr., New York, NY 10115-0089 http://www.cpancapa.org/	Every 3 years		$235–335
• Post-Anesthesia Nurse	CPAN				3,957	
• Ambulatory Perianesthesia Nurse	CAPA				1,803	
Perioperative Nursing						
• Operating Room Nurse	CNOR	2400 hours in OR practice and been employed in the last 2 years	National Certification Board of Perioperative Nursing, 2170 S. Parker Rd., Suite 295, Denver, CO 80231 http://www.certboard.org/	Every 5 years	28,700	$250–350
• RN First Assistant	CRNFA	Certified as CNOR; 2000 hours of practice as first assistant with 500 hours in past 2 years; formal RNFA program; BSN		Every 5 years	1,650	$425–550

Specialty	Abbreviation	Requirements	Certifying Organization	Recertification	Number Certified	Fee
Plastic and Reconstructive Surgical Nursing	CPSN	2 years experience in specialty within last 5 years; and have spent at least 50% of practice hours in plastic surgical nursing during 2 of the preceding 5 years.	Plastic Surgical Nursing Certification Board, East Holly Ave., Box 56, Pitman, NJ 08071 http://www.aspsn.org/	Every 3 years	425	$195–295
Rehabilitation Nursing • Rehabilitation Nurse	CRRN	Education in rehab nursing; 2 years practice in specialty in last 5 years	Rehabilitation Nursing Certification Board, 4700 West Lake Ave., Glenview, IL 60025-1485 http://www.rehabnurse.org/	Every 5 years	12,500 (both credentials)	$195–285
• Advanced	CRRN-A	Advanced practice; master's required		Every 5 years		$240–320
School Nursing	CSN	Baccalaureate degree, 3 years experience in school nursing	National Board for Certification of School Nurses, Inc., c/o National Association of School Nurses, 1416 Park Street, Suite A, Castle Rock, CO 80109 http://www.ncbsn.com/	N/A	1,800	$200–275
Urology Nursing • Urological Nurse	CURN	One year of experience in specialty	Certification Board for Urologic Nurses and Associates, East Holly Ave., Box 56, Pitman, NJ 08071-0056 http://www.suna.org/	Every 3 years	519 (all credentials)	$195–255
• NP	CUNP	Master's preparation				
• CNS	CUCNS	Master's preparation				

(continued)

Appendix 5 (continued)[a]

Specialty	Credential	Eligibility[b]	Certifying organization	Recertification	Numbers certified (2004)	Fee[c]
Wound, Ostomy, Continence Nursing		Baccalaureate degree; specialty education accredited by WOCN, or graduate-level program in nursing with clinical work in the specialty, or 1500 clinical hours and 50 CEUs in past 5 years	Wound, Ostomy, Continence, Nursing Certification Board, 555 East Wells Street, Suite 1100, Milwaukee, WI 53202-3823 http://www.wocncb.org/	Every 5 years	N/A	1 exam: $225
• Wound, Ostomy, Continence	CWOCN					2 exams: $275
• Wound	CWCN					3 exams: $300
• Ostomy	COCN					
• Continence	CCCN					

[a]Certifications offered by the American Nurses Credentialing Center (ANCC) are not included in this appendix, but presented in Exhibit 13.2 of Chapter 13. ANCC offers 39 certifications, and currently certifies over 145,000 nurses. Information on eligibility requirements can be obtained from ANCC, 8515 Georgia Avenue, Silver Spring, MD 20910-3492, http://www.nursingworld.org/.

[b]The RN is assumed for eligibility, except if noted as multidisciplinary.

[c]The fee cited here is for initial certification; renewal fees are generally less; reduced rates are commonly offered to members of specialty associations.

Appendix 6 Basics of Parliamentary Procedure

By-laws. An organization's by-laws are the basis on which it functions. They include:

- Name
- Purposes
- Functions
- Requirements for membership
- Dues
- The officers
- Governing body
- Committees
- Other organizational units and their responsibilities
- How elected or appointed
- How amendments are made
- The parliamentary authority used to conduct business (often *Robert's Rules of Order Newly Revised*)

Usual *order of business* at a meeting (may have additional parts at a convention):

1. Call to order
2. Minutes of previous meetings
3. Reports of officers, boards, standing committees
   Executive reports
   Executive announcements
   Reports of:
       President
       Vice-President
       Secretary
       Treasurer
       Board of Directors
       Standing committees
4. Reports of special committees
5. Announcements
6. Unfinished business
7. New business
8. Adjournment

Motions are proposals or suggestions that initiate action or enable the assembly to express itself. To make a motion:

1. Stand or raise your hand or go to a microphone when indicated.
2. Wait for the chair's signal to go ahead.
3. Address the presiding officer as "Madame (or Mister) Chairman," "Chairperson," "President," or "Speaker."
4. Identify yourself by name and whatever else is customary in that organization, such as office, affiliation, city, or state.
5. State the motion clearly and as briefly as possible. Write out a motion if time permits, for accuracy and the record. Frequently a written motion is given to the secretary for the minutes.
6. Ask to speak to the motion after making it. Do not speak first and then make the motion. Wait for the second before presenting your statement.
7. The chair will call for a second. (Not required if it is a committee motion.)
8. For seconding, rise, identify yourself, and say "I second the motion."
9. If no one seconds, the motion is automatically lost and not recorded.
10. If the motion is seconded, the chair says, "It has been moved and seconded that . . . Is there any discussion?"
11. If there is a discussion, it may take the form of comments and/or a motion suggesting an amendment. The maker of the motion speaks first.
12. An amendment, if any, is voted on first, then the original motion with the amendment, if it was accepted.

13. Discussion may be stopped by saying. "I move to close debate" or "I call for the question." This is not debatable and if carried, the motion on the floor is voted on immediately.
14. There may be motions to table a motion (set it aside temporarily—sometimes permanently), to postpone action, or to refer it to a committee. All avoid further action at that time.
15. If an action is taken (motion passed or rejected) that, for whatever reason, people regret, someone on the *prevailing* side may ask to bring it before the assembly again. Anyone can second. This takes precedence and is acted on at once, following the usual procedure. The result may be the same or different, usually different.

Resolutions are indications of the organization's position on key issues:

1. Resolutions are submitted to a resolutions committee by any member, committee, or other organizational entity.
2. The format usually begins with: Whereas (giving one or more reasons) and ends with Therefore be it resolved: (stating one or more resolutions related to the "whereas").
3. Resolutions are reviewed by the committee, and sometimes edited or combined with a similar resolution, with permission of the originators.
4. Resolutions usually go to the board, but do not necessarily have to be approved by them, depending on policy.
5. A rejected resolution can usually be presented from the floor.
6. At conventions, there may be an open resolutions committee hearing in which resolutions are discussed and debated without formal parliamentary procedure. They may then be changed before formal presentation at the business meeting, saving time and confusion.
7. Resolutions are voted on like motions.
8. Courtesy resolutions at the end of the meeting are usually formalities, showing appreciation to various people or groups.

Appendix 7 Distinguished Nurses of the Past: Fifty Nurses Who Made a Difference*

Names, dates, place of birth	Education and selected honors	Key events; Contributions
Alline, Anna (later Brown, 1923) 1864–1935 East Machias, ME	Normal school in Iowa; Brooklyn Homeopathic Hosp. Trng Sch for Nsg, 1893; Post-grad study Gen. Mem. Hosp. NYC 1896; Enrolled in Teachers College (TC) Columbia U, NYC, 1900.	Pioneer in nsg ed.; studied under Richards and served as her asst. One of first two students to enroll in new hospital economics courses at TC. Stayed as director and teacher; helped to ensure continuity of program. First inspector of nsg schools for NY state board. Treasurer Am Society of Superintendents of Training schools for nursing (ASSTSN) later NLNE and NLN. Life member NLNE. Numerous articles in *American Journal of Nsg (AJN)*.
Arnstein, Margaret 1904–1972 New York City	AB, Smith College, 1925; Presbyterian Hosp Sch Nsg, 1928; AM, TC, 1929; MS, Johns Hopkins U, 1934; Honorary degrees: Smith College, 1950; Wayne State U, 1964, U of Mich, 1972. Number of honors: first woman to receive Rockefeller Public Service Award (Lasker Award), USPHS Distinguished Service Award; APHA Sedgwick Mem Medal.	Leader and educator in public health nursing, US and abroad. Encouraged by Wald, close friend of family. As nurse-researcher and head of nsg div. of USPHS, increased its ability to provide statistical information. (25-year career with USPHS.) Helped launch plan to increase nsg students for WW II. Worked with WHO to prepare guide for surveying nsg services in various countries. Influential in improving health care and developing services in Balkans after WW II. Sr Advisor for intl health (AID and Rockefeller Foundation) 1945. Dean, Yale Sch of Nsg. Author: many articles; coauthor *Communicable Disease Control*, 1962.

(continued)

*For further information about these and other nursing leaders, see Chapters 1 and 2, as well as References and Bibliography for these chapters.

Appendix 7 (continued)

Names, dates, place of birth	Education and selected honors	Key events; Contributions
Barton, Clarissa (Clara) 1821–1912 N. Oxford, MA	Liberal Institute, Clinton, NY, 1850–51. No nsg ed. More than 25 honors, including Iron Cross (Germany); Medal of Intl RC; Sultan's decoration (Turkey).	Founder of Am Red Cross (ARC). Major contrib to nsg in disaster nsg. Early Civil War nurse, present at many battles, known as "Angel of the Battlefield." With support of Pres Lincoln in 1865, set up office to locate MIAs. Later, went to Europe for health, studied work of Intl Red Cross (IRC). Served as volunteer nurse in Franco-Prussian War. In 1881, was successful in persuading US govt of need for an ARC. As president, participated in numerous disaster relief activities in US and abroad. Author: reports, books, articles about RC. Kept more than 40 diaries.
Bickerdyke, Mary Ann 1817–1901 Knox Co, OH	Possibly studied under Dr. Hussey, who ran Physio-Botanic Med College, Cinn. Honors: Mother Bickerdyke Day, Kansas, 1897; statue in Galesburg, IL, "Victory freighter," WW II, named after her.	Volunteer nurse in Civil War. Known as "Mother" or "General" Bickerdyke and "cyclone in calico," as she nursed Union soldiers. Enraged Army doctors because she was advocate of soldiers; saw that they were cared for as well as possible. Became friend of Grant and Sherman, who supported her against them; e.g. campaigned for women nurses in army, physicians objected, Grant approved; found supplies for wounded not reaching them, remedied situation with Grant's support. Rode ambulance wagon with Sherman's march through Georgia, and cared for freed Union prisoners from Andersonville. Throughout war, searched battlefields for wounded. Successfully raised funds throughout North for US Sanitary Commission, between battles.

Names, dates, place of birth	Education and selected honors	Key events; Contributions
Breckenridge, Mary 1881?–1965 Memphis, TN	St. Luke's Hospital Sch Nsg, 1910; Postgrad course in pub health nsg, TC, 1921; certified nurse-midwife, and postgrad trng in London, 1923–24. Honorary LLD, U of Kentucky. Honors: French medal; NLN Nutting Award; other awards from natl and community groups. ANA Hall of Fame. Women's Hall of Fame (Seneca Falls, NY).	Best known as founder of Frontier Nsg Service of Kentucky, offering maternal-child care to people in isolated mountains. Director, 40 years. Also founded school of midwifery there. Earlier: retired from nsg in 1918 to bear children. After their death, worked for US Children's Bureau. Eventually went to France, organizing relief for pregnant women and children. Organized child hygiene and visiting nurse association (VNA) there.
Browne, Mother de Sales (Frances Browne) 1826–1910 Westmoreland, PA	Home education. No formal nsg ed.	Entered Convent of Mercy, Pgh, PA: was moved to DC to take charge of new infirmary for sick poor. Ordered to Vicksburg to establish school; organized parishioners to visit and care for sick and poor. In Civil War, cared for Confederate soldiers under harsh conditions in various hospitals, escaping as Yankees captured towns, and nursing in next place. Eventually Mother Superior for 30 yrs.
Craig, Leroy 1887–1976 Dixmont, ME	McLean Hospital Trng Sch for Nurses, Waverly, MA, 1912. Honors: PA Nurses Assn citation for contrib to psych nurs and promoting legislation affecting status of men (1956).	In vanguard of political and educational activities promoting professional recognition and opportunities for men nurses. Instrumental in federal legislation allowing male nurses to be commissioned as officers in armed services as parity with women. (Wife was Army nurse recruiter.) Appointed as founding director and supt of nurses in Men's Nursing Dept, Pa Hosp for Mental and Nervous Diseases, concurrently serving as 1st director, Pa Hosp Sch of Nsg for Men (1914), remaining active in both until retirement (1956). Established innovations in nursing curriculum; wrote several articles noting contributions of men nurses.

(continued)

Appendix 7 (continued)

Names, dates, place of birth	Education and selected honors	Key events; Contributions
Curtis, Namahyoke Gertrude (Sockum) 1861–1935 Raleigh, NC	Snell Seminary, San Francisco, 1888. No formal nsg ed. Honors: Given high official commendation for leadership of "immune nurses."	Noted for being commissioned by War Dept. to serve as contract nurse in Spanish–American War, recruiting also 30 additional "immune nurses," black women who had had yellow fever. (Later received lifetime gov't pension for this.) Descended from family of German, Afro-American, and native American stock. Married secretly at 18 to man who later graduated from Northwestern University Medical School, Chicago. There, became instrumental in efforts to found Provident Hospital; became active in local, state, and national politics and held number of politically appointed govt positions in Chicago and Washington, DC, where husband was CEO of Freedman's Hospital. Served under Clara Barton in Galveston Flood in Texas as ARC volunteer. Remained in public service during WW I. Buried in Arlington Cemetery.
Davis, Mary E.P. c. 1840–1924 New Brunswick, Canada	Mass Gen Hosp Trng School for Nurses, Boston 1878. Honors: ANA Hall of Fame.	Largely responsible, with Palmer, for planning the organization and financing of AJN. As business manager, made it self-supporting. One of the founders of ASSTSN. Previously supt. of hospital and training school, Hosp. Univ. of Penn; progressive attitude about ed. Helped found Mass Nurses Assn; wrote many journal articles.

Names, dates, place of birth	Education and selected honors	Key events; Contributions
Delano, Jane 1862–1919 Montour Falls, NY	Bellevue Trng Sch for Nurses, NYC, 1886. Honors: Disting Service Medal (US and ARC) Sculpture in ARC hdq, DC; ANA Hall of Fame.	Appointed Supt Army Nurse corps (ANC) 1910. As director of Dept. Nsg, ARC (held simultaneously with ANC position), perfected plan, with ANA, to have 9000 qualified nurses ready when US declared war on Germany (supplied 20,000 nurses). Said to have rendered greatest service of any US woman to help win WW I. Previously held major positions at U of PA and Bellevue Hospitals. Author: book on home care of sick. Died in France making final inspection of hospitals. Buried with military honors at Arlington Natl cemetery.
Dix, Dorothea 1802–1887 Hambden, ME	School in Boston, then studied privately and in libraries, public lectures. Honors: US stamp in her honor; named park in Hambden; ANA Hall of Fame.	Spearheaded national reforms in treatment of mentally ill and disabled. Opened school for small children at age 14 and continued to teach. Outraged at treatment of women in a "house of correction," most of whom were mentally ill; began campaign for improvement with varying success. Was recognized, and when volunteered, was appointed Supt of US Army Nurses for Civil War, set up infirmaries and recruited and screened nurses. Was undermined by requirement that nurses responsible only to doctors. Never regained momentum after war ended.

(continued)

Appendix 7 (continued)

Names, dates, place of birth	Education and selected honors	Key events; Contributions
Dock, Lavinia 1858–1956 Harrisburg, PA	Bellevue Trng Sch for Nurses, NY, 1886. Honors: ANA Hall of Fame.	Active in early development of nursing organizations in US, and of ICN. Edited "Foreign Dept" of *AJN* for 23 years. Militant woman suffragist and ardent crusader for rights of poor and workers; pacifist. Supported concept of "one world." Held key positions at Bellevue, Johns Hopkins, IL Trng Sch for Nurses; worked with Wald at Henry Street Settlement; also nurse in several social organizations. Held office in ASSTSN and ICN. Author of books on materia medica, nsg history, Red Cross history, "Hygiene and Morality" (about venereal disease, then very daring), and numerous articles.
Franklin, Martha 1870–1968 New Haven, CT	Women's Hosp Trng Sch for Nurses, Philadelphia, 1898. Honors: ANA Hall of Fame.	Only Afro-American graduate of her class. Over next 10 years, recognized and fought discrimination in nursing as well as society. One of earliest to pass state registration exams. Primarily did private duty, but campaigned nationally for racial equality in nsg. Founded and first president of Natl Assn Colored Grad Nurses (NACGN).
Freeman, Ruth 1906–1982 Methuen, MA	Mt. Sinai Sch Nsg NYC, 1927; BS Columbia U, NY, 1934; MA, NYU, 1939; EdD, NYU, 1951. Many honors incl: ANA McIver Award; NLN Nutting Award; APHA Bronson Award; and named award by Nsg section; IRC Nightingale Medal; honorary member, Sigma Theta Tau.	Leader in public health nsg; helped professionalize field through teachings, writings, work in prof. orgs. Worked at Henry St. Visiting Nurse Service; then taught NYU; U. Minn, Johns Hopkins. Stressed interdisciplinary practice and communication. Pres, NLN, Natl Health Council; VP; NOPHN; key positions, APHA. Several books; many articles

Names, dates, place of birth	Education and selected honors	Key events; Contributions
Gardner, Mary 1871–1961 Newton, MA	Newton Hosp Sch Nsg RI, 1905; Honorary MA, Brown U, 1918.	One of earliest directors and organizers of a visiting nurse association (VNA). One of founders of NOPHN, first secretary and second president. Key positions in Providence District Nurses Assn (RI). ARC Town and Country Nsg Service: as special advisor to ARC, surveyed public health nsg in Eastern Europe (1920). Considered intl authority on pub health nsg. Prolific writer including *Public Health Nursing*, first text on subject; translated into many languages; book on phn admin; novel, *Katherine Kent*, and numerous articles.
Goodrich, Annie 1866–1954 New Brunswick, NJ	New York Hosp Trng Sch for Nsg, NYC, 1892. Honorary Degrees: DSC, Mount Holyoke, 1921; MA, Yale, 1923; LLD Russell Sage College, 1936. Many honors incl: NLN Nutting Award; US Disting Service Award; several from France and Belgium; ANA Hall of Fame.	Distinguished educator and inspiring leader, who aroused public to need for higher educational standards for nurses. First dean, Yale University School for Nursing. Key positions in various hospitals/schools in New York City, asst professor, TC, NY, Dir of Nsg, Henry Street Settlement, Dean, Army School of Nursing. Held major offices in ANA, ASSTSN, and other US nursing organizations and ICN. Author, *Social and Ethical Significance of Nursing*, 1932
Gretter (Mrs.), Lystra 1858–1951 Bayfield, Ontario, Canada	Buffalo Gen Hosp Trng Sch for Nurses, Buffalo, NY, 1888.	Leader in many forward trends: first 8-hour day for student nurses; one of first to employ graduate nurses to supervise and teach students (instead of doctors). "Moving Spirit" of group that wrote Nightingale Pledge. Principal, Trng School, Harper Hospital, Detroit, Director, Detroit VNA. Major offices in state and national nsg org; Charter member, NOPHN.

(continued)

Appendix 7 (continued)

Names, dates, place of birth	Education and selected honors	Key events; Contributions
Hall, Lydia 1906–1969 New York City	Gettysburg College; NY Hosp Sch Nsg 1927; BS in PHN, TC, 1937; MA, TC, 1942; doctoral study TC. Honors: TC alumni Dist. Achievement Award; hospital named after her (NY); ANA Hall of Fame.	Known for professional care model, considered by some as a type of nsg theory. At Montefiore Hosp, NY, developed unit (Loeb Center) in which nurses selected pts for their potential for rehab, gave prof care, assessing pt needs on one-to-one basis. Had been at VNS of NY, Fordham Hosp Sch Nsg, and NY Heart Assn. Actively involved in ANA, NLN, NOPHN, and volunteer committees in NY. Sought-after speaker, prolific author particularly about Loeb Center concept.
Henderson, Virginia A. 1897–1996 Kansas City, MO	Army Sch of Nsg, Washington, DC, 1921; Teachers College, Columbia Univ., BSN, MA, 1934–1948; 12 honorary doctorates; Christianne Reimann Prize (ICN); ANA Hall of Fame.	A modern legend in nursing, Virginia A. Henderson has earned the title "foremost nurse of the 20th century." Her contributions are compared to those of Florence Nightingale because of their far-reaching effects on the national and international nursing communities. Henderson's most important writings were the first to emphasize science and theory as the basis for nursing practice. Currently available in 27 languages, these classic texts are credited as having changed the way nurses are educated throughout the world. Henderson spent her early career at Teachers College, and accepted a position at Yale University School of Nursing in 1953 as research associate where she stayed for the rest of her career.

Names, dates, place of birth	Education and selected honors	Key events; Contributions
Kimber, Diana (Sister Mary Diana) ?–1928 Oxfordshire, England	Bellevue Hosp Trng School, 1885; previous broad education in England and Germany.	Recognized as author of first scientific book written by a nurse for nurses (anatomy and physiology); repeated editions between 1893 and 1948. Asst supt under Robb in Ill., then Old Charity Hospital in NYC. Returned to England; joined Anglican Sisterhood, whose chief work was public health nsg. Also contributed to welfare of sick nurses.
Kuehn, Ruth Perkins 1900–1986 Sharon, WI	Children's Memorial Hosp, Chicago, 1925; BS 1931, MA 1934; PhD 1942, Ohio State U. Honors include: Sigma Theta Tau; received first mentor award 1985, from one of her protégés who was then president; also named endowed research award at Pitt.	Founder and first dean, University of Pgh. Sch of Nsg (1939), after demanding it be an autonomous school of nursing. Initiated nation's first CE workshop. First US dean to hold PhD. Developed master's and doctoral programs; pioneer in nursing research especially on method improvement and utilization of personnel. Pitt became first PA nursing school to admit Afro-American students and first to allow students to marry and complete program (was herself married to MD); mentor to future leaders. Previous positions as faculty at Ohio State. President of Sigma Theta Tau; VP; ANA; involved with ICN (had recruited international students since she became dean). Held other offices and committee assignments in nursing and nonnursing organizations; international consultant. Author, pediatric textbook, 1933, and coauthor, *Patterns of Patient Care*, first on team nursing research; also articles.

(continued)

Appendix 7 (continued)

Names, dates, place of birth	Education and selected honors	Key events; Contributions
Lambertsen, Eleanor 1915–1998	Overlook Hosp Sch of Nsg, Summit, NJ, 1938; Teachers College, Columbia, BS 1949, MA 1950, EdD 1957; R. Louise McManus Award, Teachers College; honorary recognition, ANA; membership, Institute of Medicine; honorary fellowship, AHA.	One of the most important national and international figures in nursing services of the century; pioneered the concept of team nursing and promoted professional education for leadership in nursing administration; the first Director, Division of Nursing and Assistant Secretary, Professional Services at the American Hospital Association; held the Helen Hartley chair at Teachers College and was Dean of the Cornell University–New York Hospital School of Nursing.
Maas, Clara 1876–1901 E. Orange, NJ	Newark German (Memorial) Hosp, Newark, NJ, 1895. Honors: commemorative stamp (Cuba and US) and medal (Franklin Mint); ANA Hall of Fame; NJ hospital named after her.	Young army nurse martyr who volunteered to participate in investigation of yellow fever transmission, in Cuba. Bitten by infected mosquito and died. Had offered services in Cuba and Philippines during Spanish–American War. Buried with military honors.
Mahoney, Mary 1845–1923 Boston, MA	N Eng Hosp for Women and Children, 1879, Boston. Honors: Mary Mahoney Award: named by NACGN, now given by ANA; ANA Hall of Fame.	First "Negro" nurse in US. Inspired black nurses to strive for better working conditions and facilities in "Negro" nursing schools and work toward combating racial discrimination. Primarily worked as private duty nurse in Boston. Life member of Natl Assn Colored Grad Nurses (NACGN).
Markolf, Ada (Stewart) 1870–1945 Braintree, MA	Waltham Trng Sch for Nurses, Waltham, MA, 1893. Later passed course on massage.	Best remembered as first industrial nurse hired by employer in US (VT Marble Co), followed by sister. Matron of hosp opened by Company (1896), for 2 years; then 20 years practicing massage and private duty. Retired at 47 to marry.

Names, dates, place of birth	Education and selected honors	Key events; Contributions
Maxwell, Anna 1851–1929 Bristol, NY	Boston City Hosp Trng Sch for Nurses, 1880. Many honors including: ANA Hall of Fame; Medal of Honor from France for organizing the nsg service of Presbyterian Hosp Unit in WW I. Buried with military honors in Arlington Cemetery.	Made nursing a more desirable occupation for women with high social standing, interpreting nsg to those outside the profession. Instituted standardization of nursing techniques and procedures. Active in ASSTSN, ANA, AJN; ICN. Key positions: Boston Trng School, St Luke's, and Presbyterian. NYC. In charge of Steinberg Hospital, GA, during Spanish–Am War. Coauthor of book on practical nursing.
McGarvah, Mary Eleanor 1886–1979 Windsor, Ontario, Canada	Farrand Trng Sch for Nurses, Harper Hosp, Detroit, 1911; Bachelor of Law, University of Detroit, 1929. Honors: named Humanitarian Award established by Am Assn Nurse Attorneys.	First nurse attorney; expert in public health law and regulation. After graduation from nsg school, did private duty, then joined Detroit Health Dept. Helped to establish prenatal clinics and registration of midwives. As supervisor in new special investigation division, found Health Dept needed legal/legislative clout, so became attorney. Was promoted to dir div and served Health Dept for 41 years, also maintaining private practice. Many accomplishments in public health. Coauthored 2d and 3d edition of *Jurisprudence for Nurses* (1935, 1945), believed to be first book on nursing and the law.
McIver, Pearl 1893–1976 Lowery, MN	Minn State Teacher's College, 1912; BS, U of Minn Sch Nurs, 1919; MA, in PHN admin, 1932; Hon degree, Western Reserve, 1957. Honors: APHA Lasker Award; ANA, PHN Award, later named for her; ICN: F. Nightingale Medal; Honorary member, Sigma Theta Tau; U Minn outstanding achievement award.	As chief, expanded public health nursing in USPHS into modern and extensive agency. First PHN on staff in 1933. First chief, 1944–1957. Initiated census of PHNs. Administered nsg ed program, 1941–43, and traveled extensively to other countries after WW II as part of US technical assistance program. Key roles in PH and nsg org. As pres, ANA, initiated census of all prof nurses. Pres AJN Co, later ex dir. Wrote many articles for *AJN* and *Public Health Nursing*.

(continued)

Appendix 7 (continued)

Names, dates, place of birth	Education and selected honors	Key events; Contributions
McManus, N. Louise 1906–1993 N. Smithfield, MA	Diploma, Institutional Mgt Prog, Pratt Instit (NY); Diploma, Mass Gen Hosp; Bacc, Masters, TC, NY; PhD ed res Columbia U, 1947. Many honors incl: NLN Nutting Award; first recipient of TC alumni award, named after her; CU Bicentennial Medal; Medals, Greek RC; Women's Hall of Fame (Seneca Falls, NY).	Major contrib to nsg ed, incl: first org unit for research in nsg ed (TC, 1953); leader in dev of AD nsg progs; resp for dev of natl state board lic exam pool. One of first nurses to receive PhD. Assist dir NLNE study leading to curriculum guide. At TC for 36 years, 14 as dir, nurs ed div, following Stewart. Consulted internationally in Turkey, Kenya, others, with AID and ICN. Past chair, Florence Nightingale Intl Foundation. Many benchmark publications (books, articles) primarily on nsg ed and research.
Montag, Mildred 1908–2004 Struble, IA	Hamline U, U of Minnesota, BS; Teachers Coll, Columbia, MA 1938, EdD 1948.	One of the most notable nursing influentials of the twentieth century. She restructured nursing more in her lifetime than any other personality before or yet to come. In 1952, as a doctoral candidate at Teachers College, she detailed how two-year nursing programs could benefit the nation. Her dissertation led to the creation of experimental associate-degree programs at seven community colleges around the nation. This put into motion the associate degree movement as a route for entry into nursing practice. By 1994, there were 868 such programs at community and junior colleges. Her life in academic nursing was spent at Adelphi University and Teachers College.

Names, dates, place of birth	Education and selected honors	Key events; Contributions
Nutting, Mary Adelaide 1858–1948 Waterloo, Alberta, Canada	Johns Hopkins Hosp Sch of Nsg. Baltimore, 1891. Many honors incl: medals, historical collection at TC, 4 funds, ed unit at Johns Hopkins, all named after her ANA Hall of Fame.	First nurse to hold professorship in university. First head of what was later the Dept of Nursing Education at TC. (Persuaded Dean Russell to introduce courses for nurses.) Attracted nurses from around world. Great influence on education of nurses, particularly colleges and universities. Key offices in ASSTSN, ANA, ICN, and other nursing org. Helped establish *AJN*, mem of committee that published Goldmark Report. Coauthor, *History of Nursing*, and book on economics of nursing schools.
Osborne, Estelle (Massey) Riddle 1901–1981 Palestine, TX	2 yr course at Prairie View State College, TX; City Hospital Number 2, St. Louis, MO, 1923; BS, 1930, and MA, 1931 TC, NYC; 1st black nurse as honorary fellow AAN; ANA Hall of Fame; NEF named scholarship for black nurses seeking master's degree in nsg.	Leader in nurs ed and development of nsg org. Faced prejudice throughout her education. Resigned early jobs because of discrimination. Studied part time at TC, while teaching at Lincoln Hosp and Harlem Hospitals. After MA, became 1st dir of nsg ed at Freedman's Hospital (DC); established closer relations with Howard U. Other educational positions incl NYU, then asst dir, later assoc gen director, at NLN. Retired in 1967, but continued to speak extensively on role of black nurses. Many firsts for a black nurse: NOPHN Committee, ANA Board of Directors, Rep to ICN, Director Philips Hosp, St. Louis. Active as pres, NACGN and various Afro-American organizations.

(continued)

Appendix 7 (continued)

Names, dates, place of birth	Education and selected honors	Key events; Contributions
Palmer, Sophia 1853–1920 Milton, MA	Mass Gen Hosp Trng Sch for Nurses, Boston c. 1900. Also studied journalism. Honors: several nursing libraries named after her. ANA Hall of Fame.	Helped establish *AJN*; first editor from first issue to death. Leader in movement to secure state licensure for nurses. Helped organize ASSTSN and ANA. Previously, organized St. Luke's Trng School, Bedford, MA. Reorganized Garfield Memorial, DC, and established school; supt Rochester City Hosp; first pres, NY State Bd of Nurse Examiners. Member local and national RC committees.
Peplau, Hildegard 1909–1999 Reading, PA	Pottstown, PA, Sch of Nsg, 1931; BA, Psychology, Bennington College, 1943; master's and EdD, TC; William Alanson White Institute, NYC, certificate in psychoanalysis. Honors: Fellow, AAN; ANA Hall of Fame; ICN Christiane Reimann Award Recipient; Honored as a "Living Legend" by the AAN; honorary doctorates from Duke, Indiana, Ohio State, Rutgers, and the University of Ulster in Ireland.	Universally regarded as the "mother of psychiatric nursing." Her book, *Interpersonal Relations in Nursing* (1952), was widely credited with transforming nursing from a group of skilled workers to a full-fledged profession. Created the first graduate level program for the preparation of clinical specialists in psychiatric nursing at Rutgers University. Her original book from 1952 has been translated into nine languages.
Reiter, Frances 1904–1977 Smithton, PA	Johns Hopkins Hosp Trng Sch for Nurses, 1931; BA, nsg ed TC 1941; MA, TC, 1942. Many honors include: ANA honorary membership; IRC Nightingale Medal; NLN disting service award; Honorary fellow, AAN.	Chiefly known for concept and term "nurse clinician." Strong believer in bacc ed, Chair of ANA committee that wrote "position paper." Main contrib in nsg ed and research; held key admin and teaching positions in Montefiore (Pgh), Johns Hopkins, Boston U, Mass Gen, TC, First Dean, Grad Sch Nsg, NY Med College. Proj dir, US PHS study on quality of nsg care on ex comm, *Nsg Research*; major roles in nsg orgs.

Names, dates, place of birth	Education and selected honors	Key events; Contributions
Richards, Linda 1841–1930 Near Potsdam, NY	St. Johnsburg Academy, VT, N Eng Hosp for Women and Children, Boston, 1873. Numerous honors include: Likeness engraved on corporate seal of ANA. In 1948, 63 cities and 48 states observed Linda Richards day in honor of her graduation 75 years previously. NLN named award; ANA Hall of Fame. Women's Hall of Fame (Seneca Falls, NY).	Taught school in Vermont. Entered nurse trng, inspired by Nightingale's writings. Known as America's "first trained nurse." Primarily organizer and supt of many trng schools and nursing services, usually only staying 2 years. Also pioneer in establishing trng schools for nurses in mental hospitals. Active in founding national nsg organizations: first president ASSTSN; organized first trng school for nurses in Japan, under missionary auspices. Part of committee approaching TC re courses for nurses. Wrote reminiscences on being first trained nurse, 1911.
Robb, Isabel Hampton 1860–1910 Welland, Ontario, Canada	Teaching certif: Collegiate Institute of St. Catherine's Ontario, Canada, Bellevue Trng School for Nurses, NY, 1883; course at St. Paul's House, Rome 1883–85. Honors: several scholarships and funds named after her; ANA Hall of Fame.	Brilliant leader who did much to improve and develop curriculum in early nursing schools, including lengthening program, inaugurating a regular class schedule, providing for holidays, eliminating stipend. Supt, Ill. Trng Sch for Nurses, Chicago; organizer and supt Johns Hopkins. One of founders and first pres Nurses Associated Alumni (NAA); pres ASSTSN; helped found *AJN*; ICN committee member. One of earliest nursing authors: books on practice and ethics. Continued to participate in nursing (but not practice) after marriage.
Roberts, Mary 1877–1950 Sheboygan, MI	Jewish Hosp Sch of Nsg, Cincinnati, OH, 1899; BS, TC, NYC, 1921. Honors: Bronze Medal, France; Nutting award for leadership; IRC Nightingale medal; named awards; ANA Hall of Fame.	Brilliant writer and editor of *AJN* for 28 years. Considered great teacher and investigator who had insight into nursing movements. Traveled throughout Europe visiting nsg centers under sponsorship of Rockefeller Foundation. Established trng sch for nurses, Savannah Hosp, GA. Supt of several other hosps. Dir, Army Sch of Nsg and Bureau of Nsg, Lake Denison, ARC, WW I. Many committees

(continued)

Appendix 7 (continued)

Names, dates, place of birth	Education and selected honors	Key events; Contributions
		of national nsg orgs, ICN, and Nsg Council on Natl Defense, WW I. Author of books on nsg history and ANC.
Rogers, Martha 1914–1994 Dallas, TX	U of Knoxville, 1931–33; Knoxville Genl Hosp Sch of Nurs, 1936; BSN in public health nsg, George Peabody College, Nashville, 1937; MA, public health supervision, TC, 1945; MPH, Johns Hopkins, 1952; ScD Johns Hopkins, 1953; numerous honorary degrees. Honors: many awards; Fellow, AAN; ANA Hall of Fame.	Primarily known as originator of the nursing theory, "Science of Unitary Human Beings" or "Rogerian Science." Professor and head of NYU Div Nsg Ed from 1954–1975. After retirement, continued to teach (professor emeritus). Consultant to US govt. Prolific author/speaker and nsg gadfly re "anti-educational archaisms." In nursing education, president of number of natl ed orgs plus Sigma Theta Tau. Active in nsg org committees. Prior to 1954, had been involved in public health nursing and supervision.
Sanger, Margaret 1879–1966 Corning, NY	Claverack College, NY. White Plains Hosp, NY, 1902; postgrad, Manhattan Eye and Ear, 1902; Self-study on pop problems; Hon LLD, Smith College, 1949; Hon LLD, U Ariz, 1966. Many honors incl: Am Women's Assn Medal of Achievement; Gold Medal, Emperor of Japan, 1962; Pl Parenthood, Albert and Mary Lasker Award, and medal named after her; ANA Hall of Fame.	Nurse leader of Am birth control movement; founder, Planned Parenthood. Was teacher, after postgrad course, married, had 3 children. Constant flare-ups of TB. Doing home nsg, became concerned by women on Lower East Side (NY), who died of childbirth or illegal abortions and could get no information about birth control. During years of battle for reform, was arrested for disseminating such information, much of which she had gotten in Europe. Started birth control clinics and research; got support of wealthy. Fought many court battles, wrote many books. Finally got AMA support. Retired to Arizona: new leaders of movement deemed her brand of feminism counterproductive.

Names, dates, place of birth	Education and selected honors	Key events; Contributions
Shaw, Mrs. Clara Weeks 1857–1940 Sanbarton, NH	NY Hosp Trng Sch for Nurses, 1880. Previously graduated, RI State Normal School.	Credited with being first nurse to write a nursing textbook in U.S. (1885). Became standard text for many schools. Supt, Paterson Gen Hospital, Paterson, NJ. No further nursing work after marriage in 1888.
Staupers, Mabel 1890–1989 Barbados, W. Indies	Freedman's Hosp Sch of Nsg, DC, 1917. Many honors, incl: Spingarn Medal, NAACP, NLN Linda Richards Award; ANA Mahoney Award; Medgar Evans Human Rights Award; Urban Leage Award; ANA Hall of Fame.	Strong integrationist and feminist. Through political and public pressure, and help of Eleanor Roosevelt, forced Army and Navy to accept black nurses without quotas (WW II). Helped black MD's organize first private facility in Harlem, allowing black doctors to treat pts. Served as administrator and dir of nsg. Conducted survey of health needs of Harlem; led to NYTB and Health Assn; became first ex sec (12 yrs). Became first ex sec NACGN, 1934–1946. Pres, NACGN later. Wrote significant book on integration of "Negroes" into American nursing.
Stewart, Isabel Maitland 1878–1963 Fletcher, Ontario, Canada	Normal School, Winnipeg Genl Hosp Trng Sch 1902; BS (1911), MA (1913), TC. Number of hon doctorates in US and Canada. Many honors from US, Canada, Finland. One of 23 "women of achievement," NY League of Nat Fed Bus and Prof Women, 1936. ANA Hall of Fame.	Helped shape development of 20th century nsg ed and practice. Instrumental in developing first program for preparing nurse faculty at TC; aided in educational research, promoting use of objective tests. Revived interest in study of nsg schs by outside group, resulting in valuable 1926 report (Appendix 1). Prof of Nurs Ed and Dir of Dept at TC for 22 years. Involved in natl and intl nsg ed orgs. Member Women's Board of Henry St, VNA. Coauthor, with Dock, of nsg history text, 1920. Author, *Education of Nurses*, 1943; editor, *AJN* Dept of Nsg Ed.

(continued)

Appendix 7 (continued)

Names, dates, place of birth	Education and selected honors	Key events; Contributions
Stimson, Julia 1881–1948 Worcester, MA	NY Hosp Sch of Nsg, NYC, 1908; BA, Vassar College; MA, Washington U, St. Louis, 1917. Honors: Many honors from US. Britain, Belgium, France. Also: ANA Hall of Fame; IRC Nightingale Medal.	First woman given rank of major in U.S. (Colonel, 1945). Came to natl notice through spectacular achievement of organizing and administering work of nurses at Gen Hosp in Rouen, France, WW I. Recruited nurses for ANC and ARC; longest tenure in history of ANC. Chief nurse ARC, France 1918 and dir nurs service, Am Expeditionary Forces 1918, Supt ANC 1919–37, also dean, Army Sch of Nsg. Had been supt of nurses several hosp. Pres ANA; Many ARC, army and nsg committees. Author, *Handbook of Drugs and Solutions*; many articles.
Taylor, Susie King 1848–1912 Savannah, GA	Secret tutoring to read and write.	Born a slave; escaped to area under Union control; married Union soldier at 14. Known as nurse during Civil War, having made rounds with Clara Barton at about age 15. Services never compensated after war. Started schools after war, then domestic employment. In Boston, helped organize, and involved with, Woman's Relief Corps (for Union veterans), but never nursed officially again. Wrote insightful reminiscences of camp life in Civil War, which she published herself.

Names, dates, place of birth	Education and selected honors	Key events; Contributions
Thomas, Adah c. 1870–1943 Richmond, VA	Normal School, Richmond; Woman's Infirmary and Sch of Therapeutic Massage, NYC, 1900; then Lincoln Hosp and Home Trng Sch, NYC, 1905; courses in various NYC institutions. Honors: first to receive NACGN's Mahoney Award; ANA Hall of Fame.	Known chiefly for seeking equal opportunity for black nurses, particularly getting 18 accepted in army with full rank and pay. (Surgeon General had refused, but her persistence and shortage of nurses in flu epidemic of 1918, forced him to accede.) Asst Dir, Lincoln Hosp, 18 yrs. Helped organize NACGN. Among first to add pub health nsg course to curriculum at Lincoln. Participated in intl affairs—one of first 3 black delegates to ICN. Apptd by Asst Surg Gen to key advisory council, 1921. Actively involved in many nsg and other org. Wrote first history of black nurses.
Truth, Sojourner (Isabella Von Wagener) c. 1797–1883? Hurley, NY	No formal education. Honors: Michigan Women's Hall of Fame; Nat'l Women's Hall of Fame, Seneca Falls, NY. Mars Robot (US) named Sojourner to honor her (1995).	Amazing, brave, and resourceful Afro–American, best known for her abolitionist activities and stirring speeches although she was a lifelong illiterate. Born a slave, she escaped and was given refuge by a family whose name she took. In 1843, took name of Sojourner (will travel) Truth (will tell) and began preaching, raising money for her causes. At 77, traveled to DC, met with president, eventually appointed to work with Freedman's Hospital. For 2 years, cared for black soldiers, brought order to filthy, chaotic conditions. Continued campaigning for freed slaves' rights and women's rights.

(continued)

Appendix 7 (continued)

Names, dates, place of birth	Education and selected honors	Key events; Contributions
Tubman, Harriet (Araminta) c. 1820–1913 Bricktown, MD	No formal education. Honors: commemorative stamp; monument in Auburn	Escaped abused slave known as the "conductor of the underground railroad" for the secret trips she made to lead more than 300 slaves to freedom. During Civil War served as nurse in Sea Islands and other camps, as needed, caring for sick and wounded regardless of color; was also spy and scout for Union Army (for which she later received a pension). Helped develop Freedman's Colony in SC and worked in that hosp using it as a base; also served in hospitals in NC and FL. In Auburn, NY, later used her home as shelter for needy black people. Given military funeral.
Wald, Lillian 1867–1940 Cincinnati, OH	NY Hosp Trng Sch, 1891; studied at Women's Medical College, NYC. Honorary Degrees: LLD, Mount Holyoke, 1912; Smith, 1930. Numerous honors and medals incl: recognition by Mayor LaGuardia in 1936 as "citizen rendering greatest service to NYC." Memorial tributes by Pres Roosevelt, NY governor, 2 NYC mayors and leaders of health and social service agencies; ANA Hall of Fame; Women's Hall of Fame (Seneca Falls, NY); Hall of Fame for Great Americans, NYU	Founded Henry St VNA in NYC, first nonsectarian publ health service in US. Promoted publ health and social welfare concepts entire life. Started school nsg, NYC. Fought for better housing in slums; initiated idea for U.S. Children's Bureau. Taught at TC. One of organizers and 1st pres, NOPHN. Served on numerous local, natl, intl committees. Author, 2 books about Henry St.
Yellowtail, Susie 1903–1981 Cross Agency, MT	Bacone College, OK; E. Northville Hosp Trng Sch, Springfield, MA, with internships, Boston Hosp, 1926. Honors: President's Award for Outstanding Nsg and Health Care; Mrs. Indian America.	One of the first Native American RNs. Strong effective advocate for better ed and health on reservations. Worked for USPHS, various reservations, then 30 yrs for own people (Crow Agency); nsg and midwife services. With husband, medicine man, reintroduced aspects of traditional healing ceremony. Apptd by Pres Kennedy to PH, Ed, and Welfare Board, 1961; served through several presidencies, fought for improvement of health services for her people; traveled nationally.

Index